CLINICAL UROGYNECOLOGY

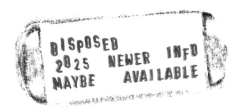
Books are to be returned on or before
the last date below.

17 JAN		
1 DEC 1996		
10	6	97		
17 FEB		
28 OCT 2002		
-5 MAY 2005		
03 NOV 2005		
28 NOV 2005		
21·4 2010		

LIBREX —

CLINICAL UROGYNECOLOGY

Mark D. Walters, MD
Director of Urogynecology
Department of Obstetrics and Gynecology
University Hospitals of Cleveland;
Associate Professor, Department of Reproductive Biology
Case Western Reserve University
Cleveland, Ohio

Mickey M. Karram, MD
Director of Urogynecology
Good Samaritan Hospital;
Assistant Professor of Obstetrics and Gynecology
University of Cincinnati
Cincinnati, Ohio

With 206 illustrations

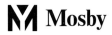

St. Louis Baltimore Boston Chicago London Philadelphia Sydney Toronto

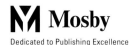

Mosby

Dedicated to Publishing Excellence

Executive Editor: Stephanie Manning
Developmental Editor: Laura DeYoung
Project Manager: Carol Sullivan Wiseman
Designer: Julie Taugner
Manufacturing Supervisor: John Babrick

Printed in the United States of America

Mosby–Year Book, Inc.
11830 Westline Industrial Drive
St. Louis, Missouri 63146

Library of Congress Cataloging in Publication Data

Walters, Mark D.
    Clinical urogynecology / Mark D. Walters, Mickey M. Karram.
       p.   cm.
    Includes bibliographical references and index.
    ISBN 0-8016-5673-7
    1. Urogynecology. I. Karram, Mickey M. II. Title.
    [DNLM: 1. Urinary Incontinence. 2. Urodynamics—Pelvis—
—physiopathology. 3. Uterine Prolapse.   WJ 190 W233c 1993]
    RG484.W35   1993
    616.6—dc20
    DNLM/DLC
    for Library of Congress   93-18612
                                                CIP

93 94 95 96 97 GW/MY 9 8 7 6 5 4 3 2 1

Contributors

J. Thomas Benson
Director, OB/GYN Education
Methodist Hospital of Indiana
Clinical Professor of Obstetrics and Gynecology
Indiana University Medical Center
Indianapolis, Indiana;
Visiting Professor of Obstetrics and Gynecology
Rush University Medical School
Chicago, Illinois

Molly C. Dougherty
Professor/Research Coordinator
University of Florida—College of Nursing
Gainesville, Florida

Thomas E. Elkins
Head of Obstetrics and Gynecology
Louisiana State University
New Orleans, Louisiana

Christopher Fitzpatrick
Coombe Lying-In Hospital
Dublin, Ireland

Mickey M. Karram
Director of Urogynecology
Good Samaritan Hospital;
Assistant Professor of Obstetrics and Gynecology
University of Cincinnati
Cincinnati, Ohio

Paul Koonings
Department of Obstetrics and Gynecology
Associate Director, Division of Gynecologic
  Oncology
Assistant Professor, Obstetrics and Gynecology
Eastern Virginia Medical School
Norfolk, Virginia

George W. Mitchell
Professor, Department of Obstetrics and
  Gynecology
University of Texas Health Science Center at San
  Antonio
San Antonio, Texas

Edward R. Newton
Associate Professor, Department of Obstetrics and
  Gynecology
Director, Maternal/Fetal Medicine Fellowship
University of Texas Health Science Center at San
  Antonio
San Antonio, Texas

Pat D. O'Donnell
Professor, Division of Urology
Director, Female Urology and Geriatric Urology
University of Cincinnati Medical Center
Cincinnati, Ohio

Linda M. Partoll
Fellow, Division of Urogynecology
Department of Obstetrics and Gynecology
Good Samaritan Hospital
University of Cincinnati
Cincinnati, Ohio

Bruce Rosenzweig
Department of Obstetrics and Gynecology
Assistant Professor of Obstetrics and Gynecology
  and Head of Urogynecology
University of Illinois
Chicago, Illinois

Laszlo Sogor
Chief of Gynecology
Department of Obstetrics and Gynecology
University Hospitals of Cleveland;
Associate Professor, Department of Reproductive
  Biology
Case Western Reserve University School of
  Medicine
Cleveland, Ohio

Carmen J. Sultana
Department of Obstetrics and Gynecology
University Hospitals of Cleveland;
Assistant Professor, Department of Reproductive
  Biology
Case Western Reserve University
Cleveland, Ohio

Mark D. Walters
Director of Urogynecology
Department of Obstetrics and Gynecology
University Hospitals of Cleveland;
Associate Professor, Department of Reproductive
  Biology
Case Western Reserve University
Cleveland, Ohio

To
Ginny,
for over 10 years of love and friendship,
and to my parents,
Margaret and Don,
for their unyielding support during my career
MARK D. WALTERS

To my father,
Mike Karram, Sr,
for his guidance
and for instilling in me the values of hard work and discipline,
and in memory of my mother,
Mary Karram,
for her love, kindness, and unselfish support
MICKEY M. KARRAM

Foreword

It is a privilege and an honor to prepare this foreword for *Clinical Urogynecology*. Old friends will understand and new colleagues perhaps will be surprised by this brief reentry into the field of urology.

My interest in this field covers a span of more than 40 years, initially stimulated by my experience as a Pediatric Surgical resident, utilizing (by present standards) primitive urodynamic recording instrumentation to evaluate bladder and urethral function. In those days, a careful clinical evaluation was supplemented by measurements often suspect because of lack of comparative data. Today, regrettably, sophisticated urodynamic testing frequently promises more than it can deliver, often in the absence of a thorough clinical evaluation. Fortunately for our patients, there is increasing recognition that disorders of micturition and symptomatic alterations in pelvic anatomy require an expertise that can best be evaluated and treated by the gynecologist appropriately trained in urogynecology.

The authors have approached this problem from the clinical standpoint but have wisely assumed that a review of anatomy and the basic principles of neurophysiology are essential for a contemporary understanding of the diagnosis and treatment of urinary incontinence and genital prolapse. This text will appeal to the gynecologist interested in disorders of micturition and the diagnosis and treatment of pelvic relaxation. It also provides sufficient information to encourage further inquiry and training in this subspecialty now available through a number of fellowship programs.

The student will be stimulated, the practicing gynecologist challenged, and the expert pleasantly surprised by the completeness and logic of the presentation. I congratulate the authors on their achievement.

Douglas J. Marchant, MD
Professor of Obstetrics and Gynecology
Professor of Surgery
Tufts University School of Medicine
Adjunct Professor of Obstetrics and Gynecology
Brown University School of Medicine
Providence, Rhode Island

Preface

The subspecialty of urogynecology, formally referred to as gynecologic urology, has benefitted from renewed interest and enthusiasm in recent years. After a period of relative disinterest in lower urinary tract complaints, gynecologists are again realizing, as did most pioneers in surgical gynecology, that lower urinary tract disorders in women are often best managed within the specialty of obstetrics and gynecology.

Renewed national interest in diseases of women and older persons in general has helped to increase awareness of the high prevalence of urinary incontinence in women. This interest led to national programs, such as the Consensus Development Conference on Urinary Incontinence in Adults, sponsored by the National Institute on Aging and the Office of Medical Applications of Research of the National Institutes of Health in conjunction with other agencies. In 1992, the American Board of Obstetrics and Gynecology also convened a conference on pelvic floor dysfunction to study curriculum enhancement in residency education in obstetrics and gynecology. Finally, in 1992, the Residency Review Committee, under the Accreditation Council for Graduate Medical Education, added knowledge of the "diagnosis and medical and surgical management of urinary incontinence" to their special requirements for residency training in obstetrics and gynecology. These programs all underscore the widespread need for education and training in urogynecology for practicing generalists and residents in obstetrics and gynecology. More physicians with special expertise in urogynecology are also needed to meet the expanding training needs within this specialty.

Clinical Urogynecology is a clinically oriented yet comprehensive textbook on the subject of urogynecology. We believe that this subject fundamentally encompasses three main topics: female urinary incontinence, urodynamic testing, and pelvic relaxation. This textbook is separated into 4 sections. Chapters 1 through 4 describe in detail basic principles and subjects that are needed to understand and treat disorders of the lower urinary tract and pelvic floor. Chapters 5 through 11 outline basic and advanced concepts of the evaluation of lower urinary tract disorders in women. Chapters 12 through 18 present management guidelines for women with genuine stress incontinence and pelvic organ prolapse. Finally, Chapters 19 through 29 discuss specific conditions and special subjects that are occasionally encountered by physicians treating patients with lower urinary tract disorders.

Special features of this book include a large number of superbly illustrated original surgical drawings on the treatment of genuine stress incontinence and pelvic organ prolapse. Using computer-generated graphic techniques, the urodynamic illustrations were created from actual drawings of patients with various urogynecologic disorders. This allows for enhanced learning free of the artifacts that are common in actual urodynamic tracings. Because female incontinence is best managed in a multidisciplinary fashion, recognized authorities in nursing, geriatric urology, maternal-fetal medicine, and gynecologic oncology have contributed chapters related to their particular areas of expertise. Innovative chapters resulted, such as those that discussed obstetric factors and geriatric issues as they affect lower urinary tract function.

We hope that this book will meet the training needs of residents in obstetrics and gynecology and other specialties and that it can be used as a reference text for generalists and urogynecologic experts alike.

ACKNOWLEDGMENTS

We would like to acknowledge the indispensable and exemplary work of Lisa Szabo and Mary Jo Crooker for performing the huge volume of secretarial and transcribing work involved in this book. We would also like to thank Gretta Small for her invaluable medical editing of our manuscripts.

Special acknowledgment goes to the medical illustrators—Michael A. Cooley; Nancy A. Burgard, MA; and Joe Chovan—for their hard work in creating particularly clear surgical and urodynamic drawings.

Mark D. Walters
Mickey M. Karram

Contents

PART ONE
Basic Science

1　Anatomy of the Lower Urinary Tract and
Pelvic Floor, 3
Mark D. Walters

2　Neurophysiology of the Lower Urinary
Tract, 17
J. Thomas Benson
Mark D. Walters

3　Epidemiology and Social Impact of Urinary
Incontinence, 29
Mark D. Walters

4　Classification of Disorders of Storage and
Evacuation of Urine, 40
Mark D. Walters

PART TWO
Evaluation

5　Evaluation of Incontinence: History, Physical
Examination, and Office Tests, 49
Mark D. Walters

6　Urodynamics: Cystometry, 62
Mickey M. Karram

7　Urodynamics: Voiding Studies, 77
Mickey M. Karram

8　Urodynamics: Urethral Pressure
Profilometry, 89
Mickey M. Karram

9　Electrophysiologic Testing, 102
J. Thomas Benson

10　Endoscopic Evaluation of the Lower Urinary
Tract, 124
Bruce A. Rosenzweig

11　Radiologic Studies of the Lower Urinary
Tract, 134
Bruce A. Rosenzweig

PART THREE
**Management of Genuine Stress Incontinence
and Pelvic Organ Prolapse**

12　Pathophysiology and Obstetrics Issues of
Genuine Stress Incontinence, 151
Mark D. Walters
Edward R. Newton

13　Genuine Stress Incontinence: Nonsurgical
Treatment, 163
Molly C. Dougherty
Mark D. Walters

14　Transvaginal Needle Suspension Procedures
for Genuine Stress Incontinence, 182
Mickey M. Karram

15   Genuine Stress Incontinence: Retropubic
Surgical Procedures, 196
Mark D. Walters

16   Surgical Correction of Genuine Stress
Incontinence Secondary to Intrinsic Urethral
Sphincter Dysfunction, 210
Mickey M. Karram

17   Pelvic Organ Prolapse: Cystocele and
Rectocele, 225
Mark D. Walters

18   Pelvic Organ Prolapse: Enterocele and Vaginal
Vault Prolapse, 236
Mickey M. Karram
Mark D. Walters

PART FOUR
Specific Conditions

19   Detrusor Instability and Hyperreflexia, 263
Mickey M. Karram

20   Frequency, Urgency, and Painful Bladder
Syndromes, 285
Mickey M. Karram

21   Voiding Dysfunction and Retention, 299
Linda M. Partoll

22   Lower Urinary Tract Infection, 310
Mickey M. Karram

23   Lower Urinary Tract Fistulas, 330
Thomas E. Elkins
Christopher Fitzpatrick

24   Suburethral Diverticula, 342
Laszlo Sogor

25   Gynecologic Injury to the Ureters, Bladder,
and Urethra: Recognition and
Management, 354
George W. Mitchell
Mark D. Walters

26   The Effects of Gynecologic Cancer and Its
Treatment on the Lower Urinary Tract, 373
Paul P. Koonings

27   The Urinary Tract in Pregnancy, 388
Edward R. Newton

28   Geriatric Issues in Female Incontinence, 409
Pat D. O'Donnell

29   Bladder Drainage and Urinary Protective
Methods, 421
Carmen J. Sultana

The Standardisation of Terminology of Lower
Urinary Tract Function Recommended by the
International Continence Society, 430

Basic Science

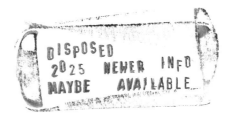

Anatomy of the Lower Urinary Tract and Pelvic Floor

Mark D. Walters

Lower Urinary Tract
    Embryology
    Anatomy
Vagina
Pelvic Organ Support
    Pelvic floor
    Endopelvic fascia
Anal Sphincter Mechanism

LOWER URINARY TRACT
Embryology
Formation of Intraembryonic Mesoderm

At approximately 15 days after fertilization, invagination and lateral migration of mesodermal cells occur between the ectodermal and endodermal layers of the presomite embryo. These migrating cells form the intraembryonic mesoderm or mesodermal germ layer. By the seventeenth day of development, the endoderm and ectoderm layers are separated entirely by the mesoderm layer, with the exception of the prochordal plate cephalically and the cloacal plate caudally. The cloacal plate consists of tightly adherent endodermal and ectodermal layers.

Formation of Allantois and Cloaca

Concomitantly, at about the sixteenth day of development, the posterior wall of the yolk sack forms a small diverticulum, the allantois, which extends into the connecting stalk. With ventral bending of the embryo cranially and caudally during somite development, the connecting stalk and contained allantois, as well as the cloacal membrane, are displaced onto the ventral aspect of the embryo.

The hindgut undergoes slight dilation to form the cloaca; it receives the allantois ventrally and the two mesonephric ducts laterally. Ventral mesodermal elevations occur forming the urethral folds (primordia of the labia minora) and genital tubercle (primordia of the clitoris).

Partitioning of Cloaca into Urogenital Sinus and Rectum

A spur of mesodermal tissue migrates from the base of the allantois toward the cloacal membrane around 28 days after fertilization, forming the urorectal septum (Fig. 1-1). This structure partitions the cloaca into a ventral urogenital sinus and a dorsal rectum. The urogenital opening (future vestibule) is formed by the independent involution of the urogenital membrane. The point at which the urorectal septum intersects the cloacal membrane will become the perineal body.

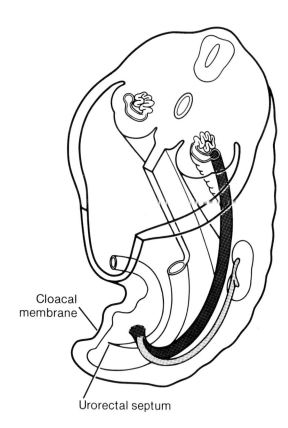

Fig. 1-1   Embryo approximately 32 days (8 mm crown-rump length) after fertilization. The urorectal septum is shown dividing the cloaca into a ventral urogenital sinus and dorsal rectum. Definitive ureter and mesonephric duct share a common opening into partially divided cloaca. Note that the ureter has induced formation of a kidney from metanephrogenic blastema. *(From Gosling JA, Dixon J, Humpherson JR:* Functional anatomy of the urinary tract, *London, 1982, Gower Medical Publishing.)*

Cloacal membrane

Urorectal septum

Fig. 1-2   By thirty-seventh day (14 mm crown-rump length), kidney has continued to ascend and undergo medial rotation, and the mesonephric duct and future ureter have separated. In addition, cloaca has been divided into ventral urogenital and dorsal elementary parts. *(From Gosling JA, Dixon J, Humpherson JR:* Functional anatomy of the urinary tract, *London, 1982, Gower Medical Publishing.)*

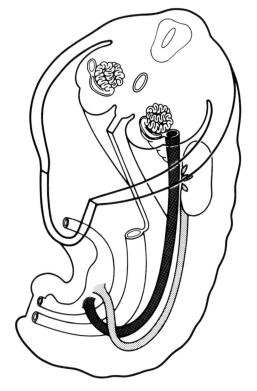

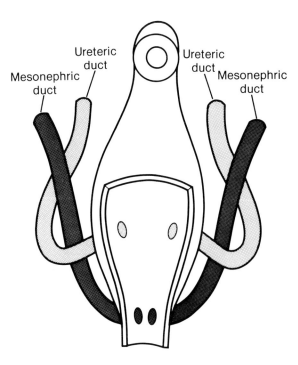

Fig. 1-3 Urogenital sinus and associated duct approximately 40 days (17 mm crown-rump length) after fertilization. Trigone lies between separated ureteric orifices and mesonephric ducts. *(From Gosling JA, Dixon J, Humperson JR: Functional anatomy of the urinary tract, London, 1982, Gower Medical Publishing.)*

Formation of Ureteric Bud and Induction of Future Kidney

By 28 days of development, the mesonephric ducts have reached and fused with the urogenital sinus. At this time, the ureteric bud appears as a diverticulum from the posteromedial aspect of the mesonephric duct at the point where the terminus of the duct bends to enter the cloaca. The free cranial end of the ureter grows dorsally, then cranially, and induces the formation of the metanephrogenic blastema (future kidney; Fig. 1-1). The presence of the developing ureter is essential for this differentiation, absence of the ureteric bud is invariably associated with renal agenesis. The ureteric bud branches and dilates to create the renal pelvis, major and minor calyces, and collecting ducts. The remaining parts of each nephron

are derived from the mesoderm of the metanephrogenic blastema. At this time in the female, the mesonephric system is undergoing degeneration.

The renal blastema originates at the level of the upper sacral segments. The final position of the kidney at the level of the upper lumbar vertebrae is attributed to "ascent" of the renal blastema. According to Maizels, the four mechanisms that lead to normal renal ascent are caudal growth of the spine, active elongation of the ureter into the metanephrogenic blastema, intrinsic growth and molding of the renal parenchyma, and axial growth of the spine after fixing of the kidney to the retroperitoneum.

Formation of Bladder, Trigone, and Urethra

At the point of its connection with the mesonephric ducts, the urogenital sinus is divided into the vesicourethral canal cranially and the definitive urogenital sinus caudally. Dilation of the cranial portion of the vesicourethral canal forms the definitive bladder, which is of endodermal origin. The vesicourethral canal communicates at its cranial end with the allantois, which becomes obliterated at about 12 weeks of fetal life, forming the urachus. This structure runs from the bladder dome to the umbilicus and is called the median umbilical ligament in the adult.

The ureteric bud begins as an outgrowth of the mesonephric duct, but with positional changes of the embryo during growth, the mesonephric duct and the ureteric bud shift positions so that the ureter comes to lie posterolaterally to the duct (Fig. 1-2). The segment of the mesonephric duct distal to the site of origin of the ureteric bud dilates and is absorbed into the urogenital sinus, forming the bladder trigone. This structure effectively gives the endodermal wall of the vesicourethral canal a mesodermal contribution. At about 42 days after fertilization, the trigone may be defined as that region of the vesicourethral canal lying between the ureteric orifices and the termination of the mesonephric ducts (Fig. 1-3). The caudal portion of the vesicourethral canal remains narrow and forms the entire urethra. A small portion of the posterior proximal urethra may be derived, like the trigone, from mesoderm of the mesonephric duct, although this theory is controversial. A timetable and schematic representation of the embryologic contributions of the various structures of the urogenital system are shown in Table 1-1 and Fig. 1-4, respectively.

The separate development of the trigone and bladder may explain why the muscle laminae of the trigone are contiguous with the muscle of the ureter, but not with the detrusor muscle of the bladder. This separate development also may account for pharmacologic responses of the musculature of the bladder neck and trigone, which differ partially from those of the detrusor.

Congenital Anomalies of the Urinary Tract

Knowledge of the embryology of the genitourinary system is necessary for understanding the causes of the multiple congenital anomalies of the upper and lower urinary tracts. Selected congenital anomalies of the urinary tract and their embryologic causes are shown in Table 1-2.

Anatomy
Bladder

The urinary bladder is a hollow, muscular organ that is a reservoir for the urinary system. The bladder is flat when empty and globular when distended. The superior surface and the upper 1 or 2 cm of the posterior aspect of the bladder are covered by peritoneum,

TABLE 1-1 Timetable of events in the development of the lower urinary tract

Time after fertilization	Event
15 days	Ingrowth of intraembryonic mesoderm
16-17 days	Allantois appears
17 days	Cloacal plate forms
28-38 days	Partitioning of cloaca by urorectal septum
28 days	Mesonephric duct reaches cloaca; ureteric bud appears
30-37 days	Ureteric bud initiates formation of metanephros (permanent kidney)
41 days	Lumen of urethra is discrete; genital tubercles prominent
42-44 days	Urogenital sinus separates from rectum; mesonephric ducts and ureters drain separately into urogenital sinus, defining boundaries of trigone
51-52 days	Kidneys in lumbar region; glomeruli appear in kidney
9 weeks	First likelihood of renal function
12 weeks	External genitalia become distinctive for sex
13 weeks	Bladder becomes muscularized
20-40 weeks	Further growth and development complete the urogenital organs

TABLE 1-2 Selected congenital anomalies of the urinary tract and their embryologic causes

Condition	Embryologic cause
Renal agenesis	Early degeneration of the ureteric bud
Pelvic kidney	Failure of kidney to ascend to the lumbar region
Horseshoe kidney	Fusion of lower poles of both kidneys; ascent to lumbar region prevented by root of inferior mesenteric artery
Urachal fistula, cyst, sinus	Variable persistence of the intraembryonic portion of allantois, from bladder to umbilicus
Double ureter	Early splitting of the ureteric bud
Ectopic ureter	Two ureteric buds develop from one mesonephric duct. One bud is in normal position; the abnormal bud moves downward with the mesonephric duct to enter into the urethra, vagina, vestibule, or uterus
Bladder exstrophy	Failure of the ventral wall of the urogenital sinus to increase to accommodate positional changes, followed by breakdown of the urogenital membrane

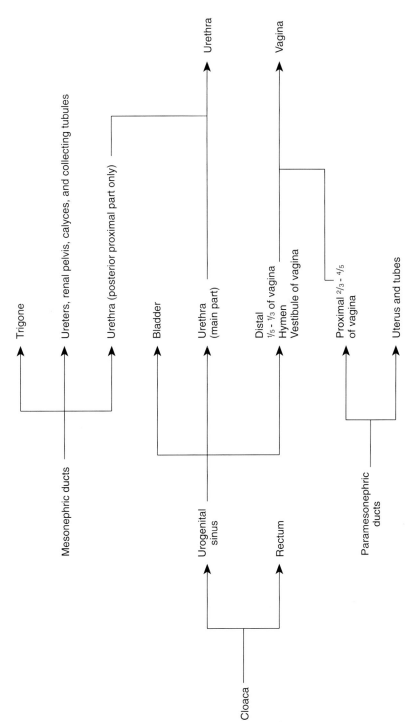

Fig. 1-4   Schematic representation of the embryologic contributions of various structures of the female urogenital system.

which sweeps off the bladder into the vesicouterine pouch. The anterior bladder wall is extraperitoneal and adjacent to the retropubic space. Between the bladder and the pubic bones lie adipose tissue, the pubovesical ligaments and muscle, and a prominent venous plexus. Inferiorly, the bladder rests on, and is firmly attached to, the anterior vagina and lower uterine segment. The bladder is enveloped in endopelvic fascia.

The epithelium lining the bladder lumen is loosely attached to its musculature over its surface area, except in the trigone, where it is firmly adherent to the underlying musculature. The bladder lining consists of transitional epithelium (urothelium) supported by a layer of loose connective tissue, the lamina propria. The internal surface of the bladder has a rugose appearance formed by mucosal folds in the contracted state. In the distended state, a variably prominent meshlike appearance is formed by mucosal-covered detrusor musculature.

The bladder wall musculature is often described as having three layers: an inner longitudinal layer, a middle circular layer, and an outer longitudinal layer. However, this layering occurs only at the bladder neck; the remainder of the bladder musculature is composed of fibers that run in many directions, both within and between layers. This plexiform arrangement of detrusor muscle bundles is ideally suited to reduce all dimensions of the bladder lumen on contraction.

The inner longitudinal layer has widely separated muscle fibers that course multidirectionally. Near the bladder neck, these muscle fibers assume a longitudinal pattern that is contiguous through the trigone and, according to Tanagho, into the inner longitudinal muscular layer of the urethra. The middle circular layer is prominent at the bladder neck where it fuses with the deep trigonal muscle, forming a muscular ring. This layer does not continue into the urethra. The outer longitudinal layer forms a sheet of muscle bundles around the bladder wall above the level of the bladder neck. Anteriorly, these fibers continue past the vesical neck as the pubovesical muscles and insert into tissues on the posterior surface of the pubic symphysis. The pubovesical muscles may act to facilitate bladder neck opening during voiding. In the female, longitudinal fibers fuse posteriorly with the deep surface of the apex of the trigone. In addition, posterior longitudinal fibers communicate with several detrusor muscle loops at the bladder base; these loops probably aid in bladder neck closure.

Trigone

In the base of the bladder is a triangular-shaped area, the trigone. The trigone has a relatively flattened appearance with a smooth mucosal covering. The corners of the trigone are formed by three orifices: the paired ureteral orifices and the internal urethral orifice. The superior boundary of the trigone is a slightly raised area between the two ureteric orifices, termed the interureteric ridge. The two ureteral openings are slitlike and, in an undistended organ, lie about 3 cm apart.

The trigone has two muscular layers: a superficial layer and a deep layer. The superficial muscular layer is directly continuous with the longitudinal fibers of the distal ureter. This layer is also continuous posteriorly with the smooth muscle of the proximal urethra. The deep trigone forms a dense, compact layer that fuses somewhat with detrusor muscle fibers. The deep layer is in direct communication with a fibromuscular sheath, Waldeyer's sheath, in the intravesical portion of the ureter (Fig. 1-5). The deep trigonal muscle has autonomic innervation identical to that of the detrusor, being rich in cholinergic (parasympathetic) nerves and relatively sparse in noradrenergic (sympathetic) nerves. In contrast, the superficial trigonal muscle possesses few cholinergic nerves, but a relatively greater number of noradrenergic nerves.

Pelvic Ureter

As it courses retroperitoneally from the renal pelvis to the bladder, the ureter is divided anatomically into abdominal and pelvic segments, which are approximately equal in length, 12 to 15 cm each. The ureter enters the pelvis by crossing over the iliac vessels where the common iliac artery divides into the external iliac and hypogastric vessels. At this point, the ureter lies medial to the branches of the anterior division of the hypogastric artery and lateral to the peritoneum of the cul de sac. It is attached to the peritoneum of the lateral pelvic wall. As it proceeds more distally, the ureter courses along the lateral side of the uterosacral

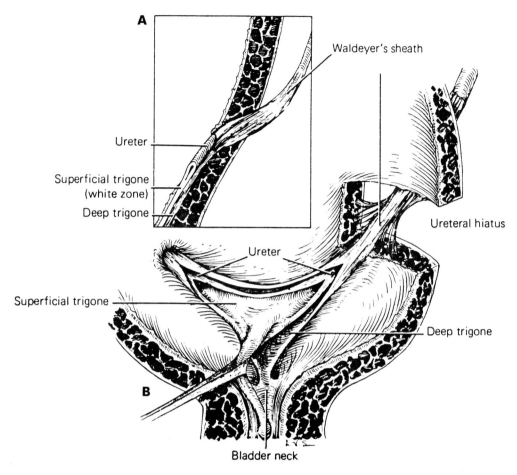

Fig. 1-5 Normal ureterovesicotrigonal complex. **A,** Side view with Waldeyer's muscular sheath surrounding vestige of the intravesical ureter and continuing downward as the deep trigone, which extends to the bladder neck. The ureteral musculature becomes the super- ficial trigone, which extends to just short of the external meatus in the female. **B,** Waldeyer's sheath connected by a few fibers to the detrusor muscle in the ureteral hiatus. This muscular sheath inferior to the ureteral orifice becomes the deep trigone. The musculature of the ureters continues downward as the superficial trigone. *(From Tanagho EA: Anatomy of the lower urinary tract. In Walsh PC, Gittes RF, Perlmutter AD, Stamey TA (eds):* Campbell's urology, *ed 5, Philadelphia, 1986, WB Saunders.)*

ligament and enters the endopelvic fascia of the peri- metrium (cardinal ligament). The ureter passes be- neath the uterine artery approximately 1.5 cm lateral to the cervix. The distal ureter then moves medially to enter the trigone of the bladder.

The ureter has only one muscular coat that forms an irregular, helical pattern of muscle bundles with fibers oriented in almost every direction. As the ureter approaches and enters the bladder wall, its helical fibers elongate and become parallel to its lumen. The intravesical ureter is about 1.5 cm long and is divided into an intramural segment, totally surrounded by the bladder wall, and a submucosal segment directly un- der the bladder mucosa. The longitudinal muscle fi- bers of the distal ureter proceed uninterrupted into the superficial trigone.

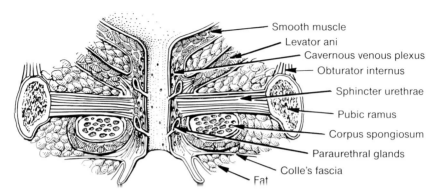

Fig. 1-6 Female urethra and surrounding structures.

The distal and intramural segments of the ureter are surrounded by Waldeyer's sheath. Waldeyer's sheath fuses proximally with the intrinsic musculature of the ureter and distally acts as an added fixation, linking the ureter proper to the detrusor muscle (Fig. 1-5). Waldeyer's sheath has been described thoroughly by Tanagho (1986) and by Woodburne (1968).

Urethra

The female urethra is about 4 cm long and averages 6 mm in diameter. Its lumen is slightly curved as it passes from the retropubic space, perforates through the perineal membrane, and ends with its external orifice in the vestibule directly above the vaginal opening. Throughout its length, the urethra is embedded in adventitia of the vaginal wall.

The urethral epithelium has longitudinal folds and many small glands, which open into the urethra throughout its entire length. The epithelium is continuous externally with that of the vulva and internally with that of the bladder. It is primarily a stratified squamous epithelium that becomes transitional near the bladder.

The epithelium is supported by a layer of loose fibroelastic connective tissue, the lamina propria. The lamina propria contains many bundles of collagen fibrils and fibrocytes, as well as an abundance of elastic fibers oriented both longitudinally and circularly around the urethra. Numerous thin-walled veins are another characteristic feature. This rich vascular supply probably contributes to urethral resistance. Fig.

1-6 demonstrates many of the structures that surround the female urethra.

Urethral Musculature

The urethral smooth muscle is composed primarily of oblique and longitudinal muscle fibers, with a few circularly oriented outer fibers. This muscle, and the detrusor muscle in the bladder base form what has been termed the internal urethral sphincter mechanism. This smooth muscle is usually noted to be under both alpha-adrenergic and cholinergic control, although Gosling found an extensive cholinergic nerve supply, with relatively few noradrenergic nerves. The longitudinally directed muscles probably act to shorten and widen the urethral lumen during micturition, whereas the circular smooth muscle (along with the striated urogenital sphincter muscle) contributes to urethral resistance to outflow at rest.

The striated urethral and periurethral muscles form the extrinsic urethral sphincter mechanism. It has two components: an inner portion, which lies within and adjacent to the urethral wall, and an outer portion, which is composed of skeletal muscle fibers of the pelvic diaphragm (see pelvic diaphragm section of Pelvic Floor). The inner portion is made up of the sphincter urethrae, a striated band of muscle that surrounds the proximal two thirds of the urethra, and the compressor urethrae and urethrovaginal sphincter (known together formerly as the deep transverse perineus muscle), which consist of two straplike bands of striated muscle that arch over the ventral surface

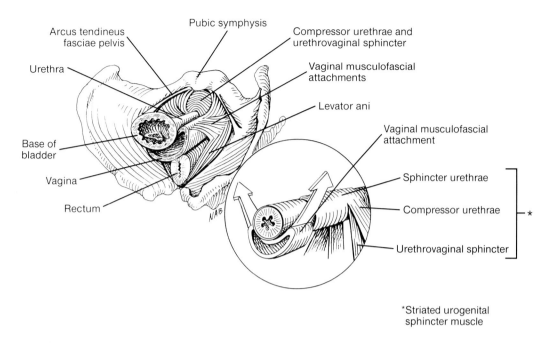

Fig. 1-7 Diagrammatic representation showing the component parts of the urethral support and sphincteric mechanisms. Note that the proximal urethra and bladder neck are supported by the anterior vaginal wall and its musculofascial attachments to the pelvic diaphragm. *Inset,* Contraction of the levator ani muscles elevates the anterior vagina and overlying bladder neck and proximal urethra, contributing to bladder neck closure. The sphincter urethrae, urethrovaginal sphincter, and compressor urethrae are all parts of the striated urogenital sphincter muscle.

of the distal one third of the urethra (Fig. 1-7, *inset*). These three muscles, which function as a single unit, have been termed by Oelrich the striated urogenital sphincter muscle. It is composed primarily of small-diameter, slow-twitch muscle, making it ideally suited to exert tone on the urethral lumen over prolonged time periods. This muscle may also contribute (along with the levator ani) to voluntary interruption of the urine stream and to urethral closure with stress, via reflex muscle contraction.

Urethral Support

Traditionally, the supporting structures of the urethra and bladder neck are thought to be formed by the interaction of the pubourethral ligaments, the urogenital diaphragm, and the muscles of the pelvic diaphragm. Numerous investigators have described the so-called pubourethral ligaments as extending from

the inferior surface of the pubic bones to the urethra. Milley and Nichols found bilaterally symmetric anterior, posterior, and intermediate pubourethral ligaments and stated that the anterior and posterior ligaments were formed, respectively, by inferior and superior fascial layers of the urogenital diaphragm. An anatomic defect of the pubourethral ligaments has been cited as a contributing factor to urinary stress incontinence in women.

Studies by DeLancey provide a more complete view of urethral support. Rather than being suspended ventrally by ligamentous structures, the proximal urethra and bladder base are supported in a slinglike fashion by the anterior vaginal wall, which is attached bilaterally to the muscles of the pelvic diaphragm (levator ani muscles) and to the arcus tendineus fasciae pelvis. Similar anatomic connections between the pelvic diaphragm and vagina have been described by

Olesen and Grau, and others. These attachments extend caudally and blend with the superior fibers of the perineal membrane (urogenital diaphragm). The tissues, described as pubourethral ligaments, are comprised of the perineal membrane and the most caudal portion of the arcus tendineus fasciae pelvis, which fix the distal urethra beneath the pubic bone. Fig. 1-7 illustrates the anatomic structures that contribute to urethral support and closure.

Anterior vaginal wall support to the pelvic diaphragm may contribute to urethral closure by providing a stable base onto which the bladder neck and proximal urethra are compressed with increases in intraabdominal pressure. These attachments also are responsible for the posterior movement of the vesical neck seen at the onset of micturition (when the pelvic floor relaxes) and for the elevation noted when a patient is instructed to arrest her urinary stream (Fig. 1-7, *inset*). Defects in these attachments probably result in proximal urethral support defects (urethral hypermobility) and displacement cystocele, conditions associated with stress urinary incontinence. These defects correspond to the paravaginal fascial defects described by Richardson et al.

VAGINA

The vagina is a hollow, fibromuscular tube that extends from the vestibule to the uterine cervix. The walls of the vagina are in contact except where its lumen is held open by the cervix. The vagina has an H-shaped lumen, with the principal dimension being transverse. The side walls are suspended by their attachments to the lateral pelvic connective tissues and pelvic diaphragm. Anteriorly, the vagina is contiguous with the bladder base, from which it is separated by loose connective tissue, and with the urethra, to which it is intimately connected. Posteriorly, the vagina is related to the cul de sac, to the rectal ampulla, and, inferiorly, to the perineal body. The rectovaginal septum and fascia intervene between the vagina and rectum. The terminal portions of the ureters pass close to the lateral fornices of the vagina.

The vagina is lined by stratified squamous epithelium with rugal folds that lie over a dense, thin layer of elastic fibers. Beneath these fibers is a well-developed fibromuscular layer. The structure of the vaginal wall and epithelium permits distention and return to normal size.

The human vagina is in a near horizontal position in a standing woman. The endopelvic fasciae support the uterus and upper vagina over the levator plate. The mid-vagina is supported by connections to the pelvic diaphragm and lower endopelvic fascia. The lower vagina is supported predominantly by connections to fibers of the pelvic diaphragm and the perineal membrane. The most posterior portion of the lower third is further attached to the perineal body.

PELVIC ORGAN SUPPORT

Pelvic Floor

With the change from plantigrade to erect posture, the pelvis and vertebral column of humans underwent various evolutionary changes that restored balance between intraabdominal pressure and visceral support. The lumbosacral curve, a specific human characteristic, directed the viscera forward onto the abdominal wall and flattened pubic bones. Downward pressure was directed backward and downward onto the sacrum and the rearranged levator ani muscles, which now filled in the pelvic cavity. These muscles formed a sphincter for the emerging urethra, vagina, and rectum.

The pelvic floor is made up of muscular and fascial structures that support the abdominal-pelvic cavity and the external opening of vagina (for parturition) and the urethra and rectum (for elimination). The pelvic floor consists of the pelvic diaphragm and perineal membrane (urogenital diaphragm).

Pelvic Diaphragm

The pelvic diaphragm consists of the levator ani and coccygeus muscles covered by superior and inferior fasciae. The diaphragm is stretched hammocklike between the pubis in front and the coccyx behind and is attached along the lateral pelvic wall to a thickened band in the obturator fascia, the arcus tendineus levatoris ani (Fig. 1-8). The levator ani muscle consists of three principal parts: puborectalis, pubococcygeus, and ileococcygeus muscles. The most medial of these muscles is the puborectalis. It arises from the inner

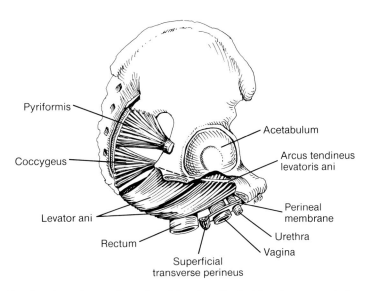

Pyriformis

Acetabulum

Coccygeus

Arcus tendineus
levatoris ani

Levator ani

Perineal
membrane

Rectum

Urethra

Vagina

Superficial
transverse perineus

Fig. 1-8 The levator ani, seen from the side when the ischium is removed. Arcus tendineus levatores ani runs from the ischial spine to the pubic bone. Note the perineal membrane that supports distal portions of the urethra and vagina.

surface of the pubic bones, proceeds backward along the edge of the genital hiatus in contact with the side of the vagina, and turns behind the rectum, joining the muscle bundle from the other side at the midline. The more lateral pubococcygeus portion of the levator ani also arises from the inner surface of the pubic bones, passes backward along the puborectalis muscle, and inserts into the anococcygeal raphe and the superior surface of the coccyx. The ileococcygeus portion of the levator ani arises from the arcus tendineus levatoris ani and the ischial spine and inserts into the anococcygeal raphe and the coccyx. The coccygeus muscle arises from the ischial spine and the sacrospinous ligament, passes backward against the posterior border of the ileococcygeus muscle, and inserts into the coccygeus and lower segment of the sacrum.

The ileococcygeus and coccygeus muscles receive their innervation from the inferior branch of the ventral ramus of the third and fourth sacral nerve. Recent work suggests that the puborectalis and pubococcygeus muscles are also supplied by sacral nerves via the pelvic plexus, not by the pudendal nerve, as formerly thought.

The muscle fibers of the pelvic diaphragm form a broad anteriorly directed U-shaped muscle layer called the urogenital hiatus (Fig. 1-9). The urethra, vagina, and rectum pass within this area. These organs are connected to the muscle and fasciae of the pelvic diaphragm, contributing to support of the anterior mid-vagina (and overlying bladder base and proximal urethra) and posterior mid-vagina and rectovaginal

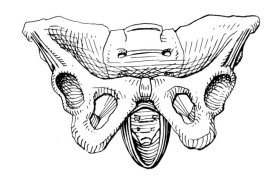

Fig. 1-9 The levator ani, with patient in the semirecumbent position. The muscle fibers of the pelvic diaphragm form a broad, anteriorly directed, U-shaped muscle layer. The pelvic organs pass within this U-shaped area, called the urogenital hiatus. *(After Dickinson RL:* Am J Obstet Dis Women Child *22:897, 1889.)*

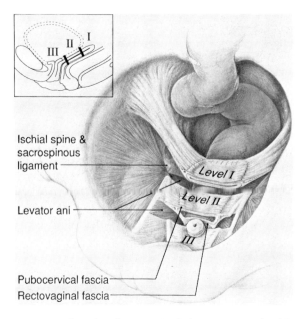

Ischial spine & sacrospinous ligament

Levator ani

Pubocervical fascia
Rectovaginal fascia

Level I

Level II

III

Fig. 1-10 Levels of support of the upper and mid-vagina. In level I (suspension), endopelvic fascia suspend vagina from lateral pelvic walls. Fibers of level I extend both vertically and also posteriorly toward sacrum. In level II (attachment), vagina is attached to arcus tendineus fascia pelvis and superior fascia of levator ani muscles. *(From DeLancey JO: Am J Obstet Gynecol 166:1717, 1992.)*

fascia (level II in Fig. 1-10). The region of the levator ani between the anus and coccyx formed by the anococcygeal raphe is clinically called the levator plate. It forms a supportive shelf on which the rectum, upper vagina, and uterus can rest and contributes to vaginal and uterine support.

Perineal Membrane

The perineal membrane is a triangular sheet of dense fibromuscular tissue that spans the anterior half of the pelvic outlet. It has previously been called the urogenital diaphragm and, according to DeLancey, this change in name reflects the appreciation that it is not a two-layered structure with muscle in between, as had previously been thought. The vagina and urethra pass through the perineal membrane and are supported by it. Cephalad to the perineal membrane lies the

striated urogenital sphincter muscle, which as already mentioned compresses the distal urethra.

Endopelvic Fascia

The endopelvic fascia invests the pelvic viscera, forming a subserous covering for them and enclosing their vascular peduncles. It is continuous with and an elaboration of extraperitoneal connective tissue. Histologically, it is made up of fibroelastic connective tissue, smooth muscle, blood vessels, nerves, and lymphatics. The bladder, rectum, lower uterus, and vagina receive an endopelvic fascial covering, and the thin-walled veins of the pelvis are contained within its meshes. The uterus and upper vagina are supported above the pelvic diaphragm to the pelvic walls by the upper portion of endopelvic fascia (level I in Fig. 1-10). These structures are identified surgically as the cardinal and uterosacral ligament complex. Cadaver studies by Mengert and by DeLancey have confirmed that these tissues are most important for support of the uterus and upper vagina.

The mid-portion of the endopelvic fascia attaches to the pelvic diaphragm at the arcus tendineus fasciae pelvis at the sides and in front of the bladder and urethra. The arcus tendineus fasciae pelvis separates from the arcus tendineus levatoris ani, as the latter turns toward the obturator canal. It continues forward to the pubococcygeus muscle and ends near the median line of the back of the lower border of the pubis. The sheet of endopelvic fascia that sweeps medialward from the arcus tendineus fasciae pelvis is termed the pubovesical ligament and contains the pubovesical muscle.

ANAL SPHINCTER MECHANISM

The anal sphincter mechanism comprises the internal anal sphincter, the external anal sphincter, and the puborectalis muscles (Fig. 1-11). The internal sphincter is a thickened, circular smooth muscle layer of the distal rectal wall that is under autonomic control. The voluntary sphincter is made up of the external anal sphincter and puborectalis muscles, which function together as a unit. As with the bladder neck and urethra, a spinal reflex causes the striated sphincter to contract during sudden increases in intraabdominal

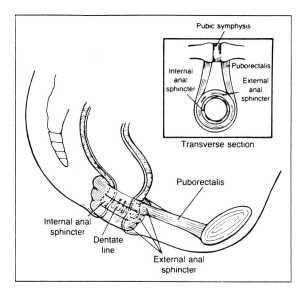

Fig. 1-11 Diagram of the rectum, anal canal, and surrounding muscles. The puborectalis muscle forms a sling posteriorly around the anorectal junction. The external anal sphincter (skeletal muscle) surrounds the anal canal and is closely associated with the puborectalis muscle. The internal anal sphincter muscle (smooth muscle) lies within the ring of external sphincter muscle and is a continuation of the inner circular layer of the smooth muscle of the rectal wall. *(From Madoff RD, Williams JG, Caushaj PF: N Engl J Med 326:1003, 1992.)*

pressure, such as coughing. The anal-rectal angle is produced by the anterior pull of the puborectalis muscles. These muscles form a sling posteriorly around the anorectal junction. The anal-rectal angle was previously thought to be important in maintaining fecal continence, but its importance has recently been questioned. More recent studies suggest that fecal incontinence in women is often related to denervation of the muscles of the pelvic diaphragm. This theory is discussed thoroughly in Chapter 12.

BIBLIOGRAPHY
Embryology

Gosling JA: Anatomy. In Stanton SL (ed): *Clinical gynecologic urology,* ed 1, St. Louis, 1984, Mosby–Year Book.

Gosling JA, Dixon J, Humpherson JR: *Functional anatomy of the urinary tract,* London, 1982, Gower Medical Publishing.

Hilton P: The mechanism of continence. In Stanton SL, Tanagho EA (eds): *Surgery of female incontinence,* ed 2, New York, 1986, Springer-Verlag.

Langman J: *Medical embryology,* Baltimore, 1976, Williams & Wilkins.

Maizels M: Normal development of the urinary tract. In Walsh PC, Gittes RF, Perlmutter AD, Stamey TA (eds): *Campbell's urology,* ed 5, Philadelphia, 1986, WB Saunders.

Muckle CW: Developmental abnormalities of the female reproductive organs. In Sciarra JJ (ed): *Gynecology and obstetrics,* vol 1, Hagerstown, Md, 1981, Harper & Row.

Snyder HMcC: Anomalies of the ureter. In Gillenwater JY, Grayhack JT, Howards SS, Duckett JW (eds): *Adult and pediatric urology,* vol 2, Chicago, 1987, Mosby–Year Book.

Anatomy

Curtis AH, Anson BJ, Ashley FL: Further studies in gynecological anatomy and related clinical problems, *Surg Gynecol Obstet* 74:709, 1942.

Curtis AH, Anson BJ, McVay CB: The anatomy of the pelvic and urogenital diaphragms, in relation to urethrocele and cystocele, *Surg Gynecol Obstet* 68:161, 1939.

DeLancey JO: Anatomy of the pelvis. In Thompson JD, Rock JA (eds): *Telinde's operative gynecology,* ed 7, Philadelphia, 1992, JB Lippincott.

DeLancey JO: Correlative study of paraurethral anatomy, *Obstet Gynecol* 68:91, 1986.

DeLancey JO: Anatomy of the female bladder and urethra. In Ostergard DR, Bent AE (eds): *Urogynecology and Urodynamics,* ed 3, Baltimore, 1991, Williams & Wilkins.

DeLancey JO: Structural aspects of the extrinsic continence mechanism, *Obstet Gynecol* 72:296, 1988.

DeLancey JO: Histology of the connection between the vagina and levator ani muscles, *J Reprod Med* 35:765, 1990.

DeLancey JO: Pubovesical ligament: a separate structure from the urethral supports ("pubo-urethral ligaments"), *Neurourol Urodyn* 8:53, 1989.

DeLancey JO: Anatomic aspects of vaginal eversion after hysterectomy, *Am J Obstet Gynecol* 166:1717, 1992.

Dickinson RL: Studies of the levator ani muscle, *Am J Obstet Dis Women Child* 22:897, 1889.

Elbadawi A: Neuromorphologic basis of vesicourethral function: I. histochemistry, ultrastructure and function of the intrinsic nerves of the bladder and urethra, *Neurourol Urodyn* 1:3, 1982.

Funt MI, Thompson JD, Birch H: Normal vaginal axis, *South Med J* 71:1534, 1978.

Gosling JA, Dixon JS, Humpherson JR: Functional anatomy of the urinary tract, an integrated text and color atlas, Baltimore, 1982, University Park Press.

Gosling JA, Dixon JS, Critchley HO, et al: A comparative study of the human external sphincter and periurethral levator ani muscles, *Br J Urol* 53:35, 1981.

Gosling JA: The structure of the female lower urinary tract and pelvic floor, *Urol Clin North Am* 12:207, 1985.

Halban J, Tandler J: *Anatomie and Atiologie der Genital-prolapse beim Weibe,* Vienna and Leipzig, 1907, Wilhelm Braumuller, (Translated by Porges RF, Porges JC: The anatomy and etiology of genital prolapse in women, *Obstet Gynecol* 15:790, 1960.

Krantz KE: The anatomy of the urethra and anterior vaginal wall, *Am J Obstet Gynecol* 62:374, 1951.

Lawson JO: Pelvic anatomy. I. Pelvic floor muscles, *Ann R Coll Surg Engl* 52:244, 1974.

Lund CJ, Fullerton RE, Tristan TA: Cinefluorographic studies of the bladder and urethra in women, *Am J Obstet Gynecol* 78:706, 1959.

Madoff RD, Williams JG, Caushaj PF: Fecal incontinence, *N Engl J Med* 326:1003, 1992.

McGuire EJ: The innervation and function of the lower urinary tract, *J Neurosurg* 65:278, 1986.

Mengert WF: Mechanics of uterine support and position, *Am J Obstet Gynecol* 31:775, 1936.

Milley PS, Nichols DH: The relationship between the pubo-urethral ligaments and the urogenital diaphragm in the human female, *Anat Rec* 170:281, 1971.

Muellner SR: The physiology of micturition, *J Urol* 65:805, 1951.

Nichols DH, Randall CL: *Vaginal surgery,* ed 3, Baltimore, 1989, Williams & Wilkins.

Oelrich TM: The striated urogenital sphincter muscle in the female, *Anat Rec* 205:223, 1983.

Olesen KP, Grau V: The suspensory apparatus of the female bladder neck, *Urol Int* 31:33, 1976.

Redman JF: Anatomy of the genitourinary system. In Gillenwater JY, Grayhack JT, Howards SS, Duckett JW (eds): *Adult and pediatric urology,* vol 1, Chicago, 1987, Mosby–Year Book.

Richardson AC, Lyon JB, Williams NL: A new look at pelvic relaxation, *Am J Obstet Gynecol* 126:568, 1976.

Tangaho EA: Anatomy of the lower urinary tract. In Walsh PC, Gittes RF, Perlmutter AD, Stamey TA (eds): *Campbell's urology,* ed 5, Philadelphia, 1986, WB Saunders.

Woodburne RT: Essentials of human anatomy, ed 5, New York, 1976, Onford University Press.

Woodburne RT: Anatomy of the bladder and bladder outlet, *J Urol* 100:474, 1968.

Zacharin RF: Pelvic floor anatomy and the surgery of pulsion enterocoele, New York, 1985, Springer-Verlag.

Zacharin RF: The suspensory mechanism of the female urethra, *J Anat* 97:423, 1963.

CHAPTER 2

Neurophysiology of the Lower Urinary Tract

J. Thomas Benson
Mark D. Walters

General Nervous System Arrangements
  Central nervous system
  Peripheral nervous system
Neural Control of the Lower Urinary Tract
  Autonomic nervous system
  Sensory innervation
  Central nervous system modulation
Mechanisms of Normal Bladder Filling, Storage, and Voiding
  Filling and storage
  Voiding
Clinical Pharmacology of the Lower Urinary Tract
  Therapy to facilitate bladder emptying
  Therapy to facilitate urine storage

The two functions of the lower urinary tract are the storage of urine within the bladder and the timely expulsion of urine from the urethra. The precise neurologic pathways and neurophysiologic mechanisms that control micturition are complex and not completely understood. The storage and expulsion of urine are part of a complex neurophysiologic function that involves autonomic and somatic nervous systems. Function is controlled by reflex pathways, which are further modulated by central voluntary control. Precise knowledge of neuroanatomy, neurophysiology, and pharmacology is important to understand and treat many diseases of the lower urinary tract. This chapter reviews normal function and neurologic control of the lower urinary tract in women.

GENERAL NERVOUS SYSTEM ARRANGEMENTS

The nervous system is arranged into the central and the peripheral systems. The central nervous system includes the brain and spinal cord. Twelve paired cranial and 31 paired spinal nerves with their ganglia compose the peripheral nervous system. The somatic component of the peripheral system innervates skeletal muscle and the autonomic division innervates cardiac muscle, smooth muscle, and glands.

Central Nervous System

Within the brain and cord, nerve cell bodies are arranged in groups of various sizes and shapes referred to as nuclei. Those fibers with a common origin and destination are called a tract; some are so anatomically distinct that they are termed *fasciculus, brachium, peduncle, column,* or *lemniscus.*

Older methods of tracing the nervous system pathways consisted of inducing cell degeneration and applying appropriate stains to identify the degenerated fibers. Newer methods that do not require nerve tissue destruction and that use chemical tracers have been available since the 1970s. Such tracers as carbon-14 labeled proline move from the cell bodies to the axon terminals (orthograde) and are identified autoradiographically. Retrograde tracers, such as horseradish peroxidase, move from axon terminals to cell bodies and are identified by light and electron microscopy.

Nerve cell bodies originating high in the central nervous system send axons to the motor nuclei in the brain stem and spinal cord to exert control over the cranial and spinal nerves. The control may be positive or inhibiting, but lesions of these tracts (upper motor neuron lesions) lead to opposite-body hyperreflexia and spastic weakness due to a net reduction of inhibiting influences.

Peripheral Nervous System

Both somatic reflex pathways and autonomic pathways compose the peripheral nervous system, particularly as it applies to the lower urinary tract. The spinal nerve, then, has functional components dealing with somatic and visceral afferent and efferent fibers.

Somatic Reflex Pathway

A segmental skeletal muscle reflex consists of nerves that activate large extrafusal muscle fibers. They are affected by regulatory afferent nerves from the muscle spindles, acting through intermediate neurons. The urethral skeletal muscle, however, has no spindles, so afferent regulatory activity is generated in some as yet undefined way.

Supraspinal afferent fibers similarly affect alpha-motor neurons. Alpha-motor neurons also innervate interneurons in the ventral horn (Renshaw cells), which act to inhibit other alpha-motor neurons, a negative feedback response allowing more rapid firing.

Typically, motor neuron size correlates with muscle fiber types. Smaller motor neurons innervate smaller units to activate slower, less fatigable muscle fibers used for tonicity, whereas larger motor neurons activate the fast twitch response muscle fibers.

Autonomic Pathways

The autonomic nervous system consists of general visceral efferent and general visceral afferent fibers, which ordinarily function at a subconscious level. Un-

like the somatic motor system, the peripheral fibers reach the effector organ by a two-neuron chain. The preganglionic neuron arises in the intermediolateral cell column of the brain stem or spinal cord and terminates at an outlying ganglion, where the postganglionic neuron continues the impulse transmission to the end organ.

Fibers arising from the intermediolateral gray column of the 12 thoracic and first two lumbar segments of the spinal cord constitute the sympathetic division of the autonomic nervous system. The parasympathetic division consists of fibers arising from the second through the fourth sacral segments and from cranial outflows.

Sympathetic nerves to the pelvic cavity originate in cord levels T5 to L2 and pass to ganglia located at roots of arteries for which they are named (for example, lumbar splanchnic nerves terminate in inferior mesenteric and hypogastric ganglia). Postganglionic fibers from these ganglia follow the visceral arteries to the organs of the lower abdomen and pelvis. Pelvic parasympathetic system preganglionic fibers originate in spinal segment S2 through S4 and extend to ganglia located within or very near the organs they supply, thus having very short postganglionic fibers.

NEURAL CONTROL OF THE LOWER URINARY TRACT

The urinary tract is controlled principally by local innervation acting under central nervous system modulation. Local innervation is chiefly by parasympathetic and sympathetic autonomic and peripheral somatic motor and sensory systems. A summary of the neural pathways involved in micturition are shown in Figs. 2-1 and 2-2.

Autonomic Nervous System

The autonomic nervous system controls the lower urinary tract by its actions on the ganglia, detrusor muscle, and smooth muscle of the trigone and urethra.

Ganglia

Sympathetic preganglionic fibers from thoracolumbar spinal segments form white rami communicants to corresponding chain ganglia. Postganglionic neurons

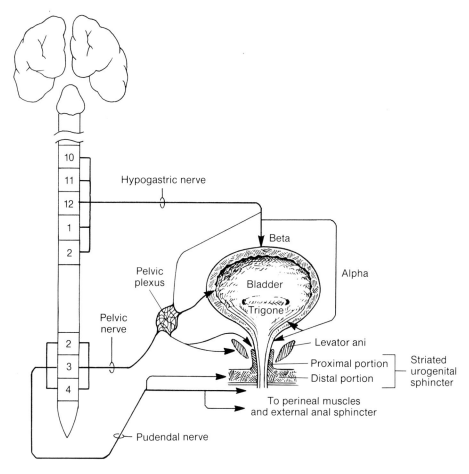

Fig. 2-1   Peripheral innervation of the female lower urinary tract.

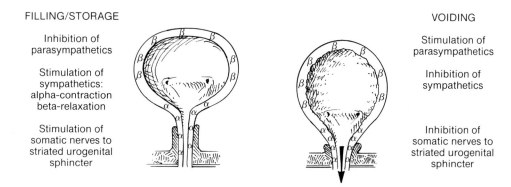

FILLING/STORAGE

Inhibition of parasympathetics

Stimulation of sympathetics:
alpha-contraction
beta-relaxation

Stimulation of somatic nerves to striated urogenital sphincter

VOIDING

Stimulation of parasympathetics

Inhibition of sympathetics

Inhibition of somatic nerves to striated urogenital sphincter

Fig. 2-2   Actions of the autonomic and somatic nervous systems during bladder filling/storage and voiding.

reach inferior mesenteric ganglia by the lumbar splanchnic nerves and continue through the *hypogastric plexus* to the presacral fascia, across the upper posterior lateral pelvic wall, 1 to 2 cm behind and below the ureter. After these neurons join the pelvic nerves, the *pelvic plexus* is formed, running below and medial to the internal iliac vessels overlying the anterior lateral lower rectum near the anorectal junction. The plexus spreads in the lateral wall of the upper one third of the vagina beneath the uterine artery, medial to the ureter, and 2 cm inferolateral to the cervix. Within the vesicovaginal space, the plexus supplies the upper vagina, bladder, proximal urethra, and lower ureter.

The parasympathetic preganglionic fibers arise from nerve roots S3 and S4 and occasionally S2. These fibers emerge from the piriformis muscle overlying the sacral foramina and enter the presacral fascia near the ischial spine at the posterior layer of the hypogastric sheath, where they contribute to the already described pelvic plexus. These parasympathetic fibers terminate in pelvic ganglia located within the wall of the bladder, a location quite vulnerable to end-organ disease, such as overstretch, infection, or fibrosis.

At the ganglia, excitatory transmission occurs from activation of nicotinic acetylcholine receptors, with some ganglionic cells having secondary muscarinic receptors. Norepinephrine also acts as a neurotransmitter, and alpha-adrenergic receptors, when stimulated, depress pelvic ganglion transmission by suppression of presynaptic cholinergic neurotransmitter release. Neuropeptide agents, especially enkephalin, probably also function at ganglia; precise knowledge of transmission regulation is not available at present.

Detrusor Innervation

Postganglionic detrusor nerve fibers diverge and store neurotransmitter agents in axonal varicosities termed *synaptic vesicles*. The agent is diffused to neuromuscular bundles of 12 to 15 smooth muscle fibers enclosed in a collagen capsule that acts similarly to the tendon insertion of a muscle. Stimulating electrical pulses produce two episodes of depolarization, suggesting the release of two neurotransmitters. The first neurotransmitter is noncholinergic and nonadrenergic,

and the second neurotransmitter is acetylcholine. This observation accounts for detrusor atropine resistance. Cholinergic receptors are present more in the body than in the base of the bladder, whereas adrenergic and neuropeptide receptors are more prevalent in the base. Neuropeptide receptors include vasoactive intestinal polypeptide and substance P. Histaminic and purinergic receptors may also be present in detrusor smooth muscle.

Trigone and Urethra

The trigone is a separate anatomic and embryologic region where muscle fibers have an almost exclusively adrenergic innervation. Norepinephrine transmitter acts on alpha-receptors, which are stimulated by higher doses and produce smooth muscle contraction, and on beta-receptors, which are stimulated by lower doses of norepinephrine and produce smooth muscle relaxation (except in cardiac muscle). Beta-receptors are thought to be more prominent in the detrusor body, whereas alpha-receptors occur chiefly in the bladder outlet and urethra. Cholinergic development in the bladder is present at birth, whereas adrenergic development occurs later. Prostaglandins act as intracellular messengers to relax trigonal muscles.

The proximal urethra is rich in alpha-adrenergic receptors. Acetylcholine, substance P, vasoactive intestinal polypeptide, and histamine are all additional potential transmitters in the urethra.

Somatic motor control is effected by segmented innervation to the intraurethral and periurethral skeletal muscle. The exact neuropathways supplying the external urethral sphincter are controversial. The proximal intramural component of the striated urogenital sphincter muscle (sphincter urethrae) probably is innervated by somatic efferent branches of the pelvic nerves, a component of the pelvic plexus. The more distal periurethral striated muscles (compressor urethrae and urethrovaginal sphincter), however, are innervated by the pudendal nerve, as is the skeletal muscle of the external anal sphincter and perineal muscles. Embryologic speculation is that pelvic caudal muscles (tail waggers), which compose the levator group in humans, are supplied from the pelvic plexus on the pelvic surface side, whereas the sphincter cloacal derivatives are supplied from the perineal aspect by the pudendal nerve.

The pudendal nerve passes between the coccygeus and piriformis muscles, leaves the pelvis through the greater sciatic foramen, crosses the ischial spine, and reenters the pelvis through the lesser sciatic foramen (see Chapter 12, Fig. 12-5). Here the nerve accompanies the pudendal vessels along the lateral wall of the ischiorectal fossa in a tunnel formed by a splitting of the obturator fascia, Alcock's canal. At the perineal membrane, the nerve divides into the inferior rectal nerve, supplying the external anal sphincter, the perineal nerve, and the dorsal nerve to the clitoris. The perineal nerve splits into a superficial branch to the labia and a deep branch to the periurethral striated muscles.

The periurethral muscles are composed mostly of slow twitch fibers (type 1) with an approximate concentration of 35% fast twitch fibers (type 2). Thus constant tonus occurs with emergency reflex activity available mainly in the distal half of the urethra.

The response of segmental spinal reflex leading to pudendal nerve function involves several spinal cord segments. Afferent fibers involved in the reflex have both segmental and supraspinal routing. This dual routing explains the bimodal response of pudendal motor neurons when pudendal sensory nerves are stimulated, and it differs from stimulation of pelvic detrusor afferents. Evoked response studies of pelvic plexus afferents to the cord demonstrate temporal durations more than twice those of pudendal afferents.

The neurotransmitter at the periurethral skeletal neuromuscular junction is acetylcholine and receptors are nicotinic type. The intimate adherence of the neuromuscular junction to the striated muscle fibers conveys a resistance to blockade by neuromuscular blocking agents.

Sensory Innervation

Detrusor proprioceptive endings exist as nerve endings in collagen bundles. They are stimulated by stretch or contraction and are responsible for the feeling of bladder fullness. Pain and temperature nerve endings are free in bladder mucosa and submucosa. The sensory endings in the detrusor probably contain acetylcholine and substance P.

Two types of bladder sensors have been postulated, the first sensor perhaps being at the trigone, the second being stretch receptors in the bladder body. Loss of

the first sensor may lead to urge incontinence as the bladder is ready to contract before sensation is noted.

Urethral sensation is carried principally by the pudendal nerve, although the pelvic nerve also contributes (Fig. 2-3). Urethral smooth muscle sensory innervation, like the detrusor, has both a contralateral and an ipsilateral supply.

Central Nervous System Modulation

The detrusor and the periurethral striated muscle mechanisms have separate cortical and other higher center regulation. The effects of such regulation are chiefly on the brain stem for the detrusor and on the sacral cord for the periurethral mechanisms.

Cortical Pathways

Cortical-reticular axons originating from pyramidal detrusor area cells in the supramedial portion of the frontal lobes and in the genu of the corpus callosum traverse the basal ganglia and terminate in the pontomesencephalic reticular formation of the brain stem on detrusor motor nuclei in the nucleus lateralis dor-

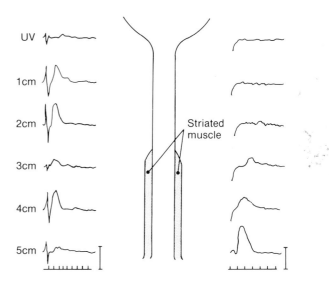

Fig. 2-3 Longitudinal sensory innervation of urethra. Column on *left* shows responses evoked in the pelvic nerve. Column on *right* shows responses evoked in the pudendal nerve. *(From Bradley WE: Physiology of urinary bladder. In Walsh PC, Perlmutter AD, Gittes RF, et al, editors: Campbell's urology, vol 1, Philadelphia, 1986, WB Saunders.)*

salis. These detrusor motor nuclei receive suppressive afferents from basal ganglia, coordinating afferents from the cerebellum, and sensory cord afferents from tension receptors in the detrusor muscle, which synapse here to constitute the so-called "long routing" detrusor reflex. Fibers from the raphe nuclei of the reticular formation may function to moderate responsiveness to different phases of the sleep-wake cycle or emotional states.

Efferents of the brain stem detrusor motor nuclei go to detrusor motor neurons in the intermediolateral cell column from the T10 to L1 and the S2 to S4 segments of the cord. It is speculated that because the detrusor reflex is a brain stem function rather than a spinal function, temporal amplification can occur, allowing for complete bladder emptying.

Pudendal cortical pathways affect periurethral striated muscle innervation by direct descending paths originating in the central vertex of the pudendal cerebral cortical area and going to pudendal nuclei in the ventromedial portion of the ventral gray matter of the S1 to S3 cord segments. At this level, the pudendal motor nuclei act as a segmental skeletal muscle reflex.

Ascending axons from periurethral striated muscle go to the pudendal cortical area, possibly synapsing in the nucleus ventralis posterolateralis of the thalamus, the brain's chief relay station. Sensory afferents from both pudendal and detrusor pelvic nerves send input to the anterior vermis of the cerebellum, which then originates an axon relay to the cortex in the dentate nucleus. Fibers for both detrusor and pudendal proprioception and exteroception (pain, temperature, and touch) ascend in posterior columns and spinothalamic tracts, respectively.

Neurotransmitters involved in these pathways include acetylcholine and peptides, especially substance P and enkephalin. Neurotransmitter agents are stored in astrocytes, which may also function to regulate extracellular concentrations.

Other Higher Centers

The basal ganglia clearly have an effect on detrusor reflex control, which is probably suppressive. The neurotransmitter dopamine, manufactured in the substantia nigra by enzymatic conversion of catecholamines, is important for the control of somatic movements related to posture. Exhaustion of dopamine

from the body is found in the 1 million patients suffering from Parkinson's disease, characterized by slowness of movement, gait disturbance, tremor, and in 45% to 75%, hyperreflexia of the bladder.

The limbic system in the temporal lobes exerts controls affecting all autonomic functions and is a favored site for epileptiform activity. Enkephalin is a notable neurotransmitter here as well as in the reticular formation.

The hypothalamus function, although poorly delineated, is known to involve beta-endorphin neurotransmitters, the opioid peptides constituting an entire class of brain neurotransmitters.

The cerebellum, where gamma-aminobutyric acid (GABA) is prominent along with standard neurotransmitters, regulates muscle tone and coordinates movement. Disease in this area produces spontaneous, high-amplitude bladder hyperreflexia.

The brain stem's importance in the lower urinary tract function has been known since 1921, when Barrington ablated this area in cats and produced permanent urinary retention. Brain stem neurotransmitters include substance P, GABA, and serotonin, which is produced from tryptophan.

Spinal Cord

By adolescence, disparity in growth of the spinal cord and the vertebral column leads to the cord's terminating around the first lumbar vertebra. The adult conus medullaris is quite short and contains the entire S1 to S5 segment. Although the thoracolumbar levels are important in sympathetic autonomic influence of the lower urinary tract, the conus medullaris has greater significance because autonomic detrusor nuclei and pudendal somatic nuclei are housed in the intermediolateral and ventromedial anterior gray matter, respectively. The conus medullaris also houses neurons involved with defecation and sexual function, with relays for cortical separation of these visceral functions (encephalization) developing after birth.

Urine storage and evacuation reflexes actively involve this area of the cord and have been classified by Mahoney et al (Table 2-1); however, the reflex pathways are mostly theoretical, few having been demonstrated in humans. In experimental animals, three pathways have been demonstrated. The first, the proximal urethra to the detrusor, facilitates detrusor

TABLE 2-1 Proposed reflexes that influence urine storage and evacuation

Pathway	Result
Reflexes involved in bladder storage	
1. Sympathetic detrusor to detrusor reflex	Inhibits detrusor in response to increased detrusor tension
2. Detrusor-urethral stimulating reflex	Increased detrusor tension stimulates urethral smooth muscle
3. Perineal-detrusor inhibition	Inhibits detrusor in response to perineal sphincter muscles
4. Urethrosphincter guarding	Contracts external striated sphincter in response to trigone tension
Micturition initiation reflexes	
5. Perineodetrusor facilitative	Decreasing pelvic floor muscle tone
	Stimulates detrusor
6. Detrusor-detrusor facilitative	Increased detrusor tension stimulates detrusor
Reflexes to maintain micturition	
7. Detrusor-urethral inhibiting	Detrusor to segmental inhibition or urethral smooth muscle
8. Detrusor-sphincter inhibiting	Detrusor to segmental inhibition of external striated sphincter
9. Urethrodetrusor facilitative	Proximal urethra segmental reflex to stimulated detrusor
10. Urethrobulbar detrusor facilitative	Proximal urethra reflex to stimulate detrusor via brain stem
11. Urethrosphincteric inhibiting	Urethra to external striated sphincter
	Segmental reflex
Micturition cessation reflex	Pelvic floor afferent fibers to brain stem to inhibit detrusor

From Benson JT: *Obstet Gynecol Clin North Am* 16:733, 1989.

reflex, which may be important when considering proximal urethral relationships to bladder instability. The second pathway, periurethral striated muscle to the detrusor for detrusor inhibition, is used for biofeedback therapy of unstable bladder conditions. The third pathway is sacral cord afferent fibers to lumbar cord efferent fibers for depression of ganglion transmission.

MECHANISMS OF NORMAL BLADDER FILLING, STORAGE, AND VOIDING

Our understanding of the neurophysiology of micturition developed from a large body of literature primarily based on animal models. Precise neural pathways involved in voiding remain controversial. The concepts presented here are primarily based on those by Bradley et al and DeGroat et al, as synthesized by Blaivas (1982) and McGuire. Fig. 2-4 is a summary of the major neurologic pathways involved in bladder filling and voiding.

Filling and Storage

During physiologic bladder filling, little or no increase in intravesical pressure is observed, despite large increases in urine volume. This process, called accommodation, is due primarily to passive elastic and viscoelastic properties of the smooth muscle and connective tissue of the bladder wall. During filling, muscle bundles in the bladder wall undergo reorganization, and the muscle cells are elongated up to four times their length. As bladder filling progresses and at a certain bladder wall tension, a desire to void is felt, although it has not been determined where in the brain this sensation is processed. Mechanoreceptors in the bladder wall are activated and action potentials run with afferent parasympathetic pelvic nerves to the spinal cord at the level of S2 to S4.

As filling increases to a critical intravesical pressure, or with rapid bladder filling, detrusor muscle contractility is probably inhibited by activation of a spinal sympathetic reflex. The sympathetic efferents that influence micturition arise at the T10 through L2

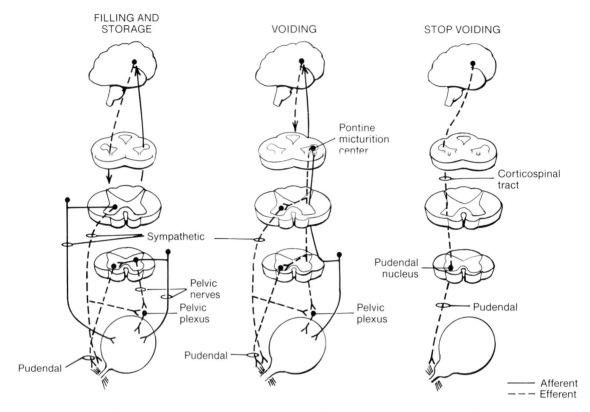

Fig. 2-4 Summary of major neurologic pathways involved in bladder function. *Storage*—bladder distention results in afferent pelvic nerve discharge. After synapse in pudendal nucleus efferent pudendal nerve impulses result in contraction of external urethral sphincter. At same time afferent sympathetic discharges traverse hypogastric nerve. After synapse in sympathetic nuclei efferent firing causes (1) inhibition of transmission of postganglionic parasympathetic neuron, which inhibits detrusor contraction and (2) increased tone at bladder neck. Net effect is that urethral pressure remains greater than detrusor pressure, facilitating urine storage. *Voiding*—afferent pelvic nerve discharges ascend in spinal cord and synapse in pontine micturition center. Descending efferent pathways cause (1) inhibition of pudendal firing, which relaxes external sphincter; (2) inhibition of sympathetic firing, which opens bladder neck and permits postganglionic parasympathetic transmission; and (3) pelvic parasympathetic firing, which causes detrusor contraction. Net result is that relaxation of external sphincter causes decrease in urethral pressure followed almost immediately by detrusor contraction and voiding ensues. *Stop*—voluntary interruption of urinary stream. Descending corticospinal pathways emanating from motor cortex synapse in pudendal nucleus, resulting in contraction of external urethral sphincter. Urethral pressure increases above detrusor pressure, interrupting stream. *(Modified from Blaivas JG: J Urol 127:958, 1982.)*

area and synapse in the inferior mesenteric and pelvic ganglia. This reflex, with sensory afferent activity through the pelvic nerve and efferent activity through the hypogastric nerve, results in inhibition of detrusor contractility and facilitation of bladder relaxation. As noted by McGuire, three sympathetic neural responses to afferent pelvic nerve firing associated with increasing bladder volume have been demonstrated experimentally: (1) beta-receptor-mediated relaxation of the detrusor musculature; (2) alpha-receptor-mediated increase in urethral smooth muscle activity and urethral pressure; and (3) inhibition of ganglionic transmission in the pelvic (vesical) ganglia, which, in effect, inhibits sacral parasympathetic outflow to the bladder. These actions are illustrated in Fig. 2-2.

During bladder filling, outlet resistance increases by reflex stimulation of alpha-adrenergic receptors within the smooth muscle of the bladder neck and proximal urethra. In addition, stimulation of the striated external sphincter occurs, resulting from increased efferent somatic (pelvic and pudendal) nerve activity. As noted earlier, innervation of the proximal intramural portion of the striated urogenital sphincter (sphincter urethrae) is from somatic components of the pelvic nerve, via the pelvic plexus. Innervation of the distal striated urogenital sphincter (compressor urethrae and urethrovaginal sphincter) is probably via the pudendal nerve. These responses have been shown to both increase intraurethral pressure and inhibit preganglionic detrusor motor neurons in the intermediolateral cell columns of the sacral spinal cord.

Voiding

Normal voiding is a voluntary act involving reflex-coordinated relaxation of the urethra and sustained contraction of the bladder until emptying is complete. In healthy women, the micturition reflex is probably not a simple segmental sacral reflex, but is modulated supraspinally in the pontine micturition center. Voluntary control of the micturition reflex is mediated by connections between the frontal cerebral cortex and the pons. Voluntary control of the external urethral sphincter is via the corticospinal pathway connecting the frontal cortex with the pudendal nucleus in the ventral horn of the sacral spinal cord. Bradley et al believe that connections between the sensorimotor cortex and the pudendal nucleus control voluntary

sphincter activity and that voiding is controlled voluntarily by complex interactions among cortical areas (frontal cortex), subcortical areas (thalamus, hypothalamus, basal ganglia, and limbic system), and brain stem (mesencephalic-pontine-medullary reticular formation).

With filling to bladder capacity, stimuli from the bladder cause afferent discharges in the pelvic nerve, which traverse pathways in the spinal cord to synapse in a supraspinal micturition center in the pontine mesencephalic reticular formation. Voiding is initiated voluntarily or when the bladder volume is so large that it is no longer possible to suppress micturition. To initiate voiding, the external urethral sphincter relaxes voluntarily via somatic motor neurons from the ventral horn. Efferent impulses from the pontine micturition center run in the reticulospinal tracts to inhibit pudendal firing (relaxing the external sphincter) and to stimulate parasympathetic neurons situated in the intermediolateral cell column at levels S2 through S4, causing detrusor contraction. During voiding, sympathetic efferents are inhibited, which opens the bladder neck and permits postganglionic parasympathetic transmission.

Urodynamically, the micturition reflex begins with sudden and complete relaxation of the striated muscles of the urethra and pelvic floor and a decrease in urethral pressure. Several seconds later, intravesical pressure increases, owing to a highly controlled coordinated contraction of the bulk of the detrusor muscle. Descent and funneling of the bladder neck and proximal urethra occur and urine flow begins.

Brain stem modulation of the micturition reflex allows for a detrusor contraction long enough to evacuate intravesical contents completely. With voluntary termination of voiding or with the "stop" test, the striated muscles of the urethra and pelvic floor contract to elevate the bladder base, increase intraurethral pressure, and empty the urethra of urine. The detrusor muscle is reflexly inhibited and intravesical pressure returns to normal.

CLINICAL PHARMACOLOGY OF THE LOWER URINARY TRACT

Thorough understanding of the neurologic control of the urinary bladder and its outlet allows one to intelligently use pharmacologic agents to manage many types of lower urinary tract dysfunction. Basic concepts of pharmacologic treatment will be summarized within a functional scheme of therapy for micturition disorders as developed by Wein et al. More specific guidelines for pharmacologic treatments of various lower urinary tract complaints and reviews of the clinical studies using these agents are found in chapters describing individual urogynecologic disorders.

Most pharmacologic agents produce their effects by combining with cell receptors. The drug-receptor interaction initiates a series of biochemical and physiologic changes that characterize the effects produced by the agent. Most drugs alter lower urinary tract function by affecting (1) synthesis, transport, storage, and release of the neurotransmitter; (2) the combination of the neurotransmitter with postjunctional receptors; or (3) the inactivation, degradation, or reuptake of the neurotransmitter.

Clinically, pharmacologic agents can be grouped into those that facilitate bladder emptying and those that facilitate urine storage (see accompanying box).

Patients with disorders of bladder emptying usually have voiding dysfunction; drugs that improve bladder emptying do so by increasing bladder contractility or by decreasing outlet resistance. Patients with disorders of urine storage often present with urinary incontinence, which is usually due either to an overactive detrusor or to an incompetent urethral sphincter mechanism. Agents that facilitate urine storage act by inhibiting bladder contractility, thereby increasing bladder capacity, or by increasing outlet resistance. The most effective and commonly used agents act on either the parasympathetic or sympathetic systems.

Therapy to Facilitate Bladder Emptying
Increasing Intravesical Pressure

A major portion of the final common pathway in a physiologic bladder contraction is stimulation of the muscarinic cholinergic receptor sites at the postganglionic, parasympathetic neuromuscular junction. Parasympathetic nerve stimulation causes the release of acetylcholine (Ach) at postsynaptic, parasympathetic receptor sites. Ach release produces muscarinic

---

Drug Effects on Lower Urinary Tract Function

Therapy to Facilitate Bladder Emptying

Increasing intravesical pressure/bladder contractility
  Parasympathomimetic agents
  Prostaglandins
  Blockers of inhibition
    Alpha-adrenergic antagonists
    Opioid antagonists
Decreasing outlet resistance
  At the level of the smooth sphincter
    Alpha-adrenergic antagonists
    Beta-adrenergic agonists
  At the level of the striated sphincter
    Skeletal muscle relaxants
      Centrally acting relaxants
      Dantrolene
      Baclofen
    Alpha-adrenergic antagonists

Therapy to Facilitate Urine Storage

Inhibiting bladder contractility/decreasing sensory input/increasing bladder capacity
  Anticholinergic agents
  Musculotropic relaxants
  Polysynaptic inhibitors
  Calcium antagonists
  Beta-adrenergic agonists
  Alpha-adrenergic antagonists
  Prostaglandin inhibitors
  Tricyclic antidepressants
  Dimethyl sulfoxide (DMSO)
  Bromocriptine
Increasing outlet resistance
  Alpha-adrenergic agonists
  Tricyclic antidepressants
  Beta-adrenergic antagonists
  Estrogen

Modified from Wein AJ, Arsdalen KV, Levin RM: Pharmacologic therapy. In Krane RJ, Siroky MB, editors: *Clinical neurology*, ed 2, Boston, 1991, Little, Brown.

and nicotinic effects; one of the muscarinic effects is contraction of the detrusor muscle and relaxation of the trigone. Ach itself cannot be used for therapeutic purposes because of actions at central and ganglionic levels and because of its rapid hydrolysis by acetyl-cholinesterase and by nonspecific cholinesterase.

Bethanechol chloride exhibits a relatively selective Ach-like action on the urinary bladder and gut with little or no action at therapeutic doses on ganglia or on the cardiovascular system. It is cholinesterase-resistant and causes a contraction of smooth muscle from all areas of the bladder in vitro. Although its clinical effectiveness has been questioned, it has been used extensively for treatment of postoperative and postpartum urinary retention.

Other pharmacologic methods of achieving a cho-linergic effect include the use of cholinesterase agents, dopamine antagonists (metoclopramide), and alpha-adrenergic blocking agents (to block the inhibitory effect of sympathetics on pelvic parasympathetic gan-glionic transmission). In addition, prostaglandins may facilitate bladder emptying by inducing detrusor con-traction and maintaining smooth muscle tone.

Decreasing Outlet Resistance

The lower urinary tract has alpha- and beta-adrenergic receptor sites, the functions of which have been dis-cussed. Facilitation of bladder emptying could be achieved by the use of alpha-adrenergic antagonists, which decrease outlet resistance by smooth muscle relaxation of the bladder neck and proximal urethra. Some investigators have suggested that these agents may affect striated sphincter tone as well. Alpha-sym-pathetic blocking agents have thus been used to treat both smooth sphincter dyssynergia and detrusor-striated sphincter dyssynergia. Wein et al has pub-lished a review of the effectiveness of these agents.

Therapy to Facilitate Urine Storage
Decreasing Bladder Contractility

Hyperactivity of the bladder during filling may present as involuntary detrusor contractions, decreased blad-der compliance, or sensory urgency. The pathophys-iology and treatment of detrusor instability and hy-perreflexia is thoroughly discussed in Chapter 19. Pharmacologic agents used to treat detrusor overac-tivity are directed toward inhibiting bladder contrac-tility or decreasing sensory input during filling. Atro-pine and atropine-like agents depress detrusor overactivity of any etiology by inhibiting muscarinic cholinergic receptor sites. Propantheline bromide is the most commonly used oral agent with this mech-anism of action; however, side effects limit its use.

Smooth muscle relaxing drugs are commonly used to treat detrusor overactivity and tend to have fewer side effects. These agents reportedly act directly on smooth muscle at a site that is metabolically distal to the cholinergic receptor mechanism. The drugs most commonly used in clinical practice include oxybu-tynin chloride, dicyclomine hydrochloride, and fla-voxate hydrochloride. In addition to being musculo-tropic relaxants, these agents all possess variable antimuscarinic and local anesthetic properties.

Tricyclic antidepressants, particularly imipramine hydrochloride, have prominent systemic anticholin-ergic effects, weak antimuscarinic effects on bladder smooth muscle, antihistaminic effects, and local an-esthetic properties. Imipramine also appears to in-crease bladder outlet resistance due to a peripheral blockade of noradrenalin uptake. Thus it may be ef-fective for the treatment of urine storage disorders by both decreasing bladder contractility and by increasing outlet resistance.

Other drugs that have been used to decrease bladder contractility include calcium antagonists, beta-adren-ergic agonists, alpha-adrenergic antagonists, polysy-naptic inhibitors, prostaglandin inhibitors, and di-methyl sulfoxide.

Increasing Outlet Resistance

Because of the preponderance of alpha-adrenergic re-ceptor sites in the bladder neck and proximal urethra, alpha-adrenergic agonists have been used to produce urethral smooth muscle contraction, thereby increas-ing resting urethral pressure and resistance to outflow. The pharmacologic actions and clinical uses of these agents are discussed in Chapter 13. Beta-adrenergic blocking agents may be expected to increase urethral resistance as well by potentiating an alpha-adrenergic effect. Few studies, however, have tested this hy-pothesis and clinical effects are likely to be small.

Estrogens affect adrenergic nerves by influencing

excitability, neuronal influences on the muscle, receptor density and sensitivity, and transmitter metabolism. The clinical use of estrogen to augment lower urinary tract function is also discussed in Chapter 13.

REFERENCES

Barrington FJ: The relation of the hindbrain to micturition, *Brain* 44:23, 1921.

Barrington FJ: The nervous mechanism of micturition, *Q J Exp Physiol* 8:33, 1914.

Beck RP: Neuropharmacology of the lower urinary tract in women, *Obstet Gynecol Clin North Am* 15:753, 1989.

Benson JT: Neurophysiologic control of lower urinary tract, *Obstet Gynecol Clin North Am* 15:733, 1989.

Blaivas JG: The neurophysiology of micturition: a clinical study of 550 patients, *J Urol* 127:958, 1982.

Blaivas JG: Pathophysiology of lower urinary tract dysfunction, *Urol Clin North Am* 12:216, 1985.

Bradley WE: Physiology of urinary bladder. In Walsh PC, Perlmutter AD, Gittes RF, et al., editors: *Campbell's urology,* vol 1, Philadelphia, 1986, WB Saunders.

Bradley WE: Cerebro-cortical innervation of the urinary bladder, *Tohoku J Exp Med* 131:7, 1980.

Bradley WE, Timm GW, Scott FB: Innervation of the detrusor muscle and urethra, *Urol Clin North Am* 1:3, 1974.

DeGroat WC, Booth AM, Krier J, et al: Neural control of the urinary bladder and large intestine. In Brooks C McC, Koizumi K, Sato A, editors: *Integrative functions of the autonomic nervous system,* Amsterdam, 1979, Elsevier/North Holland, Biomedical Press.

DeGroat WC, Ryall RW: Recurrent inhibition in sacral parasympathetic pathways to the bladder, *J Physiol* 196:579, 1968.

DeGroat WC: Nervous control of the urinary bladder in the cat, *Brain Res* 87:201, 1975.

Downie JW, Armour JA: Relation of afferent nerve activity in the pelvic plexus with pressure, length, and wall strain in the urinary bladder of the cat, *Soc Neurosci Abstr* 8:858, 1982.

Edvardsen P: Changes in urinary-bladder motility following lesions in the nervous system in cats, *Acta Neurol Scand* 42:25, 1966.

Elbadawi A: Neuromorphologic basis of vesicourethral function. I. Histochemistry, ultrastructure, and function of intrinsic nerves of the bladder and urethra, *Neurourol Urodyn* 1:3, 1982.

Finkbeiner A, Welch L, Bissada N: Uropharmacology. IX. Direct acting smooth muscle stimulants and depressants, *Urology* 12:18, 1978.

Fletcher TF, Bradley WE: Neuroanatomy of the bladder-urethra, *J Urol* 119:153, 1978.

Gibson A: The influence of endocrine hormones on the autonomic nervous system, *J Auton Pharmacol* 1:331, 1981.

Gosling JA, Dixon JS: The structure and innervation of smooth muscle in the wall of the bladder neck and proximal urethra, *Br J Urol* 47:549, 1975.

Gosling JA, Dixon JS, Critchley HOD: A comparative study of the human external sphincter and periurethral levator ani muscles, *Br J Urol* 53:35, 1981.

Kelin LA: Urge incontinence can be a disease of bladder sensors, *J Urol* 139:1010, 1988.

Kulseng-Hanssen S, Klevmark B: Continence mechanism. In Drive JO, Hilton P, Stanton SL, editors: *Micturition,* London, 1990, Springer-Verlag.

Mahoney DT, Laberte RO, Blais DJ: Integral storage and voiding reflexes: neurophysiologic concept of continence and micturition, *Urology* 10:95, 1977.

McGuire EJ: The innervation and function of the lower urinary tract, *J Neurosurg* 65:278, 1986.

Mundy AP: Clinical physiology of the bladder, urethra and pelvic floor. In Mundy AP, Stephenson TP, Wein AJ, editors: *Urodynamics: principles, practice and application,* New York, 1984, Churchill Livingstone.

Ostergard DR: Neurological control of micturition and integral voiding reflexes. In Ostergard DR, editor: *Gynecologic urology and urodynamics,* ed 2, Baltimore, 1985, Williams & Wilkins.

Pernow B: Substance P, *Pharmacol Rev* 35:85, 1983.

Raezer D, Wein AJ, Jacobowitz D, et al: Autonomic innervation of canine urinary bladder: cholinergic and adrenergic contributions and interaction of sympathetic and parasympathetic systems in bladder function, *Urology* 2:211, 1973.

Sillen U: Central neurotransmitter mechanisms involved in the control of urinary bladder function, *Scand J Urol Nephrol* 58(suppl):1, 1980.

Swash M: Innervation of the bladder, urethra and pelvic floor. In Drive JO, Hilton P, Stanton SL, editors: *Micturition,* London, 1990, Springer-Verlag.

Tanagho EA, Miller ER: Initiation of voiding, *Br J Urol* 42:175, 1970.

Taylor P: Cholinergic agonists. In AG Gilman et al, editors: *Goodman and Gilman's The pharmacological basis of therapeutics,* ed 7, New York, 1985, Macmillan.

Torrens M: Human physiology. In Torrens M, Morrison JFB, editors: *The physiology of the lower urinary tract,* London, 1987, Springer-Verlag.

Tulloch AG: Sympathetic activity of internal urethral sphincter in empty and partially filled bladder, *Urology* 5:353, 1975.

Uvelius B, Gabella G: Relation between cell length and force production in urinary bladder smooth muscle, *Acta Physiol Scand* 110:357, 1980.

Walters MD: Mechanisms of continence and voiding, with International Continence Society classification of dysfunction, *Obstet Gynecol Clin North Am* 16:773, 1989.

Wein AJ, Barrett DM: *Voiding function and dysfunction,* Chicago, 1988, Year Book Medical Publishers.

Wein AJ, Arsdalen KV, Levin RM: Pharmacologic therapy. In Krane RJ, Siroky MB, editors: *Clinical neurourology,* ed 2, Boston, 1991, Little, Brown.

Winter DL: Receptor characteristics and conduction velocities in bladder efferents, *J Psychiatr Res* 8:225, 1971.

CHAPTER **3**

Epidemiology and Social Impact of Urinary Incontinence

Mark D. Walters

Prevalence and Incidence
Risk Factors for Incontinence
    Sex
    Age
    Race
    Childbirth
    Menopause
    Smoking
    Obesity
Psychosocial Impact of Incontinence
    Social changes
    Psychological changes
    Sexual changes
Economic Issues

Urinary incontinence is a common disease that has long been ignored by patients and physicians. It has frequently been considered to be a natural result of aging and an inevitable problem with which women must contend. Many studies however, have now shown that urinary incontinence has multiple and broad-reaching effects that influence daily activities, social interactions, and self-perceptions of health. This chapter reviews epidemiologic issues related to urinary incontinence, including prevalence and the social, psychologic, sexual, and economic effects of urinary incontinence in community-dwelling and nursing home women.

PREVALENCE AND INCIDENCE

Estimates of the prevalence of urinary incontinence in women vary widely, probably because of differences in populations studied, in the methods used to collect data, and in definitions of disease. Incorrect estimates may result from biases in sample surveys and because incontinence is embarrassing and tends to be underreported. Herzog and Fultz found an 83% agreement between self-reported data and the clinician's assessment of incontinence. Because of these issues, estimates from the literature should be considered only as close approximations.

Considerable variation in estimates of prevalence of "any" urinary incontinence, i.e., any urine loss during a 12-month period, has been reported. Early studies found that up to half of young nulliparous women said that they occasionally leak urine associated with coughing, laughing, and sneezing. The prevalence of more frequent stress incontinence in this group was 2% to 5%, although one study reported daily incontinence in 16% of nulliparous female students. The reported prevalence of "any" urinary incontinence among older persons ranges from 8% to 34%. Herzog and Fultz believe that the higher figures are probably more accurate because cognitive problems associated with forgetting and motivational problems associated with the embarrassing nature of the condition would both tend to produce underreporting. These authors suggest that a 30% prevalence of any urine loss during a 12-month period is a plausible estimate.

Studies addressing the prevalence of more severe loss of urine—defined variably as "daily," "weekly," or "most of the time"—range from between 3% and 11%, with the majority between 4% and 6%. This estimate probably corresponds more to the clinical estimate of disease because it more likely identifies women who consider the involuntary urine loss to be a social or hygienic problem.

Incidence of incontinence is defined as the probability of becoming incontinent during a defined period of time, given continence at the onset of the time period. Because few long-term longitudinal studies have been performed, little information about the incidence of urinary incontinence is available. Several studies of elderly people showed that about 10% of originally continent adults developed urinary incontinence over a 3-year period. These estimates include both chronic and acute causes of urinary incontinence.

Urine loss is transient in approximately a third of all elderly incontinent persons. The acute, transient causes, such as urinary infection, drug use, and delirium, frequently regress after treatment. Thus, there appears to be a yearly fluctuation of development and regression of incontinence among individuals. We still do not know the incidence of chronic progression from continent to incontinent and from mild to more severe incontinence.

RISK FACTORS FOR URINARY INCONTINENCE
Sex

Incontinence is two to three times more common among women than men. The sex difference appears to be most pronounced among adults under 60 years of age, probably because of the very low prevalence of incontinence among younger men. In an interview study of 1955 senior citizens aged 60 years or more, 18% of men and 38% of women reported uncontrolled urine loss. These sex differences appear to be consistent whether the measure is "any" incontinence, "severe" incontinence, or irritative bladder symptoms. The symptom of stress incontinence is relatively uncommon in men, but relatively common in women. Voiding problems are probably more common in elderly men.

Age

The prevalence of urinary incontinence appears to increase with advancing age. In a postal survey of community-dwelling women in Great Britain, Thomas et al found that the percentage of women reporting urinary leaking at least twice monthly rose steadily from 4% of women aged 15 to 24, to 16% aged 75 and greater (Fig. 3-1). Stress incontinence was a more common complaint before age 65; urgency and mixed stress/urge incontinence were more common thereafter. Yarnell et al noted that 28% of women aged 17 to 34 reported some incontinence, compared to 51% of women aged 35 and greater, and 59% of women 75 years old and older. However, no significant differences in prevalence rates were noted by decades after age 35.

Reasons for the increase in prevalence of urinary incontinence with age are unknown. Normal aging is characterized by decline in the reserve capacity of all organ systems. Lower urinary tract function probably parallels changes seen throughout the body, although few data address this possibility. Bladder capacity, the ability to postpone voiding, bladder compliance, and urinary flow rate probably decrease with advancing age in both sexes. In addition, the prevalence of uninhibited bladder contractions and postvoid residual urine volume increase with age. Maximal urethral closure pressure and functional urethral length decrease in women. These changes in bladder and urethral function probably are related directly to aging and to the development of various medical conditions that affect bladder function.

Another important age-related change is an alteration in the pattern of fluid excretion. Whereas younger individuals excrete the bulk of their daily ingested

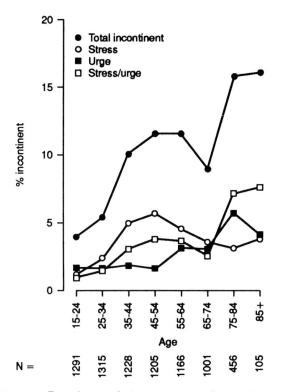

Fig. 3-1 Prevalence of stress, urge, and stress/urge incontinence in women by age. *(From Thomas TM: Epidemiology of micturition disorders. In Stanton SL (ed): Clinical gynecologic urology, St Louis, 1984, Mosby–Year Book.)*

Race

Very little epidemiologic information is available regarding racial differences of incontinence. Genital prolapse, enterocele, and stress incontinence apparently are uncommon in Chinese, Eskimo, and black women. A study of 30 Chinese female cadavers revealed that the general anatomic relationship of the levator ani muscles and urethra was similar to that found in Western women. The levator ani muscle bundles in the Chinese cadavers, however, were judged to be thicker and to extend more laterally on the arcus tendineus than in white cadavers. Furthermore, the fascia of the pelvic diaphragm, extending from the levator ani muscles to the posterior pubourethral ligaments, was particularly dense. Although this work was uncontrolled and subjective, it provides one explanation for a possible racial difference in the prevalence of pelvic support defects and incontinence.

Childbirth

Thomas et al reported a significant association between incontinence and parity (Fig. 3-2). Incontinence was reported less commonly by nulliparous than by parous women at all ages; but no difference in rates of incontinence was noted for women who had had one, two, or three births. Women who had had four or more babies were most likely to report regular incontinence. The rise in prevalence of incontinence with parity is mainly due to a rise in the prevalence of stress and mixed incontinence; little or no association is found between urge incontinence and parity. The effects of parity on prevalence of urinary incontinence are independent of the effects of age.

Childbirth injury has been implicated as the major etiologic factor leading to pelvic support abnormalities and stress incontinence. It has been theorized that vaginal delivery directly damages pelvic fascial supports and may cause partial denervation of the pelvic floor and urethral muscles. Vaginal delivery leads to weakening of pelvic muscle strength in the immediate postpartum period, although most or all of this strength may be recovered with aggressive pelvic muscle exercises. Women who have had cesarean births demonstrate greater pelvic muscle strength during and after the postpartum period than women who have had vaginal births.

fluid before bedtime, the pattern reverses with age so that one or two episodes of nocturia per night may be normal.

Urinary symptoms are found in over half of institutionalized elderly persons. In addition to the various urologic diagnoses of incontinence, nonurologic causes of incontinence, such as behavioral problems, immobility, medication, and diabetes, frequently are present. Jirovec and Wells observed that, when multiple variables were examined together, mobility emerged as the best predictor of the patient's urinary control, followed by cognitive impairment. Therapy should always include a combination of urologic treatments with nonurologic, behavioral treatments in dealing with urinary incontinence in nursing homes.

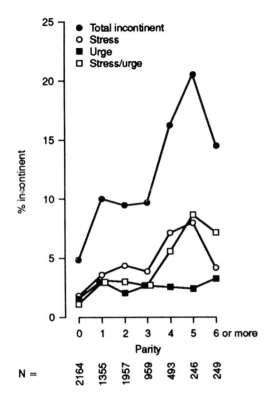

Fig. 3-2 Prevalence of stress, urge, and stress/urge incontinence in women by parity. *(From Thomas TM: Epidemiology of micturition disorders. In Stanton SL (ed): Clinical gynecologic urology, St Louis, 1984, Mosby–Year Book.)*

Urethral pressure studies have shown that vaginal delivery is associated with a reduction in functional urethral length, urethral closure pressure, and maximum urethral pressure. No changes in these variables were observed in women who delivered by cesarean section. One case-control study showed that although the parity was similar in subjects with genuine stress incontinence and in continent controls, urodynamic evidence of distal urethral sphincter impairment was associated with vaginal delivery in the controls.

These data suggest that childbirth adversely affects lower urinary tract function. Childbirth per se, however, does not explain all cases of genuine stress incontinence, which can begin during pregnancy and is found occasionally in up to a third of nulliparous women. Further research is needed to define the roles of pregnancy and childbirth in the cause of pelvic support defects and urinary incontinence.

Menopause

The vagina and urethra have similar epithelial linings due to their common embryologic origin. Urinary cytologic changes are similar to those of vaginal cytology during the menstrual cycle, during pregnancy, and after menopause. High affinity estrogen receptors have been identified in nuclear and cytoplasmic fractions of rabbit and rat urethra. Estrogen receptors have been observed in animal bladder preparations in some, but not all, studies. In women, several studies identified high affinity estrogen receptors in surgically removed urethral tissue and pubococcygeal muscle. Receptors appear to be present in the bladder trigone, but are found infrequently in the bladder body.

Normal urethral function in the female is affected by age and estrogen status. Maximum urethral pressure and urethral length increase from infancy to 25 years and then decrease with advancing age. A further decrease in functional urethral length occurs after menopause, possibly because of estrogen deprivation. Urinary incontinence is maintained under resting conditions by a complex interaction of urethral smooth muscle, urethral wall elasticity and vascularity, and periurethral striated muscle. Under stress conditions, such as with coughing or lifting, urethral closure is augmented by intraabdominal pressure transmission and with a rapid striated muscle contraction from the urogenital diaphragm and possibly the levator ani muscle.

Many studies have shown that genitourinary symptoms are a common complaint after menopause. Vaginal symptoms include dryness and dyspareunia; urinary symptoms include frequency, urgency, dysuria, and incontinence. Lack of estrogen results in cytologic changes of the distal urethra similar to those found in the vagina. These changes may be at least partially responsible for the sensory symptoms and decreased resistance to infection frequently found after menopause. Decreased urethral vascularity and abnormal smooth and skeletal muscle efficiency results in low resting urethral pressure and an abnormal stress response. Finally, age- and estrogen-induced changes in the collagen of the endopelvic fascia allows for the development and progression of urethral detachment and pelvic prolapse.

Several lines of evidence question whether estrogen has an independent clinical effect on lower urinary tract function. One study of the effect of aging on urethral function failed to find specific menopause-related deterioration in urethral pressures, although significantly shorter functional urethral length was noted after menopause. Estrogen replacement therapy in young continent nulliparous women who are hypoestrogenemic due to premature ovarian failure results in little change in urethral function.

In a study of 72 postmenopausal women with genuine stress incontinence, Fantl et al compared the clinical and urodynamic parameters between subjects who were given estrogen supplementation with those who were not. Estrogen-supplemented women had more estrogen-related cytologic changes of the vagina and urethra, but no differences in urodynamic parameters of urethral sphincter function were noted between groups. The only beneficial effect of estrogen was on the proprioceptive sensory threshold of the lower urinary tract. Examined together, these studies suggest that independent of aging and underlying urethral pathology, estrogen has little measurable effect on urethral function.

Smoking

In a large retrospective, case-controlled study of incontinent women, Bump and McClish noted a significant association between cigarette smoking and the development of all forms of urinary incontinence. Smoking was associated with a twofold to threefold increase in relative risk of urinary incontinence. Knowledge of this association may help discourage some women from starting to smoke or to encourage smoking women to stop.

Obesity

Obesity is common in women with urinary incontinence. In a large study of incontinent women, Dwyer et al found that obesity (greater than 20% above average weight, for height and age) was significantly more common in women with genuine stress incontinence and detrusor instability than in the normal population. Obesity was related to age, parity, and previous incontinence operations. However, there were no significant differences between obese and nonobese incontinent women for any of the urodynamic variables measured. Thus, it remains unknown whether obesity is an independent factor in the development of incontinence.

Surgical treatment of genuine stress incontinence is technically more difficult, and postoperative complications are more common in obese patients, especially when retropubic procedures are performed. Obesity may also decrease the long-term effectiveness of incontinence surgery, although this possibility has not been consistently reported.

PSYCHOSOCIAL IMPACT OF INCONTINENCE
Social Changes

Loss of urine control can have a significant impact on the social well-being of the affected individual. Indeed, use of the International Continence Society's definition of urinary incontinence—"a condition in which involuntary loss of urine is a social or hygienic problem . . . "—requires that all women with urinary incontinence have some degree of social distress. Obviously, urinary incontinence and related psychosocial distress constitute a spectrum related to the actual severity of the leaking and to the women's perception of her disability. A summary of possible psychosocial consequences of urinary incontinence is shown in Table 3-1.

Many techniques have been used to measure psychosocial impact of urinary incontinence. In an excellent review, Wyman et al examined epidemiologic and clinical studies addressing the psychosocial impact of urinary incontinence on community-dwelling women. They noted wide variations among studies regarding patient populations surveyed, methods of evaluation, and definitions used. Reports of interference with social activities ranged from 8% to 52%. Areas affected included social, domestic, physical, occupational, and leisure activities. Sufferers may give up or restrict certain household chores, church attendance, shopping, traveling, vacations, physical recreation, entertainment events outside the home, and hobbies. They may also avoid activities outside the

TABLE 3-1 Summary of consequences of urinary incontinence

Individual	Family	Health care professional
Psychological symptoms	Care-giver burden and emotional stress	Negative feelings and behaviors toward patients with urinary incontinence
Insecurity	Impaired interpersonal relationships	Reaction formation
Anger	Economic worries	Overindulgence
Apathy	Health deterioration of primary care giver	Excessive permissiveness
Dependence	Potential for abuse or neglect	Excessive caring
Guilt	Decision to institutionalize	Extra care responsibilities
Indignity	Delay discharge from institutional care	Staff frustration, depression, and guilt
Feeling of abandonment		Reduction in staff morale
Shame		"Burn-out" syndrome
Embarrassment		
Depression		
Denial		
Sense of self		
Loss of self-confidence/self-esteem		
Sexual difficulties		
Lack of attention to personal hygiene		
Social interaction		
Reduction in social activities		
Socially disengaged		
Socially isolated		
Psychologic and functional decline		
Potential for institutionalization		

From Ory MG, Wyman JF, Yu L: *Clin Geriatr Med* 2:657, 1986.

home if they are unsure of rest room locations. Some incontinent individuals become increasingly isolated as they limit social activities and social contacts. Even incontinent homebound women, when compared with continent homebound women, have significantly fewer social interactions, particularly with family members. Spousal relationships appear to be most impaired, perhaps because of an additional adverse effect on sexual relationships.

Urinary incontinence among very old persons can lead to such disability and dependency that family or home care givers may have difficulty coping and responding to increased demands. Thus incontinence is thought to be a major factor leading to institutionalization of the elderly.

Studies relating measures of perceived social impact with objective measures of incontinence have yielded inconsistent results. Norton noted that the degree of disability as reported on questionnaire does not correlate with the amount of incontinence. In contrast, Wyman et al found significant, although modest, positive relationships between psychosocial impact scores and the number of incontinent episodes reported in a diary, as well as the amount of fluid lost with a perineal pad test. Some studies noted more social restriction with stress compared to urge incontinence, whereas others reported more abnormal psychosocial impact with detrusor instability. These inconsistencies in the literature indicate that the patient's threshold for tolerance of urinary incontinence and perceived disability/distress may be wide and is probably influenced by other, still undefined, factors.

Urinary incontinence appears to be generally underrecognized and undertreated. In a survey of community-dwelling elderly women, Diokno et al reported that only 41% of those suffering from urinary incontinence told their physicians about their condition. In a study of 1442 randomly selected women in the Netherlands, 22.5% reported some incontinence, although fewer than one fourth of them considered it to be a problem. Only 32% of the incontinent women were identified as incontinent by their general practitioner; however, only a small minority of the women who felt severely restricted were not identified by their physician.

Several studies have documented a significant delay in the treatment of incontinent individuals. Norton et al observed that length of delay did not directly correlate with reported distress. Reasons for delaying reflected lack of information, such as acceptance of symptoms as normal and fear that surgery was the only treatment. Delay was also related to embarrassment and reluctance to discuss the problem with their general practitioner.

Psychologic Changes

Urinary incontinence is a complex phenomenon with multiple causative factors including psychogenic causes. Early studies, perhaps because of insufficient understanding of the pathophysiology, stressed the psychosomatic aspects of urinary complaints. Psychiatric analyses of women with lower urinary tract symptoms described somatization, hysteria, depression, anxiety, and abnormal levels of situational life stresses. Such disorders have been considered to be etiologic of lower urinary tract dysfunction, specifically urethral syndrome, unstable bladder, and urinary retention. Urinary incontinence has been implicated as one expression of "masked depression," seen frequently in gynecologic patients. Most of these studies were methodologically flawed by biases in patient selection and interview techniques, lack of appropriate control groups, and little application of statistical analyses.

More recent studies used personality testing in patients with urinary incontinence. Using the Eysenck Personality Inventory questionnaire, Morrison et al recorded significantly increased scores in the Neuroticism-Stability scale for incontinent patients as compared with controls. However, no association was found between neuroticism and detrusor overactivity. Macaulay et al assessed the mental state of 211 incontinent patients using three standardized, self-rating questionnaires. All incontinent patients were more anxious and depressed than normal controls. Com-

pared to those with genuine stress incontinence, patients with detrusor instability had higher scores on anxiety and hysteria scales. Regardless of urologic diagnosis, however, patients with the most severe disease (judged on a self-rated scale) were most abnormal on psychologic testing. Walters et al found that compared to matched continent controls, many incontinent women had Minnesota Multiphasic Personality Inventory profiles that were clinically significant, reflecting moodiness, feelings of helplessness and sadness, pessimism, and general hypochondriasis/somatization. No differences in profile scores were found between women with detrusor instability and those with genuine stress incontinence.

Taken together, these studies suggest that anxiety, depression, and other psychologic abnormalities may be related to urinary incontinence. Because most objective studies report similar test results with the various diagnoses of incontinence, it is more likely that psychologic changes are related to the symptom and related disability/distress than to specific urogynecologic conditions. This possibility is consistent with literature that correlates significant declines in the frequency of once-pleasurable activities with depression. Because most studies are retrospective, however, the direction of any cause-and-effect relationship remains to be determined.

It is unknown whether the psychologic changes described in incontinent patients are amenable to treatment. In patients with sensory urgency and detrusor instability, bladder-retaining drills and pharmacotherapy with propantheline bromide result in significant reductions in state anxiety on follow-up testing. Psychotherapy in patients with detrusor instability result in fewer somatic symptoms, but no reduction in state anxiety. In a study of bladder retaining for the treatment of detrusor instability, Oldenburg and Millard reported improvement in psychologic symptoms regardless of urologic response. Although preliminary and somewhat conflicting, these studies suggest that psychologic factors associated with urinary incontinence can be modified with therapy.

Sexual Changes

The close anatomic proximity of the bladder and urethra with the vagina allows for an association between lower urinary tract dysfunction and sexual difficulties.

The effects can be bidirectional; sexual activity can cause or aggravate bladder problems and bladder problems can lead to sexual dysfunction. Examples of conditions in which vaginal intercourse affects the lower urinary tract are the increase in risk of urinary tract infection with intercourse, especially in vaginal diaphragm users, and the pain experienced during intercourse by women with urethral diverticula. In addition, many women experience urgency to void during or immediately after sexual intercourse. This latter symptom is felt by Masters and Johnson to be due to irritation of the posterior wall of the bladder during penile thrusting.

Lower urinary tract dysfunction can have a profound effect on sexual function. Urine loss occurs during vaginal intercourse in 24% to 46% of incontinent women. This complaint is volunteered infrequently, probably because of embarrassment. Approximately two thirds of sufferers report leaking urine with penetration; the remaining patients complain of leaking urine with orgasm. Hilton demonstrated that 70% of those who became incontinent on penetration had genuine stress incontinence and 4% had detrusor instability, whereas of those who complained of incontinence at orgasm, 42% had genuine stress incontinence and 35% had detrusor instability.

Sexual dysfunction occurs commonly in women with detrusor instability and with urinary incontinence in general. The association between urologic symptoms and sexual problems may occur in several ways. Urinary symptoms may be a direct cause of sexual difficulties, where none previously existed. Alternatively, urinary symptoms may be used (consciously or unconsciously) as an excuse to avoid sexual contact in the presence of a preexisting, but unacknowledged, sexual problem. Further, confounding factors may aggravate sexual dysfunction. Conditions common in incontinent women, such as advanced age and the climacteric, can lead to physical and physiologic changes that adversely affect sexual response. These conditions include vaginal mucosal atrophy, decreased lubrication and vaginal secretions, and fewer orgasmic contractions. Declining general health of the woman and her partner with advancing age also may affect a woman's sexual activity. Thus many complex factors can affect the quality of sexual function.

Sexual function may be positively or negatively affected by the surgical treatment of urinary incontinence. Francis and Jeffcoate found that about half of sexually active women had some sexual problems after anterior and posterior colpoperineorrhaphy with or without hysterectomy. Fifty-five percent of these patients reported loss of sexual desire or impotence (male or female), which frequently predated the vaginal surgery. Shortened or stenotic vaginas, dyspareunia, or fear of injury was the cause of sexual difficulties in the remaining women.

Haase and Skibsted studied 55 sexually active women who underwent a variety of operations for stress incontinence or genital prolapse. Postoperatively, 24% of the patients experienced improvement in their sexual satisfaction, 67% experienced no change, and 9% experienced deterioration. Improvement often resulted from cessation of urinary incontinence. Deterioration was always due to dyspareunia after posterior colporrhaphy. These authors concluded that the prognosis for an improved sexual life is good after surgery for stress incontinence but that posterior colpoperineorrhaphy causes dyspareunia in some patients.

ECONOMIC ISSUES

Urinary incontinence is one of the most prevalent conditions experienced by elderly women. As noted earlier, approximately 5% to 10% of community-dwelling women experience some urinary incontinence, and 40% to 50% of elderly people in nursing homes suffer from the problem. Studies of the economic impact of urinary incontinence are scarce, however, primarily because of the absence of reliable prevalence, risk factor, and cost data and because of wide diversification of treatment methods. Most available economic studies have focused on the cost of caring for elderly incontinent people in nursing homes because the data are relatively easier to obtain there than in a private home setting.

In 1986, Hu studied the direct and indirect costs of urinary incontinence in the United States. Direct costs were defined as those resources from the economy used to diagnose, treat, care for, and rehabilitate incontinent patients. Indirect costs were defined as resources such as the value of lost productivity and time and resources that are not fully used as a result of illness or premature death. Indirect costs of incontinence include the cost of time spent by unpaid care givers who take patients to seek medical treatment, the loss of productivity resulting from urinary incontinence, and mortality. The accompanying box illustrates the direct and indirect cost categories of urinary incontinence. The sum of direct and indirect costs of urinary incontinence would reflect the total economic burden of the entire economy. Not every incontinent patient would incur all of these costs, and data describing the precise frequency and amount of medical intervention as a result of urinary incontinence are not available.

Based on multiple assumptions regarding incontinence prevalence rate and cost information, Hu estimated that the total direct and indirect economic cost of urinary incontinence for the entire economy in 1984 was $8.1 billion: $6.6 billion in direct costs and $1.5 billion in indirect costs. Community-dwelling incontinent persons incurred $4.8 billion in direct costs and $1.5 billion in indirect costs. Costs incurred by nursing homes, which are all direct costs, totaled about $1.8 billion, which represents about 10% of total nursing home care costs. This figure is roughly similar to a 1984 study that estimated that the costs of supplies, laundry, and labor for incontinent nursing home patients ranged from $3.00 to $11.00 per patient per day or $0.5 billion to $1.5 billion overall per year.

In spite of the large economic burden of urinary incontinence in nursing homes, whether therapies decrease or actually increase the overall cost of urinary incontinence remains unknown. In their analysis, Ouslander and Kane demonstrated that more active evaluation and treatment of incontinence in nursing homes could result in considerable cost savings for both patients and caregivers. In studies of behavioral therapy for incontinent nursing home residents, however, Hu et al noted that whereas residents receive the benefits of reduced incontinence and the nursing home realizes some cost savings in laundry and supplies, the nursing aides will have increased work load and thus incur the cost of treatment. It appears that, at least for the short term, behavioral therapy to improve incontinence in institutionalized elderly may cost

---

Costs of Urinary Incontinence

Direct Costs

Diagnostic and evaluation costs
    Physician consultation and examination
    Laboratory
    Diagnostic procedures
Treatment costs
    Surgery
    Drugs
Routine care costs
    Nursing labor
    Supplies
    Laundry
Rehabilitation costs
    Nursing labor
    Supplies
Incontinence consequence costs
    Skin breakdowns
    Urinary tract infections
    Falls
    Additional nursing home admissions
    Longer hospital stays

Indirect Costs

Time costs of unpaid caregivers for treating and
    caring for incontinent elderly persons
Loss of productivity because of morbidity
Loss of productivity because of mortality

From Hu TW: *Clin Geriatr Med* 2:673, 1986.

---

more than the direct cost normally incurred by the nursing home. Quality of life and other second-order benefits must be considered if continence rehabilitation is to be cost-effective.

BIBLIOGRAPHY
Prevalence and Incidence

Campbell AJ, Reinken J, McCosh L: Incontinence in the elderly: prevalence and prognosis, *Age Ageing* 14:65, 1985.

Diokno AC, Brock BM, Brown MB, et al: Prevalence of urinary incontinence and other urological symptoms in the noninstitutionalized elderly, *J Urol* 136:1022, 1986.

Herzog AR, Fultz NH: Prevalence and incidence of urinary incontinence in community-dwelling populations, *J Am Geriatr Soc* 38:273, 1990.

Nemir A, Middleton RP: Stress incontinence in young nulliparous women, *Am J Obstet Gynecol* 68:1166, 1954.

Ouslander JG: Diagnostic evaluation of geriatric urinary incontinence, *Clin Geriatr Med* 2:715, 1986.

Ouslander JG, Kane RL, Abrass IB: Urinary incontinence in elderly nursing home patients, *JAMA* 248:1194, 1982.

Pannill FC, Williams TF, Davis R: Evaluation and treatment of urinary incontinence in long term care, *J Am Geriatr Soc* 36:902, 1988.

Thomas TM, Plymat KR, Blannin J, et al: Prevalence of urinary incontinence, *Br Med J* 281:1243, 1980.

Thomas TM: Epidemiology of micturition disorders. In Stanton SL (ed): *Clinical gynecologic urology*, St Louis, 1984, Mosby–Year Book.

Wolin LH: Stress incontinence in young, healthy nulliparous female subjects, *J Urol* 101:545, 1969.

Yarnell JWG, St Leger AL: The prevalence, severity and factors associated with urinary incontinence in a random sample of the elderly, *Age Aging* 8:81, 1979.

Yarnell JWG, Voyle GJ, Richards CJ, et al: The prevalence and severity of urinary incontinence in women, *J Epidemiol Community Health* 35:71, 1981.

Risk Factors

Anderson RS: A neurogenic element to urinary genuine stress incontinence, *Br J Obstet Gynaecol* 91:141, 1984.

Batra S, Björk P, Sjögren C: Binding of estradiol-17β and estriol in cytosolic and nuclear fractions from urogenital tissues, *J Steroid Biochem* 21:163, 1984.

Bump RC, McClish DK: Cigarette smoking and urinary incontinence in women, *Am J Obstet Gynecol* 167:1213, 1992.

Carlile A, Davies I, Rigby A, et al: Age changes in the human female urethra: a morphometric study, *J Urol* 139:532, 1988.

Cosner KR, Dougherty MC, Bishop KR: Dynamic characteristics of the circumvaginal muscles during pregnancy and postpartum, *J Nurse Midwifery* 36:221, 1991.

Dwyer PL, Lee ETC, Hay DM: Obesity and urinary incontinence in women, *Br J Obstet Gynaecol* 95:91, 1988.

Fantl JA, Wyman JF, Anderson RL, et al: Postmenopausal urinary incontinence: comparison between non-estrogen-supplemented and estrogen-supplemented women, *Obstet Gynecol* 71:823, 1988.

Francis WJA: The onset of stress incontinence, *J Obstet Gynaecol Br Emp* 67:899, 1960.

Ingelman-Sundberg A, Rosen J, Gustafsson SA, et al: Cytosol estrogen receptors in the urogenital tissues in stress-incontinent women, *Acta Obstet Gynecol Scand* 60:585, 1981.

Iosif CS, Batra S, Ek A: Estrogen receptors in the human female lower urinary tract, *Am J Obstet Gynecol* 141:817, 1981.

Jirovec MM, Wells TJ: Urinary incontinence in nursing home residents with dementia: the mobility-cognition paradigm, *Appl Nurs Res* 3:112, 1990.

Karram MM, Yeko TR, Sauer MV, et al: Urodynamic changes following hormonal replacement therapy in women with premature ovarian failure, *Obstet Gynecol* 74:208, 1989.

Lindskog M, Sjögren C, Andersson KE, et al: Oestrogen binding sites in nuclear fractions from the rat urogenital tract, *Acta Pharmacol Toxicol* 50:238, 1982.

McCallin PF, Taylor ES, Whitehead RW: A study of the changes in the cytology of the urinary sediment during the menstrual cycle and pregnancy, *Am J Obstet Gynecol* 60:64, 1950.

Nichols DH, Randall CL: *Vaginal surgery,* ed 2, Baltimore, 1983, Williams & Wilkins.

Punnonen R, Lukola A, Puntala P: Lack of estrogen and progestin receptors in the urinary bladder of women, *Horm Metab Res* 15:464, 1983.

Resnick NM: Diagnosis and treatment of incontinence in the institutionalized elderly, *Semin Urol* 7:117, 1989.

Rud T: Urethral pressure profile in continent women from childhood to old age, *Acta Obstet Gynecol Scand* 59:335, 1980.

Saez S, Martin PM: Evidence of estrogen receptors in the trigone area of human urinary bladder, *J Steroid Biochem* 15:317, 1981.

Samples JT, Dougherty MC, Abrams RM, et al: The dynamic characteristics of the circumvaginal muscles, *J Obstet Gynecol Neonatal Nurs* 17:194, 1988.

Sampselle CM: Changes in pelvic muscle strength and stress urinary incontinence associated with childbirth, *J Obstet Gynecol Neonatal Nurs* 19:371, 1990.

Semmelink HJF, de Wilde PCM, van Houwelingen JC, et al: Histomorphometric study of the lower urogenital tract in pre- and post-menopausal women, *Cytometry* 11:700, 1990.

Semmens JP, Wagner G: Estrogen deprivation and vaginal function in postmenopausal women, *JAMA* 248:445, 1982.

Snooks SJ, Swash M, Henry MM, et al: Risk factors in childbirth causing damage to the pelvic floor innervation, *Int J Colorectal Dis* 1:20, 1986.

Solomon C, Panagotopoulos P, Oppenheim A: The use of urinary sediment as an aid in endocrinological disorders in the female, *Am J Obstet Gynecol* 76:56, 1958.

Tapp A, Cardozo L, Versi E, et al: The effect of vaginal delivery on the urethral sphincter, *Br J Obstet Gynaecol* 95:142, 1988.

Urner F, Weil A, Herrmann WL: Estradiol receptors in the urethra and the bladder of the female rabbit, *Gynecol Obstet Invest* 16:307, 1983.

Van Geelen JM, Lemmens WAJG, Eskes TKAB, et al: The urethral pressure profile in pregnancy and after delivery in healthy nulliparous women, *Am J Obstet Gynecol* 144:636, 1982.

Zacharin RF: "A Chinese anatomy": the pelvic supporting tissues of the Chinese and Occidental female compared and contrasted, *Aust NZ J Obstet Gynaecol* 17:1, 1977.

Psychosocial Changes

Abrams P, Blaivas JG, Stanton SL, et al: The standardization of terminology of lower urinary tract function, *Scand J Urol Nephrol* 114(suppl):5, 1988.

Andrews K: Relevance of readmission of elderly patients discharged from a geriatric unit, *J Am Geriatr Soc* 34:5, 1986.

Barnick C, Cardozo L: Sexual and bladder dysfunction—how are they related? *The Female Patient* 14:63, 1989.

Cardozo LD: Sexually induced urinary incontinence, *Br J Sex Med* 14:154, 1987.

Carson CC III, Osborne D, Segura JW: Psychologic characteristics of patients with female urethral syndrome, *J Clin Psychol* 35:312, 1974.

Epstein S, Jenike MA: Disabling urinary obsessions: an uncommon variant of obsessive-compulsive disorder, *Psychosomatics* 31:450, 1990.

Francis WJA, Jeffcoate TNA: Dyspareunia following vaginal operations, *Br J Obstet Gynaecol* 68:1, 1961.

Haase P, Skibsted L: Influence of operations for stress incontinence and/or genital descensus on sexual life, *Acta Obstet Gynecol Scand* 67:659, 1988.

Hafner FJ, Stanton S, Guy J: A psychiatric study of women with urgency incontinence, *Br J Urol* 49:211, 1977.

Herzog AR, Diokno AC, Fultz NH: Urinary incontinence: medical and psychosocial aspects, *Annu Rev Gerontol Geriatr* 9:74, 1989.

Herzog AR, Fultz NH: Urinary incontinence in the community: prevalence, consequences, management, and beliefs, *Top Geriatr Rehabil* 3:1, 1988.

Herzog AR, Fultz NH, Brock BM, et al: Urinary incontinence and psychological distress among older adults, *Psychol Aging* 3:115, 1988.

Hilton P: Urinary incontinence during sexual intercourse: a common, but rarely volunteered, symptom, *Br J Obstet Gynaecol* 95:377, 1988.

Holst K, Wilson PD: The prevalence of female urinary incontinence and reasons for not seeking treatment, *NZ Med J* 101:756, 1988.

Iosif S, Henriksson L, Ulmsten U: The frequency of disorders of the urinary tract, urinary incontinence in particular, as evaluated by a questionnaire survey in a gynecologic health control population, *Acta Obstet Gynecol Scand* 60:71, 1981.

Lagro-Jansenn TLM, Smits AJA, Van Weel C: Women with urinary incontinence: self-perceived worries and general practitioners' knowledge of problem, *Br J Gen Pract* 40:331, 1990.

Macaulay AJ, Stern RS, Homes DM, et al: Micturition and the mind: psychological factors in the aetiology and treatment of urinary symptoms in women, *Br Med J* 294:540, 1987.

Masters WH, Johnson VE: *Human sexual response*, London, 1966, Churchill Livingstone.

Molinski H: Masked depressions in obstetrics and gynecology, *Psychother Psychosom* 31:283, 1979.

Morrison LM, Eadie AS, McAlister ES, et al: Personality testing in 226 patients with urinary incontinence, *Br J Urol* 58:387, 1986.

Norton C: The effects of urinary incontinence in women, *Int Rehabil Med* 4:9, 1982

Norton PA, MacDonald LD, Sedgwick PM, et al: Distress and delay associated with urinary incontinence, frequency and urgency in women, *Br Med J* 297:1187, 1988.

Oldenburg B, Millard RJ: Predictors of long term outcome following a bladder re-training programme, *J Psychosom Res* 30:691, 1986.

Ory MG, Wyman JF, Yu L: Psychosocial factors in urinary incontinence, *Clin Geriatr Med* 2:657, 1986.

Stanley EMG, Ramage MP: Sexual problems and urological symptoms. In Stanton SL (ed): *Clinical gynecologic urology*, St Louis, 1984, Mosby–Year Book.

Sutherst J, Brown M: Sexual dysfunction associated with urinary incontinence, *Urol Int* 35:414, 1980.

Walters MD, Taylor S, Schoenfeld LS: Psychosexual study of women with detrusor instability, *Obstet Gynecol* 75:22, 1990.

Wyman JF, Harkins SW, Fantl JA: Psychosocial impact of urinary incontinence in the community-dwelling population, *J Am Geriatr Soc* 38:282, 1990.

Wyman JF, Harkins SW, Choi SC, et al: Psychosocial impact of urinary incontinence in women, *Obstet Gynecol* 70:378, 1987.

Economic Issues

Hu TW: The economic impact of urinary incontinence, *Clin Geriatr Med* 2:673, 1986.

Hu TW, Kaltreider L, Igou JF, et al: Cost effectiveness of training incontinent elderly in nursing homes: a randomized clinical trial, *Health Serv Res* 25:455, 1990.

Hu TW, Igou JF, Kaltreider L, et al: A clinical trial of a behavioral therapy to reduce urinary incontinence in nursing homes, *JAMA* 261:2656, 1989.

Ouslander JG, Kane RL: The cost of urinary incontinence in nursing homes, *Med Care* 22:69, 1983.

Schnelle JF, Sowell VA, Hu TW, et al: Reduction of urinary incontinence in nursing homes: does it reduce or increase costs? *J Am Geriatr Soc* 34:34, 1988.

CHAPTER 4

Classification of Disorders of Storage and Evacuation of Urine

Mark D. Walters

Classification Systems of Lower Urinary Tract Dysfunction
    International Continence Society classification
    Functional classification
Classification of Genuine Stress Urinary Incontinence
Differential Diagnosis

CLASSIFICATION SYSTEMS OF LOWER URINARY TRACT DYSFUNCTION

The purpose of any classification system is to facilitate understanding of the etiology and pathophysiology of disease, to use this information to establish treatment guidelines, and to avoid confusion among those who are concerned with the problem. A number of classification systems for micturition disorders and stress urinary incontinence have been developed. These classifications have been based on various anatomic, radiographic, and urodynamic findings. The advantages, disadvantages, and applicability of the various classification systems of voiding dysfunction have been described previously by Wein and Barrett. This chap-

ter reviews two practical systems for the classification of voiding dysfunction in women. In addition, the classifications for stress urinary incontinence and their clinical usefulness are discussed. Based on these classifications, various surgical and nonsurgical treatments have been advocated. It is hoped that the nomenclature used in these classification systems will become more widely understood and that further research will be aimed at defining their clinical applicability.

International Continence Society Classification

In 1973, the International Continence Society (ICS) established a committee for the standardization of terminology of lower urinary tract function. Five of the six reports from this committee were published. These reports have since been revised, extended, and collated in a monograph. Following is a summary of their findings.

The lower urinary tract is composed of the bladder and urethra, which work together as a functional unit to promote storage and emptying of urine. Although a complete urodynamic investigation is not necessary for all symptomatic patients, some clinical or uro-

---

The International Continence Society Classification of Lower Urinary Tract Dysfunction

I. Storage Phase
   A. Bladder Function During Storage
      1. Detrusor activity
         a. normal
         b. overactive
      2. Bladder sensation
         a. normal
         b. increased (hypersensitivity)
         c. reduced (hyposensitivity)
         d. absent
      3. Bladder capacity
      4. Bladder compliance
   B. Urethral Function During Storage
      1. Normal
      2. Incompetent
II. Voiding Phase
   A. Detrusor Function During Voiding
      1. Normal
      2. Underactive
      3. Acontractile
   B. Urethral Function During Voiding
      1. Normal
      2. Obstructive
         a. overactive
         b. mechanical

---

dynamic assessment of the filling and voiding phases is essential for each patient. It is useful to examine bladder and urethral activity separately in each phase. If urodynamic studies are performed, results should clearly reflect the patient's symptoms and signs.

Filling and Storage Phase

The ICS classification of abnormalities of the storage and voiding phases is outlined in the accompanying box. Cystometry is used to examine the bladder during filling and storage. Function should be described in terms of bladder (detrusor) activity, sensation, capacity, and compliance.

Detrusor activity may be normal or overactive. Overactive detrusor function is characterized by involuntary detrusor contractions during filling. They may be spontaneous or provoked and cannot be completely suppressed. Overactive detrusor function in the absence of a known neurologic abnormality is called *unstable detrusor;* overactivity due to disturbance of the nervous control mechanisms is termed *detrusor hyperreflexia.* These conditions are frequently associated with the symptom of urinary urgency. Urgency associated with overactive detrusor function is termed *motor urgency;* urgency associated with bladder hypersensitivity is termed *sensory urgency.*

Urethral function during storage can be assessed clinically (direct observation of urine loss with cough or Valsalva maneuver), urodynamically (urethral closure pressure profilometry), or radiographically (cystourethrography). The urethral closure mechanism may be normal or incompetent. An incompetent urethral closure mechanism is one that allows leakage of urine in the absence of a detrusor contraction. Leakage may occur whenever intravesical pressure exceeds intraurethral pressure (genuine stress incontinence) or when there is an involuntary fall in urethral pressure (unstable urethra). The definition and significance of this latter condition await additional data.

Urinary incontinence is an involuntary (urethral or extraurethral) loss of urine that can be demonstrated objectively and constitutes a social or hygienic problem for the patient. Urinary incontinence is a symptom, a sign, and a condition. Urinary incontinence as a symptom means that the patient states she has involuntary urine loss. Examples of types of symptoms of incontinence include stress incontinence, urge incontinence, enuresis, postmicturition dribble, and continuous incontinence. The sign of stress incontinence denotes the observation of urine loss from the external urethral meatus synchronously with physical exertion such as a cough or Valsalva maneuver. Postmicturition dribble and continuous leakage are other signs of incontinence. Because symptoms and signs of urinary incontinence are sometimes misleading, accurate diagnosis often requires urodynamic investigation in addition to careful history and physical examination.

The ICS defines the following conditions of urinary incontinence:

  1. *Genuine stress incontinence* is the involuntary loss of urine that occurs when, in the absence

of a detrusor contraction, the intravesical pressure exceeds the maximum urethral pressure.

2. *Reflex incontinence* is the loss of urine due to detrusor hyperreflexia, involuntary urethral relaxation, or both in the absence of the sensation usually associated with the desire to void. This condition is seen only in patients with neuropathic bladder or urethral disorders.

3. *Overflow incontinence* is any involuntary loss of urine associated with overdistention of the bladder.

Voiding Phase

During the voiding phase, the detrusor muscle may be normal, acontractile, or underactive. Normal voiding usually is achieved by a voluntarily initiated detrusor contraction that is sustained and can be suppressed. An underactive detrusor during micturition implies that the detrusor contraction is of inadequate magnitude or duration (or both) to effect bladder emptying within a normal time span. Detrusor areflexia is defined as acontractility due to an abnormality of nervous control and denotes the complete absence of centrally coordinated contraction.

During voiding, urethral function may be normal or obstructed. Obstruction may be due to urethral overactivity, as in detrusor-external sphincter dyssynergia, or to mechanical obstruction, such as with a urethral stricture or tumor.

Simultaneous measurement of intravesical or detrusor pressure and urine flow is necessary to determine whether the patient's voiding is obstructive. In general, high detrusor pressures with low flow rates suggest an obstructive problem, whereas low detrusor pressures with low flow rates imply that the problem is one of detrusor underactivity or acontractility. Simultaneous external urethral sphincter electromyography is necessary to determine whether an obstructive voiding pattern is secondary to urethral overactivity or to mechanical obstruction.

Functional Classification

Wein classified voiding dysfunction on a functional basis, describing the dysfunction simply in terms of whether the deficit is primarily one of the filling/

storage phase or of the voiding phase of micturition. Each section is then subcategorized into whether the deficit is one of the bladder or of the outlet. The expanded functional classification, as suggested by Wein and Barrett, is shown in the accompanying box.

The Expanded Functional Classification

I. Failure to store
   A. Because of the bladder
      1. Detrusor hyperactivity
         a. involuntary contractions
            (1) suprasacral neurologic disease
            (2) bladder outlet obstruction
            (3) idiopathic
         b. decreased compliance
            (1) fibrosis
            (2) idiopathic
      2. Sensory urgency
         a. inflammatory
         b. infectious
         c. neurologic
         d. psychologic
         e. idiopathic
   B. Because of the outlet
      1. Genuine stress incontinence
      2. Nonfunctional bladder neck/proximal urethra (type III)
II. Failure to empty
   A. Because of the bladder
      1. Neurologic
      2. Myogenic
      3. Psychogenic
      4. Idiopathic
   B. Because of the outlet
      1. Anatomic
         a. prostatic obstruction
         b. bladder neck contracture obstruction
         c. urethral stricture
      2. Functional
         a. smooth sphincter dyssynergia
         b. striated sphincter dyssynergia

Modified from Wein AJ, Barrett DM: Classification of voiding dysfunction. In *Voiding function and dysfunction*, Chicago, 1988, Mosby–Year Book.

A reasonably accurate urodynamic description is required for proper use of this system for a given voiding problem, but an exact diagnosis is not required for treatment. Several deficits can be present in the same patient and all of them should be recognized to properly use this classification system.

CLASSIFICATION OF GENUINE STRESS URINARY INCONTINENCE

Green was one of the first investigators to attempt to classify stress incontinence. Based on his clinical experience, he noted that stress incontinence resulted from loss of the posterior urethrovesical angle. Patients were divided into two categories based on the presence or absence of anatomic support of the urethrovesical junction: type I defect was defined as loss of posterior urethrovesical angulation with a well-supported urethra; type II defects represented loss of posterior urethrovesical angulation in conjunction with urethral and bladder neck hypermobility. Based on this classification, Green advocated treating type I defects with anterior colporrhaphy and type II defects with retropubic bladder neck suspension. Subsequent studies, in which bead chain cystourethrograms were performed on both stress incontinent and continent patients, revealed that some women who were completely continent of urine, or were incontinent secondary to detrusor instability, also had loss of posterior urethrovesical angulation and urethral hypermobility. Because posterior urethrovesical angulation is not believed to be an important factor in genuine anatomic stress incontinence, Green's classification system is no longer valid.

Currently, the most accepted theory to explain the development of genuine stress incontinence is based on work by Enhorning, Hodgkinson, and McGuire et al. Hydrodynamically, continence is achieved because maximum urethral pressure is greater than intravesical pressure during bladder filling and during increases in intraabdominal pressure. Continence during straining occurs because intraabdominal pressure is transmitted equally to the bladder body and to the bladder neck/ proximal urethra. Genuine stress incontinence occurs when intraabdominal pressure transmission to the

bladder is greater than that to the bladder neck/proximal urethra or when the urethral sphincteric mechanism fails to function at rest.

If the patient has a relatively normally functioning urethral sphincteric mechanism at rest, but has loss of support of the proximal urethra with straining, so that it descends outside of the sphere of abdominal pressure transmission, the patient frequently develops stress incontinence. This form of anatomic stress incontinence has been classified by McGuire et al and Blaivas and Olsson as types I, IIa, and IIb, depending on the amount of descent of the bladder base at rest and with straining. In these types, the bladder neck is always closed at rest in the absence of a detrusor contraction, as determined by video-urodynamic studies. During periods of increased intraabdominal pressure, the proximal urethra opens and incontinence ensues. These patients are usually treated with simple elevation and stabilization of the bladder neck via numerous types of operations.

The second mechanism by which stress incontinence occurs is when the urethra no longer functions as a sphincter. Even at rest, it looses the ability to maintain a watertight seal. This has been termed type III urethra by McGuire et al and Blaivas and Olsson. On video-urodynamic studies, the vesical neck and proximal urethra are open at rest in the absence of a detrusor contraction. On urethral closure pressure profile, the maximal urethral closure pressure may be very low (e.g., <20 cm H_2O) and/or the functional urethral length may be shortened. In its most severe form, the urethra is a fixed, rigid, nonfunctioning tube, known as a *lead pipe urethra*.

Although various tests may be used to identify patients with type III genuine stress incontinence, investigators have not agreed that any single modality is diagnostic. This condition may be secondary to previous bladder neck surgery, radiation, or advanced age. These patients generally require surgical procedures aimed at obstructing the urethra, such as a suburethral sling procedure, collagen injection, or artificial sphincter placement. Typical characteristics of anatomic and type III genuine stress incontinence are shown in Table 4-1, although overlap of these characteristics between groups frequently occurs.

TABLE 4-1   Typical characteristics of two types of genuine stress urinary incontinence in women

Characteristic	Anatomic stress incontinence	Poorly or non-functioning urethra
Anterior vaginal wall on pelvic examination	Descent at rest and/or with straining	Fixed, scarred
Urethral mobility	Hypermobile	Nonmobile
Maximal urethral closure pressure	Normal to low (usually >20 cm H_2O)	Low to very low (usually <20 cm H_2O)
Bladder neck on video-urodynamic tests	Closed at rest	Open at rest
Classification type*	I, IIa, IIb	III

*As defined by McGuire et al and Blaivas and Olsson.

DIFFERENTIAL DIAGNOSIS

Among women complaining of urinary incontinence, the differential diagnosis includes genitourinary and nongenitourinary conditions (see accompanying box). As previously mentioned, genitourinary disorders include problems of bladder filling and storage, as well as extraurethral disorders, such as fistula and congenital abnormalities. Nongenitourinary conditions that cause urinary incontinence generally are functional conditions that occur simultaneously with normal or abnormal urethral and bladder function. These conditions are found most commonly in elderly women.

The most common urine storage disorder in women is genuine stress incontinence. Bladder filling disorders due to overactive detrusor function are the second most common cause of urinary incontinence. Underactive or acontractile detrusor function may result in voiding dysfunction or urinary incontinence. As previously mentioned, involuntary loss of urine associated with overdistention of the bladder is termed overflow incontinence. This condition is less prevalent in women and is usually associated with diabetes, neurologic diseases, severe genital prolapse, or postsurgical obstruction.

Functional incontinence is associated with cognitive, psychologic, or physical impairments that make it difficult to reach the toilet or that interfere with appropriate toileting. With these conditions, continent persons may not have enough time to avoid an acci-

---

Differential Diagnosis of Urinary Incontinence in Women

Genitourinary Etiology
Filling/storage disorders

Genuine stress incontinence
Detrusor instability (idiopathic)
Detrusor hyperreflexia (neurogenic)
Mixed types
Overflow incontinence

Fistula

Vesical
Ureteral
Urethral

Congenital

Ectopic ureter
Epispadias

Nongenitourinary Etiology

Functional
Neurologic
Cognitive
Environmental
Pharmacologic
Metabolic

dent. Functional causes also may act synergistically with other urinary problems. For example, persons with manageable detrusor instability may become incontinent if another disease or physical problem keeps them from reaching the toilet. Physical conditions that may cause functional incontinence include joint abnormalities, arthritic pain, or muscular weakness. An unfamiliar setting, lack of convenient toilet facilities, or other environmental factors can aggravate this condition. Psychologic difficulties and other repressed or hostile behavior may be related to incontinence, especially in the institutionalized elderly. Finally, iatrogenic factors, such as drugs, can cause or aggravate incontinence (see Chapter 5).

The relative likelihood of each condition causing incontinence varies with the age and health of the individual (Fig. 4-1). Among ambulatory, adult incontinent women, the most common condition is genuine stress incontinence, which represents 50% to 70% of cases. Detrusor abnormalities and mixed forms (usually genuine stress incontinence and detrusor instability) account for 20% to 40% of incontinence cases. Among elderly, noninstitutionalized incontinent patients evaluated in referral centers, genuine stress incontinence is found less frequently (30% to 46%) and detrusor abnormalities and mixed disorders are relatively more common, occurring in 29% to 61% of cases. However, in a urodynamic study of elderly community dwelling women with incontinence, Diokno et al reported a prevalence of detrusor abnormalities of only 12%, probably reflecting a healthier group of women. Institutionalized elderly women who are incontinent have detrusor overactivity (with or without impaired bladder contractility) in 38% to 61% of cases and genuine stress incontinence in only 16% to 21% of cases.

BIBLIOGRAPHY

Abrams P, Blaivas JG, Stanton SL, et al: Sixth report on the standardization of terminology of lower urinary tract function. Procedures related to neurophysiological investigations: electromyography, nerve conduction studies, reflex latencies, evoked potentials and sensory testing. *World J Urol* 4:2, 1986; *Scand J Urol Nephrol* 20:161, 1986.

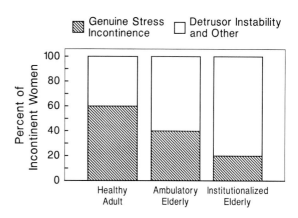

Fig. 4-1 Estimated likelihood of conditions causing incontinence in women, in various age categories.

Abrams P, Blaivas JG, Stanton SL, et al: The standardization of terminology of lower tract function, *Scand J Urol Nephrol* 114(suppl):5, 1988.

Bates P, Bradley WE, Glen E, et al: First report on the standardization of terminology of lower urinary tract function. Urinary incontinence. Procedures related to the evaluation of urine storage: cystometry, urethral closure pressure profile, units of measurement, *Br J Urol* 48:39, 1976; *Eur Urol* 2:274, 1976; *Scand J Urol Nephrol* 11:193, 1976; *Urol Int* 32:81, 1976.

Bates P, Glen E, Griffiths D, et al: Second report on the standardization of terminology of lower urinary tract function. Procedures related to the evaluation of micturition: flow rate, pressure measurement, symbols, *Acta Urol Jpn* 27:1563, 1977; *Br J Urol* 49:207, 1977; *Scand J Urol Nephrol* 11:197, 1977.

Bates P, Bradley WE, Glen E, et al: Third report on the standardization of terminology of lower urinary tract function. Procedures related to the evaluation of micturition: pressure flow relationships, residual urine, *Br J Urol* 52:348, 1980; *Eur Urol* 6:170, 1980; *Acta Urol Jpn* 27:1566, 1980; *Scand J Urol Nephrol* 12:191, 1980.

Bates P, Bradley WE, Glen E, et al: Fourth report on the standardization of terminology of lower urinary tract function. Terminology related to neuromuscular dysfunction of lower urinary tract, *Br J Urol* 52:333, 1981; *Urology* 17:618, 1981; *Scand J Urol Nephrol* 15:169, 1981; *Acta Urol Jpn* 27:1568, 1981.

Bent AE, Richardson DA, Ostergard DR: Diagnosis of lower urinary tract disorders in postmenopausal patients, *Am J Obstet Gynecol* 145:218, 1983.

Blaivas JG, Olsson CA: Stress incontinence: classification and surgical approach, *J Urol* 139:727, 1988.

Blaivas JG: Classification of stress urinary incontinence, *Neurourol Urodyn* 2:103, 1983.

Castleton CM, Duffin HM, Asher MJ: Clinical and urodynamic studies in 100 elderly incontinent patients, *Br Med J* 282:1103, 1981.

Diokno AC, Brown MB, Brock BM, et al: Clinical and cystometric characteristics of continent and incontinent non-institutionalized elderly, *J Urol* 140:567, 1988.

Enhorning G: Simultaneous recording of intravesical and intra-urethral pressure, *Acta Chir Scand* (suppl) 276:1, 1961.

Green TH: Development of a plan for the diagnosis and treatment of urinary stress incontinence, *Am J Obstet Gynecol* 83:632, 1962.

Green TH: The problem of urinary stress incontinence in the female, *Obstet Gynecol Surv* 23:603, 1968.

Hodgkinson CP: Relationships of the female urethra and bladder in urinary stress incontinence, *Am J Obstet Gynecol* 65:650, 1953.

McGuire EJ, Lytton B, Pepe V, et al: Stress urinary incontinence. *Am J Obstet Gynecol* 47:255, 1976.

McGuire EJ: Urodynamic findings in patients after failure of stress incontinence operations. In Zinner NR, Sterling AM (eds); *Female incontinence,* New York, 1981, Alan R Liss.

Ouslander J, Staskin D, Raz S, et al: Clinical versus urodynamic diagnosis in an incontinent female geriatric population, *J Urol* 37:68, 1987.

Quigley GJ, Harper AC: The epidemiology of urethral-vesical dysfunction in the female patient, *Am J Obstet Gynecol* 151:220, 1985.

Resnick NM, Yalla SV, Laurino E: The pathophysiology of urinary incontinence among institutionalized elderly persons, *N Engl J Med* 320:1, 1989.

Walters MD, Shields LE: The diagnostic value of history, physical examination, and the Q-tip cotton swab test in women with urinary incontinence, *Am J Obstet Gynecol* 159:145, 1988.

Wein AJ: Classification of neurogenic voiding dysfunction, *J Urol* 125:605, 1981.

Wein AJ, Barrett DM: Voiding function and dysfunction, Chicago, 1988, Mosby–Year Book.

Williams ME, Pannill FC: Urinary incontinence in the elderly. *Ann Intern Med* 97:895, 1982.

PART TWO

Evaluation

CHAPTER 5

Evaluation of Incontinence: History, Physical Examination, and Office Tests

Mark D. Walters

History and Physical Examination
   History
   Urinary diary
   Gynecologic examination
   Neurologic examination
Techniques for Measuring Urethral Mobility
   Bead-chain cystourethrography
   Q-tip test
   Ultrasonography
Perineal Pad Tests
Office Diagnostic Tests
   Laboratory
   Evaluation of bladder filling and voiding
   Bladder neck elevation test
Making the Diagnosis
Diagnostic Accuracy of Office Evaluations
Indications for Urodynamic Tests

Urinary incontinence can be a symptom of which patients complain, a sign demonstrated on examination, or a condition (i.e., diagnosis) that can be confirmed by definitive studies. When a woman complains of urinary incontinence, appropriate evaluation includes exploring the nature of her symptoms and looking for physical findings. The history and physical examination are the first and most important steps in the evaluation. A preliminary diagnosis can be made with simple office and laboratory tests, with initial therapy based on these findings. If complex conditions are present, if the patient does not improve after initial therapy, or if surgery is being considered, definitive, specialized studies are necessary.

HISTORY AND PHYSICAL EXAMINATION
History

Early in the interview, one should elicit a description of the patient's main complaint including duration and frequency. A clear understanding of the severity of the problem or disability and its effect on quality of life should be sought. The accompanying box lists questions that are helpful in evaluating incontinent women. The first question is designed to elicit the symptom of stress incontinence, i.e., urine loss with events that increase intraabdominal pressure. The symptom of stress incontinence is usually (but not always) associated with the diagnosis of genuine stress incontinence. Questions 2 through 9 help elicit the symptoms associated with the condition of detrusor instability. The symptom of urge incontinence is present if the patient answers question 3 affirmatively. Frequency (questions 4 and 5), bedwetting (question 6), leaking with intercourse (question 8), and a sense of urgency (questions 2 and 7) are all associated with

Helpful Questions in the Evaluation of Female Urinary Incontinence

1. Do you leak urine when you cough, sneeze, or laugh?
2. Do you ever have such an uncomfortably strong need to urinate that if you don't reach the toilet you will leak?
3. If "yes" to No. 2, do you ever leak before you reach the toilet?
4. How many times during the day do you urinate?
5. How many times do you void during the night after going to bed?
6. Have you wet the bed in the past year?
7. Do you develop an urgent need to urinate when you are nervous, under stress, or in a hurry?
8. Do you ever leak during or after sexual intercourse?
9. Do you find it necessary to wear a pad because of your leaking?
10. How often do you leak?
11. Have you had bladder, urine, or kidney infections?
12. Are you troubled by pain or discomfort when you urinate?
13. Have you had blood in your urine?
14. Do you find it hard to begin urinating?
15. Do you have a slow urinary stream?
16. Do you have to strain to pass your urine?
17. After you urinate, do you have dribbling or a feeling that your bladder is still full?

From Walters MD, Realini JP: The evaluation and treatment of urinary incontinence in women: a primary care approach, *J Am Board Fam Pract* 5:289, 1992.

TABLE 5-1   Medications that can affect lower urinary tract function

Type of medication	Lower urinary tract effects
Diuretics	Polyuria, frequency, urgency
Anticholinergic agents	Urinary retention, overflow incontinence
Alcohol	Sedation, impaired mobility, diuresis
Psychotropic agents	
antidepressants	Anticholinergic actions, sedation
antipsychotics	Anticholinergic actions, sedation
sedatives/hypnotics	Sedation, muscle relaxation, confusion
Alpha-adrenergic blockers	Stress incontinence
Alpha-adrenergic agonists	Urinary retention
Beta-adrenergic agonists	Urinary retention
Calcium-channel blockers	Urinary retention, overflow incontinence

more, strong coughing associated with chronic pulmonary disease can markedly worsen symptoms of stress incontinence. A bowel history should be noted because chronic severe constipation has been associated with voiding difficulties, urgency, stress incontinence, and increased bladder capacity. A past history of hysterectomy, vaginal repair, pelvic radiotherapy, or retropubic surgery should alert the physician to the possibility of prior surgical trauma to the lower urinary tract.

A complete list of the patient's medications should be sought to determine if individual drugs might influence the function of the bladder or urethra, leading to urinary incontinence or voiding difficulties. A list of drugs that commonly affect lower urinary tract function is shown in Table 5-1. In these cases, altering drug dosage or changing to a drug with similar therapeutic effectiveness, but with fewer lower urinary tract side effects, will often "cure" the offending urinary tract symptom. In addition, diuretic use may worsen preexisting symptoms of incontinence.

detrusor instability. Questions 9 and 10 help to define the severity of the problem. Questions 11 through 13 screen for urinary tract infection and neoplasia, and questions 14 through 17 are designed to elicit symptoms of voiding dysfunction.

After the urologic history, thorough medical, surgical, gynecologic, neurologic, and obstetric histories should be obtained. Certain medical and neurologic conditions, such as diabetes, stroke, and lumbar disc disease, may cause urinary incontinence. Further-

Urinary Diary

Patient histories regarding frequency and severity of urinary symptoms are often inaccurate and misleading. Urinary diaries are more reliable and require the patient to record volume and frequency of fluid intake and of voiding, usually for a 1- to 7-day period. Episodes of urinary incontinence and associated events or symptoms such as coughing or urgency are noted. The number of times voided each night and any episodes of bedwetting are recorded the next morning. The maximum voided volume also provides a relatively accurate estimate of bladder capacity. The physician should review the frequency/volume charts with the patient and corroborate or modify the initial diagnostic impression. If excessive frequency and volume of fluid intake are noted, restriction of excessive oral fluid intake (combined with scheduled voiding) may improve symptoms of stress and urge incontinence by keeping the bladder volume below the threshold at which urinary leaking results.

Gynecologic Examination

General, gynecologic and lower neurologic examinations should be performed on every incontinent woman. The pelvic examination is of primary importance. Vaginal discharge is known to mimic incontinence, so evidence of this problem should be sought and, if present, treated. Vulvar and vaginal atrophy consistent with hypoestrogenemia suggests that the urethra and periurethral tissues are also atrophic. The presence and severity of anterior vaginal relaxation, including cystocele and proximal urethral detachment and mobility, or anterior vaginal scarring, are estimated. Associated pelvic support abnormalities, such as rectocele, enterocele, and uterovaginal prolapse, are noted. A bimanual examination is performed to rule out coexistent gynecologic pathology, which can occur in up to two thirds of patients. The rectal examination further evaluates for pelvic pathology and for fecal impaction, the latter of which may be associated with voiding difficulties and incontinence in elderly women. Urinary incontinence has been shown to improve or resolve after the removal of fecal impactions in institutionalized geriatric patients.

Neurologic Examination

Urinary incontinence may be the presenting symptom of neurologic disease. The screening neurologic examination should evaluate mental status as well as sensory and motor function of both lower extremities. Mental status is determined by noting the patient's level of consciousness, orientation, memory, speech, and comprehension. Disorders associated with mental status aberrations that may produce neurourologic abnormalities include senile and presenile dementia, brain tumors, and normal pressure hydrocephalus.

Evaluation of the motor and sensory systems may identify an occult neurologic lesion or can help determine the level of a known lesion. Common diseases associated with motor abnormalities that can produce urologic disturbances include Parkinson's disease, multiple sclerosis, cerebrovascular disease, infections, and tumors. Sacral segments 2 through 4, which contain the important neurons controlling micturition, are particularly important (Fig. 5-1). To test motor function, the patient extends and flexes the hip, knee, and ankle and inverts and everts the foot. The strength and tone of the bulbocavernosus muscle and external anal sphincter are estimated digitally. The patellar, ankle, and plantar reflex responses are tested. Sensory function along the sacral dermatomes is tested by using light touch and pinprick on the perineum and around the thigh and foot.

Two reflexes may help in the examination of sacral reflex activity. In the anal reflex, stroking the skin adjacent to the anus causes reflex contraction of the external anal sphincter muscle. The bulbocavernosus reflex involves contraction of the bulbocavernosus and ischiocavernosus muscles in response to tapping or squeezing of the clitoris. Unfortunately, these reflexes can be difficult to evaluate clinically and are not always present, even in neurologically intact women.

TECHNIQUES FOR MEASURING URETHRAL MOBILITY

Examination of the anterior vaginal wall is relatively inaccurate in predicting the amount of urethral mobility. It is difficult with physical examination to differentiate between cystocele and rotational descent of

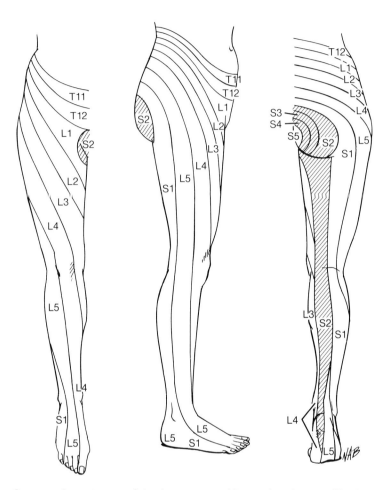

Fig. 5-1 Sensory dermatomes of the lower extremities and perineum. Shaded area represents sacral segments 2, 3, 4. *(Modified from Boileau Grant JC:* Grant's atlas of anatomy, *ed 6, Baltimore, 1972, Williams & Wilkins.)*

the urethra and the two frequently coexist. Many tools are available for estimating the amount of urethral mobility in women. Videocystourethrography probably is the standard by which all other modalities should be judged. This technique allows a dynamic assessment of the anatomy and function of the bladder base and urethra during retrograde filling with contrast material and during voiding. It is also the most invasive, most expensive, and probably least available diagnostic procedure used in the evaluation of incontinence. For these reasons, other methods are usually used to measure urethral mobility in incontinent women.

Bead-chain Cystourethrography

Bead-chain cystourethrography provides a radiologic view of the relationships among the urethra, bladder, vagina, and bony pelvis. Its use was popular more than two decades ago when emphasis of the relationship between the urethral axis and the bladder base was thought to be the sole basis of the diagnosis of stress incontinence. Lateral roentgenograms obtained with the patient at rest and straining demonstrate urethrovesical relationships without distorting the urethral configuration or impairing urethral mobility. Unfortunately, wide interobserver variations occur in the measurement of specific radiologic landmarks, and strict criteria for reproducible interpretations have not been established. Nevertheless, bead-chain cystourethrography remains a viable method of viewing the general configuration and anatomic relationships of the urethra, bladder, and vagina as compared with the bony pelvis at rest and during maximum straining.

Q-tip Test

Placement of a cotton swab in the urethra to the level of the vesical neck and measurement of the axis change with straining can be used to demonstrate urethral mobility. The Q-tip test was described initially as an aid in differentiating type I (loss of posterior urethrovesical angle with normal urethral axis) from type II (loss of posterior urethrovesical angle with rotational descent of the urethra) anatomic defects in women with stress incontinence. It was noted that the swab deflection correlated with the amount of urethral axis rotation on bead-chain cystourethrography and that rotation >20 degrees from the horizontal indicated that a type II defect was present.

To perform the Q-tip test, a sterile, lubricated cotton-tipped applicator is inserted transurethrally into the bladder, then withdrawn slowly until definite resistance is felt, indicating that the cotton tip is at the bladder neck. This is best accomplished with the patient in the supine lithotomy position during a pelvic examination. The resting angle of the applicator stick in relation to the horizontal is measured with a goniometer or protractor. The patient is then asked to cough and perform a Valsalva maneuver and the maximum straining angle from the horizontal is measured. Results are not affected by the amount of urine in the bladder. Care should be taken to ensure that the cotton tip is not in the bladder or at the mid-urethra because this results in a falsely lower measurement of urethral mobility.

Although maximum straining angle measurements greater than 30 degrees are generally considered to be abnormal, few data are available to differentiate normal from abnormal measurements. Urethral mobility in continent women is probably related to age, parity, and support defects of the anterior vaginal wall. Walters and Diaz noted that asymptomatic women with a mean parity of two and a mean age of 32 years had an average resting Q-tip angle of 18 degrees and an average maximum straining angle of 54 degrees. Women with genuine stress incontinence had a significantly higher maximum straining angle of 73 degrees, although there was wide overlap in measurements between the continent and incontinent women. These data indicate that arbitrary cut-off values around 30 degrees are too low to define "normal" urethral mobility for parous women.

Ultrasonography

More recently, ultrasonography was introduced as an alternate method of evaluating the urethrovesical anatomy. When compared to bead-chain cystourethrography, fluoroscopy, and the Q-tip test, perineal and vaginal ultrasonography accurately displays the descent of the urethrovesical junction, opening of the bladder neck, and detrusor contractions. This technique appears to hold promise as a relatively noninvasive and accurate method of evaluating the mobility of the urethrovesical junction and proximal urethra in incontinent women.

PERINEAL PAD TESTS

Perineal pad weighing may be used when one wishes to objectively document the presence and amount of urine loss. The test should approximate activities in daily life and should evaluate as long a period as possible, yet be practical. A 1-hour period of testing is currently recommended by the International Continence Society. This test can be extended for additional 1-hour periods if the result of the first test is not considered representative of the symptoms by either the patient or the physician. Alternatively, the test can be repeated after filling the bladder to a defined volume.

The total amount of urine lost during the test period is determined by weighing a collecting device such as an absorbent pad. The pad should be worn inside waterproof underpants or should have a waterproof backing. Care should be taken to use a collecting device of adequate capacity. Immediately before the test begins the collecting device is weighed to the nearest gram. A typical test schedule is as follows:

1. Test is started without the patient voiding.
2. Preweighed collecting device is put on and first 1-hour test period begins.
3. Subject drinks 500 ml sodium-free liquid within a short period (maximum 15 min), then sits or rests.
4. Half-hour period: subject walks, including stair climbing equivalent to one flight up and down.
5. During the remaining period the subject performs the following activities:
   a. Standing up from sitting, 10 times.
   b. Coughing vigorously, 10 times.
   c. Running on the spot for 1 minute.
   d. Bending to pick up small object from floor, 5 times.
   e. Washing hands in running water for 1 minute.
6. At the end of the 1-hour test the collecting device is removed and weighed.
7. If the test is regarded as representative, the subject voids and the volume is recorded.
8. If the test is not regarded as representative, the test is repeated, preferably without voiding.

If the collecting device becomes saturated or filled during the test, it should be removed, weighed, and replaced. The total weight of urine lost during the test period is taken to be equal to the gain in weight of the collecting device(s). In interpreting the results of the test, it should be remembered that a weight gain of up to 1 g may be due to weighing errors, sweating, or vaginal discharge.

Two critical variables determine the sensitivity of pad weighing: the amount of fluid in the bladder during exercise and the type of activity used to generate increased intraabdominal pressure. Lose et al found that pad weight correlated significantly with the fluid load on the bladder, i.e., the initial volume plus diuresis. Pad weighing has acceptable test-retest reliability and is easy to perform in a clinical setting. However, it has low sensitivity and poor correlation between pad gain and videographic assessment of incontinence severity. These shortcomings have limited acceptance of pad weighing as a routine part of the evaluation of incontinence.

Phenazopyridine hydrochloride (Pyridium) is sometimes used to aid clinicians in differentiating urinary continence from incontinence in women with disturbing vaginal wetness. Patients are given Pyridium tablets and are instructed to wear a sanitary pad for a given time. The pad is then removed and examined. Red-orange staining is taken as evidence that urine loss has occurred. Although this test may occasionally be useful, Wall et al demonstrated that although all incontinent women had pad staining, 52% of healthy continent women also had staining, reflecting a high rate of false-positive tests.

OFFICE DIAGNOSTIC TESTS
Laboratory

Few laboratory tests are necessary for the evaluation of incontinence. A clean midstream or catheterized urine sample should be obtained for urinalysis and culture. Acute cystitis can present with multiple irritative symptoms, such as dysuria, frequency, urgency, incontinence, and voiding difficulty. In these cases, treatment of the infection will usually eradicate the symptoms. Bacteriuria, however, is frequently asymptomatic, especially in the elderly. Boscia et al demonstrated that no differences in urinary symptoms were found when elderly bacteriuric subjects were compared with themselves when they were nonbacteriuric. In view of these conflicting data, it seems reasonable to examine the urine for infection in all incontinent patients and, if bacteriuria is found, to prescribe appropriate antibiotics and reevaluate the patient in several weeks.

Patients with hematuria or with recurrent or persistent urinary tract infections should undergo appropriate evaluation and urologic consultation. Diabetes should be ruled out in patients with frequency, nocturia, voiding difficulties, or chronic urinary tract infection. Tests of renal function, urine cytology, and radiographic procedures are necessary only for specific medical and urologic indications.

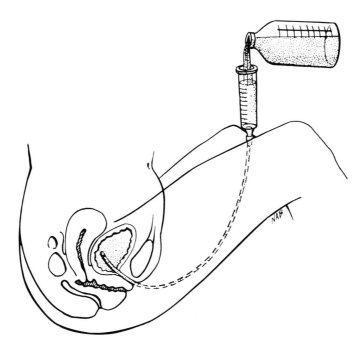

Fig. 5-2 Office evaluation of bladder filling function. In sitting or standing position with a catheter in the bladder, the bladder is filled by gravity by pouring sterile water into the syringe.

Evaluation of Bladder Filling and Voiding

The office evaluation of incontinence should involve some assessment of voiding, of detrusor function during filling, and of competency of the urethral sphincteric mechanism. During the assessment, one should try to determine specifically the circumstances leading to the involuntary loss of urine. If possible, such circumstances should be reproduced and directly observed during clinical evaluation. The examination is most easily initiated with the patient's bladder comfortably full. The patient is allowed to void as normally as possible in private. The time to void and the amount of urine voided are recorded. The patient then returns to the examination room and the volume of residual urine is noted by transurethral catheterization or ultrasound examination. If a sterile urine sample has not yet been obtained for analysis and culture, it can be obtained at this time. A 50 ml syringe without its piston or bulb is attached to the catheter and held above the bladder. The patient is then asked to sit or

stand and the bladder is filled by gravity by pouring 50 ml aliquots of sterile water into the syringe (Fig. 5-2). The patient's first bladder sensation, first urge to void, and maximum bladder capacity are noted. The water level in the syringe should be closely observed during filling, as any rise in the column of water can be secondary to a detrusor contraction. Unintended increases in intraabdominal pressure by the patient should be avoided.

The catheter is then removed and the patient is asked to cough in a standing position. Loss of small amounts of urine in spurts simultaneous with the coughs strongly suggests a diagnosis of genuine stress incontinence. Prolonged loss of urine, leaking 5 to 10 seconds after coughing, or no urine loss with provocation indicates that other causes of incontinence, especially detrusor instability, may be present. Interpretation of these office tests can, at times, be difficult because of artifact introduced by rises in intraabdominal pressure due to straining or patient movement.

Borderline or negative tests should be repeated to maximize their diagnostic accuracy.

Bladder Neck Elevation Test

Examination of the perineum with manual or instrumented elevation of the bladder neck, as proposed by Bonney and later Marshall et al, has long been used to aid in the evaluation of urinary incontinence. Marshall et al believed that cessation of urine loss with coughing after elevation of the bladder neck was predictive that the Marshall-Marchetti-Krantz procedure would cure the incontinence. These authors also noted that pulling the vesical base downward toward the introitus with Allis clamps caused increased loss of urine in women with stress incontinence; this observation could be used as accessory evidence that the Marshall-Marchetti-Krantz procedure would be curative. More modern studies of the bladder neck elevation test used microtip transducers and urethral pressure profilometry before and during the test. These studies demonstrated that digital or instrumented bladder neck elevation restores continence during coughing by obstructing the urethra and urethrovesical junction and not by simple reestablishment of equal pressure transmission to the bladder neck and urethra. Because this test causes extrinsic compression of the urethra, it should not be relied on as a prognostic test for selection of patients suitable for incontinence surgery. Furthermore, as with tests for urethral mobility, bladder neck elevation should not be used in place of simple or complex urodynamic testing to determine the cause of urinary incontinence.

MAKING THE DIAGNOSIS

Based on the clinical evaluation, the physician can formulate a presumptive diagnosis and initiate treatment, using the algorithm in Fig. 5-3 as a guide. Similar guidelines for evaluation of incontinence have been used with success in elderly individuals. The initial goal should be to diligently seek out and treat

---

Conditions That Can Cause Transient Urinary Incontinence

Delirium
Restricted mobility
Drugs
Urinary retention
Urinary infection
Urethritis
    Infectious
    Atrophic
Fecal impaction
Spinal cord compression
Polyuria
Psychological

Modified from Ouslander JG, *Clin Geriatr Med* 2:715, 1986.

Situations That Warrant Consultation for the Evaluation and Treatment of Lower Urinary Tract Dysfunction

History
    Neurologic disease
    Surgery to treat urinary incontinence
    Pelvic malignancy
    Radiation therapy
Physical examination and office evaluation
    Persistent urinary infection after treatment
    Hematuria
    Abnormal neurologic examination
    Difficulty passing urethral catheter
    Signs of voiding difficulty or retention
        absent bladder sensation with filling
        large bladder capacity
        high postvoid residual urine volume
    Small bladder capacity
    Fistula
    Urethral diverticula
Failure to improve after treatment of incontinence based on clinical evaluation
Whenever objective clinical findings do not correlate with or reproduce the patient's symptoms and/or concerns

From Walters MD, Realini JP: The evaluation and treatment of urinary incontinence in women: a primary care approach, *J Am Board Fam Pract* 5:289, 1992.

URINARY INCONTINENCE IN WOMEN

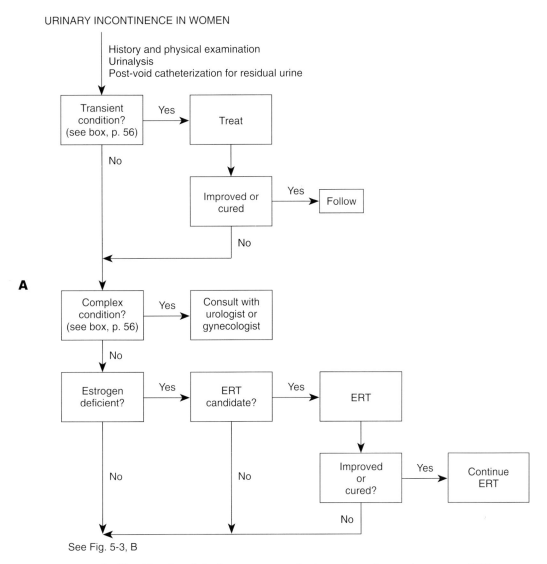

Fig. 5-3   A, Algorithm for clinical assessment of urinary incontinence in women. *ERT,* Estrogen replacement therapy.   *Continued.*

all transient causes of urinary incontinence and voiding difficulty (see accompanying box). Complex causes of incontinence are triaged for urodynamic testing or for consultation (see accompanying box).

After the evaluation, patients can be categorized as having probable genuine stress incontinence or probable detrusor instability (with or without coex-

istent stress incontinence). For either diagnosis, appropriate behavioral or medical therapy can be given and a substantial percentage of patients expected to respond. Even patients with mixed disorders (coexistent genuine stress incontinence and detrusor instability) respond to various forms of conservative therapy in about 60% of cases.

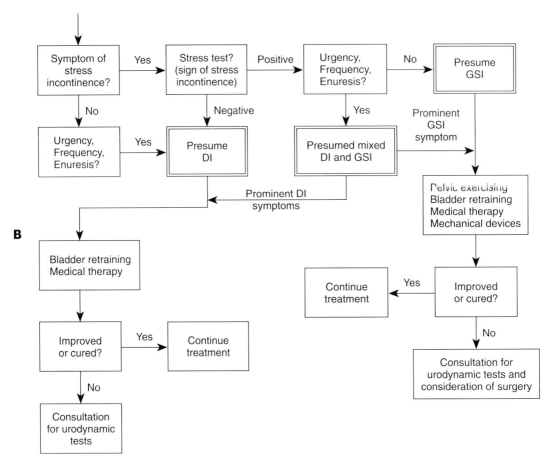

Fig. 5-3, cont'd.   **B**, Algorithm for clinical assessment of urinary incontinence in women. *GSI,* Genuine stress incontinence, *DI,* detrusor instability.

DIAGNOSTIC ACCURACY OF OFFICE EVALUATIONS

The findings of a careful history and physical examination predict the actual incontinence diagnosis with reasonable accuracy. Women who have the symptom of stress incontinence as their only complaint have a 64% to 90% chance of having genuine stress incontinence confirmed on diagnostic urodynamic testing. Ten percent to thirty percent of these patients will be found to have detrusor instability (alone or coexistent with genuine stress incontinence). Other rare conditions that can cause the symptom of stress incontinence are urethral diverticulum, genitourinary fistula, ectopic ureter, and urethral instability. Physical find-

ings associated with genuine stress incontinence are anterior vaginal relaxation and urethral hypermobility.

Sensory urgency, urge incontinence, diurnal and nocturnal frequency, and bedwetting all have been associated with unstable bladder. The more of these abnormal urinary symptoms the patient has, the greater the chance that she has an unstable bladder. Cantor and Bates observed that 81% of patients with three or more of these symptoms had detrusor instability on cystometry. The physical findings of abnormal neurologic examination and absent urethral hypermobility have been associated with overactive detrusor function.

Is the determination of urethral mobility useful in

diagnosing the cause of urinary incontinence? Urethrocystographic findings, such as the posterior urethrovesical angle, funneling of the proximal urethra on straining, and angle of urethral inclination, do not differ between continent and incontinent women with pelvic relaxation. Numerous authors have shown that although the bead-chain cystourethrogram and Q-tip test accurately reflect the amount of urethral mobility with stress, they are of little value in differentiating genuine stress incontinence from detrusor instability. Furthermore, serial addition of the measurement of urethral inclination with a Q-tip to the history and pelvic examination does not appreciably change the sensitivity or specificity for diagnosing genuine stress incontinence. However, because most women with primary genuine stress incontinence have urethral hypermobility, a negative test should cause one to question that diagnosis, perhaps indicating the need to perform urodynamic testing. Clearly, the measurement of urethral mobility should not be used to differentiate urethral sphincter incompetence from abnormalities of voiding or detrusor function, as these diagnoses require the measurement of detrusor pressure during filling and emptying.

Although the determination of urethral mobility is not useful in the diagnosis of urinary incontinence, it may provide some information about which surgical therapy is most appropriate. In patients with genuine stress incontinence, anterior colporrhaphy, needle urethropexy or a retropubic suspension procedure are used when urethral hypermobility is found to coexist with relatively normal intrinsic urethral sphincteric function. When the urethra is nonmobile and/or intrinsically functionless, a sling procedure, artificial urinary sphincter, or injection of bulk-enhancing agents are likely to provide better results. Thus measurement of urethral mobility can aid the surgeon in choosing one group of surgical procedures over another, but cannot determine which procedures yield the best results in each clinical situation.

Retrograde bladder filling provides an assessment of bladder sensation and an estimate of bladder capacity. Patients without urgency and frequency who note a sensation of bladder fullness and have an estimated bladder capacity that is within normal range probably have normal bladder filling function. There seems to be no clear consensus about the definition of normal bladder capacity. Values range from 300 to 750 ml. However, large bladder capacities are not always pathologic. Weir and Jaques showed that 33% of women with bladder capacities greater than 800 ml were urodynamically normal and only 13% had true bladder atony.

In the absence of symptoms of voiding difficulty, patients usually have normal voiding function. The incidence of asymptomatic voiding dysfunction among women with other urologic complaints is only about 3%. Normal values for postvoid residual urine measurements have not been established. Volumes less than 50 ml indicate adequate bladder emptying and volumes greater than 200 ml can be considered inadequate emptying. Clinical judgment must be exercised in interpreting the significance of postvoid residual urine volumes, especially in the intermediate range of 50 to 200 ml. Because isolated instances of elevated residual urine volume may not be significant, the test should be repeated when abnormally high values are obtained. Among women with symptoms of voiding difficulty and those who appear to void abnormally or have retention, more sophisticated testing is required to determine the etiology and the mechanism of the voiding dysfunction.

INDICATIONS FOR URODYNAMIC TESTS

The physician must recognize that even under the most typical clinical situations, the diagnosis of incontinence based only on clinical evaluation may be uncertain. This diagnostic uncertainty may be acceptable if medical or behavioral treatment (as opposed to surgery) is planned because of the relatively low morbidity and cost of these treatments and because the ramifications of noncure (continued incontinence) are not severe. When surgical treatment of stress incontinence is planned, urodynamic testing is recommended to confirm the diagnosis.

As noted, consultation should be considered for complex cases that may require urodynamic testing, surgical treatment, or both. Whenever objective clinical findings do not correlate with or reproduce the patient's symptoms, urodynamic testing is indicated for diagnosis. Finally, when trials of therapy are used, patients must be followed up periodically to evaluate response. If the patient fails to improve, appropriate further testing is indicated.

BIBLIOGRAPHY

History and Physical Examination

Bannister JJ, Laurence WT, Smith A, et al: Urological abnormalities in young women with severe constipation, *Gut* 29:17, 1988.

Benson JT: Gynecologic and urodynamic evaluation of women with urinary incontinence, *Obstet Gynecol* 66:691, 1985.

Blaivas JG, Zayed AAH, Kamal BL: The bulbocavernosus reflex in urology: a prospective study of 299 patients, *J Urol* 126:197, 1981.

Diokno AC, Wells TJ, Brink CA: Comparison of self-reported voided volume with cystometric bladder capacity, *J Urol* 137:698, 1987.

Fantl JA, Wyman JF, Wilson MS, et al: Diuretics and urinary incontinence in community-dwelling women, *Neurourol Urodyn* 9:25, 1990.

Hilton P, Stanton SL: Algorithmic method for assessing urinary incontinence in elderly women, *Br Med J* 282:940, 1981.

Julian TM: Pseudoincontinence secondary to unopposed estrogen replacement in the surgically castrate premenopausal female, *Obstet Gynecol* 70:382, 1987.

Ostergard DR: Effect of drugs on the lower urinary tract. In Ostergard DR (ed): *Gynecologic urology and urodynamics,* ed 2, Baltimore, 1985, Williams & Wilkins.

Walters MD, Realini JP: The evaluation and treatment of urinary incontinence in women: a primary care approach, *J Am Board Fam Pract* 5:289, 1992.

Wyman JF, Choi SC, Harkins SW, et al: The urinary diary in evaluation of incontinent women: a test-retest analysis, *Obstet Gynecol* 71:812,1988.

Techniques for Measuring Urethral Mobility

Bergman A, Koonings PP, Ballard CA: Negative Q-tip test as a risk factor for failed incontinence surgery in women, *J Reprod Med* 34:193, 1989.

Bergman A, McCarthy TA, Ballard CA, et al: Role of the Q-tip test in evaluating stress urinary incontinence, *J Reprod Med* 32:273, 1987.

Bergman A, McKenzie C, Ballard CA, et al: Role of cystourethrography in the preoperative evaluation of stress urinary incontinence in women, *J Reprod Med* 33:372, 1988.

Bhatia NN, Ostergard DR, McQuown D: Ultrasonography in urinary incontinence, *Urology* 29:90, 1987.

Crystle CD, Charme LS, Copeland WE: Q-tip test in stress urinary incontinence, *Obstet Gynecol* 38:313, 1971.

Fantl JA, Beachley MC, Bosch HA, et al: Bead-chain cystourethrogram: an evaluation, *Obstet Gynecol* 58:237, 1981.

Fantl JA, Hurt WG, Bump RC, et al: Urethral axis and sphincteric function, *Am J Obstet Gynecol* 155:554, 1986.

Gordon D, Pearce M, Norton P: Comparison of ultrasound and lateral chain urethrocystography in the determination of bladder neck position and descent, *Neurourol Urodyn* 5:181, 1987.

Karram MM, Narender N, Bhatia MD: The Q-tip test: standardization of the technique and its interpretation in women with urinary incontinence, *Obstet Gynecol* 71:807, 1988.

Kohorn EI, Scioscia AL, Jeanty P, et al: Ultrasound cystourethrography by perineal scanning for the assessment of female stress urinary incontinence, *Obstet Gynecol* 68:269, 1986.

Montz FJ, Stanton SL: Q-tip test in female urinary incontinence, *Obstet Gynecol* 67:258, 1986.

Walters MD, Diaz K: Q-tip test: a study of continent and incontinent women, *Obstet Gynecol* 70:208, 1987.

Perineal Pad Tests

Abrams P, Blaivas JG, Stanton SL, et al: The standardization of terminology of lower urinary tract function recommended by the International Continence Society, *Int Urogynecol J* 1:45, 1990.

Christensen SJ, Colstrup H, Hertz JB, et al: Inter- and intradepartmental variations of the perineal pad weighing test, *Neurourol Urodyn* 5:23, 1986.

Fantl JA, Harkins SW, Wyman JF, et al: Fluid loss quantitation test in women with urinary incontinence: a test-retest analysis, *Obstet Gynecol* 70:739, 1987.

Haylen BT, Frazer MI, Sutherst JR: Diuretic response to fluid load in women with urinary incontinence: optimum duration of pad test, *Br J Urol* 62:331, 1988.

Jakobsen H, Vedel P, Andersen JT: Which pad-weighing test to choose: ICS one hour test, the 48 hour home test or a 40 min test with known bladder volume? *Neurourol Urodyn* 4:23, 1987.

Jorgensen L, Lose G, Anderson JT: One hour pad-weighing test for objective assessment of female urinary incontinence, *Obstet Gynecol* 69:39, 1987.

Kinn A-C, Larsson B: Pad test with fixed bladder volume in urinary stress incontinence, *Acta Obstet Gynecol Scand* 55:369, 1987.

Klarskov P, Hald T: Reproducibility and reliability of urinary incontinence assessment with a 60 min test, *Scand J Urol Nephrol* 18:293, 1984.

Lose G, Gammelgaard J, Jorgenson TJ: The one-hour pad-weighing test: reproducibility and the correlation between the test result, the start volume in the bladder, and the diuresis, *Neurourol Urodyn* 5:17, 1986.

Richmond DH, Sutherst JR, Brown MC: Quantification of urine loss by weighing perineal pads. Observation on the exercise regimen, *Br J Urol* 59:224, 1987.

Sutherst JR, Brown MC, Shawer M: Assessing the severity of urinary incontinence in women by weighing perineal pads, *Lancet* 1 (8230):1128, 1981.

Sutherst JR, Brown MC, Richmond D: Analysis of the pattern of urine loss in women with incontinence as measured by weighing perineal pads, *Br J Urol* 58:273, 1986.

Versi E, Cardozo L: Perineal pad weighing versus videographic analysis in genuine stress incontinence, *Br J Obstet Gynaecol* 93:364, 1986.

Wall LL, Want K, Robson I, et al: The pyridium pad test for diagnosing urinary incontinence, *J Reprod Med* 35:682, 1990.

Walters MD, Dombroski RA, Prihoda TJ: Perineal pad testing in the quantitation of urinary incontinence, *Int Urogynecol J* 1:3, 1990.

Office Diagnostic Tests

Abrams P: The practice of urodynamics. In Mundy AR, Stephenson, TP, Wein AJ (eds): *Urodynamics*, Edinburgh, 1984, Churchill Livingstone.

Abrams P, Feneley R, Torrens M: The clinical contribution of urodynamics. In Chism DG (ed): *Urodynamics*, New York, 1983, Springer-Verlag.

Bergman A: Invalidity of the Bonney stress test. In Ostergard D (ed): *Gynecologic urology and urodynamics*, ed 2, Baltimore, 1985, Williams & Wilkins.

Bhatia NN, Bergman A: Urodynamic appraisal of the Bonney test in women with stress urinary incontinence, *Obstet Gynecol* 62:696, 1983.

Bonney V: On diurnal incontinence of urine in women, *J Obstet Gynaecol Br Emp* 30:358, 1923.

Boscia JA, Kobasa WD, Abrutyn E, et al: Lack of association between bacteriuria and symptoms in the elderly, *Am J Med* 81:979, 1986.

Brocklehurst JC, Dillane JB, Griffiths L, et al: The prevalence and symptomatology of urinary infection in an aged population, *Gerontol Clin* 10:242, 1968.

Eastwood HDH, Warrell R: Urinary incontinence in the elderly female: prediction in diagnosis and outcome of management, *Age Ageing* 13:230, 1984.

Marshall VF, Marchetti A, Krantz K: The correction of stress incontinence by simple vesicourethral suspension, *Surg Gynecol Obstet* 88:509, 1949.

Migliorini GD, Glenning PP: Bonney's test—fact or fiction? *Br J Obstet Gynaecol* 94:157, 1987.

Poston G, Joseph A, Riddle P: The accuracy of ultrasound and the measurement of changes in bladder volume, *Br J Urol* 55:361, 1983.

Sourander LB: Urinary tract infection in the aged. An epidemiological study, *Ann Med Intern Fenn* 55(suppl 45):1, 1966.

Stanton SL: Voiding difficulties and retention. In Stanton SL (ed): *Clinical gynecologic urology*, St Louis, 1984, Mosby–Year Book.

Stanton SL, Ozsoy C, Hilton P: Voiding difficulties in the female: prevalence, clinical and urodynamic review, *Obstet Gynecol* 61:144, 1983.

Wein AJ, Barrett DM: Voiding function and dysfunction, Chicago, 1988, Mosby–Year Book.

Weir J, Jaques PF: Large capacity bladder, *Urology* 4:544, 1974.

Diagnostic Accuracy of Office Evaluation and Indications for Urodynamic Testing

Arnold EP, Webster JR, Loose H, et al: Urodynamics of female incontinence: factors influencing the results of surgery, *Am J Obstet Gynecol* 117:805, 1973.

Byrne DJ, Hamilton Stewart PA, Gray BK: The role of urodynamics in female urinary stress incontinence, *Br J Urol* 59:228, 1987.

Cantor TJ, Bates CP: Comparative study of symptoms and objective urodynamic findings in 214 incontinent women, *Br J Obstet Gynaecol* 87:889, 1980.

Drutz HP, Mandel F: Urodynamic analysis of urinary incontinence symptoms in women, *Am J Obstet Gynecol* 134:789, 1979.

Fantl JA: Genuine stress incontinence: pathophysiology and rationale for its medical management, *Obstet Gynecol Clin North Am* 16:827, 1989.

Farrar DJ, Whiteside CG, Osborne JL, et al: A urodynamic analysis of micturition symptoms in the female, *Surg Gynecol Obstet* 144:875, 1975.

Fischer-Rasmussen W, Hansen RI, Stage P: Predictive values of diagnostic tests in the evaluation of female urinary stress incontinence, *Acta Obstet Gynecol Scand* 65:291, 1986.

Kadar N: The value of bladder filling in the clinical detection of urine loss and selection of patients for urodynamic testing, *Br J Obstet Gynaecol* 95:698, 1988.

Karram MM, Bhatia NN: Management of coexistent stress and urge urinary incontinence, *Obstet Gynecol* 73:4, 1989.

Korda A, Krieger M, Hunter P, et al: The value of clinical symptoms in the diagnosis of urinary incontinence in the female, *Aust NZ J Obstet Gynaecol* 27:149, 1987.

Moolgaoker AS, Ardran GM, Smith JC, et al: The diagnosis and management of urinary incontinence in the female, *J Obstet Gynaecol Br Commonw* 79:481, 1972.

Ouslander JG: Diagnostic evaluation of geriatric urinary incontinence, *Clin Geriatr Med* 2:715, 1986.

Ouslander J, Staskin D, Raz S, et al: Clinical versus urodynamic diagnosis in an incontinent female geriatric population, *J Urol* 37:68, 1987.

Quigley GJ, Harper AC: The epidemiology of urethral-vesical dysfunction in the female patient, *Am J Obstet Gynecol* 151:220, 1985.

Sand PK, Hill RC, Ostergard DR: Incontinence history as a predictor of detrusor stability, *Obstet Gynecol* 71:257, 1988.

Urinary Incontinence Guideline Panel. Urinary incontinence in adults: clinical practice guideline. AHCPR Pub. No. 92-0038. Rockville, MD: Agency for Health Care Policy and Research, Public Health Service, US Department of Health and Human Services, March 1992.

Walters MD, Shields LE: The diagnostic value of history, physical examination, and the Q-tip cotton swab test in women with urinary incontinence, *Am J Obstet Gynecol* 159:145, 1988.

Webster GD, Sihelnik SA, Stone AR: Female urinary incontinence: the incidence, identification, and characteristics of detrusor instability, *Neurourol Urodyn* 3:235, 1984.

CHAPTER 6

Urodynamics: Cystometry

Mickey M. Karram

Background
Normal Cystometry
Video-Urodynamic Testing
Ambulatory Monitoring
Cystometry: Abnormal Studies
Summary

The term *urodynamics* means observation of the changing function of the lower urinary tract over time. Urodynamic tests have been slow to achieve acceptance and are by no means universally used; however, in recent years there has been a resurgence of interest in the hydrodynamic and neurophysiologic aspects of the storage and evacuation of urine. An abundance of new diagnostic procedures, methodologies, and testing equipment have made it exceedingly difficult for the clinician to decide what tests are necessary to adequately evaluate lower urinary tract dysfunction in women.

To understand the fundamental value of urodynamics, one should realize that the female bladder responds similarly to a variety of pathologies. Symptoms do not always reflect accurately the physiologic state of the bladder. For example, a patient may feel that her bladder is full, when in reality it is nearly empty, or that her bladder is contracting when it is not. Nevertheless, the evaluation of a woman with lower urinary tract complaints should not neglect the basic history and physical examination. The validity of any urodynamic diagnosis is linked to the patient's symptoms and the reproduction of these symptoms during the testing session. To obtain the most accurate, clinically relevant interpretation of urodynamic studies, the urodynamicist should clearly understand lower urinary tract function and correlate urodynamic data with other clinical information. The urodynamicist should be the physician who takes the history, performs the physical examination, interprets other tests, explains the diagnosis, and develops a reasonable management plan.

It is desirable that results of urodynamic investigations be recorded in a way that can be communicated among physicians and other health care personnel. For this reason, the recommendations detailed in the standardization reports of the International Continence Society (ICS) should be followed (see Appendix).

Chapters 6 through 8 will discuss urodynamic modalities used in the evaluation of filling, storage, and evacuation of urine. The intent is to give the reader a clear understanding of the rationale, technique, utility, and limitations of each test.

BACKGROUND

The first cystometer dates back to 1872 when Schatz accidentally discovered a crude technique for measuring bladder pressure while trying to record intraabdominal pressure. Shortly thereafter, DuBois studied the effects of changes in body position on intravesical and intrarectal pressures and observed that the desire to void was associated with contraction of the detrusor muscle. The currently popular water cystometer was designed by Lewis in 1939. The later use of air and carbon dioxide as filling media further simplified the procedure.

Cystometry is a urodynamic test that measures the pressure and volume relationship of the bladder. It is used to assess detrusor activity, sensation, capacity, and compliance. Every factor has unique implications, and before any definitive conclusions can be reached, each parameter must be examined in association with symptoms and clinical findings.

A normal bladder has the power of accommodation; it can maintain an almost constant low intravesical pressure throughout filling, regardless of volume. A normal woman should be able to suppress voiding even at maximum capacity. Then, in an acceptable environment, she should be able to initiate a voiding reflex of sufficient magnitude to empty her bladder.

NORMAL CYSTOMETRY

The basic principle of cystometry is the coupling of a manometer to the bladder lumen. A filling medium is instilled into the bladder and, as it fills, intravesical pressure is measured against volume. Testing apparatuses range from simple single-channel methods, which are performed manually or electronically, to complex methods combining electronic measurements of bladder, abdominal, and urethral pressure, together with electromyography and fluoroscopy.

A cystometrogram has two phases: a filling / storage phase and an emptying (voiding) phase (Fig. 6-1). The filling phase is subdivided into a brief initial rise in pressure to achieve resting bladder pressure, followed by a tonus limb that reflects vesicoelastic properties of accommodation of the smooth muscle and collagen of the bladder wall. There may be a third increase in the pressure, which is attributed to stretch-

ing of detrusor muscle and collagenous elements of the bladder wall beyond their limits at bladder capacity. During this third stage, the patient is still able to suppress voiding. A detrusor contraction then is initiated voluntarily and the patient voids.

A female bladder normally experiences a first sensation of bladder filling at a volume of approximately 150 ml, a first urge to void at 200 to 300 ml, and a severe urge to void at 400 to 550 ml. During filling, an initial pressure rise between 2 and 8 cm H_2O usually occurs. The average pressure rise is approximately 6 cm H_2O and never exceeds 15 cm H_2O. Provocation of a normal bladder by rapid filling, change of posture, coughing or catheter movement should not incite any abnormal rises in detrusor pressure.

Despite the widespread use of cystometry, the optimal technique for performing the test is unknown. Controversy remains regarding type of cystometry, filling media, temperature of fluid, technique of bladder filling, rate of bladder filling, types of catheters, and indications for and technique of cystometry.

Cystometers

It is beyond the scope of this chapter to discuss all commercially available cystometers, but recent reviews by

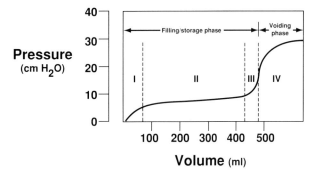

Fig. 6-1 Normal cystometrogram. Note filling phase is divided into an initial slight rise in bladder pressure (phase I), followed by a tonus limb reflecting bladder accommodation (phase II). At maximum capacity, the detrusor muscle and elastic bladder wall tissue are stretched to their limits causing a rise in bladder pressure (phase III). A detrusor contraction then is initiated voluntarily and the patient voids (phase IV). *(Modified from Wein AJ, Barrett DM:* Voiding function and dysfunction, *Chicago, 1988, Mosby–Year Book.)*

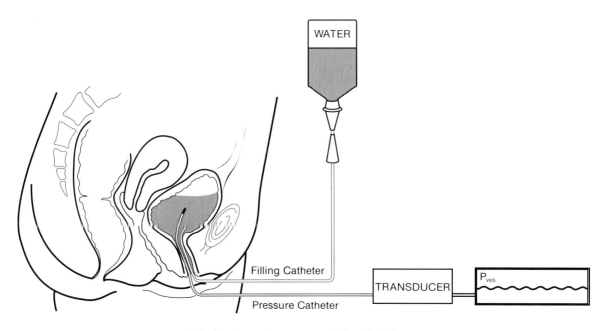

Fig. 6-2 Single-channel cystometry. (P_{ves}, Bladder pressure.)

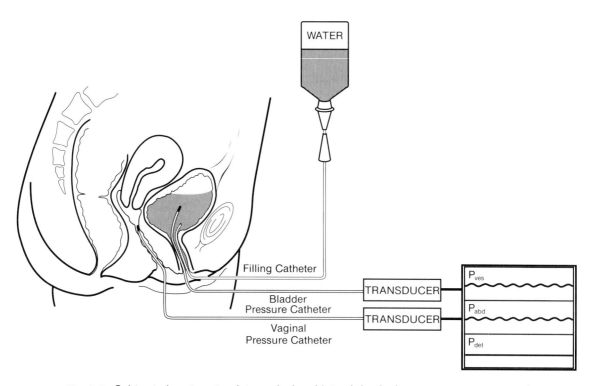

Fig. 6-3 Subtracted cystometry. Intravesical and intraabdominal pressures are measured and true detrusor pressure is electronically derived ($P_{ves} - P_{abd}$). (P_{ves}, Bladder pressure; P_{abd}, abdominal pressure; P_{det}, detrusor pressure.)

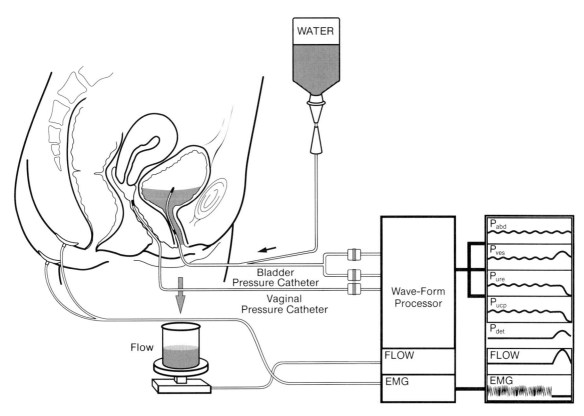

Fig. 6-4 Multichannel urodynamics. Intravesical, intraabdominal and intraurethral pressures are measured. True detrusor pressure (P_{det}) and urethral closure pressure (P_{ucp}) are electronically derived. EMG and flow studies are also performed. (P_{ves}, Bladder pressure; P_{abd}, abdominal pressure; P_{det}, detrusor pressure; P_{ure}, urethral pressure; P_{ucp}, urethral closure pressure; *EMG*, electromyography.)

Blavias and Rowan et al give current information. The simplest cystometer is a water manometer connected by a Y tube to both a reservoir and a catheter. A variation of this technique is discussed in Chapter 5.

Commercially available cystometers can be broadly classified into single-channel and multichannel machines (subtracted cystometry). Single-channel cystometry involves the placement into the bladder of a pressure-measuring catheter that produces an electronic signal, creating a graph on a recording device (Fig. 6-2). Multichannel cystometry relies on the measurement of both abdominal (P_{abd}) and intravesical pressures (P_{ves}), thereby making one able to distinguish changes in intraabdominal pressure from changes in intravesical pressure (Fig. 6-3). Abdom-

inal pressure can be measured via either transrectal or transvaginal catheters. We prefer vaginally placed catheters, as they are more comfortable, easier to clean and maintain, and measurements are not cluttered by rectal peristalsis. Electronic subtraction of intraabdominal from intravesical pressure allows for the calculation of true detrusor pressure (P_{det}).

Subtracted cystometry may be enhanced further by additional measurement of urethral pressure (P_{ure}). This measurement allows for the calculation of urethral closure pressure (P_{ucp}), which is the difference between urethral and bladder pressures. Certain machines also allow for the simultaneous measurement of electromyographic (EMG) activity and the performance of flow studies (Fig. 6-4).

Filling Media

The commonly used infusants for cystometry include water, carbon dioxide, and radiographic contrast material. In 1971, Merrill et al introduced the use of carbon dioxide, which has become popular in North America. It is particularly suitable for office studies because it is relatively clean, quick, and can be instilled at rates of up to 300 ml/min. Nevertheless, the following reservations about the use of gas during cystometry exist: it further decreases the physiologic nature of the test; (2) if gas is used, the bladder volume cannot be assessed because CO_2 is compressible; (3) CO_2 dissolves in urine to form carbonic acid, which irritates and reduces functional bladder capacity; (4) abdominal pressure is not usually measured during CO_2 cystometry making interpretation more difficult; and (5) when CO_2 is used for filling cystometry, it is impossible to perform a stress test or voiding studies. For these reasons, we believe that gas cystometry should be used only if water cystometry is unavailable.

Position of the Patient and Provoking Maneuvers

Cystometry should mimic everyday stresses on the bladder as much as possible. Thus it is preferable to perform the test with the patient in the sitting or standing position. During cystometry, the bladder should be provoked by a series of tests that usually include coughing, heel bouncing, walking in place, and listening to running water. These maneuvers may provoke uninhibited detrusor contractions or induce stress incontinence. If the patient continues to demonstrate a stable cystometrogram despite these maneuvers, yet is strongly suspected of having an overactive detrusor, she can be restudied 15 to 30 minutes after the subcutaneous injection of 2.5 mg of bethanechol chloride. This approach should not significantly alter the activity of a normal detrusor, but may unmask occult detrusor overactivity.

Physical factors may influence the positioning of patients during urodynamic tests, e.g., in elderly patients or those with neurologic disease, it may be difficult to undertake cystometry in any position other than supine.

Temperature of Fluid

Most laboratories use fluid at room temperature, although some investigators believe that the instillation of warm or cold fluid may provoke abnormal bladder activity. In addition, varying the temperature of the fluid may help evaluate for sensation abnormalities secondary to neurologic dysfunction.

Technique of Bladder Filling

Theoretically, the most physiologic method of filling is by diuresis, combined with a suprapubically placed pressure line. The long time needed to investigate the patient prohibits natural filling as a practical method of performing cystometry in most centers. Therefore, cystometry is usually performed through a transurethrally placed catheter. Filling is accomplished using either simple gravity or a water pump. The bladder is filled through either a small catheter or, preferably, a separate channel on the pressure-measuring catheter.

Rate of Bladder Filling

The ICS attempted to standardize filling rates by describing three ranges: slow fill is less than 10 ml/min, medium fill is 10 to 100 ml/min, and rapid or fast fill is greater than 100 ml/min. Patients with normal lower urinary tract function can tolerate most fast-fill rates. The effect of the filling rate on an unstable bladder is still poorly understood, but fast-fill methods may be more effective in provoking detrusor overactivity. For this reason, medium- or fast-fill techniques are more widely used.

Types of Catheters

A variety of catheters have been used for cystometry. Simple or manual cystometry can be performed with a transurethral Foley catheter. Electronically monitored studies require more sophisticated balloon or microtransducer catheters. Water-filled balloon catheters or water perfusion catheters have been used with moderate success. These catheters are inexpensive, disposable, and relatively easy to use. More sophisticated laboratories, however, usually use sensitive microtransducer catheters (Fig. 6-5). These catheters are available with one to six microtransducers on the catheter. They have small diameters, are flexible, and can measure rapid changes in pressure accurately during repetitive coughing or other provoking maneuvers. Disadvantages include their expense, their need to be replaced after approximately 100 studies, and their

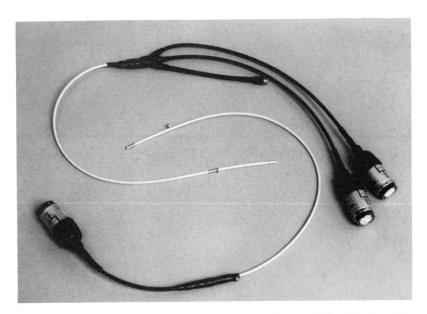

Fig. 6-5 Two microtransducer catheters. One catheter has a single microtransducer and is used for estimating abdominal pressure. The other catheter has two microtransducers approximately 6 cm apart used to measure intravesical and intraurethral pressure. This catheter also contains a fluid filling port.

tendency to produce rotational artifacts, as pressure readings may vary depending on the orientation of the transducer to the bladder or urethral wall.

Indications for and Technique of Cystometry

The indications for cystometry, as well as the various techniques used in performing the test, are somewhat controversial. Each patient must be evaluated individually. Based on clinical findings and planned treatments, the physician must decide if cystometry is indicated and, if it is, whether it should be performed via a simple office test or with more sophisticated electronic testing. In our opinion, an electronic single-channel study does not offer any more information than does a carefully performed nonelectronic test. We believe the only reason to perform electronic urodynamic testing is to measure pressures from several anatomic sites, thus obtaining subtracted pressures of importance.

Indications for single-channel cystometry versus subtracted or multichannel cystometry have been debated extensively; however, few comparisons exist in the literature. One study by Ouslander et al reported a sensitivity of 75% in geriatric patients undergoing simple supine cystometry when compared to multichannel testing. Sutherst and Brown compared single-channel and multichannel urodynamics in a blinded crossover study of 100 incontinent women. They noted single-channel studies to be 100% sensitive and 89% specific compared to multichannel studies. Multichannel cystometry may have a higher sensitivity for recognizing low pressure detrusor contractions, which have sometimes been termed "subthreshold detrusor instability." Multichannel techniques also improve the specificity of cystometry by avoiding false positive test results created by increases in abdominal pressure. Whether the cost of multichannel testing is justified for most patients remains to be proved. The accompanying box lists suggested indications for subtracted cystometry.

The technique of multichannel subtracted urethrocystometry used in our laboratory is as follows:

1. The patient presents with a symptomatically full bladder. She voids spontaneously in a uroflow

---

Indications for Multichannel Subtracted Cystometry
Complicated history Single-channel studies are inconclusive Stress incontinence before surgical correction Urge incontinence not responsive to therapy Recurrent urinary loss after previous surgery for stress incontinence Frequency, urgency, and pain syndromes not responsive to therapy Nocturnal enuresis not responsive to therapy Lower urinary tract dysfunction after pelvic radiation or radical pelvic surgery Neurologic disorders Continuous leakage

chair. A postvoid residual urine volume is obtained via a transurethral catheter. With the catheter in place, approximately 100 ml of sterile, room-temperature saline or water is placed into the bladder to facilitate placement of the microtransducer catheters and to decrease the amount of initial artifact secondary to the bladder wall collapsing around the microtip.

2. The microtransducer catheters are connected to the appropriate cables and to the tubing from the water pump. The machine is calibrated with the catheters in water and all channels are set at zero. A small amount of water is flushed through the tubing to remove any air.

3. With the patient in the supine position on a birthing or urodynamic chair, the abdominal catheter is placed into the vagina and taped to the inside of the leg. If the patient has severe vaginal prolapse or has undergone previous vaginal surgery resulting in a narrowed vagina, the catheter is placed into the rectum. A dual microtransducer catheter with a filling port is then placed into the bladder. The patient is moved to a sitting position and the catheter secured to a mechanical puller (if urethral pressure studies are anticipated) or to the inside of the leg, so

that the proximal transducer is near the mid-urethra (area of maximum urethral closure pressure).

4. After the catheters are appropriately placed, the subtraction is checked by asking the patient to cough. Cough-induced pressure spikes should be seen on the P_{ves}, P_{abd}, and P_{ure} channels, but not on the true detrusor pressure channel. If there is an inappropriate deflection on P_{det}, it is usually secondary to inaccurate placement of the vaginal (or rectal) catheter. If repositioning the catheter does not correct the problem, all connections and calibration techniques should be rechecked.

5. Bladder filling is begun. First sensation, initial urge to void, and maximum capacity are recorded. Throughout the filling portion of the examination, the patient is asked to perform provocative activities, such as coughing and straining. The external urethral meatus is constantly observed for any involuntary urine loss. Any abnormal rise in true detrusor pressure is noted. If the patient's symptoms are reproduced during filling, then the test can be completed in the sitting position. If they are not, the patient should be asked to stand and provocative maneuvers performed in an attempt to reproduce her symptoms.

6. At the completion of filling, urethral pressure and flow studies can be performed, if indicated. These tests are discussed in Chapters 7 and 8. Fig. 6-6 illustrates an example of normal urethrocystometric and voiding studies.

VIDEO-URODYNAMIC TESTING

Video-urodynamic studies of the lower urinary tract represent a combination of video-cystourethrography and standard urodynamic techniques. Video-urodynamics requires equipment for cystometry, plus an image intensifier and a videotape recorder. In addition, various interface modules are necessary, depending on the exact design of the system. A television camera positioned above the recorder with a mixing device projects the recording channels on a television monitor

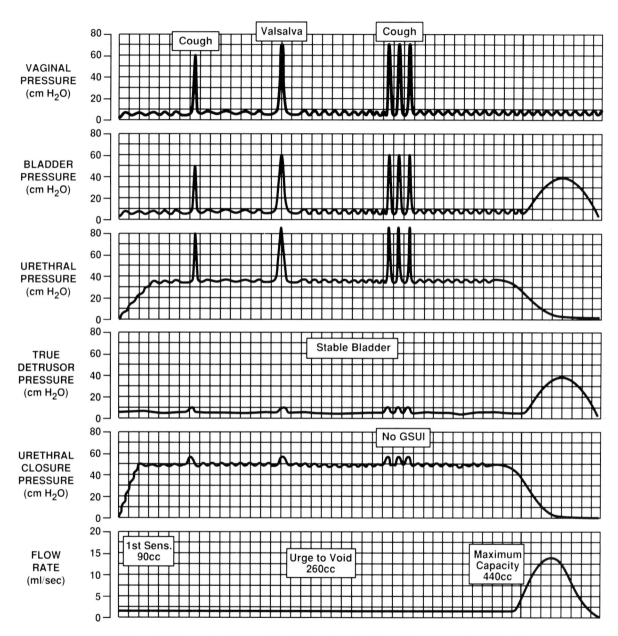

Fig. 6-6 Normal filling and voiding subtracted cystometry. Note that provocation in the form of coughing and straining does not provoke any abnormal rise in true detrusor pressure. At maximum capacity on command, a detrusor contraction is generated and voiding is initiated. (*GSUI*, Genuine stress urinary incontinence.)

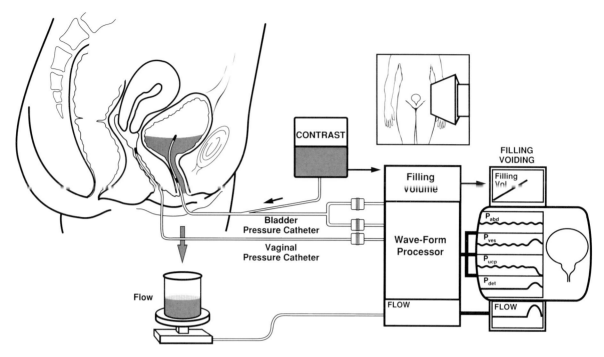

Fig. 6-7 Video-urodynamic testing. Multichannel urodynamic tests are performed under fluoroscopy, thus allowing simultaneous visualization of the lower urinary tract during recording of pressures. (P_{ves}, Bladder pressure; P_{abd}, abdominal pressure; P_{det}, detrusor pressure; P_{ucp}, urethral closure pressure.)

alongside the radiographic image of the bladder (Fig. 6-7). Radio-opaque filling medium is used for video-urodynamic studies. As with all other urodynamic studies, every effort must be made to limit the inhibitory effect of the additional machinery and personnel imposed on the patient.

Potential advantages of video-urodynamic studies include the consolidation of multiple evaluation modalities into one examination, thereby providing information about lower urinary tract anatomy and function under various provocative environments. Descent of the bladder neck, milk-back of urine from the urethra to the bladder, and bladder neck funneling all may be visualized during simultaneous recording and imaging of bladder, urethral, and abdominal pressures. Asymptomatic abnormalities such as urethral or bladder diverticula also may be noted. The major disadvantages of video-urodynamic testing are the ra-

diation exposure, cost, and technical expertise and support necessary for its use.

The indications for video-urodynamic studies are controversial. Some authorities believe that no additional information is obtained when these studies are compared to more conventional nonimaged multichannel studies; however, others believe that valuable additional information can be obtained from simultaneous imaging, especially in recurrent cases of incontinence or complicated neurologic conditions. The preoperative assessment of patients complaining of stress incontinence may be improved by video-urodynamic studies, particularly in patients who complain of stress incontinence, but this finding cannot be visualized objectively during clinical examination and standard urodynamic tests. In addition, visualizing bladder neck opening at rest and during straining may help differentiate anatomic from type III urethral incompetence.

AMBULATORY MONITORING

The largest deficiency of currently available urodynamic techniques is that laboratory observations may not always represent accurately physiologic behavior of the bladder and urethra. At times, the urodynamicist cannot reproduce the patient's symptoms in the laboratory setting. Theoretically, at these times ambulatory monitoring is indicated. Instruments for ambulatory monitoring have become commercially available only recently and are certain to become more popular in the future.

Continuous ambulatory monitoring studies often reveal a higher incidence of unstable bladder contractions than do standard cystometrograms. One study demonstrated detrusor instability in 16 of 21 patients by continuous ambulatory monitoring, whereas only 4 of 21 had been diagnosed using sitting cystometry. In another study, continuous ambulatory cystometric monitoring revealed detrusor contractions in 8 of 26 patients who had stable bladders at the time of initial urodynamic testing. Conversely, four patients were found to have normal ambulatory studies after having had previous unstable cystometrograms.

CYSTOMETRY: ABNORMAL STUDIES

Abnormalities of bladder filling are categorized into abnormal detrusor activity, compliance, sensation, and capacity. If urethral pressure is being measured simultaneously, the urethral response to filling and provocation can be elicited. For descriptive purposes, these abnormalities tend to be compartmentalized; however, no single urodynamic finding should be taken in isolation. Many patients have more than one cystometric abnormality (Fig. 6-8).

Any significant rise that occurs in true detrusor pressure during filling or provocation should be interpreted as abnormal detrusor activity or compliance. A pressure increase of 15 cm H_2O has been used previously by the ICS to differentiate between normal and abnormal. It has recently become apparent that this cut-off is too arbitrary and any pressure rise must be assessed in terms of the patient's symptoms. The most recent ICS recommendations have redefined detrusor overactivity to be any rise in true detrusor pressure that is felt not to be due to normal bladder compliance.

Although it is useful to categorize pressure changes during cystometry, the different patterns that occur are not mutually exclusive. Examples of the various cystometric findings in detrusor overactivity are shown in Fig. 6-9. Detrusor overactivity may present as phasic contractions that return to baseline after each contraction or as phasic contractions in which there is a gradual rise in pressure. A steady rise in true detrusor pressure is best termed a low-compliance bladder. When this type of pattern is noted, an organic reason for the poor bladder compliance, such as interstitial cystitis, should be ruled out. The clinical relevance of these various patterns is not fully understood. However, once intravesical pathology is ruled out, all of these abnormalities, regardless of the cause, are managed similarly with anticholinergic therapy and bladder retraining (see Chapter 19).

Sensory abnormalities are classified as either hypersensitive or hyposensitive. Hypersensitive bladder behavior is similar whether there is a definable cause, such as interstitial cystitis, or whether the cause is unknown. In these patients, catheterization is often painful. Volumes at first sensation of bladder filling, first desire to void, and maximum capacity are reduced. The condition of sensory urgency is present when the patient experiences a strong desire to void at abnormally low bladder volumes in the absence of any rise in true detrusor pressure (Fig. 6-10, *A*). Bladder overactivity may be associated with hypersensitivity from causes such as radiation therapy and interstitial cystitis. This condition may affect the results of treatment. Therapy may result in bladder stability; however, the symptoms of frequency and urgency may persist if the bladder remains hypersensitive.

Urodynamically, the hyposensitive bladder behaves similarly, whatever the cause. The bladder has a large capacity and a flat cystometrogram (Fig. 6-10, *B*). At maximum capacity, there may rarely be a rise in pressure as the limits of compliance are reached. This rise does not represent a detrusor contraction and there may be little or no sensation to filling up to this point. Weir and Jaques noted that 30% of patients with bladder capacities in excess of 800 ml were able to generate a normal detrusor contraction and void to completion on command. A hyposensitive, overdistended bladder, in itself, is not necessarily an indication of pathology.

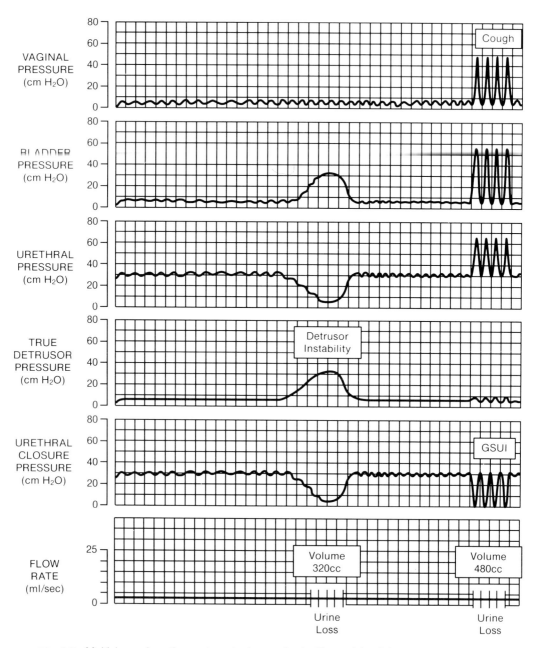

Fig. 6-8 Multichannel urethrocystometry in a patient with combined detrusor instability and genuine stress incontinence. (*GSUI*, Genuine stress urinary incontinence.)

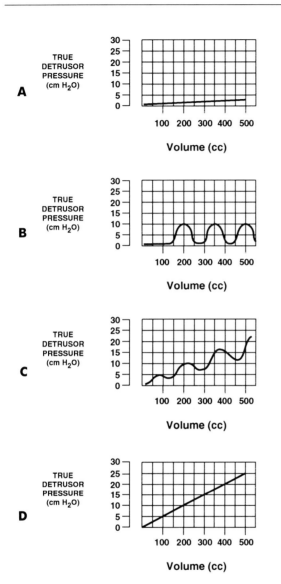

Fig. 6-9 Various detrusor responses to filling: **A**, normal filling cystometry; **B**, phasic contractions that return to baseline; **C** phasic contractions with gradual rise in true detrusor pressure; **D**, steady rise in true detrusor pressure (low-compliance bladder).

During cystometry, functional and cystometric bladder capacity should be differentiated. Maximum cystometric capacity is a somewhat subjective measure of the total volume of fluid the patient can tolerate comfortably during bladder filling. Functional bladder

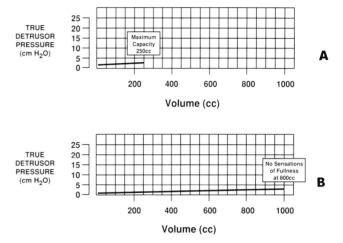

Fig. 6-10 A, Urodynamic diagnosis of sensory urgency. Patient experiences severe urgency at abnormally low bladder capacity in the absence of any significant rise in true detrusor pressure. **B**, Urodynamic diagnosis of hyposensitive bladder. Patient experiences no sensation of fullness at abnormally high bladder volume.

capacity is the amount of urine the bladder can hold under natural conditions. This amount can be checked easily by asking the patient to drink a large amount of water and hold it until she feels a maximum sensation to void. She then urinates and a postvoid residual urine volume is measured. The sum of the volumes of urine voided plus the residual urine provides the maximal functional bladder capacity. The artifacts of catheter insertion, the environment of cystometric examination, and the presence of medical personnel may change the patient's bladder capacity. Thus it is important to interpret bladder capacity data as derived from cystometry on a comparative basis with the patient's functional capacity as determined on frequency volume charts.

Both local and systemic conditions can result in abnormal bladder capacity. The accompanying box reviews the differential diagnosis of low-volume and high-volume bladder capacity.

When urethral pressure is measured simultaneously during filling cystometry, several abnormal urethral responses may be seen. The most common is an in-

---

Differential Diagnosis of Low-Volume and High-Volume Bladder

Low Volume

Detrusor instability (idiopathic)
Detrusor hyperreflexia (neurogenic)
Genuine stress incontinence
Hypersensitive bladder (sensory urgency)
Interstitial cystitis
Radiation cystitis or fibrosis
Bladder tumor
Urinary tract infection
Emotional factors

High Volume

Chronic outlet obstruction
Uterovaginal prolapse
Urethral stricture
Urethral tumor
Neuropathy
Diabetes mellitus
Hypothyroidism
Tabes dorsalis
Pernicious anemia
Lumbospinal disk disease
Previous radical pelvic surgery
Multiple sclerosis
Habitual infrequent voiding

---

competent urethral sphincter (Fig. 6-11). This finding is usually due to genuine stress incontinence; rarely it is due to uninhibited urethral relaxation. The term *urethral instability* has been used by some investigators to describe abnormal fluctuations in urethral pressure during filling. The clinical significance of this finding is controversial and is discussed in more detail in Chapter 8.

SUMMARY

Cystometry is the most important and most commonly performed urodynamic test. It assesses bladder filling and storage and is also important in evaluating bladder emptying, when used in conjunction with the other urodynamic and radiologic tests. Although clinically useful, its limitations should be recognized. Gynecologists should become familiar with cystometry so that they can perform and interpret basic office tests and work with urogynecologic or urologic consultants when more sophisticated tests are indicated.

BIBLIOGRAPHY

Abrams P, Blaivas JG, Stanton SL, et al: The standardization of terminology of lower urinary tract function, *Scand J Urol Nephrol* 114(suppl):5, 1988.

Arnold EP: Cystometry—postural effects in incontinent women, *Urol Int* 29:185, 1974.

Arnold EP, Webster JR, Loose H, et al: Urodynamics of female incontinence: factors influencing the results of surgery, *Am J Obstet Gynecol* 117:805, 1973.

Barnick CG, Cardozo LD, Benness C: Use of routine videocystourethrography in the evaluation of female lower urinary tract dysfunction, *Neurourol Urodyn* 8:447, 1989.

Bates CP, Whiteside CG, Turner-Warwick R: Synchronous cine/pressure/flow cystourethrography with special reference to stress and urge incontinence, *Br J Urol* 42:714, 1970.

Bates P, Bradley WE, Glen E, et al: First report on the standardization of terminology of the lower urinary tract function. Urinary incontinence. Procedures related to the evaluation of urine storage: cystometry, urethral closure pressure profile, units of measurement, *Br J Urol* 48:39, 1976; *Eur Urol* 2:274, 1976; *Scand J Urol Nephrol* 11:193, 1976; *Urol Int* 32:81, 1976.

Bhatia NN, Bradley WE, Haldeman S: Urodynamics: continuous monitoring, *J Urol* 128:963, 1982.

Bhatia NN, Bradley WE, Haldeman S, et al: Continuous ambulatory urodynamic monitoring, *Br J Urol* 54:357, 1982.

Blaivas JG: Machines for measuring urodynamics, *Contemp Obstet Gynecol* 35:99, 1990.

Blaivas JG: Multichannel urodynamic studies, *Urology* 23:421, 1984.

Bradley WE, Timm GW, Scott FB: Cystometry: III. Cystometers, *Urology* 5:843, 1975.

Bradley WE, Timm GW, Scott FB: Cystometry: V. Bladder sensation, *Urology* 6:654, 1975.

Bump RC: The urodynamic laboratory, *Obstet Gynecol Clin North Am* 16:795, 1989.

Cass AS, Ward BD, Markland C: Comparison of slow and rapid fill cystometry using liquid and air, *J Urol* 104:104, 1970.

Colstrup H, Andersen JT, Walter S: Detrusor reflex instability in male intravesical obstruction. Fact or artefact? *Neurourol Urodyn* 1:183, 1982.

Coolsaet BL, Blok C, Van Venrooij GE, et al: Subthreshold detrusor instability, *Neurourol Urodyn* 4:309, 1985.

DuBois P: Über den Druck in der Harnblase, *Arch Klin Med* 17:248, 1876.

Enhorning G: Simultaneous recording of intravesical and intraurethral pressure, Acta Chir Scand (Suppl) 276:1, 1961.

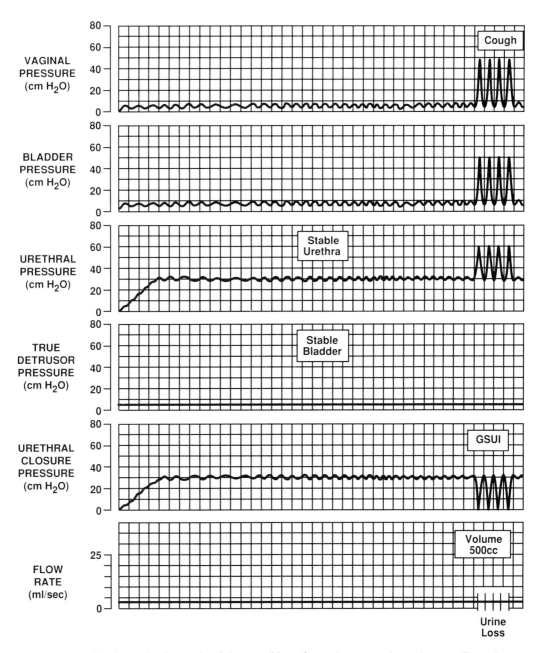

Fig. 6-11 Urodynamic diagnosis of the condition of genuine stress incontinence. There is visual loss of urine in the absence of any rise in true detrusor pressure with complete pressure equalization. (*GSUI*, Genuine stress urinary incontinence.)

Fossberg E, Beisland HO, Sauder S: Sensory urgency in females.Treatment with phenylpropanolamine, *Eur Urol* 7:157, 1981.

Gleason DM, Bottaccini MR, Reilly RJ: Comparison of cystometrograms and urethral profiles with gas and water media, *Urology* 9:155, 1977.

Jorgensen L, Lose G, Andersen JT: Cystometry: H_2O or CO_2 as filling medium? A literature survey of the influence of the filling medium on the qualitative and the quantitative cystometric parameters, *Neurourol Urodyn* 7:343, 1988.

Lapides J, Friend CR, Ajemian EP: Denervation supersensitivity as a test for neurogenic bladder, *Surg Gynecol Obstet* 114:141, 1962.

Lewis LG: A new clinical recording cystometer, *J Urol* 41:638, 1939.

Massey A, Abrams P: Urodynamics of the female lower urinary tract, *Urol Clin North Am* 12:231, 1985.

McCarthy TA: Validity of rectal pressure measurements as indication of intraabdominal pressure changes during urodynamic evaluation, *Urology* 20:657, 1982.

McGuire EJ, Savastano JA: Stress incontinence and detrusor instability/urge incontinence, *Neurourol Urodyn* 4:313, 1985.

Melzer M: The urecholine test, *J Urol* 108:729, 1972.

Merrill DC, Bradley WE, Markland C: Air cystometry. I. Technique and definition of terms, *J Urol* 106:678, 1971.

Merrill DC, Bradley WE, Markland C: Air cystometry. II. A clinical evaluation of normal adults, *J Urol* 108:85, 1972.

Merrill DC, Rotta JA: A clinical evaluation of detrusor denervation supersensitivity using air cystometry, *J Urol* 111:27, 1974.

Ouslander JG, Staskin D, Raz S, et al: Clinical versus urodynamic diagnosis in an incontinent geriatric female population, *J Urol* 137:68, 1987.

Penders L, De Leval J: Simultaneous urethrocystometry and hyperactive bladders: a manometric differential diagnosis, *Neurourol Urodyn* 4:89, 1985.

Rowan D, James ED, Kramer AE, et al: Urodynamic equipment: technical aspects. Produced by the International Continence Society Working Party on Urodynamic Equipment, J Med Eng Technol 1:57, 1987.

Sand PK, Bowen LW, Ostergard DR: Uninhibited urethral relaxation: an unusual cause of incontinence, *Obstet Gynecol* 68:645, 1986.

Sand PK, Hill RC, Ostergard DR: Supine urethroscopic and standing cystometry as screening methods for the detection of detrusor instability, *Obstet Gynecol* 70:57, 1987.

Sutherst JR, Brown MC: Comparison of single and multichannel cystometry in diagnosing bladder instability, *Br Med J* 288:1720, 1984.

Torrens M, Abrams P: Cystometry: symposium on clinical urodynamics, *Urol Clin North Am* 6:71, 1979.

Wein AJ, Barrett DM: Voiding function and dysfunction, Chicago, 1988, Mosby–Year Book.

Weir J, Jacques PF: Large-capacity bladder: a urodynamic survey, *Urology* 4:544, 1974.

CHAPTER 7

Urodynamics: Voiding Studies

Mickey M. Karram

Uroflowmetry
    Flow curve patterns
    Residual urine measurement
    Factors influencing uroflow parameters
    Clinical usefulness of uroflowmetry
Pressure-flow Studies
    Interpretation of pressure-flow studies
    Clinical usefulness of pressure-flow studies
Combined Studies
Summary

The process of normal micturition depends on a multitude of complex factors that must be coordinated to facilitate bladder emptying. Voiding consists of a combination of bladder contraction and outlet relaxation so that emptying is rapid and complete. The neurophysiologic mechanisms involved in the process of micturition are complex and have been discussed elsewhere. Disturbances in any of the connections within the voiding mechanism have the potential to produce abnormal micturition.

Various urodynamic techniques have been devised to study voiding. Uroflowmetry is the simplest and most commonly used of these investigations. Drake described one of the first clinically useful urinary flow meters in 1948. By using a kymograph that was attached to a receptacle for the voided urine and by rotating the kymograph at a known speed, a tracing of voided urine volume against time was obtained.

Drake was the first to record average flow rates in men and noted that flow rates significantly increased with increasing volumes. Von Garrelts, in 1956, described the first of the electronic urine flow meters, which consisted of a tall urine collecting cylinder with a pressure transducer in the base. The pressure transducer measured the pressure exerted by an increase in the column of urine as the patient voided. Because of the direct relationship between the volume voided and the pressure recorded, von Garrelts was able to produce electronically a direct recording of urine flow rate.

UROFLOWMETRY

Uroflowmetry, the measure of urine volume voided over time, is simple and noninvasive. It is performed by asking the patient to void in a special commode. Urine is funnelled into a flow meter that records volume versus time (Fig. 7-1). It is important to get a representative flow pattern; this pattern depends on a number of factors. First, the patient should understand the simple nature of the test and be as relaxed as possible to have a normal desire to void at the time of the study. Second, the patient should be allowed to void in private because tension and embarrassment can artificially reduce the maximum flow achieved. Third, if there is doubt about the accuracy of the test, it is important to ask the patient whether he or she felt it was representative. If the patient believed that the test was not typical, it should be repeated.

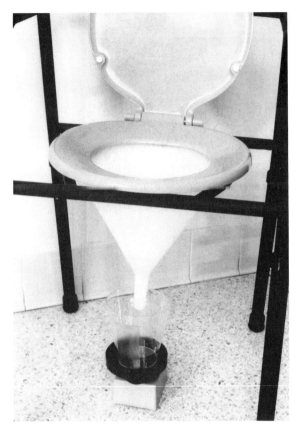

Fig. 7-1 Special commode and flowmeter used for spontaneous uroflowmetry.

The following parameters can be obtained from a uroflowmetric evaluation: (1) flow rate (Q), which is the volume of urine passed in milliliters per second; (2) maximum flow rate (Q_{max}); (3) total flow time (Q_{time}); (4) total volume voided; (5) average flow rate (Q_{ave}); and (6) postvoid residual urine volume. It is currently not known what represents normal values for these parameters. Drach et al observed that the mean maximum flow rate in asymptomatic women was 26 ± 14 ml/sec with an average voided volume of 224 ml. Flow time, maximum flow rate, and average flow rate all increase with corresponding increases in volume voided. Flow rates are higher in women than in men and in pregnant versus nonpregnant women. Little variation in flow rates with menstrual cycles, menopause, or increasing age has been reported.

Most experts would agree that one can consider a study normal if the patient voids at least 200 ml over 15 to 20 seconds and it is recorded as a smooth single curve with a maximum flow rate greater than 20 ml/sec (Fig. 7-2). Maximum flow rates of less than 15 ml/sec with a voided volume of greater than 200 ml are generally considered abnormal. However, because flow rate is determined by the relationship between detrusor force and urethral resistance, and because these factors may vary considerably and still produce adequate bladder emptying, a precise definition of a

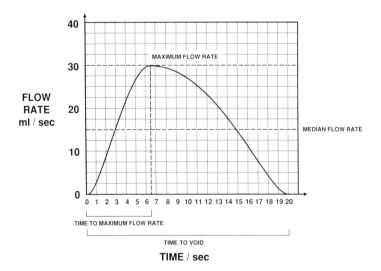

Fig. 7-2 Graphic representation of normal uroflow curve.

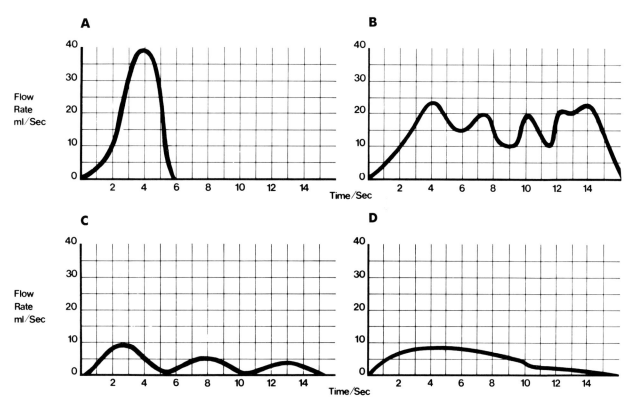

Fig. 7-3 Graphic representation of various uroflow patterns. **A,** Superflow commonly seen with poor urethral resistance. **B,** Intermittent multiple peak pattern. **C,** Intermittent interrupted pattern. **D,** Abnormal flow rate characteristic of detrusor outlet obstruction. *(From Karram MM: Urodynamics. In Benson JT (ed): Female pelvic floor disorders: investigation and management, New York, 1992, Norton Medical Books.)*

normal or a low flow rate cannot be made. In general, depending on the clinical situation, borderline low flow rates require further urodynamic testing.

Flow Curve Patterns

Curve patterns refer to the configuration of the uroflowmetric curve. Continuous flow showing a rapidly increasing flow rate reaching the maximum within one third of the total voiding time is usually considered normal (Fig. 7-2).

Flow is considered intermittent when the flow rate drops and subsequently increases (Fig. 7-3, *B* and *C*). Intermittent flow rates are described as "multiple peak" patterns when there is a downward deflection of the flow rate, which does not reach 2 ml/sec (Fig. 7-3, *B*). If the downward deflection of the flow rate reaches 2 ml/sec or less, it is termed "interrupted"

pattern (Fig. 7-3, *C*). Uroflowmetric parameters can be obtained from multiple peak patterns by reconstructing the curve as shown in Fig. 7-4. The peak flow rate is determined by the highest horizontal segment that has a duration of at least 1 second. The peak flow rate then is connected to an ascending and descending limb. Deflections from the reconstructed curve are analyzed individually. Uroflowmetric parameters on curves with interrupted flow patterns are usually not estimated.

Obstructed voiding patterns are much less common in women than in men and usually produce a low, flat tracing (Fig. 7-3, *D*). Abnormal flow tracings due to detrusor underactivity with abdominal straining or to intermittent urethral sphincter activity are characterized by slow changes in flow rate producing a wave-like tracing. Each rise or fall in flow rate represents

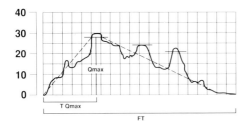

Fig. 7-4 Uroflowmetric curve with multiple peak pattern. Q_{max}, Maximum flow rate; TQ_{max}, time to maximum flow rate; *FT*, flow time. *(Adapted from Fantl AJ, Smith PJ, Schneider V, et al: Am J Obstet Gynecol 145:1017, 1983.)*

either a contraction of the abdominal and diaphragmatic muscles or a contraction of the external striated sphincter (Fig. 7-3, *B* and *C*).

A patient that voids very quickly can produce what has been termed a *super-flow* pattern in which there is very little outlet resistance. This pattern can be seen in patients with severe stress incontinence (Fig. 7-3, *A*).

Residual Urine Measurement

Residual urine is the volume of urine remaining in the bladder immediately after the completion of micturition. It is most accurately measured via a transurethral catheter, but also can be estimated by radiographic studies or ultrasound examination. A consistently high residual urine volume generally indicates increased outlet resistance, decreased bladder contractility, or both. Absent postvoid residual urine is compatible with normal urinary tract function, but also can exist in the presence of significant filling/storage disorders (incontinence) or with disorders of emptying in which the intravesical pressure is sufficient to overcome increased outlet resistance.

What constitutes an abnormally high residual urine volume is not universally established. Previous investigators empirically have chosen volumes of 50 or 100 ml to indicate normal residual urine volumes. It is best, however, to state the residual urine volume only in the context of the total voided volume. Normality should be described as a percentage of the total voided volume. We believe that most asymptomatic

women should void spontaneously at least 80% of their total intravesical volume.

Factors Influencing Uroflow Parameters

Abnormal uroflowmetric parameters can occur secondary to factors that affect detrusor contractility, urethral resistance, or both.

Detrusor contractility can be affected by neuropathic lesions, pharmacologic manipulation, instrinsic detrusor muscle or bladder wall dysfunction, or psychogenic inhibition.

Urethral resistance can be altered by tissue trophic changes producing atrophy or fibrosis, drug effects such as alpha-adrenergic stimulators, neuropathic striated muscle contraction, pain or fear, and urethral axis distortion secondary to severe pelvic relaxation. Outlet obstruction secondary to an intraurethral lesion or stricture is exceedingly rare in women. Extraurethral lesions, such as vaginal masses or cysts, and large enterocele or rectocele may compress the urethra resulting in obstructed voiding.

Detrusor-external sphincter dyssynergia is a condition in which there is lack of coordination between the detrusor muscle and the external striated sphincter. This leads to obstructed voiding and is always secondary to a neurologic lesion, most classically, high spinal cord trauma.

Clinical Usefulness of Uroflowmetry

Flow studies are much less useful in women than in men. Over half of cases of lower urinary tract dysfunction in men are related to outflow obstruction, whereas only about 4% of cases of lower urinary tract dysfunction in women are related to voiding problems. Nevertheless, uroflowmetry is a simple urodynamic investigation that is useful as a preliminary screening test to distinguish those patients who need more extensive studies from those who do not. It is also an integral part of the full urodynamic studies performed for more complex problems. Some clinical situations in which spontaneous uroflowmetry may be useful are briefly discussed here.

1. Symptoms suggestive of voiding dysfunction—If uroflow measures are normal in patients complaining of symptoms consistent with voiding difficulty, further investigation is unnecessary.

Abnormal flow rates would require further urodynamic testing.

2. Frequency/urgency syndromes—It is often necessary to find the urodynamic abnormality responsible for the symptom complex of frequency, nocturia, urgency, and urge incontinence. Flow studies are only preliminary to cystometry in this situation. Flow studies also can be used to evaluate treatment response. One study by Bergman et al on patients with urethral syndrome noted a significant improvement in uroflow parameters after urethral dilation in patients who were subjectively improved, whereas no significant change was observed in patients who remained symptomatic.

3. Before pelvic surgery—Stanton et al have shown that symptoms are an unreliable guide to the presence of voiding difficulty. They recommend that women undergoing pelvic surgery, particularly suprapubic procedures for incontinence and radical pelvic surgery, and those who are elderly, have neurologic disease, or have had past pelvic surgery should have uroflowmetry performed. On the other hand, Bhatia and Bergman (1986) noted that neither abnormal peak flow rates (defined as less than 20 ml/sec during uroflowmetry with voided volumes greater than 200 ml) nor high postvoid residual urine volumes were predictive of prolonged postoperative voiding difficulties in patients undergoing surgery for stress incontinence.

4. Neurologic disease—When neurologic disease affects the lower urinary tract, various degrees of voiding dysfunction can result. Uroflowmetry is preliminary to more detailed urodynamic tests and at times can be helpful in the diagnosis, management, and prognosis of these patients.

PRESSURE-FLOW STUDIES

A normal flow rate in women does not necessarily indicate a normal voiding mechanism. For example, some women have normal flow rates in the absence of detrusor contraction because sphincteric relaxation is assisted by increased intraabdominal pressure from straining. To define voiding mechanisms and objectively establish the basis of a patient's voiding dysfunction, pressure-flow studies can be performed.

These studies are usually performed after a cystometric evaluation. At maximum cystometric capacity in the sitting position, the patient is asked to void with an intravesical pressure catheter in place (Fig. 7-5). An intravaginal or intrarectal catheter records intraabdominal pressure to assess whether the patient uses a Valsalva maneuver to void and to electronically derive true detrusor pressure. Thus these studies involve the monitoring of abdominal, intravesical, and true detrusor pressure synchronously with flow. External sphincter electromyographic (EMG) activity, as well as urethral pressure, also may be measured. Once flow is initiated, the patient is asked to suddenly interrupt her stream (stop test). This test establishes voluntary control of micturition and also obtains isometric detrusor pressure.

The specific parameters in ICS-recommended terms are shown in Fig. 7-6. Several attempts have been made to integrate the parameters of pressure-flow studies into a single model. These models, however, do not take into account urethral shape, distensibility, or voided volume and thus await clinical verification.

Interpretation of Pressure-Flow Studies

Pressure-flow studies are invasive because the patient is asked to void around catheters, sometimes with electromyographic needles in place. Some normal patients will be unable to void secondary to psychogenic inhibition. In addition, instrumented urinary flow may be completely different from the flow the patient is able to generate without instrumentation. Thus, noninvasive spontaneous uroflowmetry should always be performed initially for purposes of comparison.

During the voiding phase, the detrusor muscle may be normal, acontractile, or underactive. Normal voiding is usually achieved by a voluntarily initiated detrusor contraction that is sustained and can be suppressed. An underactive detrusor during micturition implies that the detrusor contraction is of inadequate magnitude or duration (or both) to effect bladder emptying within a normal time span. Detrusor areflexia is

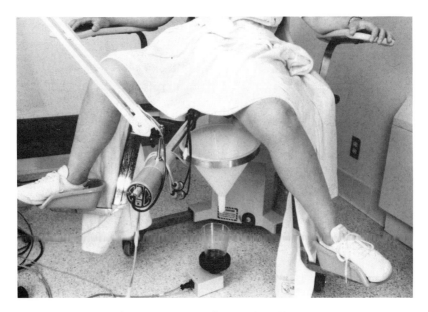

Fig. 7-5 Technique for performing pressure-flow studies. The patient must be able to void around the catheters.

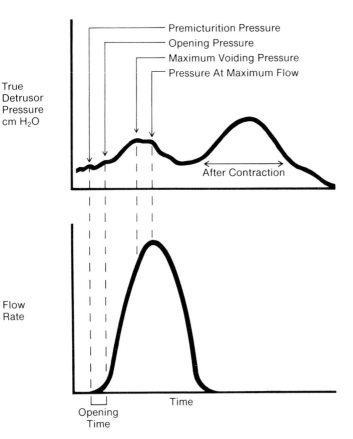

Fig. 7-6 International Continence Society terminology and specific parameters for pressure-flow studies. *(From Karram MM: Urodynamics. In Benson JT (ed): Female pelvic floor disorders: investigation and management, New York, 1992, Norton Medical Books.)*

TABLE 7-1   Potential voiding mechanisms on pressure/flow studies in neurologically intact women

Urethral relaxation	Bladder contraction	Abdominal straining
Present	Absent	Absent
Present	Present	Absent
Present	Absent	Present
Present	Present	Present

defined as acontractility due to an abnormality of nervous control and denotes the complete absence of a centrally coordinated contraction.

During voiding urethral function may be normal or obstructed. Obstruction may be due to urethral overactivity, as in detrusor-external sphincter dyssynergia, or mechanical obstruction, such as with a urethral stricture or tumor.

Depending on age, menopausal status, total voided volume, and the presence or absence of lower urinary tract dysfunction, women void by any combination of a detrusor contraction, abdominal straining, and urethral relaxation (Table 7-1, Figs. 7-7 and 7-8).

Although pressure-flow studies are an established and accepted urodynamic modality, what constitutes a normal voiding mechanism is incompletely understood as is the normal range for detrusor pressure during voiding in women. Most of the previously published literature has been derived from male subjects in which pressures are abnormally high secondary to more frequent outflow obstruction.

As previously mentioned, to better evaluate the detrusor during voiding, one may perform a "stop flow" test (Fig. 7-9). In many patients, if voiding is suddenly interrupted by sphincter action, the detrusor pressure rapidly rises. This behavior reflects a fundamental myogenic property of the contracting detrusor—a trade-off between the pressure generated and the flow delivered. The detrusor pressure attained on stopping (isometric detrusor pressure) should be a more reliable measure of detrusor contractions than the detrusor pressure during voiding, which also depends on flow rate and urethral resistance.

The routine clinical use of the "stop test" has some

disadvantages. A high isometric detrusor pressure implies a good detrusor contraction, but a low or absent rise in pressure does not necessarily imply lack of a detrusor contraction. The detrusor contraction may be reflexly inhibited when the urethra is closed, or flow may be interrupted by inhibiting the detrusor instead of increasing outlet resistance. In addition, the patient may be unable to completely interrupt her stream on command. These situations can lead to a falsely low isometric detrusor pressure. For these reasons, the test is probably more accurate when the urethra is physically occluded with a catheter or by elevation of the anterior vaginal wall.

Clinical Usefulness of Pressure-Flow Studies

The main clinical use of pressure-flow studies is to document the mechanism of abnormal voiding. If a patient has symptoms and signs of abnormal voiding, has low flow rates, and voids with a high detrusor pressure, she is probably voiding against an obstruction. On the other hand, if a patient has low flow rates and voids with minimal or no rise in detrusor pressure, then her voiding dysfunction is probably secondary to an acontractile or underactive detrusor (Fig. 7-10). The limiting factor is that there is no clear cutoff between normal and abnormally high detrusor pressure during voiding.

The clinical setting in which pressure-flow studies are most useful in gynecologic practice is in the patient who has undergone pelvic surgery or bladder neck surgery and has developed postoperative voiding dysfunction. The dysfunction may be secondary to denervation, resulting in an underactive or acontractile detrusor, or the dysfunction may be secondary to increased outlet resistance produced from the surgery. If pressure-flow studies show normal or increased detrusor pressure, then therapy such as urethral dilation can be directed toward decreasing outlet resistance. If the patient voids with no detrusor pressure, then one can assume that the outlet is normal and therapy is directed toward increasing detrusor contractility.

Bhatia and Bergman (1984) performed pressure-flow studies on 30 patients with stress incontinence before retropubic urethropexy. They noted that no patient who voided with a detrusor contraction of greater

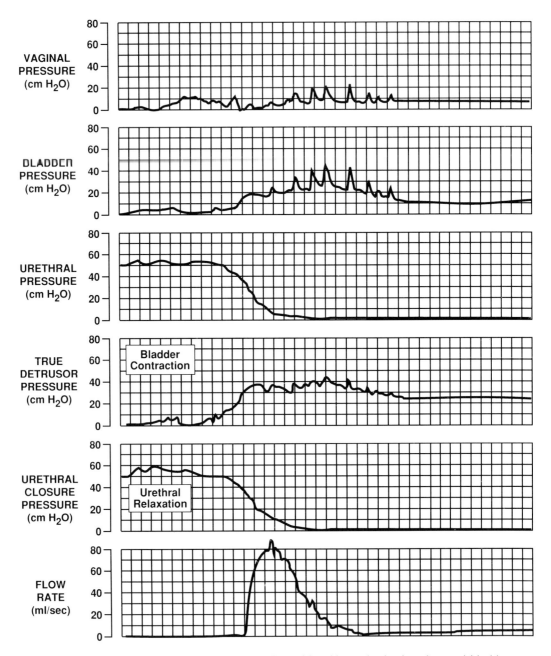

Fig. 7-7 Pressure-flow study in a patient who voids with urethral relaxation and bladder contraction. Note minimal Valsalva effort.

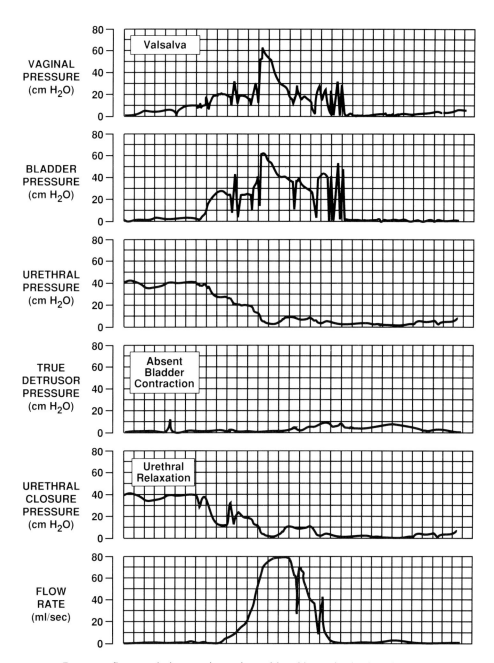

Fig. 7-8 Pressure-flow study in a patient who voids with urethral relaxation and Valsalva maneuver. Note absent bladder contraction.

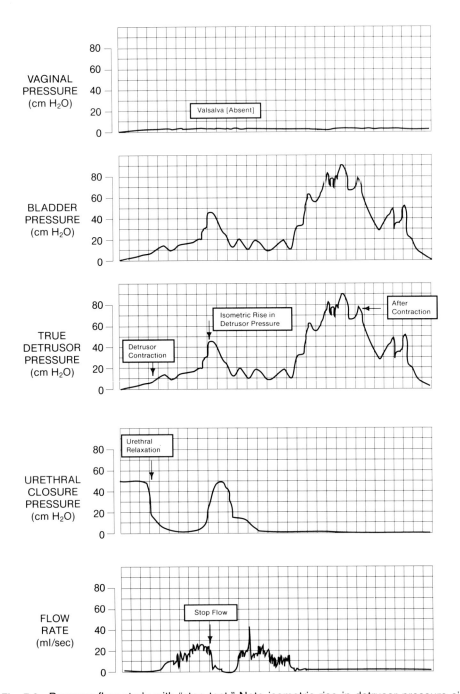

Fig. 7-9 Pressure-flow study with "stop test." Note isometric rise in detrusor pressure simultaneous with stoppage of flow.

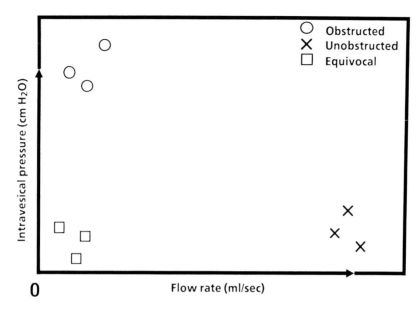

Fig. 7-10 Recommended presentation of pressure-flow relationships for normal and abnormal voiding. *(From Walters MD:* Obstet Gynecol Clin North Am *16:773, 1989.)*

than 15 cm H$_2$O preoperatively required prolonged bladder drainage (greater than 7 days). Eighty-four percent of patients who used significant abdominal straining in addition to urethral relaxation during voiding required prolonged postoperative catheterization. Thus these studies may be useful prognostically to predict postoperative voiding difficulty in patients undergoing antiincontinence surgery.

COMBINED STUDIES

Pressure-flow studies performed under fluoroscopy can be a useful diagnostic urodynamic procedure. The size of the bladder and the presence of trabeculations, bladder diverticula, and vesicoureteral reflux can be visualized. Competence of the sphincter can be assessed and the patient's ability to initiate and stop micturition can be observed. The site of significant outflow obstruction usually can also be detected. The technique of these studies is discussed in Chapter 6.

When neurogenic voiding dysfunction is present or suspected, EMG activity of the external striated sphincter should be recorded. These studies are discussed in Chapter 9.

SUMMARY

Any condition that affects detrusor contractility and/or urethral resistance can impair micturition. Uroflowmetry is a simple noninvasive test that can be used to objectively document voiding dysfunction. Because it does not provide direct information on expulsive forces or outlet resistance, it is probably best considered a screening test.

Pressure-flow studies provide information on detrusor and abdominal pressure. They are helpful in differentiating voiding dysfunction secondary to obstruction from that secondary to an underactive detrusor. They also may give useful information to predict postoperative voiding dysfunction after urethropexy. These tests, however, are invasive and unpredictable; 20% to 30% of patients are not able to void around the catheters and artifacts are difficult to assess. More research is needed to define normal voiding parameters and to determine the value of these tests in clinical practice.

BIBLIOGRAPHY

Abrams P: Uroflowmetry. In Stanton SL (ed): *Clinical gynecologic urology,* St Louis, Mosby–Year Book, 1984.

Abrams P, Blaivas JG, Stanton SL, et al: Sixth report on the standardization of terminology of lower urinary tract function. Procedures related to neurophysiological investigations: electromyography, nerve conduction studies, reflex latencies, evoked potentials and sensory testing, *World J Urol* 4:2, 1986; *Scand J Urol Nephrol* 20:161, 1986.

Abrams P, Torrens M: Urine flow studies, *Urol Clin North Am* 6:71, 1979.

Backman KA: Urinary flow during micturition in normal women, *Acta Chir Scand* 130:357, 1965.

Barnick CG, Cardozo LD, Benness C: Use of routine videocystourethrography in the evaluation of female lower urinary tract dysfunction, *Neurourol Urodyn* 8:447, 1989.

Bates P, Bradley WE, Glen E, et al: Fourth report on the standardization of terminology of lower urinary tract function. Terminology related to neuromuscular dysfunction of lower urinary tract, *Br J Urol* 52:333, 1981; *Urology* 17:618, 1981; *Scand J Urol Nephrol* 15:169, 1981; *Acta Urol Jpn* 27:1568, 1981.

Bergman A, Bhatia NN: Uroflowmetry for predicting postoperative voiding difficulties in women with stress urinary incontinence, *Br J Obstet Gynaecol* 92:835, 1985.

Bergman A, Bhatia NN: Uroflowmetry: spontaneous versus instrumented, *Am J Obstet Gynecol* 150:788, 1984.

Bergman A, Karram M, Bhatia N: Urethral syndrome: a comparison of different treatment modalities, *J Reprod Med* 34:157, 1989.

Bhatia NN, Bergman A: Urodynamic predictability of voiding following incontinence surgery, *Obstet Gynecol* 63:85, 1984.

Bhatia NN, Bergman A: Use of preoperative uroflowmetry and simultaneous urethrocystometry for predicting risk of prolonged postoperative bladder drainage, *Urology* 28:440, 1986.

Bradley WE: Urologically oriented neurological examination. In Ostergard DR, ed: *Gynecologic urology and urodynamics,* ed 2, Baltimore, 1985, Williams & Wilkins.

Drach GW, Ignatoff J, Layton T: Peak urinary flow rate: observations in female subjects and comparison to male subjects, *J Urol* 122:215, 1979.

Drake WM: The uroflowmeter: an aid to the study of lower urinary tract. *J Urol* 59:650, 1948.

Enhorning G: Simultaneous recording of intravesical and intraurethral pressure, *Acta Chir Scand* 276 (suppl):4, 1961.

Fantl AJ: Clinical uroflowmetry. In Ostergard DR, ed: *Gynecologic urology and urodynamics,* ed 2, Baltimore, 1985, Williams & Wilkins.

Fantl AJ, Smith PJ, Schneider V, et al: Fluid weight uroflowmetry in women, *Am J Obstet Gynecol* 145:1017, 1983.

Griffiths DJ: Uses and limitations of mechanical analogies in urodynamics, *Urol Clin North Am* 6:143, 1979.

Karl C, Gerlach R, Hannappel J, et al: Uroflow measurements: their information yield in a long-term investigation of pre- and postoperative measurements, *Urol Int* 41:270, 1986.

Massey A, Abrams P: Urodynamics of the female lower urinary tract, *Urol Clin North Am* 12:231, 1985.

Meunier P: Study of micturition parameters in healthy young adults using a uroflowmetric method, *Eur J Clin Inv* 13:25, 1983.

Muellner SR: The physiology of micturition, *J Urol* 65:805, 1951.

Mundy AP: Clinical physiology of the bladder, urethra and pelvic floor. In Mundy AP, Stephenson TP, Wein AJ, (eds): *Urodynamics: principles, practice and applications,* New York, 1984, Churchill Livingstone.

Stanton SL, Ozsoy C, Hilton P: Voiding difficulties in the female: prevalence, clinical and urodynamic review, *Obstet Gynecol* 61:144, 1983.

Susset JG, Brissot RB, Regnier CH: The stop-flow technique: a way to measure detrusor strength, *J Urol* 127:489, 1982.

Susset JG, Picker P, Kretz M, et al: Critical evaluation of uroflowmeters and analysis of normal curves, *J Urol* 109:874, 1983.

Tanagho EA: Urodynamics: uroflowmetry and female voiding patterns. In Ostergard DR, ed: *Gynecologic urology and urodynamics,* ed 2, Baltimore, 1985, Williams & Wilkins.

Tanagho EA, McCurrey E: Pressure and flow rate as related to lumen caliber and entrance configuration, *J Urol* 105:583, 1971.

Tanagho EA, Miller ER: Initiation of voiding, *Br J Urol* 42:175, 1970.

Tanagho EA, Miller ER, Meyers, FH, et al: Observations on the dynamics of the bladder neck, *Br J Urol* 38:72, 1966.

von Garrelts B: Analysis of micturition: a new method of recording the voiding of the bladder, *Acta Chir Scand* 112:326, 1956.

von Garrelts B, Strandell P: Continuous recording of urinary flowrate, *Scand J Urol Nephrol* 6:224, 1972.

Walter S, Olesen KP, Nordling J, et al: Bladder function in urologically normal middle aged females, *Scand J Urol Nephrol* 13:249, 1979.

Walters MD: Mechanisms of continence and voiding, with International Continence Society classification of dysfunction, *Obstet Gynecol Clin North Am* 16:773, 1989.

Yalla SV, Blunt KJ, Fam BA, et al: Detrusor-urethral sphincter dyssynergia, *J Urol* 118:1026, 1977.

CHAPTER 8

Urodynamics: Urethral Pressure Profilometry

Mickey M. Karram

Methodology
    History
    Catheter types
    Technique of urethral pressure profilometry
Interpretation
Clinical Applications of Urethral Pressure
Measurements
    Genuine stress incontinence
    Urethral instability
    Suburethral diverticula
Summary

Urinary continence depends on the pressure in the urethra exceeding the pressure in the bladder at all times, even with increases in intraabdominal pressure. Attempts to evaluate and quantify the urethra's role in lower urinary tract dysfunction have led to the development and use of urethral pressure studies. Urethral pressure profilometry is a graphic representation of pressure within the urethra at successive points along its length. Contributing to normal urethral compliance and pressure are smooth and striated urethral muscles; fibroelastic tissue of the urethral wall; vascular tension due to the rich, spongy network around the urethra; and extrinsic compression from surrounding pelvic floor musculature.

METHODOLOGY

History

A report of the first attempt to measure urethral pressure was published in 1923 by Victor Bonney who used the technique of retrograde sphincterometry. This method was replaced by a balloon catheter in 1936. Karlson introduced the technique of simultaneous measurement of intraurethral and intravesical pressure (urethrocystometry). This was refined by Tanagho et al and by Enhorning et al who used membrane catheters. In 1969, the fluid profusion method was described and popularized by Brown and Wickman. More recent technology has introduced the use of microtransducer catheters. With these catheters, sensitive receptors are placed inside the urethral lumen, thus allowing for the assessment of urethral response during stress, such as coughing and straining.

Catheter Types

Currently the most commonly used techniques for the measurement of urethral pressure involve balloon or membrane catheters, perfusion techniques, or microtransducers.

Balloon Catheters

Balloon catheters use a cylindrical balloon mounted concentrically on a catheter. It is inflated with fluid to just above atmospheric pressure and inserted into the urethra. A true hydrostatic pressure is obtained, which approximates that of the fluid-filled urethra. As the balloon is pulled through the urethra, a pressure profile is obtained. Unfortunately, over short distances along the urethra, there are significant pressure variations and the balloon technique averages these pressure variations. Therefore, the profile obtained can at times be distorted. The system has a rise time of about 40 msec and, therefore, is probably not able to give an accurate indication of urethral response to physiologic stresses. Despite these shortcomings, several workers have attempted to use the technique for stress profiles. Other disadvantages of this method are difficulties in construction of the catheters and in calibration of the equipment. It is also difficult to free the system of air bubbles.

Perfusion Techniques

The perfusion technique involves the use of a one- or two-channel catheter with side holes through which saline or gas is perfused with a motorized syringe pump. The pressure registered by the transducer represents the resistance to outflow from the catheter side hole. Urethral pressure profiles measured by gas perfusion techniques are subject to considerable variation during repetitive testing. In addition, because carbon dioxide can be infused at rates up to 300 ml/min, marked changes in intravesical volume occur while the urethral pressure profile is performed. Because bladder distention normally increases urethral pressure, results are more difficult to interpret. For these reasons, most investigators prefer saline to CO_2 as the infusing medium.

Microtransducers

Microtransducers are currently the most widely used catheters for urethral pressure studies in the United States. These catheters have two microtransducers mounted 6 cm apart. The distal transducer remains in the bladder and measures bladder pressure while the more proximal catheter is manually or mechanically withdrawn through the urethra. The major advantage of the microtransducer system over other techniques is its high frequency response time. Frequency response has been calculated at over 2000 Hz, which allow the system to record any physiologic event, in

particular, the pressure changes involved in the voiding cycle, rapid cough sequences, and pelvic floor contractions. This technique also has been shown to be more reproducible than other techniques; the fine caliber of the catheters limits errors caused by urethral distention. The disadvantages of these catheters are that they are fragile and expensive.

Microtransducer catheters have been developed with as many as six microtransducers to measure urethral pressure. These catheters simultaneously measure pressures at multiple points along the urethra. Unfortunately, the cost and rigidity of these catheters increase in proportion to the number of microtransducers. Currently these catheters should be considered only as research tools.

Technique of Urethral Pressure Profilometry

Certain other factors must be taken into consideration to assure the reproducibility of urethral pressure studies. Bladder volume should be standardized because urethral pressure increases with increasing bladder volume. The position of the patient is also important: Measurements in the supine position are not the same as those in an upright position. When performing cough urethral pressure profiles, Schick showed that pressure transmission ratios decrease as the strength of cough increases; therefore, reproducibility requires comparable strength of coughs during dynamic urethral pressure profiles.

Orientation of the microtransducer within the urethral lumen also must be taken into account. The pressure is highest when the transducer is placed anteriorly and the lowest when it is placed posteriorly. Most investigators prefer to place the transducer in the lateral position to provide a more standardized measurement.

Another point of consideration relates to the biophysics of the test. Urethral pressure is measured by inserting a transducer, mounted on a catheter, into a normally coapted lumen. In reality, what is being measured is the force exerted by the walls of the urethra on the transducer. If the urethra were a tube with a circular lumen, the occlusive forces would be equal around its circumference; but because the urethra is a collapsed tube with the anterior and posterior walls in opposition, the occlusive forces are unequally dis-

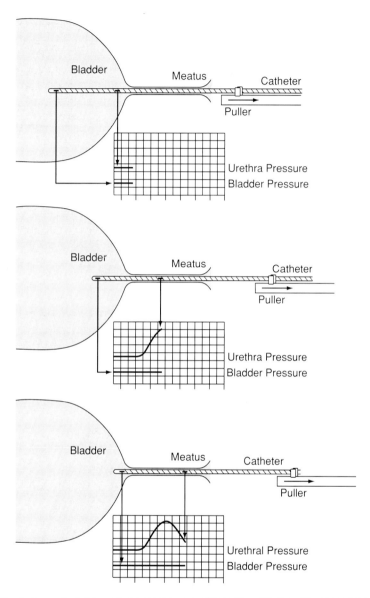

Fig. 8-1 Technique of static urethral pressure profilometry with simultaneous measurement of bladder pressure. Study begins with both microtransducers in the bladder *(top)*. As the catheter is mechanically withdrawn through the urethra *(middle and bottom)*, urethral and bladder pressures are recorded.

tributed around the urethra. In addition, the pressure measurement has been shown to depend on the size and stiffness of the catheter, as well as on the form of the pressure sensor.

In 1983, Hilton and Stanton suggested a standard technique for performing urethral pressure profiles, which has been adopted by many centers. We use a similar technique (Fig. 8-1).

1. With the patient in sitting position at maximum cystometric capacity (usually after filling cystometry), the catheter is secured to a mechanical puller and connected to a polygraph recorder.

2. With both microtransducer sensors in the bladder, the catheter is mechanically withdrawn so that the orientation of the transducer is directed laterally at the 9 o'clock position.

3. As the proximal transducer passes through the urethra, the resting (static) urethral pressure is recorded on graph paper that is moving at the same speed as the catheter. Urethral closure pressure (urethral pressure minus vesical pressure) is recorded on a separate channel. The proximal sensor is then mechanically reinserted into the bladder and a second resting pressure profile is obtained to ensure consistency of results.

4. The same procedure is repeated with the patient coughing repeatedly while the catheter is withdrawn through the urethra, thus obtaining a dynamic or cough urethral pressure profile. The patient should cough at a consistent intensity every 2 to 3 seconds, which corresponds approximately to every 2 to 3 mm of urethral length. It is important that the recorder be set so that the entire amplitude of each cough spike in the bladder and urethra remains on the chart paper. The external urethral meatus is visualized for any involuntary loss of urine.

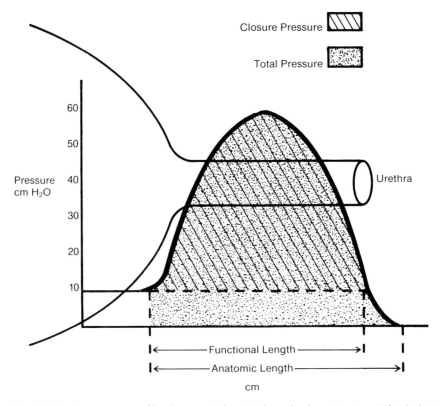

Fig. 8-2 Urethral pressure profile demonstrating total urethral pressure, urethral closure pressure, and anatomic and functional urethral length. *(From Karram MM: Urodynamics. In Benson JT (ed): Female pelvic floor disorders: investigation and management, New York, 1992, Norton Medical Books.)*

INTERPRETATION

Standardized nomenclature for urethral pressure profilometry has been recommended by the International Continence Society (ICS). The most frequently measured parameters are (1) maximum urethral pressure (MUP); (2) maximum urethral closure pressure (MUCP), which is the difference between MUP and bladder pressure; and (3) functional urethral length (FUL), which is the length of the urethra along which urethral pressure exceeds bladder pressure (Fig. 8-2). Other parameters, such as anatomic or total urethral length and area underneath the profile, can also be calculated.

Simultaneous measurement of urethral and vesical pressures during coughing allows calculation of the relative amounts of abdominal pressure transmitted to each structure. This *pressure transmission ratio* can be used to quantitate urethral closure during stress. It is calculated by dividing the cough-induced urethral pressure increase by the bladder pressure increase, then multiplying by 100 $[(\Delta P_{urethra}/\Delta P_{vesical}) \times 100]$ (Fig. 8-3).

In continent women, increased intraabdominal pressure generated by coughing or lifting increases intraurethral pressure roughly equal to the rise in bladder pressure. The simultaneous pressure rises tend to offset each other, allowing closure pressure (and continence) to be maintained. In women with weakness of the urethral sphincteric mechanism, unequal pressure transmission causes a rapid cough-related drop in urethral closure pressure, which sometimes leads to stress incontinence (Figs. 8-4 and 8-5). It is not known whether deficient pressure transmission is due to urethral hypermobility, abnormal reflex periurethral muscle contraction, or other undefined factors.

Normal values of urethral pressure measurements vary slightly among different techniques, and tend to be higher with microtransducers. Urethral closure pressure shows a downward trend with age. Rud noted a mean urethral closure pressure of 90 cm H_2O in women less than 25 years old and a mean pressure of 65 cm H_2O in women older than 64 years. Average functional urethral length was 2.4 to 2.8 cm and increased up to 50 years of age, with a decline thereafter. Menopause was associated with a significant shortening of functional urethral length. There is no variation in any parameter during the menstrual cycle.

A normal urethral pressure profile is usually symmetric. It is not uncommon to see vascular pulsations at the peak of the profile as blood pressure accounts for a significant portion of urethral closure pressure. Rarely, a twin-peak urethral pressure profile can be seen, which may be associated with previous bladder neck surgery or urethral diverticulum.

CLINICAL APPLICATIONS OF URETHRAL PRESSURE MEASUREMENTS

The clinical application of urethral pressure studies currently is controversial. Some investigators believe that urethral pressure profiles are diagnostically helpful in certain conditions; others believe that they should be considered only as a research tool. The following section discusses various clinical situations in which urethral pressure measurements may be clinically useful.

Genuine Stress Incontinence

The potential clinical applications of urethral pressure studies in relation to genuine stress incontinence are twofold: they may be helpful in making the diagnosis of the condition of genuine stress incontinence and in choosing the appropriate surgical therapy for genuine stress incontinence.

Diagnosis

Over the years, many investigators have attempted to use urethral pressure studies to explain the pathogenesis of urinary incontinence and to diagnose urethral sphincteric incontinence. In general, total loss of urethral closure pressure and urine loss coexisting with intraabdominal pressure elevations, but without a detrusor pressure increase, confirm the diagnosis of genuine stress incontinence. However, the lack of consistent associations of urethral pressure profile variables with diagnosis confirmed by video-urodynamics have limited its acceptance. Versi examined 24 urethral pressure variables and used kappa statistical analysis to determine which variables were the most discriminatory. Although there was a statistically significant difference in maximal urethral closure pressure between patients with genuine stress incon-

Abdominal Pressure

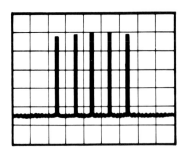

Vesical Pressure

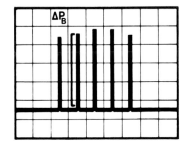

ΔP_B

Urethral Pressure

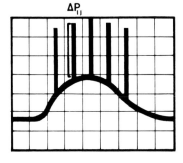

ΔP_U

ΔP_B = Intravesical Pressure

ΔP_U = Urethral Pressure

$$\frac{\Delta P_U}{\Delta P_B} \times 100 = PTR\,(\%)$$

PTR = Pressure Transmission Ratio

Urethral Closure Pressure

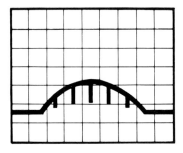

True Detrusor Pressure

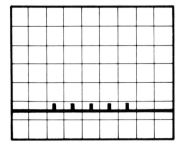

Fig. 8-3 Method of calculation of pressure transmission ratio during cough pressure profile. *(From Karram MM: Urodynamics. In Benson JT (ed): Female pelvic floor disorders: investigation and management,* New York, 1992, *Norton Medical Books.)*

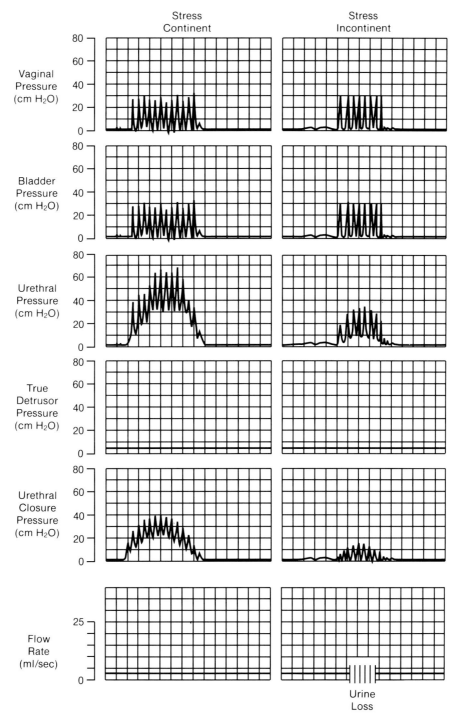

Fig. 8-4 Dynamic (cough) pressure profile in continent patient *(left)* (note good pressure transmission) and in incontinent patient *(right)* (note poor pressure transmission).

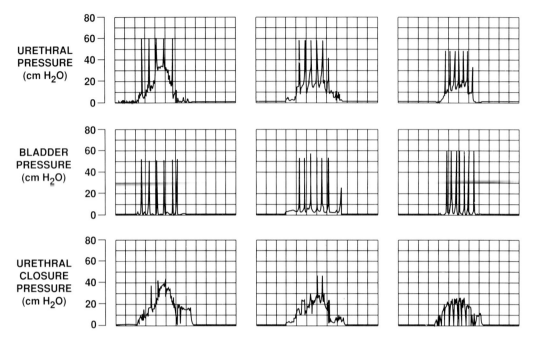

Fig. 8-5 Dynamic (cough) pressure profile showing negative profile *(left)* as closure pressure is augmented; equivocal profile *(middle)* as closure pressure is decreased but does not reach zero; and positive profile *(right)* as closure pressure reaches zero. *(Modified from Fantl AJ, Hurt WG, Bump RC, et al: Am J Obstet Gynecol 155:554, 1986.)*

tinence and continent women, there was a large overlap between the two groups. The area under the stress urethral pressure profile was the most discriminatory; however, the overlap was too great to allow this variable to be used diagnostically to differentiate women with competent versus incompetent sphincteric mechanisms. Versi concluded that no single parameter within a urethral pressure study could be used to diagnose genuine stress incontinence.

Bump et al performed pressure transmission ratios in 110 subjects and noted that women with genuine stress incontinence had significantly lower mean pressure transmission ratios when compared with continent women. The finding of a pressure transmission ratio less than 90% in the proximal half of the urethra had a sensitivity of 97%, a specificity of 56%, an abnormal predictive value of 53%, and a normal predictive value of 97% in a population of incontinent women with a genuine stress incontinence prevalence rate of 34%. Pressure transmission ratios less than

90% were more sensitive for diagnosing genuine stress incontinence and had higher predictive values than urethral closure pressures less than 50 cm H_2O or maximum straining angles of greater than 30 degrees on a cotton swab test.

More recently, Rosenzweig et al performed pressure transmission ratios on 63 patients before and after Burch colposuspensions. They observed no difference in preoperative pressure transmission ratios between urethral pressure profiles associated with and without leakage of urine. They could not determine a threshold pressure transmission ratio that was associated with urine loss. However, they did note that the higher the postoperative pressure transmission ratio, the more likely surgical success.

Choice of Surgery

Another potential use of urethral pressure profiles in patients with genuine stress incontinence is in the preoperative evaluation of those undergoing incontinence surgery. McGuire et al reported on urodynamic findings following unsuccessful incontinence surgery and found that a urethral closure pressure less than 20 cm H_2O was present in 75% of patients who had undergone multiple failed operations. More recently, Sand et al reported on 86 women undergoing Burch colposuspension and noted that the failure rate was three times higher in patients with preoperative urethral closure pressures less than 20 cm H_2O compared with those who had urethral closure pressures greater than 20 cm H_2O. Other studies have noted the failure rate with various stress incontinence surgeries to be higher in patients with low urethral closure pressures. Some of these studies have used a cutoff point of 20 cm H_2O; in other studies no cutoff point was stated. Based on this data some investigators feel that patients with genuine stress incontinence and a low urethral closure pressure should undergo an incontinence procedure aimed at obstructing the urethra (such as a sling procedure) because simple elevation and stabilization of the bladder neck may not improve sphincteric function adequately and thus lead to an unacceptable failure rate. To date, the subject of low urethral pressure as a risk factor for failure of standard incontinence procedures is controversial and awaits a randomized, prospective study to further evaluate its significance.

Evaluation Before Physiotherapy for Stress Incontinence

Physiotherapy is a successful method to treat certain patients with genuine stress incontinence. Objective success rates for this type of therapy range from 20% to 85%. Despite the widespread advocacy of pelvic muscle exercises for this condition, few data address which subgroup of patients benefit the most. In a recent study by Tapp et al, 45 women with a diagnosis of genuine stress incontinence based on video-urodynamic studies underwent a 3-month trial of pelvic muscle exercises. They noted that the group most likely to benefit from this therapy were premenopausal and had a shorter duration of symptoms, a lower visual analog score for symptoms of stress incontinence, and better urethral function during stress. When analysis was performed to determine predictor variables, women with pretreatment stress functional urethral lengths of greater than 5 mm and stress mean urethral pressures greater than 9.4 cm H_2O had greatly en-

hanced success rates. If urethral pressure profile studies could be used to predict which patients would benefit from physiotherapy, the treatment would become more effective.

Urethral Instability

When measurements of urethral pressure are performed during filling cystometry, it is not uncommon to note fluctuations in urethral pressure. Normally, fluctuations can be synchronous with the heart beat due to normal urethral vascular pulsation. Abnormal pressure fluctuations can be caused by urethral instability (uninhibited urethral relaxation associated with incontinence) or by unstable urethral pressures (large fluctuations in urethral pressure, without incontinence). Finally, artifactual pressure fluctuations due to urethral catheter movement are common and should not be confused with the preceding conditions.

Urethral instability or uninhibited urethral relaxation is the involuntary loss of urethral closure pressure, resulting in incontinence, without any rise in detrusor pressure (Figs. 8-6 and 8-7). Although this condition is well documented, it is a rare cause of urinary incontinence and its management is currently controversial. It has been argued by some that urethral instability is actually a form of detrusor instability in which urethral pressure loss occurs, but the detrusor contraction is not perceived because the urethra is open and a urethrovesical equilibrium exists.

Urethral instability should not be confused with large fluctuations in urethral pressures (variations in maximum urethral pressure during filling cystometry that exceed 10, 15, 20, or even 25 cm H_2O, depending on the definition) (Fig. 8-7). Large fluctuations in urethral pressures have been noted by some authors as being abnormal; however, the actual definition of normal and abnormal is controversial. Using outlier analysis, Versi and Cardozo demonstrated that the statistical cutoff point of normal fluctuation in urethral pressure should be 25 cm H_2O. They argued, however, that rather than have an absolute cutoff, it might be more appropriate to examine the ratio of fluctuations in relation to the resting mean urethral pressure. They concluded that any fluctuation greater than 33% of the resting mean urethral closure pressure should be regarded as abnormal. This idea was later supported by Hilton.

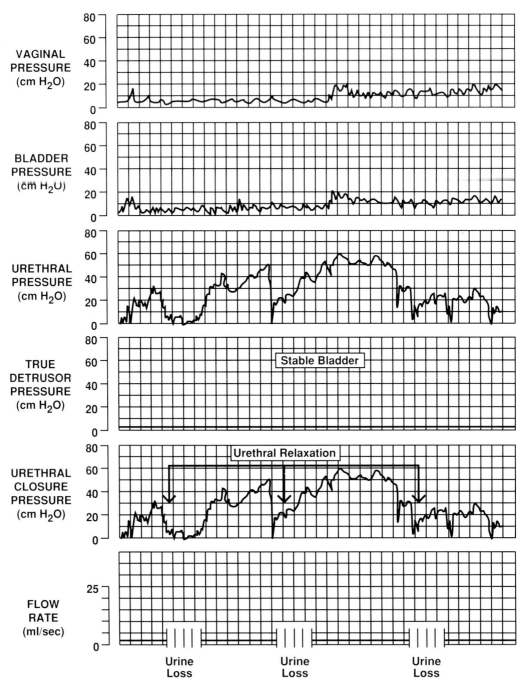

Fig. 8-6 Multichannel urodynamic tracing of a patient with urethral instability (uninhibited urethral relaxation). Note bladder pressure remains stable and there is visual loss of urine, simultaneous with drop in urethral pressure.

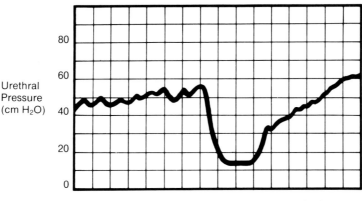

Urethral Instability (Uninhibited Urethral Relaxation)

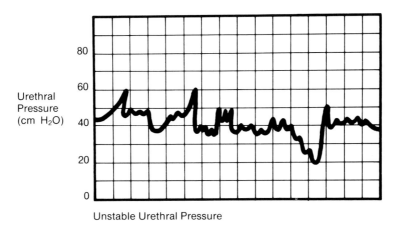

Unstable Urethral Pressure

Fig. 8-7 Graphic representation to show difference between urethral instability (uninhibited urethral relaxation) and unstable urethral pressure. *(From Karram MM: Urodynamics. In Benson JT (ed):* Female pelvic floor disorders: investigation and management, *New York, 1992, Norton Medical Books.)*

More recently, however, Tapp et al found no difference in clinical symptoms when comparing women with significant versus nonsignificant variations in mean urethral closure pressure. This analysis was carried out for absolute cutoff points and also for the ratio of change in mean urethral pressure to resting mean urethral pressure. Other investigators have used 15 and 20 cm H_2O as arbitrary levels to define abnormal. It becomes apparent that the actual significant level of fluctuation in mean urethral pressure, as well

as the overall clinical relevance of this entity, is subject to much debate.

Suburethral Diverticula

Although suburethral diverticula are best diagnosed by radiologic techniques, a few studies have suggested using urethral pressure profilometry in the management of this condition. The typical urethral pressure profile in patients with suburethral diverticulum shows a loss of urethral pressure at the level of the diverticular ostium. Bhatia et al recommended that if the diverticulum is proximal to the maximum urethral pressure, the operation of choice is diverticulectomy; however, if it is distal to this point, marsupialization (Spence procedure) is indicated.

SUMMARY

Numerous research advances have been made with the use of urethral pressure studies, thus improving understanding of lower urinary tract function and dysfunction. The routine use of these studies, however, remains controversial, and more data are needed to substantiate their clinical value and cost-effectiveness.

BIBLIOGRAPHY

Abrams P, Blaivas JG, Stanton SL, et al: The standardization of terminology of lower tract function, *Scand J Urol Nephrol* 114(suppl):5, 1988.

Asmussen M, Ulmsten U: Simultaneous urethrocystometry and urethral pressure profile measurement with a new technique, *Acta Obstet Gynecol Scand* 54:385, 1975.

Asmussen M, Ulmsten U: The role of urethral pressure profile measurement in female patients with urethral carcinoma, *Ann Chir Gynecol* 71:122, 1982.

Baker KR, Drutz HP: Retropubic colpourethropexy: clinical and urodynamic evaluation in 289 cases, *Int Urogynecol J* 2:196, 1991.

Bhatia NN, McCarthy TA, Ostergard DR: Urethral pressure profiles of women with diverticula, *Obstet Gynecol* 58:375, 1981.

Blaivas JG, Olsson CA: Stress incontinence: classification and surgical approach, *J Urol* 139:727, 1988.

Bonney V: On diurnal incontinence of urine in women, *J Obstet Gynaecol Br Emp* 30:358, 1923.

Bowen LW, Sand PK, Ostergard DR: Unsuccessful Burch retropubic urethropexy: a case controlled urodynamic study, *Am J Obstet Gynecol* 160:452, 1989.

Brown M, Wickham JEA: The urethral pressure profile, *Br J Urol* 41:211, 1969.

Bump RC, Copeland WE, Hurt WG, et al: Dynamic urethral pressure profilometry pressure transmission ratio determinations in stress-incontinent and stress-continent subjects, *Am J Obstet Gynecol* 159:749, 1988.

Bump RC, Fantl JA, Hurt WG: Dynamic urethral pressure profilometry pressure transmission ratio determinations after continence surgery: understanding the mechanism of success, failure, and complications, *Obstet Gynecol* 72:870, 1988.

Edwards L, Malvern J: The urethral pressure profile: theoretical considerations and clinical application, *Br J Urol* 46:325, 1974.

Enhorning G, Miller ER, Hinman F: Urethral closure studies with cine roentgenography and bladder urethral recording, *Surg Gynecol Obstet* 118:507, 1964.

Fantl AJ, Hurt WG, Bump RC, et al: Urethral axis and sphincteric function, *Am J Obstet Gynecol* 155:554, 1986.

Farghaly SA, Shah J, Worth P: The value of transmission-pressure ratio in the assessment of female stress incontinence, *Arch Gynecol (Suppl)* 237:366 (abst 14.42.01), 1985

Ghoneim MA, Gottembourg JL, Freton J, et al: Urethral pressure profile. Standardization of technique and study of reproducibility, *Urology* 5:632, 1975.

Hilton P: Unstable urethral pressure: toward a more relevant definition, *Neurourol Urodyn* 6:411, 1988.

Hilton P, Stanton SL: A clinical and urodynamic evaluation of the Burch colposuspension for genuine stress incontinence, *Br J Obstet Gynaecol* 90:934, 1983.

Horbach NS, Blanco JS, Ostergard DR, et al: A suburethral sling procedure with polytetrafluorethylene for the treatment of genuine stress incontinence in patients with low urethral closure pressure, *Obstet Gynecol* 71:648, 1988.

Karlson S: Experimental studies in functioning of the female urinary bladder and urethra, *Acta Obstet Gynecol Scand* 32:285, 1953.

Kauppila A, Penttinen J, Häggman V: Six-microtransducer catheter connected to computer in evaluation of urethral closure function of women, *Urology* 33:159, 1989.

Koonings PP, Bergman A, Ballard CA: Low urethral pressure and stress urinary incontinence in women: risk factor for failed retropubic surgical procedure, *Urology* 36:245, 1990.

Kujansuu E: The effect of pelvic floor exercises on urethral function in female stress urinary incontinence, an urodynamic study, *Ann Chir Gynecol* 72:28, 1982.

Kulseng-Hanssen S: Prevalence and pattern of unstable urethral pressure in one hundred seventy-four gynecologic patients referred for urodynamic investigation, *Am J Obstet Gynecol* 146:895, 1983.

McGuire EJ: Urodynamics findings in patients after failure of stress incontinence operations, *Prog Clin Biol Res* 78:351, 1981.

McGuire EJ, Lytton B, Pepe V, et al: Stress urinary incontinence. *Obstet Gynecol* 47:255, 1976.

Millar HD, Baker LE: Stable ultraminiature catheter-tip pressure transducer, *Med Biol Eng* 11:86, 1973.

Plevnik S: Model of the proximal urethra; measurement of the urethral stress profile, *Urol Int* 31:23, 1976.

Richardson DA: Value of the cough pressure profile in the evaluation of patients with stress incontinence, *Am J Obstet Gynecol* 155:808, 1986.

Rosenzweig BA, Bhatia NN, Nelson AL: Dynamic urethral pressure profilometry pressure transmission ratio: what do the numbers really mean? *Obstet Gynecol* 77:586, 1991.

Rud T: Urethral pressure profile in continent women from childhood to old age, *Acta Obstet Gynecol Scand* 59:331, 1980.

Sand PK, Bowen LW, Ostergard DR: Uninhibited urethral relaxation: an unusual cause of incontinence, *Obstet Gynecol* 68:645, 1986.

Sand PK, Bowen LW, Panganiban R, et al: The low pressure urethra as a factor in failed retropubic urethropexy, *Obstet Gynecol* 69:399, 1987.

Schick E: Objective assessment of resistance of female urethra to stress, *Urology* 26:518, 1985.

Tanagho EA, Meyers FH, Smith DR: Urethral resistance: its components and implications, *Invest Urol* 7:135, 1969.

Tapp AJS, Cardozo L, Hills B, et al: Who benefits from physiotherapy? *Neurourol Urodyn* 7:259, 1988.

Tapp AJS, Cardozo L, Versi E, et al: The prevalence of variation of resting urethral pressure in women and its association with lower urinary tract function, *Br J Urol* 61:314, 1988.

Tapp AJS, Hills B, Cardozo L: Randomized study comparing pelvic floor physiotherapy with the Burch colposuspension, *Neurourol Urodyn* 8:356, 1989.

Toews H: Intraurethral and intravesical pressure in normal and stress incontinent women, *Obstet Gynecol* 29:6137, 1967.

Ulmsten U, Hendriksson L, Iosif S: The unstable female urethra, *Am J Obstet Gynecol* 144:93, 1982.

Versi E: Discriminant analysis of urethral pressure profilometry data for the diagnosis of genuine stress incontinence, *Br J Obstet Gynaecol* 97:251, 1990.

Versi E, Cardozo L: Urethral instability: diagnosis based on variations of the maximum urethral pressure in normal climacteric women, *Neurourol Urodyn* 5:535, 1986.

Versi E, Cardozo L, Brincat M, et al: Correlation of urethral physiology and skin collagen in postmenopausal women, *Br J Obstet Gynaecol* 95:147, 1988.

Versi E, Cardozo L, Studd J: Distal urethral compensatory mechanisms in women with an incompetent bladder neck who remain continent, and the effect of the menopause, *Neurourol Urodyn* 9:579, 1990.

Ward GH, Hosker GL: The anisotropic nature of urethral occlusive forces, *Br J Obstet Gynaecol* 92:1279, 1985.

Weil A, Reyes H, Bischoff P, et al: Modification of urethral rest and stress profiles after different types of surgery for urinary stress incontinence, *Br J Obstet Gynaecol* 91:46, 1984.

CHAPTER 9

Electrophysiologic Testing

J. Thomas Benson

Electrophysiologic Studies
    Electromyography
    Conduction studies
    Evoked response
    Reflex response and sensory study
    "Supersensitivity" testing
Clinical Conditions
    Cortical lesions
    Suprasacral cord areas
    Sacral cord area
    Caudal equina
    Pelvic plexus injury
    Distal pudendal neuropathy

In the patient presenting with urinary incontinence or a voiding disturbance, it is important to consider the possible neurologic etiologies that may be associated with the symptoms. When the history and physical and urodynamic findings suggest the possibility of nervous system impairment, the adjunctive use of electrophysiologic testing is useful (1) to determine if neuropathy is a significant component of the patient's problem and (2) if it is, to localize the area of the central, peripheral, or autonomic nervous system chiefly affected. Thus the older patient with urge incontinence and headaches, the younger patient with incontinence and difficulty voiding, the patient with low back pain and overflow incontinence, and the patient with stress urinary and anal incontinence may

have the respective underlying disorders of brain tumor, multiple sclerosis, intervertebral disk disease, and pudendal neuropathy diagnosed and treated appropriately.

This chapter describes pelvic floor electrodiagnostic techniques including surface and needle electromyography (EMG), nerve conduction and terminal latency studies, evoked potentials, and reflex response studies. The clinical, urodynamic, and electrophysiologic findings to be expected with neuropathy in various areas, from the cerebral cortex to the peripheral pelvic floor nerves, are also described.

Because of the widespread technical advances and great increase in the amount of information about human neurourology, concepts are continually undergoing modification and change. This presentation will concentrate on the present aspects of clinically useful knowledge, although modification of many of the concepts will soon be required.

ELECTROPHYSIOLOGIC STUDIES

Electrical activity is produced by intracellular and intercellular neuronal activity. Within the nerve cell and its processes are semipermeable, lipoprotein, bi-layered membranes with irregular distributions of ions on either side. This ionic distribution leads to a difference in "resting" electrical potential across the membrane (inside negative, outside positive). An impulse can be transmitted (action potential), causing change in these potentials with a resultant ionic current flow that can be recorded electrically.

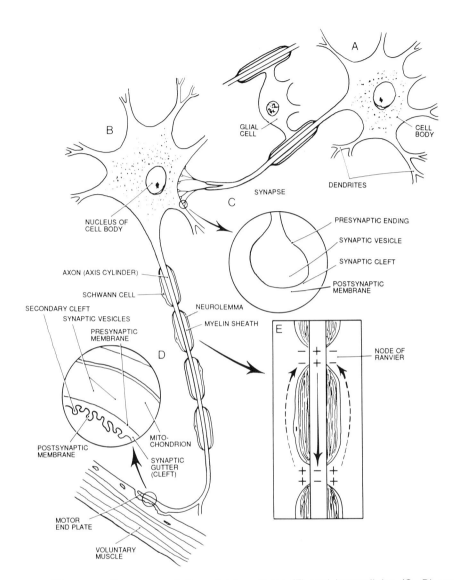

Fig. 9-1 Diagrammatic representation of intracellular *(E)* and intercellular *(C, D)* nerve conduction. *(From Manter JT:* Essentials of clinical neuroanatomy and neurophysiology, *ed 7, Philadelphia, 1987; FA Davis.)*

Many nerve cell axons have a myelin sheath, capacitating this current flow, which is interrupted at intervals referred to as nodes of Ranvier (Fig. 9-1). The amount of myelinization determines the diameter of the nerve, and the greater sized nerves with more myelinization have greater conduction speeds (Table 9-1). The conduction velocity along the axon is pro-

portional to the internodal distance. The internodal distance is decreased in neuropathy of axonal degeneration or demyelination origin. The velocity of the current flow is recorded in nerve conduction studies.

Interneuronal conduction occurs at nerve synapses and at neuroeffector junctions such as muscle fibers. Interneuronal communication is performed chemically

TABLE 9-1 Classification of nerve fibers

Sensory and motor fibers	Sensory fibers	Largest fiber diameter	Fastest conduction velocity (M/sec)	General comments
A-alpha	Ia	22	120	Motor: The large alpha motor neurons of lamina IX, innervating extrafusal muscle fibers Sensory: The primary afferent fibers of muscle spindles
A-alpha	Ib	22	120	Sensory: Golgi tendon organs, touch and pressure receptors
A-beta	II	13	70	Motor: The motor neurons innervating both extrafusal and intrafusal (muscle spindle) 110 le fibers Sensory: The secondary afferent fibers of muscle spindles, touch and pressure receptors, and pacinian corpuscles (vibratory sensors)
A-gamma		8	40	Motor: The small gamma motor neurons of lamina IX, innervating intrafusal fibers (muscle spindles)
A-delta	III	5	15	Sensory: Small, lightly myelinated fibers; touch pressure, pain, and temperature
B		3	14	Motor: Small, lightly myelinated preganglionic autonomic fibers
C	IV	1	2	Motor: All postganglionic autonomic fibers (all are unmyelinated) Sensory: Unmyelinated pain and temperature fibers

From Manter JT: *Essentials of clinical neuroanatomy and neurophysiology,* ed 7, Philadelphia, 1987, FA Davis.

by neurotransmitters, which either excite (depolarize) or inhibit (hyperpolarize) the postsynaptic membrane. Specific receptor proteins for each neurotransmitter are in the membranes on both sides of the synapse, and binding opens channels for the current flow.

Electromyography

In a muscle the fibers innervated by branches emanating from the motor neuron of a single anterior horn cell are called a *motor unit*. The electrical activity of motor units in a muscle is recordable as motor unit action potentials (MUAPs) (Fig. 9-2). The study of electrical potentials generated by the depolarization of muscle is termed electromyography (EMG).

EMG is primarily used to study striated muscle, which is relatively easy because of sodium-mediated high current flow. Smooth muscles, being phylogenetically earlier, are dependent upon calcium ion exchange with low current generation. This smaller current density is more difficult to study, requiring microelectrode intracellular recording devices.

Motor unit territories within skeletal muscles are variable in size ranging from 2 to 10 mm. Their electrical activity may be recorded by surface electrodes, which cover relatively large areas and show aggregate effects of many MUAPs, or by various types of needle electrodes, which record smaller areas of activity. The EMG potentials must be amplified and filtered and

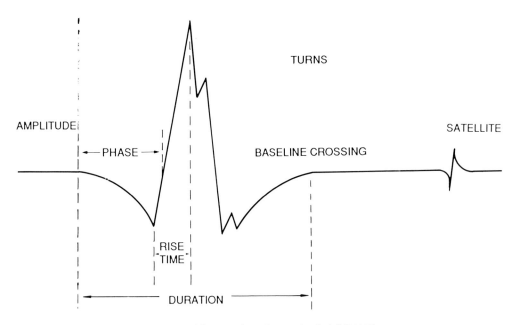

Fig. 9-2   Motor unit action potential (MUAP).

may be visualized on an oscilloscope screen or heard through audio amplifiers, which is more sensitive than visualization. These potentials are of small amplitude (20 to 2,000 μV) and are very brief (3 to 15 msec). To be recorded, therefore, the amplifiers and recording device must have wide-frequency response capabilities, from 30 to 10,000 Hz.

Surface Electrodes

The most precise way to record EMG is with a needle inserted into the muscle. In pelvic floor studies, however, especially those involving the urethra and anal sphincter, needles are uncomfortable and produce greater precision than is usually necessary. Therefore, surface electrodes may be used. Two electrodes are placed: the active placed close to the muscle under study and a "remote" electrode placed at a more distant site. If necessary, both recording electrodes can be placed over the active muscle. The EMG recording apparatus amplifies, filters, and displays the voltage changes. It is often desirable to record simultaneously low-frequency urodynamic data (e.g., cystometrics, uroflow) and high-frequency EMG data. This capability is made possible by an analog convertor, which records the EMG activity in a semiquantitative estimation of the EMG potentials per second.

Skin surface electrodes are frequently used to record perineal EMG (Fig. 9-3). Monopolar-type electrodes are placed on either side of the anal orifice. A disposable surface recording electrode, such as a silver chloride disk, can be mounted on a self-adhesive sticker. It is extremely important to reduce the electrical resistance of the skin by washing and drying the area and applying electrode paste to ensure firm adherence between electrode and skin. Other surface electrodes useful in pelvic floor studies are depicted in Figs. 9-4 to 9-7.

With surface electrodes, electromyographic pattern recordings depict the net electrical activity occurring in the muscle. Surface electrodes, therefore, demonstrate electronically generated summation of muscular electrical activity, but are incapable of distinguishing abnormal from normal individual motor unit potentials.

When surface electrodes are used in conjunction with the cystometrogram, a gradual increase in EMG activity is usually seen as the bladder is filled. Normally when a detrusor contraction occurs, the EMG

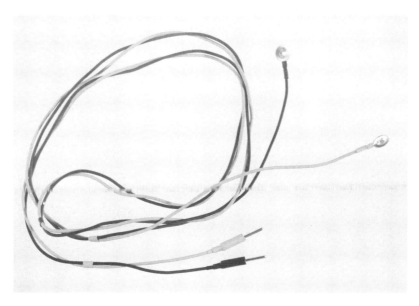

Fig. 9-3 Surface electrodes.

activity of the pelvic floor ceases. Two subgroups of abnormal coordination between electrical activity in the perineal musculature and bladder pressure record-

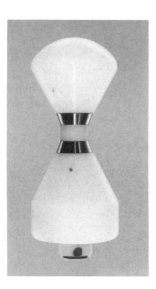

Fig. 9-4 Anal plug electrode with bipolar concentric recording surfaces mounted on a Teflon, hour-glass-shaped plug.

ings are (1) uninhibited involuntary sphincter relaxation and (2) detrusor-sphincter dyssynergia where the sphincter and detrusor contract *involuntarily* at the same time.

There are problems with the diagnosis of detrusor-sphincter dyssynergia and with terminology. True detrusor-sphincter dyssynergia occurs with a neurologic lesion, generally located between the pons and the sacral outflow to the lower urinary tract. Many times examiners will find increased EMG activity during detrusor contractions, which is behaviorally caused and not attributable to neurologic lesions (e.g., Valsalva action causes increase in perineal EMG activity and must be monitored). Activity of other surrounding musculature (such as gluteal) can contribute to the overall electrical activity measured when using surface electrodes. Simultaneous detrusor-perineal activity without cord defects has been designated as nonneurogenic neurogenic bladder. Precise recordings can distinguish features present in nonneurogenic neurogenic bladder and patients with true detrusor-sphincter dyssynergia. In the latter, dyssynergic EMG activity augments before and concomitant with the detrusor contraction, diminishing before the contraction subsides, whereas the nonneurogenic discrepancy tends

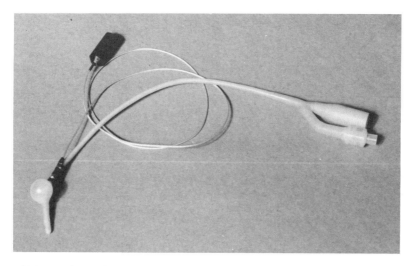

Fig. 9-5   Foley catheter ring electrode: two lengths of platinum wire protected by a plastic coating and positioned 1 cm distal to the Foley balloon.

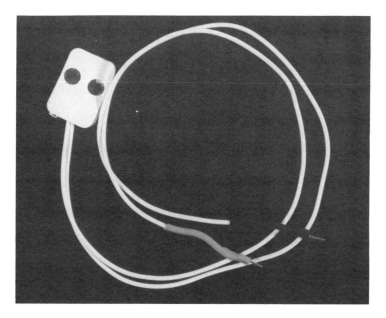

Fig. 9-6   Vaginal silver chloride electrodes attached to a disposable, flexible vinyl foam tampon.

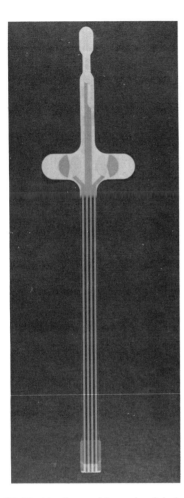

Fig. 9-7 St. Mark's disposable pudendal electrodes to be placed over index finger of a disposable glove. Stimulating anode and cathode are located at finger tip, recording electrodes at base of finger.

to have quiet EMG activity before the beginning of the detrusor contraction, which augments as the contraction subsides.

Needle EMG

Inserting a needle electrode into skeletal musculature allows analysis of individual motor units and is the superior technique used by the electromyographer for studying peripheral skeletal neuromuscular disease. The needle electrodes by design may be monopolar, concentric, or "single-fiber" in type, varying in dimensions and in the metal used in the device.

Monopolar Needle EMG

The monopolar needle electrode is made of solid stainless steel wire, 0.3 to 0.5 mm in diameter, which is insulated with Teflon except at its sharp tip. A second electrode used as a remote reference may be a surface disk or a subcutaneous needle. The monopolar electrode is less painful for the subject and less expensive. Compared with concentric needles, the recorded MUAPs have higher amplitudes, although durations are similar. The monopolar electrode is less selective, however, which may be a disadvantage when trying to isolate single recruited motor unit action potentials; and they have more recording artifact.

Artifacts create considerable difficulty for the novice electromyographer. Sixty-cycle voltage patterns may arise from appliances (even when turned off) or fluorescent lights. Improper grounding or defective needle insulation may cause markedly distorted tracings. The ground plate should be clean and applied over bone, e.g. the iliac crest, using conductive paste. Needle insulation may be examined under a microscope.

Concentric Needle EMG

Concentric electrodes have a hollow cannula, which serves as the reference electrode; extending down the shaft to the tip is an insulated fine wire with a beveled tip, which is the active electrode. The advantage of the concentric electrode is its more predictable surface area, which produces more reliable measurements of MUAP variables.

Amplifier settings influence recorded electrical activity. Gain settings determine the size of the electrical activity, which will be observable, and by convention the MUAP is recorded at a standard 100 μV per division. Filters are set at a low and high end, usually 2 to 3 Hz and 8 kHz or higher, respectively. The sweep speed determines the spread of the potential on the oscilloscope screen. A sweep of 10 msec/cm is used for most displays, although it is frequently easier to observe the characteristics of a MUAP when it is recorded at 5 msec/cm.

Concentric needle study of sphincter musculature

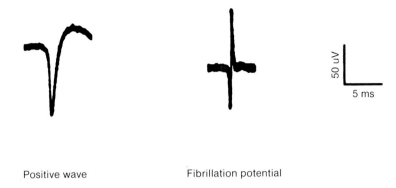

Positive wave   Fibrillation potential

50 uV

5 ms

Fig. 9-8 Positive wave (by convention, downward is positive) and fibrillation potential. Signs of abnormal increased insertional activity.

begins as soon as the needle is inserted into the muscle. Characteristic noise occurs when a muscle is penetrated (insertional activity), normally quieting soon after insertion. In the early period after denervation of skeletal muscle, increased membrane electrical sensitivity is typically seen as fibrillation potentials (small and short MUAPs) or positive waves (increased insertional activity) (Fig. 9-8). However, sphincter EMG is problematic because tonic activity of small motor units cannot be suppressed, and unlike other skeletal muscle in the body, complete electrical silence is not possible. Consequently, it is virtually impossible to identify fibrillations with certainty. In addition to fibrillations, spontaneous, abrupt onset and cessation potentials called complex repetitive discharges, and random fasciculation potentials are found in denervated muscle.

As a person increases voluntary effort, the firing rate of activated motor units is increased and finally, more motor units are recruited. This recruitment pattern describes the relationship of the rate of firing of individual motor units to the number of active motor units recorded with the EMG electrode. In denervating states with loss of some motor units, the recruitment pattern is reduced; with increasing effort there is a reduction in the number of newly recruited motor units, and those already activated discharge at a greater frequency than expected. Normally, at full contraction, there is so much recruitment that individual motor unit action potentials can no longer be identified; this phenomenon is termed *interference*

pattern. Coughing will typically produce a dramatic interference pattern in pelvic floor musculature. With dropout of motor units, a full interference pattern is not found. Care must be taken to ensure the patient is expending maximal voluntary effort.

Observation of tonic firing of motor units in the sphincter is ideal for individual motor unit analyses. To observe the firing, the equipment must have a trigger delay, which allows a motor unit to appear repeatedly at the same point on the oscilloscope screen. The duration, amplitude, and number of turns can then be assessed (Fig. 9-2).

Analyses of motor units from the normal urethral sphincter reveal durations less than 6 msec, amplitudes between 0.15 and 0.5 mV, and no more than 5 turns of 100 μV or more amplitude. More turns represent polyphasia. The number of phases in a MUAP is equal to the number of baseline zero crossings plus 1, and MUAPs having greater than four phases are considered *polyphasic*.

After nerve damage, muscle becomes reinnervated by regrowth of the axon from the site of the lesion or by collateral axonic regrowth. With the latter, the surviving motor axons sprout within the muscle, sending out branches to denervated muscle fibers. Hence, a single axon supplies a larger number of fibers, and the motor unit develops a more complex wave form with each new muscle fiber, giving rise to a new "phase" in the MUAP.

The immature axon conducts impulses slowly, which increases the duration of the motor unit poten-

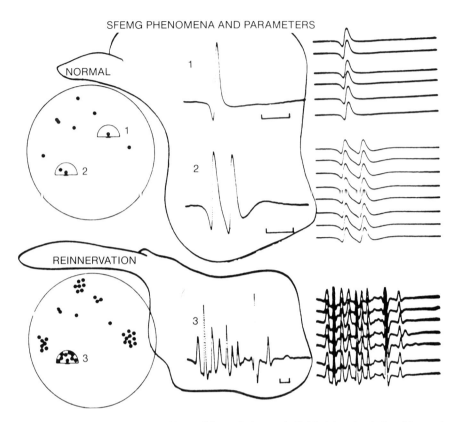

Fig. 9-9 Single fiber phenomena: Normal *(1 and 2)* muscle field pickup in circle with resultant MUAPs. Reinnervation *(3)* muscle field pickup of "bunched" muscle fibers supplied by single axon with resultant MUAPs.

tial. Thus the EMG pattern seen in established reinnervation is characterized by a reduced number of high amplitude, longer duration, polyphasic motor units firing at a rapid rate. The amplitude of a motor unit action potential is dependent on the size of the muscle fiber, being proportional to the square of the diameter. Hence, a 100 μm diameter muscle fiber produces an action potential roughly four times larger than a 50 μm fiber. The amplitude also relates to the distance from the electrode to the muscle fiber, decreasing exponentially as the distance increases. The rise time, which determines the steepness of the potential (see Fig. 9-2), also decreases with distance.

Single Fiber EMG

Single fiber EMG (SFEMG) is a selective recording technique that uses a concentric needle electrode to identify and record action potentials from individual muscle fibers. The technique is quite selective because of the small recording surface (25 μm in diameter) exposed at a port at the side of the electrode 3 mm from the tip. This distance allows examination of an area of approximately 350 μm diameter. In our laboratory, the high filter setting is 10,000 Hz and the low setting is 350 Hz. The images are triggered and delayed using a gain setting of 100 μV to trigger. In other skeletal muscle work, 200 μV is used as the triggering potential, but in sphincter work measuring smaller muscle fibers, 100 μV as a trigger is now standard. The number of fibers supplied by a branch axon (hence, firing essentially simultaneously) is observed, as each fiber creates an action potential (Fig. 9-9).

Measurements are made visually from the oscilloscope screen. At least 20 sites within the muscle are studied, usually requiring four needle insertions, which analyze five different action potentials with each insertion. The time base of the amplifier is set at 2 to 5 msec/division. All potentials with a component greater than 100 μV must be included in the calculation of the mean derived from the 20 recordings. The fiber density in SFEMG recordings increases after the age of about 60 years, so that average fiber density in a normal 30-year-old is approximately 1.4, at age 65 about 1.5, and at age 75, 1.75.

Conduction Studies

Electrical activity traveling through a nerve process can be measured by stimulating the nerve to depolarize it, thereby achieving a propagated action potential traveling away from the site of the stimulus. One may record the traveling potential directly from the nerve or when the impulse reaches a muscle, at which point the compound muscle action potential (CMAP) may be recorded. Propagation of the impulse along a nerve fiber in the same direction as occurs physiologically is referred to as *orthodromic conduction;* propagation in the opposite direction is referred to as *antidromic conduction.* Nerve conduction rates vary directly with the size of the nerve. Conduction velocities are also affected by temperature, with cooling slowing superficial nerve velocity by 0.7 to 2.4 m/sec for each degree centigrade. Generally, age has little significance or effect on conduction velocities until after age 60. One may not conclude that there is no peripheral neuropathy merely because nerve conduction velocities are normal.

The stimulation is accomplished by using two electrodes, a cathode and an anode. The cathode depolarizes the nerve and the anode hyperpolarizes it. The cathode should be located closer to the recording electrode along the pathway of the propagated action potential so that the action potential does not have to cross a hyperpolarized portion, thus avoiding the possibility of anodal block. The electrodes can be surface electrodes or monopolar needles.

The CMAP generated is referred to as the M wave. The stimulus must be supramaximal; that is, all nerve fibers to the muscle must be depolarized simultaneously. Supramaximal stimulation is achieved when increasing the stimulus no longer increases the re-

sulting amplitude of the M wave. The recording parameters are the latency in milliseconds from the nerve stimulation until the initial deflection, the amplitude of the CMAP in millivolts, and the duration in milliseconds and the configuration, which is normally a smooth curve with an initial negative component (upward deflection) followed by a terminal positive component.

Recording is accomplished with both active and reference electrodes. When studying the CMAP generated after stimulation of a nerve, the resultant latency includes the time for the nerve conduction plus the time for neuromuscular junction transmission and muscle fiber depolarization; hence it is not nerve conduction alone, but rather a terminal latency. Only a small stimulus intensity is required to achieve supramaximal stimulation of a nerve, and it is generally below the threshold regarded as painful. The stimulus pulse width must be standardized, as it affects the latency, and the sweep speed must be adjusted to visualize the resulting potentials.

Stimulus artifact is a reaction from the stimulus that may interfere with the recorded response, especially when studying latencies of short distance. The stimulus artifact can be minimized by keeping the stimulus intensity and duration as low as possible. Other techniques to maximize stimulus artifact include reducing current leakage across the skin surface by proper preparation, keeping the receptive electrodes in proximity to each other, separating the stimulator wires from the recording system to avoid induction currents, and rotating the stimulating anode to either side of the cathode.

Placement of the ground electrode on the patient is necessary, but position is not extremely critical. If convenient, the electrode is positioned between the stimulating and recording electrodes. Amplifier settings must be constant, as increasing the sensitivity of the amplifier may shorten the latency value. Motor responses (CMAPs) are usually of greater amplitude and of longer duration than sensory responses recorded from the nerve itself.

Pudendal Nerve Terminal Motor Latency (PNTML)

Kiff and Swash, in 1984, devised a method for stimulating the pudendal nerve transrectally using electrodes mounted on a disposable glove (Fig. 9-7). The

```
G= 200 H=10000 L=10.00
PW= 50  S= 2.01  RR= 0.70
AVE=  10/10    SC= 1

T= 2.68  0.00 DELTA= 2.68
```

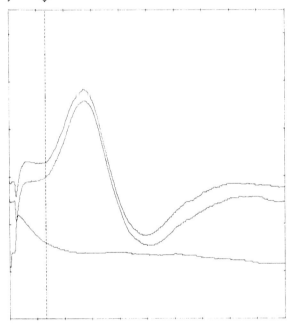

```
G=  50 H=10000 L=10.00
PW= 50  S= 2.01  RR= 0.70
AVE=  10/10    SC= 2

T= 2.10  0.00 DELTA= 2.10
```

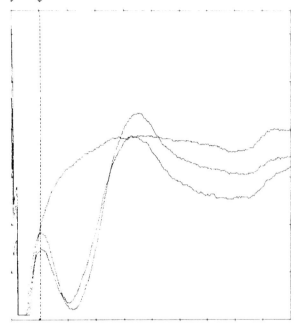

Fig. 9-10 Pudendal nerve motor terminal latency (PNTML). *G*, Gain in microvolts per (vertical) division; *H*, high frequency filter setting in hertz, *L*, low frequency filter setting in hertz; *PW*, pulse width of stimulus in microseconds; *S*, sweep speed of display in milliseconds per (horizontal) division; *RR*, repetition rate of stimulus (per second); *Ave*, number of responses averaged; *SC*, scale; *T*, time in milliseconds (determined by vertical marker placement); *Delta*, time from stimulus to vertical marker. Top two responses are with pudendal nerve stimulated (replicated response); bottom line a "control" with stimulation not applied to pudendal nerve.

Fig. 9-11 Perineal nerve motor terminal latency (PeNTML). Parameters as in Fig. 9-10. Gain setting of 50 μsec as response has lower amplitude than PNTML.

stimulating electrodes are located on the finger tip and the recording electrodes are found at the base of the finger. The pudendal nerve is stimulated transrectally near its passage in Alcock's canal by the ischial spine, and the response is obtained from the inferior hemorrhoidal division of the pudendal nerve supply-ing the anal sphincter (Fig. 9-10). Both right and left nerves may be tested. Our laboratory PNTML mean is 2.1 ± 0.2 msec, comparable to results of other laboratories.

Perineal Nerve Terminal Motor Latency (PeNTML)

Stimulating the pudendal nerve as previously described for PNTML and recording with the Foley catheter ring electrode (see Fig. 9-5) enable one to obtain the right and left PeNTML to the urethral sphincter (Fig. 9-11). This nerve branch of the pudendal nerve supplies the area of anatomic distribution, which is even more affected by vaginal delivery than is the PNTML. Our laboratory reports a mean PeNTML of 2.29 ± 0.3 msec.

G= 200 H=10000 L=10.00
PW= 50   S= 5.00   RR= 0.70
AVE= 25/10   SC= 1

T=18.51   7.28 DELTA=11.23

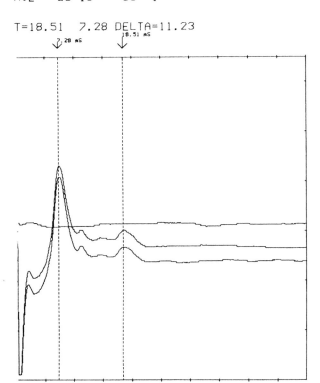

Fig. 9-12 F wave. Parameter definitions as in Fig. 9-10. Vertical marker lines at peaks of M wave and F wave. Delta is time of transmission of stimulus antidromically to cord and return orthodromically to receptor electrodes.

Late Responses

The more proximal segment of peripheral nerves can be studied using techniques of late responses. These late waves are potentials that occur after the M wave produced by the volley of electric current from the site of stimulation moving proximally and then returning distally along the nerve. The two commonly studied types are H reflexes and F waves. The H reflex is a true reflex, with orthodromic afferent sensory conduction synapsing to an outward-going wave orthodromically in motor fibers. The F wave (Fig. 9-

12) is not a reflex and is produced by antidromic impulse conduction in motor fibers rebounding off the anterior horn cell, then returning orthodromically to produce an action potential in distal muscles. The H reflex is blocked by supramaximal stimulus, whereas the F wave is produced only with supramaximal stimulus. When the F wave is obtainable, an estimation of the conduction time in the proximal nerve can be made by measuring the nerve length, subtracting arbitrary turnaround time and dividing by two (for the antidromic and orthodromic travel time). When determining the PNTML, an F wave occasionally can be obtained by changing the sweep speed. Due to the short distance of the nerve, however, this is difficult when there is prolongation of the PNTML because the nerve is still in a refractory status for the returning nerve volley. Therefore the use of this late response is limited in patients demonstrating prolonged PNTML.

Evidence of more proximal peripheral neuropathy in pelvic floor disorders has been obtained with direct spinal cord stimulation and recording the latency of response in the anal and urethral sphincters. The large voltage stimulus required for this procedure, however, precludes its approval for use by the Food and Drug Administration. Magnetic stimulators are now being developed that may provide direct stimulation tests to evaluate more effectively the proximal pelvic floor nerves.

Evoked Response

An evoked response is the summation of potentials recorded from central nervous tissue (spinal cord or cortex) that have been stimulated from a peripheral site. Because electrical activity is occurring throughout the body tissues and can be detected by the recording electrodes, it is necessary to obtain multiple responses so that the evoked potential, which is usually only a few microvolts in amplitude, can be identified against the background activity. Computer averaging within the recording system allows the individual responses, which occur in a time-locked relationship to the stimulus, to be increased in clarity against the background; the randomly occurring background activity progressively lessens in prominence.

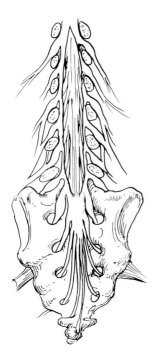

Fig. 9-13 Cauda equina: Note the relationship to first and fifth lumbar vertebra where electrodes may be placed.

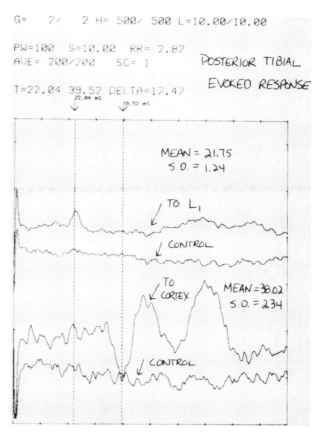

Fig. 9-14 Evoked response from stimulation of posterior tibial nerve. Top two lines represent response at L1 vertebra (and control) and bottom two lines the response at cerebral cortex (and control). (*G*, Gain; *H*, high frequency filter; *L*, low frequency filter settings for lumbar and cortical responses, respectively.) Parameter definitions as in Fig. 9-10.

Cortical evoked responses, obtained by stimulation of the dorsal nerve of the penis in men, have been difficult to obtain by clitoral stimulation in women. Now, however, the St. Mark's pudendal electrode makes this procedure possible by stimulating the pudendal nerve at the ischial spine. Further, by being able to stimulate either right or left pudendal nerve, the responses may be lateralized. The two cortical recording electrodes are placed as follows: the active electrode is placed midline, 2 cm posterior to the halfway mark between the inion and the nasion, and the reference electrode is placed in the upper mid-forehead. Recording electrodes may also be placed over the vertebral column at levels L1 (active electrode) and L5 (reference electrode), which correspond to the cord levels of the cauda equina (Fig. 9-13). Then, using two channels, the evoked responses can be simultaneously recorded from the cortex and the lumbar spine.

Similar recordings may be obtained by stimulating

posterior to the medial malleolus at the posterior tibial nerve (Fig. 9-14). These evoked responses are frequently given the name *somatosensory,* but it must be emphasized that these responses have nothing to do with examining sensory functioning. Thus sensory evoked responses do not offer objective means of assessing bladder sensory function and are only useful for indicating indirectly that tracts are intact from the point of stimulation to the point of response. This same information can be obtained for the area of the cauda equina and spinal cord by the more commonly used posterior tibial nerve. These studies determine

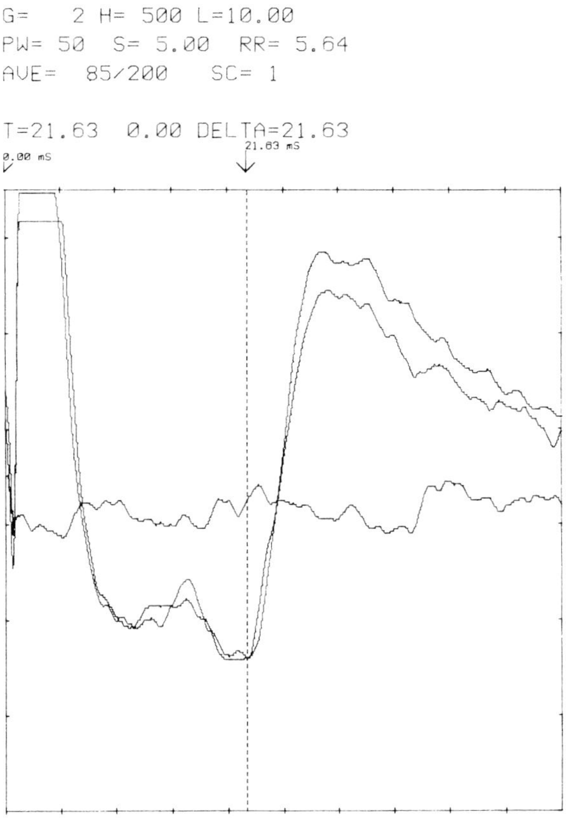

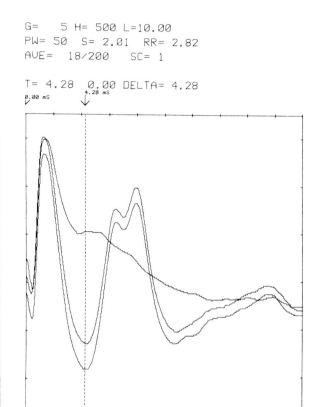

```
G=   2 H= 500 L=10.00
PW= 50  S= 5.00  RR= 5.64
AVE=  85/200    SC= 1

T=21.63   0.00 DELTA=21.63
0.00 mS         21.63 mS
```

```
G=   5 H= 500 L=10.00
PW= 50  S= 2.01  RR= 2.82
AVE=  18/200    SC= 1

T= 4.28   0.00 DELTA= 4.28
0.00 mS         4.28 mS
```

Fig. 9-15 Evoked response at L1 vertebra with stimulation at proximal urethra. Parameter definitions as in Fig. 9-10.

Fig. 9-16 Evoked response at L1 vertebra with stimulation at pudendal nerve in Alcock's canal. Parameter definitions as in Fig. 9-10.

conduction times as peripheral (from stimulus to L1), central (L1 to cortex), or total (stimulus to cortex). Localization of lesions is suggested as peripheral (delayed peripheral and total) or cord (normal peripheral, delayed central and total). Cortical lesions may have absent response.

Evoked responses to the lumbar vertebrae may also be obtained from the proximal urethra using the Foley catheter ring electrodes for stimulation (Fig. 9-15). Afferent pathways are of a slower visceral type (conduction velocity of 18 to 22 m/sec) and the latency is longer, averaging 20.24 ± 0.5 msec in our laboratory. Pudendal stimulation at the ischial spine has an evoked potential response to the lumbar vertebrae (Fig. 9-16) averaging 5.80 ± 0.99 msec, tracking the faster pudendal somatic afferent pathway, which has a shorter, less synaptic course. Finding unilateral abnormality in this evoked response suggests nerve root injury, as systemic peripheral neuropathies (e.g., with diabetes) generally have bilateral changes.

Reflex Response and Sensory Study

Stimulation delivered by the Foley catheter ring electrode produces a reflex response at the external anal sphincter, which Bradley has called *electromyelography* (myelo referring to the spinal cord) (Fig. 9-17). This reflex incorporates detrusor and urethral sensory afferents, conus medullaris synapses, and pudendal motor neurons. The stimulus has a pulse duration of 50 µsec and can be increased by increments

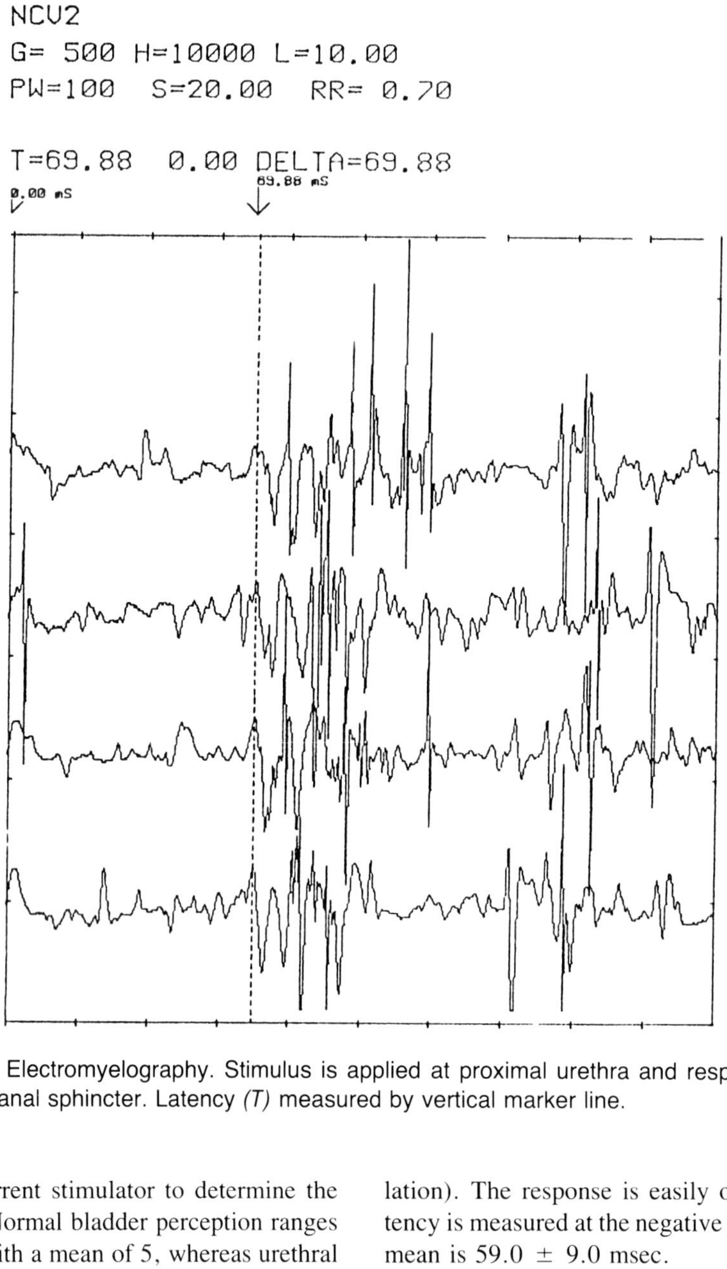

NCV2
G= 500 H=10000 L=10.00
PW=100   S=20.00   RR= 0.70

T=69.88   0.00 DELTA=69.88
                 69.88 mS
0.00 mS

Fig. 9-17 Electromyelography. Stimulus is applied at proximal urethra and response obtained at anal sphincter. Latency (T) measured by vertical marker line.

using a constant current stimulator to determine the sensory threshold. Normal bladder perception ranges from 3 to 10 mA, with a mean of 5, whereas urethral perception is considerably lower with a mean of 1.5 mA. Using a constant voltage stimulator, the stimulus may be increased until the reflex threshold (reproducible response) is obtained. Then, to determine latency, the stimulation is increased until no further change occurs in the response (supramaximal stimu-

lation). The response is easily obtained, and the latency is measured at the negative peak. Our laboratory mean is 59.0 ± 9.0 msec.

Amplitude may also be recorded and has a laboratory mean of 53.27 ± 15.25 µV. The stimulus duration affects latency and must be standardized.

Cauda equina injury is characterized by diminished amplitude or absence of this response. If the sensory threshold and evoked response from proximal urethra to lumbar spine are normal, a motor neuron lesion is implied and sphincter EMG is indicated. If the sensory threshold is elevated and the proximal urethral evoked response to the lumbar vertebrae absent, the lesion involves at least the sensory pathway, and pudendal nerve evoked response to the lumbar vertebrae may indicate proximal pudendal lesion presence or absence. If reflex response is present but the patient has lost sensation, the lesion is in the sensory cortex or ascending spinal cord tracts. The patient can usually voluntarily change the response amplitude, and failure to suppress an exaggerated response may suggest a suprasacral tract disorder. Finding normal electromyelography and normal sphincter EMG effectively *excludes* a lower motor neuron lesion of S2 through S4.

Reflex response may also be obtained when stimulating at the clitoris and picking up with electrodes at the anal sphincter. The stimulus at the clitoris may be either right or left sided, and the pick up at the anal sphincter can be performed with concentric needles that are placed into the right and left external anal sphincter musculature. In placing the needles, EMG is used to make certain that the needles are placed within the muscle. Stimulating at the clitoris creates pudendal nerve afferent stimulus, which reflexly goes to the cord and results in response contraction in the external anal sphincter that can be lateralized, either right or left. Using auditory response in conjunction is helpful. This allows lateralization of both afferent and efferent response to test dorsal and ventral roots in the sacral portion of the cord. These roots may frequently be affected in cauda equina disease. In our laboratory this reflex has a latency of 33 ± 4 msec. Sensory values can be obtained as well, since most patients perceive sensation between 3 and 12 mA. As with all reflex responses, the response must be supramaximal, and this usually requires a stimulus that is approximately twice the threshold of perception.

"Supersensitivity" Testing

Cannon's law of denervation states that once an organ is deprived of its efferent nerve supply, it develops supersensitivity to its neuromuscular transmitter. In cases of detrusor hypoactivity, a neurogenic etiology (detrusor areflexia) may be documented by injection of bethanechol chloride (Urecholine, 5 mg subcutaneously) after baseline cystometry, followed by rapid gas cystometric studies at 5-minute intervals. A positive test is indicated by a rise in intravesical pressure more than 15 cm H_2O.

Bladders that demonstrate such denervation have damage to the peripheral autonomic nerve fibers. Denervation implies loss of intermediate nerve function between the central nervous system and the muscle, and the term *decentralization* is preferable to denervation, as the actual nerves still have a presence.

CLINICAL CONDITIONS

The nervous system relationship to the lower urinary tract is extremely complex, and simplification, although clinically useful, will never be totally accurate. Every nervous system physiologic control over the urinary tract has positive and negative aspects, and either can dominate in a given clinical situation. Although the following suggestions can be useful in clinical evaluation, they do not describe situations that are always present. A schematic representation as presented by Torrens and Morrison is given in the box on p. 118.

The lower urinary tract has to accomplish storage without increased pressure so that upper tract damage does not occur. Storage must occur in a closed outlet. In emptying, a complex reflex mechanism must be mediated under autonomic, central, and peripheral nervous system control. The Barrington's center in the anterior pontine region of the brain stem acts as the detrusor reflex coordinating and augmenting center. This reflex of bladder emptying can be thought of as being facilitated or inhibited by various components of the nervous system. That concept will be applied in the following clinical descriptions.

Cortical Lesions

The only region of the cerebral cortex consistently associated with detrusor dysfunction when damaged is the superior frontal gyrus-septal area. Lesions in this area interfere with voluntary inhibition of the pontine detrusor reflex center. Urodynamic and electrophysiologic testing show detrusor hyperreflexia with contractions, which are coordinated with urethral re-

Simplified Scheme of Interaction of Various Levels of the Nervous System in Micturition

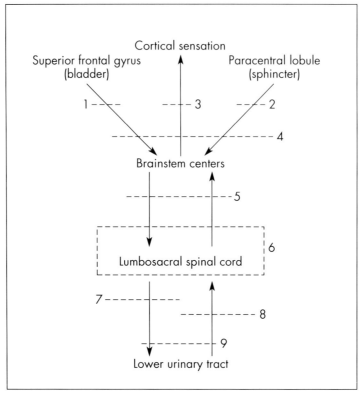

The locations of certain possible nervous lesions are denoted by numbers and explained as follows:

1, Lesions isolating the superior frontal gyrus prevent voluntary postponement of voiding. If sensation is intact this produces urge incontinence. If the lesion is larger there will be additional loss of social concern about incontinence.

2, Lesions isolating the paracentral lobule, sometimes associated with a hemiparesis, will cause spasticity of the urethral sphincter and retention. This will be painless if sensation is abolished. Minor degrees of this syndrome may cause difficulty in the initiation of micturition.

3, Pathways of sensation are not known accurately. In theory, an isolated lesion of sensation above the brainstem would lead to unconscious incontinence. Defective central conduction of sensory information would explain nocturnal enuresis.

4, Lesions above the brainstem centers lead to involuntary voiding that is coordinated with sphincter relaxation.

5, Lesions below brainstem centers but above the lumbosacral spinal cord lead, after a period of bladder paralysis associated with spinal shock, to involuntary reflex voiding that is not coordinated with sphincter relaxation (detrusor/sphincter dyssynergia).

6, Lesions destroying the lumbosacral cord or the complete nervous connections between the central and peripheral nervous system result in a paralyzed bladder that contracts only weakly in an autonomous fashion because of its remaining ganglionic innervation. However, if the lumbar sympathetic outflow is preserved in the presence of conus and/or cauda equina destruction, then there may be some residual sympathetic tone in the bladder neck and urethra that may be sufficient to be obstructive.

7, A lesion of the efferent fibers alone leads to a bladder of decreased capacity and decreased compliance associated experimentally with an increased number of adrenergic nerves.

8, A lesion confined to the afferent fibers produces a bladder that is areflexic with increased compliance and capacity.

9, As there are ganglion cells in the bladder wall it is technically impossible to decentralize the bladder completely, but congenital absence of bladder ganglia may exist producing megacystis.

From Torrens M. Morrison JFB (eds): *The physiology of the lower urinary tract,* London, 1987, Springer-Verlag.

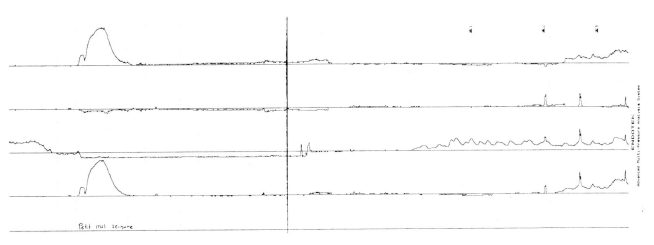

Petit mal seizure

Fig. 9-18 Multichannel cystometric study. Lines (top to bottom) vesical pressure, abdominal pressure, urethral pressure, detrusor pressure.

laxation and decreased surface EMG activity. Fig. 9-18 shows a coordinated detrusor contraction occurring simultaneously with a petit mal seizure. The contraction is of large magnitude, with the pons augmentation intact.

Such cortical lesions prevent voluntary postponement of voiding. Urge incontinence results when sensation is intact. If sensation is not intact, involuntary voiding (enuresis) occurs. With larger lesions, social concern about incontinence is lost.

A separate cortical area regulates upper motor neuron control of the pudendal nerve. This pudendal nucleus is located in paracentral lobule cortical areas. Lesions here may be involved with hemiparesis and may produce upper motor neuron findings with contralateral extensor planter reflexes and increased deep tendon reflexes. These lesions can be characterized electrophysiologically by inability to quiet electrical activity in the pelvic floor, as measured either by loss of voluntary influence on electromyelography amplitude reflex, or more simply by exaggerated surface EMG perineal musculature activity. This exaggeration and spasticity may be associated with difficulty in initiating micturition. This paracentral lobule syndrome is relatively uncommon.

The perineal sphincter is an example of a muscle that does not have a fully crossed relationship with the motor cortex because stimulation of the motor cortex on either side can cause contractions on both sides of the sphincter musculature. Cortical inhibition of sphincteric activity is partly aided by inhibition of spinal origin.

Suprasacral Cord Areas

The nature of a voiding or urinary storage disturbance that occurs with spinal cord disease depends on the site and extent of the injury, type of recovery, and presence or absence of other neurologic or urogynecologic disorders.

Lower urinary tract neurons with long ascending axons reach the pons micturition area to mediate chiefly facilitative effects. These axons enter sacral posterior roots and pass in the spinothalamic tracts. Lesions affecting these compartments can lead to detrusor areflexia and increased compliance. Correspondingly, intentional sectioning (sacral dorsal rhizotomy) prevents bladder contractions and increases capacity. Effector pathways from the pons to the lower cord are chiefly inhibitory, and lesions affecting these cord areas lead to small non-amplified, poorly coordinated detrusor contractions of short duration, with resultant increased residual urine. Hence, higher cord lesions vary in clinical manifestation.

The usual response to spinal cord injury is complete bladder paralysis followed by return of some lower urinary tract function within months. This return of reflexes is, perhaps, in response to demand, a demonstration of the body's neuroplasticity. Many patients develop automatic bladder in which the bladder contracts in response to distention. This intrinsic power is less than normal so that residual volumes generally increase.

Lesions below the pons, with resultant loss of bladder and sphincter activity coordination, generally lead to detrusor-sphincter dyssynergia, further complicating residual urine problems. These problems can be severe enough to affect the upper urinary system. Generally, this complication occurs when the bladder pressure reaches levels above 40 cm H_2O. Almost all suprasacral cord injuries produce dysfunction of both the bladder and the outlet, the detrusor becoming hyperreflexic and the outlet demonstrating varying degrees of dyssynergia. When the bladder becomes trabeculated and fibrotic, the small detrusor contractions may empty the bladder (hence no residual urine), but upper tract deterioration may continue to progress secondary to high intravesical pressure.

Neurophysiologic studies in patients with suprasacral spinal cord disease may demonstrate normal peripheral and prolonged total and central conduction times. Urodynamic studies document detrusor hyperreflexia, with or without detrusor-sphincter dyssynergia, depending on the lesion. Electromyelography and sphincter EMG studies frequently do not show abnormalities, although facilitation of the electromyelographic reflex response and lack of volitional control over it could be expected. Deep tendon hyperreflexia and impaired lower extremity sensation may be found on physical examination.

Sacral Cord Area

Lesions involving the sacral cord lead to lower motor neuron disorders with possible absence of both detrusor and urethral sphincteric activity. Lesions involving S1 and S2, however, may retain sphincter activity with loss of detrusor function. The detrusor activity may be further reduced by a block of long routing detrusor afferent nerves, compounding the areflexia. This type of bladder decentralization may result in loss of subjective sensation to large volumes, but poor compliance and increased pressure is more common. When the bladder pressure exceeds urethral closing pressure,

incontinence occurs. This incontinence usually is due to poor bladder volume tolerance, coupled with abnormal urethral function. Obstruction to the incontinence may place the upper tracts in jeopardy.

Findings in these patients include trabeculation on cystoscopy, positive bethanechol supersensitivity test, abnormal sphincter EMG (lower motor neuron disease), occasionally abnormal electromyelography, decreased sensation, and prolonged peripheral and total conduction times.

Cauda Equina

Because the cauda equina conveys the afferent and efferent nerves from the sacral cord, the findings with injury here are similar to those found with sacral cord injury. Clinically, however, they differ because in most patients cauda equina injury is a result of vertebral injury below T12 or intervertebral disk protrusion usually in the L4-L5 or L5-S1 spaces. The majority of these patients have autonomic parasympathetic interruption with decreased urinary streams as measured by uroflowmetry. Elevated postvoid residual urine volumes and occasional urinary retention are common. Urinary incontinence may be due to urine overflow, which is frequently accentuated by maintained alpha-adrenergic activity or loss of urethral competency secondary to lower motor neuron disease of the striated external urethral sphincter.

Sensory losses are prominent in cauda equina injury and may be detected by S2-S4 dermatome sensory loss. This accentuation of the sensory loss mechanism may be responsible for the high degree of areflexia and increased bladder capacity secondary to loss of afferent facilitory pathway to the pons. Urodynamic studies show abdominal-type voiding, absent detrusor activity, abnormal sphincter EMG, and abnormal electromyelography with prolonged peripheral conduction times. Bethanechol supersensitivity test is usually positive.

Neuropathy in the cauda equina may be produced from systemic disease such as diabetes and nerve root problems. Generally, systemic neuropathy shows symmetric abnormalities; on electrophysiologic testing, evoked potentials from the pudendal nerve to L1 show symmetric abnormalities (right and left). Nerve root injuries show abnormalities localized to the side

SSEP1
G=   5 H= 500 L=10.00
PW= 50   S= 2.01   RR= 2.80
AVE=   26/500   SC= 1

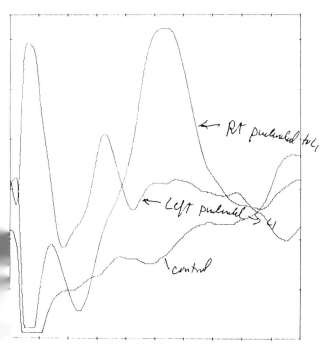

← Rt pudendal to L₁

← Left pudendal

control

Fig. 9-19 Evoked response study to L1 spine. Result of stimulating right pudendal nerve having significantly greater amplitude than from left pudendal. This patient had an infiltrating tumor of the left sacral and third sacral nerve root.

with the deficit. Fig. 9-19 shows an example of unilateral difference produced by nerve root injury. With either type of neuropathy, motor weakness in the sphincters is observed. Sensation is normally affected on the dermatome of the affected side in nerve root injury patients; more symmetric distribution occurs in cauda equina neuropathy due to diabetes.

Pelvic Plexus Injury

The pelvic plexus may be affected by surgical procedures involving the lower colorectal or gynecologic systems. Patients may present with micturition disturbances after pelvic surgery, and distinction between

damage in the pelvic plexus and damage in the cauda equina may be assisted with electrophysiologic techniques.

Generally, pelvic plexus involves damage to the sympathetic autonomic system, whereas cauda equina does not. Patients with pelvic nerve injury do not have noticeable perineal sensory loss. Sensory disturbances may be seen in the bladder when damage occurs to the afferent innervation through sympathetic nerves in the hypogastric portion of the pelvic plexus, thus increasing the micturition threshold. Generally, pudendal afferent nerves from the urethra decrease the micturition threshold, and those from the colon and perineum increase the threshold, accounting for the mixed clinical picture seen with pelvic plexus injury. The resultant decentralization that occurs with pelvic plexus injury may lead to parasympathetic denervation and detrusor areflexia, frequently with markedly decreased compliance; the block in beta-adrenergic nerves add to the likelihood of this outcome. Complicating this situation, alpha-adrenergic denervation, leads to incompetency at the bladder neck so that incontinence may be associated with the frustrating difficulty in initiating urination. Thus there is decreased bladder compliance, detrusor hypoactivity, incompetence of the bladder neck, and diminished urethral closure pressures.

Electromyelography may show changes, often of less magnitude than with cauda equina lesions. Perineal and pudendal motor terminal latencies generally are unaffected, being distal to the area of injury. Evoked responses from pudendal and bladder base to lumbar spinal cord may be affected. Posterior tibial evoked response to lumbar spine is frequently unaffected, a finding helpful in differentiating pelvic plexus from cauda equina injury. Pelvic nerve injury may be associated with hyposensitivity in the bladder and urethra. Sphincter EMG is usually abnormal.

Distal Pudendal Neuropathy

With the advent of pudendal and perineal nerve terminal motor latency studies, single fiber density studies, and other sphincter EMG studies, there is increased appreciation of the significance of distal pudendal nerve injury. It is strongly related both to urinary and fecal incontinence and to pelvic floor pro-

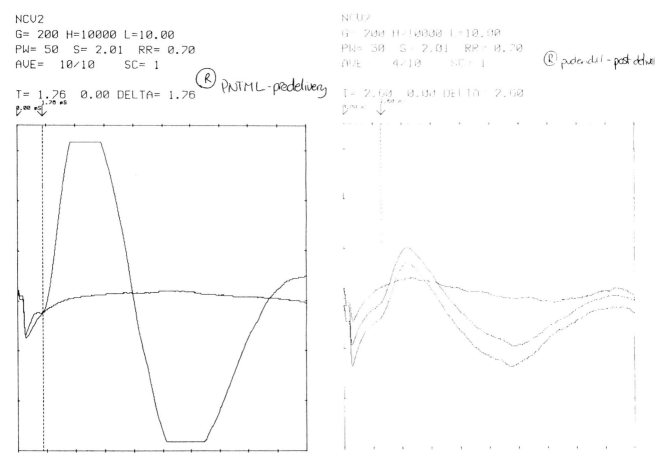

NCV2
G= 200 H=10000 L=10.00
PW= 50 S= 2.01 RR= 0.70
AVE= 10/10   SC= 1

T= 1.76 0.00 DELTA= 1.76 (R) PNTML-predelivery
0.00 mS 1.76 mS

NCV2
G= 200 H=10000 L=10.00
PW= 50 S= 2.01 RR= 0.70
AVE= 4/10   SC= 1

(R) pudendal - post delive

T= 2.00 0.00 DELTA= 2.00

Fig. 9-20 Pudendal nerve terminal motor latency. Before vaginal delivery.

Fig. 9-21 Pudendal nerve motor terminal latency. Same patient as in Fig. 9-20, after vaginal delivery.

lapse. The association of changes in latency with EMG changes in the sphincters can demonstrate peripheral neuropathy. Twenty percent of women show such changes after vaginal delivery (Figs. 9-20 and 9-21). The strong relationship between neuropathy and genuine stress urinary incontinence and anal incontinence suggests possible methods for prevention of these disorders. In patients demonstrating persistence of this neurophysiologic abnormality after vaginal delivery, change in route of subsequent deliveries may be considered to prevent the profound sequelae of pelvic floor neuropathy in later years.

BIBLIOGRAPHY

Electrophysiologic Studies

Benson JT: Neurophysiologic control of lower urinary tract, *Obstet Gynecol Clin North Am* 16:733, 1989.

Benson JT: Electrodiagnosis. In Benson JT (ed): Female pelvic floor disorders, New York, 1992, WW Norton & Co.

Blaivas JG, Singha HP, Zayed AA, et al: Detrusor-external sphincter dyssynergia, *J Urol* 125:542, 1981.

Bradley WE, Timm GW, Rockswold GL, et al: Detrusor and urethral electromyography, *J Urol* 114:69, 1975.

Cannon WB: A law of denervation, *Am J Med Sci* 198:737, 1959.

Haldeman S, Bradley WE, Bhatia NN, et al: Pudendal evoked responses, *Arch Neurol* 39:280, 1982.

Haldeman S, Bradley WE, Bhatia N: Evoked responses from the pudendal nerve, *J Urol* 12:974, 1982.

Hinman F: Non-neurogenic neurogenic bladder (the Hinman Syndrome)—15 years later, *J Urol* 136:769, 1986.

Lapides J, Friend CR, Ajemian EP, et al: A new test for neurogenic bladder, *J Urol* 88:245, 1962.

Powell PH, Feneley RCL: The role of urethral sensation in clinical urology, *Br J Urol* 52:539, 1980.

Ruby DC, Woodside JR: Non-neurogenic neurogenic bladder: the relationship between intravesical pressure and the external sphincter myogram. Neurourol Urodynam 10:169, 1991.

Snooks SJ, Swash M: Pudendal nerve terminal motor latency and spinal stimulation. In Henry MM, Swash M (eds): Coloproctology and the pelvic floor, London, 1985, Butterworth.

Snooks SJ, Swash M: Perineal nerve and transcutaneous spinal stimulation: new methods for investigation of the urethral striated sphincter musculature, *Br J Urol* 56:406, 1984.

Kiff ES, Swash M: Normal proximal and delayed distal conduction in the pudendal nerves of patients with idiopathic (neurogenic) faecal incontinence, *J Neurol Neurosurg Psychiatry* 47:820, 1984.

Percy JP: A neurogenic factor in faecal incontinence in the elderly, *Age Ageing* 11:175, 1982.

Smith ARB, Hosker GL, Warrell DW: The role of partial denervation of the pelvic floor in the aetiology of genitourinary prolapse and stress incontinence of urine. A neurophysiological study, *Br J Obstet Gynaecol* 96:24, 1989.

Snooks SJ, Barnes PRH, Swash M: Damage to the innervation of the voluntary anal and periurethral musculature in incontinence, *J Neurol Neurosurg Psychiatry* 47:406, 1984.

Snooks SJ, Henry MM, Swash M: Anorectal incontinence and rectal prolapse: differential assessment of the innervation to puborectalis and external anal sphincter muscles, *Gut* 26:470, 1984.

Clinical Conditions

Benson JT: Clinical application of electrodiagnostic studies of female pelvic floor neuropathy, *Int Urogynecol J* 1:3, 1990.

CHAPTER 10

Endoscopic Evaluation of the Lower Urinary Tract

Bruce A. Rosenzweig

History of Endoscopy/Cystoscopy
Equipment
    Endoscope
    Light sources and cables
    Distention media
    Delivery systems
    Ancillary equipment: biopsy forceps, diathermy
      instruments, and ureteral catheter-deflecting bridge
    Care and maintenance of equipment
    Sterilization of instruments
Basic Technique For Outpatient Urethrocystoscopy
    Indications and contraindications
    Prepping the patient
    Performing urethrocystoscopy
Operative Urethrocystoscopy
Pathology of the Urethra
Pathology of the Bladder
Complications and Posturethrocystoscopy Care

HISTORY OF ENDOSCOPY/CYSTOSCOPY

Bozzini, in 1805, was the first to visualize the interior of the urethra using a cumbersome urethroscope and candlelight as the light source. Segalas later refined urethroscopy by adding a cannula tube around the endoscope, which allowed easier introduction and a system of reflective mirrors to increase illumination.

Desormeaux is credited as being the father of cystoscopy; in 1835, he developed the first urethroscope and cystoscope using mirrors to reflect light from a kerosene lamp. Nitze, in 1877, added a lens system to the endoscopic tube, which increased magnification of the viewing area. This lens system is the forerunner of the modern early cystoscope. Nitze used a platinum wire loop as the source of illumination for his cystoscope. The bladder was filled with ice water to prevent burns.

In 1889, Boisseau de Rocher separated the ocular parts of the cystoscope from the outer sheath. This modification made it possible to use multiple telescopes with the same sheath, thus making possible operative manipulation through the sheath. That year Poirer successfully catheterized both ureters in a living subject using the instrumentation developed by Boisseau de Rocher.

Howard Kelly at The Johns Hopkins Hospital established the first residency training program in gynecology and became a genitourinary surgeon for women. Kelly developed an air cystoscope, which consisted of a simple open speculum (a tube with a handle) that was illuminated by light reflected from a head mirror. He found that he could fill the bladder with air by placing the patient in the knee-chest position. The bladder filled by virtue of the negative intraabdominal pressure created by this position.

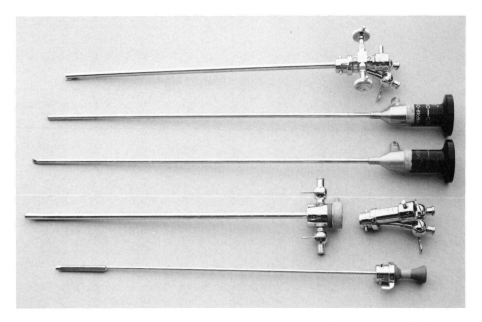

Fig. 10-1 Rigid endoscopes in urology and urogynecology. *Top to bottom*, Catheter-deflecting bridge; 30-degree telescope; 70-degree telescope; cystoscope sheath with bridge; obturator.

Kelly was the first person to pass ureteral catheters under direct vision.

Ridley described the technique of indirect air cystoscopy, which combined the use of direct (air) method of bladder distention (patient in knee-chest position), with an indirect cystoscope, which used a lens magnification system.

Hopkins reversed the typical design of the transmission medium of the telescope. He switched the air space of the telescope with glass rods and used air space as lenses. The effect of these changes was to increase light transmission and resolution while making the viewing angle larger.

In the late 1960s, Robertson modified the air cystoscope and popularized office urethrocystoscopy. Robertson used carbon dioxide as the distention medium, which allows simultaneous urethrocystoscopy and cystometry for evaluation of lower urinary tract dysfunction.

Fiberoptic lighting was also introduced in the 1960s. This system allows the transmission of high intensity light to the tip of the endoscope.

EQUIPMENT

Endoscope

The endoscope consists of a telescope and an outer sheath that has at least one channel through which distention medium can be passed and possibly other channels to evacuate fluids from the bladder or to allow the introduction of operative equipment. The rigid telescope is the mainstay of cystoscopic equipment (Fig. 10-1). It allows the operator to interchange telescopes without removing the outer sheath. A rigid telescope may look straight ahead, such as with a zero-degree lens, or it may have the field offset by viewing through different angles (30 to 120 degrees). The field of vision can be standard or have a wide angle affect. Unfortunately, the wide angle has less magnification, which means that one must get closer to an object to get a clear view. The most frequently used telescopes are the 30- and 70-degree standard lenses. The zero-degree lens is used mainly for urethroscopy (Fig. 10-2).

The tip of the outer sheath used with conventional cystoscopes has a fenestration along the lower border

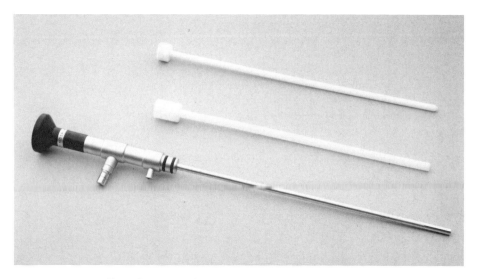

Fig. 10-2 Zero-degree urethroscope with plastic sheath and obturator.

and a beak on the anterior border. This makes cystoscopes difficult for urethroscopy because the distal urethra cannot be examined due to leakage of fluid from the fenestration, which causes the walls of the urethra to collapse around the end of the cystoscope. These sheaths must be used with an obturator for introduction into the bladder. For most diagnostic work, a sheath diameter between 17 and 21 French is adequate. For operative procedures, however, an outer sheath diameter of 24 to 27 French is needed. Newer outer sheaths for urethroscopy have omitted the fenestration along the lower border to allow visualization of the entire urethra from meatus to urethrovesical junction.

A recent innovation in endoscopic equipment is the flexible fiberoptic cystoscope. This instrument passes through the urethra more comfortably and is well suited for office urethrocystoscopy under local anesthesia. Another advantage is that the entire bladder and the inner surface of any urethral or bladder diverticula can be visualized because of the ability to deflect the telescope 180 degrees. The main disadvantage is that it is difficult to perform operative procedures because the operative channel is only 5 French in diameter. In addition, because the view afforded through the flexible urethrocystoscope is not as clear as that obtained through the rigid urethrocytoscope, greater operator skill is required to perform the procedure. There is no difference in postprocedural morbidity, including infection, as compared with the rigid urethrocystoscope.

Light Sources and Cables

Light sources are an integral part of endoscopic equipment. In general, most light sources are adequate. A light source with a built-in spare bulb that can be changed readily is advantageous because light failure during endoscopic procedure is a nuisance. Sophisticated light sources are available with brighter light for use with video and photographic equipment.

Light cables are either fiberoptic or fluid-filled. The fluid-filled cables tend to be more expensive and stronger, although they add a slight tint to the light. The fiber cables should be strong and in good condition, as broken fibers decrease the amount of light transmission. Broken fiberoptic fibers are easy to recognize because one can see light shining sideways along the length of the light cable or dark fibers when the cable is viewed straight on at low light levels.

Distention Media

Distention media can be divided into three different classifications: nonconductive fluids, conductive fluids, and gases such as air or carbon dioxide. Liquid distention media are the usual choice for cystoscopy. These solutions distend the lumen of the structure being examined and irrigate if blood or debris is encountered. The media used to distend the bladder or urethra must be transparent (so that the field of view is not obscured) and should not be irritating to the bladder. The media choice depends on the urethrocystoscopic procedure for which it will be used. For office diagnostic urethrocystoscopy, sterile water is an ideal medium in that it is relatively inexpensive and readily available. However, systemic absorption of large amounts of water can cause red blood cell hemolysis and electrolyte abnormalities. If absorption of a large volume of fluid into the vascular space is anticipated, an isosmotic solution, such as normal saline or glycine, should be used. Finally, if one expects to use electrocautery, as with a bladder biopsy, a nonconducting solution, such as water or glycine, should be used.

Delivery Systems

It is best not to use a distention pressure over 60 cm H_2O. Therefore, one should avoid hanging a fluid system higher than 60 cm above the bladder. Avoiding excessive infusion pressures limits the amount of fluid forced into the circulation and also prevents retrograde flow of fluid from the bladder up the ureters. The preferred temperature of infusion fluid for urethrocystoscopy is body temperature and should be no less than room temperature. The usual infusion delivery system is a simple 1-liter container of irrigant connected by tubing to the urethrocystoscope.

Ancillary Equipment: Biopsy Forceps, Diathermy Instruments, and Ureteral Catheter-Deflecting Bridge

The two basic types of biopsy forceps are flexible forceps and rigid forceps. The flexible forceps are used in areas more difficult to reach. However, they have a smaller bite capacity, making it more difficult to obtain the biopsy specimen. The rigid forceps allows

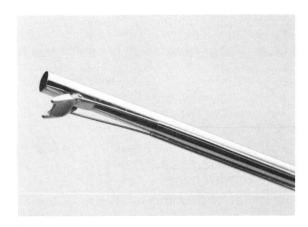

Fig. 10-3 Deflector at the tip of a catheter-deflecting bridge.

one to take repeated bites with much more accuracy. Rigid cup forceps are available in a larger angulated forceps and a smaller straight forceps. In addition, a variety of diathermy instruments can be used for both resection of the biopsy specimen and coagulation of bleeding areas.

The ureteral catheter-deflecting bridge (see Fig. 10-1, *top*) fits into a cystoscopic sheath, and the telescope fits through the bridge. Flexible ureteral catheters fit through the catheterizing port in the bridge. A deflector at the tip (Fig. 10-3) bends the catheter and is activated by the wheel control at the proximal end of the bridge.

Care and Maintenance of Equipment

Blood and other debris must be removed from the equipment to avoid both pitting of metal surfaces and their accumulation in crevices, which decrease the function of stopcocks and locking mechanisms. Cleansing of the equipment also decreases the build-up of opaque debris on the lens and light transmitting surfaces.

Sterilization of Instruments

Sterilization should not damage the delicate equipment and, particularly in an office setting, must be rapid. The most common method of sterilization is immersion of the equipment in 2% activated glutaraldehyde solution (Cidex; Surgikos, Inc, Arlington, Tx). The instruments are completely immersed in the Cidex solution for a minimum of 10 minutes between cases. The equipment must be completely rinsed after the sterilization because Cidex can build up inside the lumen of equipment and irritate the skin of both surgeon and patient. One must be careful to remove all Cidex from the lens to avoid eye irritation.

BASIC TECHNIQUE FOR OUTPATIENT URETHROCYSTOSCOPY

Indications and Contraindications

Urethrocystoscopy may be useful to evaluate many conditions in urogynecology. A list of suggested indications is shown in the accompanying box. It should always be performed when lower urinary tract malignancy is suspected, such as in the presence of microscopic or macroscopic hematuria or abnormal urinary cytology. Cystoscopy is also indicated in the evaluation of certain gynecologic malignancies, such as cervical or endometrial cancer, to assess for bladder involvement and to assist staging.

Women who have recurrent (more than three per year) or persistent urinary tract infections require an endoscopic examination to rule out an anatomic abnormality or intravesical calculus. It should be performed in patients who have frequency-urgency syndromes or painful bladder conditions of unknown etiology. Cystoscopy under anesthesia is required to make the diagnosis of interstitial cystitis.

Although urethrocystoscopy is routinely performed by many physicians to evaluate urinary incontinence, no data are currently available to justify its routine use. It probably should be performed in all recurrent cases of incontinence after surgical repairs to rule out stitch penetration or fistula formation. It may be beneficial in differentiating recurrent anatomic stress incontinence from urethral sphincteric (type III) incontinence. One can also perform an endoscopy in selected primary cases of incontinence if, after physical examination and urodynamic evaluation, the diagnosis is still in doubt, or other factors are thought to be possibly contributing to the patient's symptoms.

There are relatively few contraindications to performing urethrocystoscopy. Acute cystitis should be treated before elective cystoscopy is performed.

Suggested Indications for Urethrocystoscopy in Women

Hematuria
Abnormal urine cytology
Persistent or recurrent urinary tract infection (greater than three documented infections in 1 year)
Staging of gynecologic malignancies
Lower urinary tract fistula
Urethral or bladder diverticula
Painful bladder syndrome (including interstitial cystitis and urethral syndrome)
Selected cases of urinary incontinence, especially postsurgical recurrences

---

Prepping the Patient

Office cystoscopy can be performed safely using aseptic technique instead of full sterile surgical precautions. Fozard et al showed that there was no increased risk of postoperative urinary tract infection in patients who underwent outpatient urethrocystoscopy under aseptic technique. The patient's genital area should be thoroughly cleaned with an aqueous antiseptic solution. It is not necessary to shave the patient. The majority of patients can undergo urethrocystoscopy under topical anesthesia. A topical 2% lidocaine gel is placed on the sheath for anesthesia. It must be remembered that local anesthetic agents can cause a reddening of the urethra, making it difficult to assess the degree of inflammation. In patients who continue to have discomfort, a local anesthetic agent can be injected into the bladder pillars. Alternatively, the patient can be given oral or parenteral analgesia.

Occasionally, one encounters a patient who has stenosis of the distal urethra, which does not allow the passage of the endoscope. If the patient is postmenopausal and has urogenital atrophy, vaginal estrogen cream can be given for 3 weeks to try to decrease the amount of distal urethral stenosis. Some patients, however, require mechanical dilation to open the distal urethra to an adequate diameter to allow passage of an endoscope. In patients who fail urethral dilation, CO_2 laser can be used to vaporize the fibroelastic connective tissue band associated with distal urethral stenosis.

Performing Urethrocystoscopy

The technique for performing outpatient urethrocystoscopy begins by running the distention solution before inserting the urethrocystoscope into the distal urethra. This technique will distend the distal urethra and act as an obturator for the passage of the endoscope. The endoscope is advanced slowly through the entire length of the urethra noting the amount of inflammation, the presence of exudative material coming from the periurethral glands, or defects suggesting suburethral diverticulum. Anterior vaginal wall massage facilitates the expression of exudative material from either the periurethral glands or the orifice of a suburethral diverticulum. At the urethrovesical junction, the presence of inflammatory polyps or fronds is noted.

The endoscope then is advanced into the bladder. The infusion fluid can be turned off to avoid overdistending the bladder. The bladder is inspected systematically, beginning at the bladder neck and trigone. The ureteral orifices are inspected and bilateral passage of urine are documented. The bladder base, lateral and posterior walls, and dome of the bladder are inspected. The presence and location of bladder trabeculations, diverticula, bladder tumors, and other abnormalities are noted.

The endoscope is then withdrawn back into the proximal urethra so that the open bladder neck occupies approximately 30% of the field of vision. The sphincteric function of bladder neck is evaluated dynamically while the patient coughs and performs a Valsalva maneuver. One can observe failure or sluggish closing or even opening of the bladder neck in patients with incompetent urethral sphincter function. Funneling of the vesical neck, which the patient cannot inhibit, may occur in women with detrusor instability. Finally, the urethrovesical junction is occluded and the distending medium is turned on at a high flow rate to evaluate the urethra under pressure. This ma-

neuver often will reveal the orifice of a suburethral diverticulum.

Robertson described a technique of carbon dioxide urethrocystometry to visually evaluate the dynamic function of the bladder neck, while measuring intravesical and intraurethral pressures. This technique allows one not only to identify urethral pathology but to dynamically evaluate urethral sphincter and detrusor function during filling and in response to stressful maneuvers. Although the combination of urethrocystoscopy and urethrocystometry appears attractive, studies have not found it to be sensitive or specific in determining the etiology of urinary incontinence in women.

OPERATIVE URETHROCYSTOSCOPY

The usual indication for inpatient urethrocystoscopy is the evaluation of a bladder lesion that requires biopsy. Although biopsy sometimes can be performed in the office, it usually requires a large diameter sheath to allow the passage of a biopsy instrument, which adds to patient discomfort. One also must have the capability to coagulate the base of the biopsy site if bleeding is encountered; therefore, it is usually prudent to perform biopsies of bladder pathology in an operating room setting.

Endoscopy is an integral part of surgical procedures for stress incontinence, particularly during the performance of needle-suspension procedures. Urethrocystoscopy is performed to assure that no bladder entry has occurred and that the needles or sutures have not been passed inadvertently through the bladder or urethra. One can also evaluate the degree of elevation of the bladder neck during the tying of the suspensory sutures. Finally, intravenous indigo carmine (5 ml) can be given to evaluate ureteral patency.

PATHOLOGY OF THE URETHRA

A variety of soft tissue lesions, including urethral condylomata, caruncles, polyps, and tumors, can be present at the urethral meatus. These lesions should be evaluated by biopsy to rule out the rare case of urethral carcinoma. The normal caliber of the female

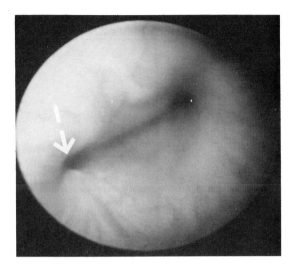

Fig. 10-4 Urethroscopic view of the orifice of a sub-urethral diverticulum *(arrow)*. The proximal urethral orifice is at the upper right side.

urethra is 18 to 28 French, although it is not uncommon to find an asymptomatic woman who has a smaller distal urethal caliber. Patients with meatal stenosis can present with complaints of difficult or irritative voiding; these symptoms may be related to stenosis caused by a fibroelastic connective tissue band between the urethral and vaginal epithelia. These patients can usually be treated with a variety of modalities including topical estrogens, urethral dilations, or laser excision of the fibroelastic connective tissue band.

Suburethral diverticula are found in approximately 3% of women. Patients present with a variety of symptoms including dysuria, dyspareunia, anterior vaginal wall mass or tenderness, incontinence, and postvoid dribbling. Diverticula can be caused by repeated infections of the periurethral glands and obstruction of their ducts. Relatively few are congenital. Diverticula are usually located in the posterior wall of and in the mid to distal segment of the urethra. Urethroscopically, one can see either the orifice to the diverticulum (Fig. 10-4) or a dropping out of the urethral floor at the level of the diverticulum. Multiple diverticula are not uncommon and a single diverticulum can have several orifices. In about half the cases, one can express pus from the diverticulum by massaging the urethra; however, this maneuver also may express fluid or exudate from the openings of the periurethral glands along the posterior aspect of the urethra or even from the Skene's glands.

The normal female urethra has a pinkish appearance. However, due to postmenopausal mucosal atrophy, or chronic irritation from either repeated urethral infections or urethral syndrome, the urethra may appear hyperemic or inflamed. Chalky exudate may be expressed from periurethral glands, and inflammatory polyps may be present at the bladder neck. The diagnosis of urethral syndrome is made by excluding other causes of acute cystitis and acute urethritis (see Chapter 20). Women with urethral syndrome present with a myriad of symptoms including urinary urgency, frequency, dysuria, suprapubic or low back pain, and voiding difficulties. Urine cultures are negative, as frequently are the urethral cultures for chlamydia or *Neisseria gonorrhoeae*. Postmenopausal patients with urethral mucosal atrophy usually exhibit other signs of estrogen deficiency of the lower genital tract.

PATHOLOGY OF THE BLADDER

In about half of women, the bladder trigone can be covered by an atypical-appearing epithelium, which has the appearance of a pearly gray-white granular epithelium known as squamous metaplasia (Fig. 10-5). This appearance has been referred to in the past as pseudomembranous trigonitis. The etiology of squamous metaplasia of the trigone is not completely understood. It has not been found to be premalignant; therefore, biopsy is not indicated.

Interstitial cystitis was first described in 1914 by Hunner who reported an unusual bladder ulcer in women. Patients with this disease can present with urinary frequency, urgency, nocturia, and pain on bladder distention. Patients also complain of suprapubic pain, which is relieved or diminished by voiding. If a diagnosis of interstitial cystitis is being considered, patients should undergo urethrocystoscopy under general anesthesia because they may not tolerate bladder filling and because biopsies may be necessary. The bladder needs to be initially filled and emptied. Occasionally, pinpoint petechial hemorrhages are de-

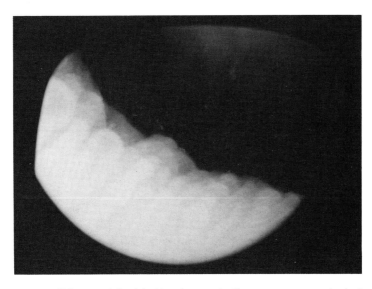

Fig. 10-5 Trigone of the bladder demonstrating squamous metaplasia.

tected on first filling. On second distention, two urethrocystoscopic patterns become evident. The minority of patients have the classic Hunner ulcers (defined as deeply red areas with a granulating base and congested vessels surrounding the area) or linear cracks and scars along the bladder mucosa. The majority of patients have urethrocystoscopic findings described by Walsh as mucosal glomerulations with red strawberry-like dots, which often coalesce to become hemorrhagic spots that ooze blood from the bladder mucosa. Occasionally, the hemorrhage forms a checkerboard pattern. Glomerulations tend to be more prominent on the bladder dome and are rarely present on the trigone. The quantity of glomerulation is variable and does not correlate with severity of disease. A reduced bladder capacity is another characteristic cystoscopic finding.

Bladder biopsies are usually performed to confirm the diagnosis. Characteristic histologic findings include inflammation, fibrosis, mastocytosis, submucosal edema, and an increased number of capillaries in the lamina propria.

Hemorrhagic cystitis is an entity with a similar urethrocystoscopic appearance. Hemorrhagic cystitis can be caused by radiation therapy, viral infection, drug therapy (particularly cyclophosphamide), and trauma. The amount of hemorrhage varies from slight to severe. Urethrocystoscopy reveals blood vessel telangiectasias, mucosal ulcerations, mucosal edema, and submucosal hemorrhage. Bladder capacity is characteristically reduced. Bleeding can be controlled with lavage, cystoscopic fulguration, installation of sclerosing agents, or hyperbaric oxygen therapy.

The bladder can also be chronically inflamed by a variety of infectious disorders, including viruses and tuberculosis. Rarely does one see condylomata in the bladder. Small bladder tumors also can be seen during urethrocystoscopy and need to be evaluated by biopsy.

Patients who have an anatomic bladder outlet obstruction need to generate high intravesical pressures in order to void. This need can be important in the genesis of bladder trabeculations, which are thickenings of the interdigitating detrusor musculature. Patients that have detrusor instability also can have bladder trabeculations.

Bladder diverticula also can be caused by bladder outlet obstruction. Bladder diverticula are diagnosed by the presence of an outpouching of a small area of the bladder wall with an ostium of varying size. Urine cytology should be performed, as a neoplasm sometimes arises within the diverticulum.

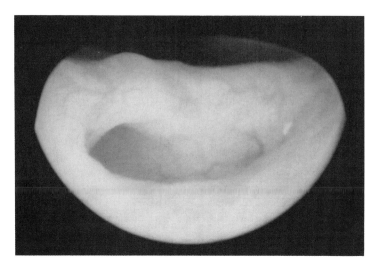

Fig. 10-6 A vesicovaginal fistula *(bottom)*.

Endoscopy is useful in the evaluation of lower urinary tract fistulas including vesicovaginal (Fig. 10-6), urethrovaginal, and ureterovaginal. Bladder fistulas also can occur to other structures, such as vesicocutaneous fistulas. Large fistulas can be easily diagnosed by the leakage of infusing fluid, thus preventing adequate distention of the bladder. The mucosal edges of a fistula caused by surgery are often edematous or hyperemic secondary to irritation or infection. Fistulas related to malignancy are often surrounded by a necrotic mass and friable mucosa.

Patients with bladder stones can present with a variety of symptoms, particularly irritative voiding symptoms or bladder instability. Bladder stones are of varying sizes and have a shaggy appearance due to the accumulation of debris on their surface.

COMPLICATIONS AND POSTURETHROCYSTOSCOPY CARE

The incidence of bacteriuria following outpatient office urethrocystoscopy is approximately 2%. Manson prospectively compared the incidence of cystitis in a group of patients who received a 3-day course of postcystoscopy antibiotics with a group who did not receive antibiotic treatment. There was no statistically significant increase in the incidence of posturethro-cystoscopy infections in patients not treated with antibiotics. Other studies, however, have shown a higher incidence of bacteriuria in untreated patients. The risk of posturethrocystoscopy bacteriuria may be highest in women with a history of multiple lower urinary tract infections. It is not unreasonable to give the patient a short course of antibiotics after urethrocystoscopy. Patients commonly complain of dysuria after urethrocystoscopy and should receive a short course of a urinary analgesic (phenazopyridine).

If difficulty is encountered in passing the cystoscope into the urethra, one can traumatize the urethra and possibly create false passages. If one is not visualizing introduction of the urethrocystoscope into the bladder, bladder perforation can occur. Nevertheless, because the incidence of complications from office urethrocystoscopy is exceeding low, office urethrocystoscopy should remain a valid tool in the armamentarium of the urogynecologist.

BIBLIOGRAPHY
History

Gunning JE, Rosenzweig BA: Evolution of endoscopic surgery. In White RA, Klein SR (eds): *Endoscopic surgery,* St Louis, 1991, Mosby–Year Book.
Ridley JH: Indirect air cystoscopy, *South Med J* 44:114, 1951.

Robertson JR: Gynecologic urethroscopy, *Am J Obstet Gynecol* 115:986, 1973.

Robertson JR: Air cystoscopy, *Obstet Gynecol* 32:328, 1968.

Robertson JR: Office cystoscopy—substituting the culdoscope for the Kelly cystoscope, *Obstet Gynecol* 28:219, 1966.

Equipment

Aso Y, Yokoyama M, Fukutani K, et al: New trial for fiberoptic cystourethroscopy—the use of metal sheath, *J Urol* 115:99, 1976.

Bagley DH, Huffman JL, Lyon ES: *Urologic endoscopy—a manual and atlas*, Boston, 1985, Little, Brown.

Fowler CG: Fiberscope urethrocystoscopy, *Br J Urol* 56:304, 1984.

Fowler CG, Badenoch DF, Thakar DR: Practical experience with flexible fiberscope cystoscopy in out-patients, *Br J Urol* 56:618, 1984.

Hargreave TB: Practical urological endoscopy, Oxford, 1988, Blackwell Scientific Publications.

Matthews PN, Bidgood KA, Woodhouse RJ: CO_2 cystoscopy using a flexible fiberoptic endoscopy, *Br J Urol* 56:188, 1984.

Matthews PN, Skewes DG, Kothari JJ, et al: Carbon dioxide versus water for cystoscopy: a comparative study, *Br J Urol* 55:364, 1983.

Basic Technique

Aldridge CW, Beaton JH, Nanzig RP: A review of office urethroscopy and cystometry, *Am J Obstet Gynecol* 131:432, 1978.

Green LF, Khan AU: Cystourethroscopy in the female, *Urology* 10:461, 1977.

O'Donnell P: Water endoscopy. In Raz S (ed): *Female urology*, Philadelphia, 1983, WB Saunders.

Robertson JR: Gas endoscopy. In Raz S (ed): *Female urology*, Philadelphia, 1983, WB Saunders.

Robertson JR: Dynamic urethroscopy. In Ostergard DR (ed): *Gynecologic urology and urodynamics*, ed 2, Baltimore, 1985, Williams and Wilkins.

Romero RE, Hicks TH, Galindo GH, et al: Evaluation of the importance of cystoscopy in staging gynecologic carcinomas, *J Urol* 121:64, 1979.

Rosenzweig BA, Bhatia NN: The use of carbon dioxide laser in female urology, *J Gynecol Surg* 7:11, 1991.

Sand PK, Hill RC, Ostergard DR: Supine urethroscopic and standing cystometry as screening methods for the detection of detrusor instability, *Obstet Gynecol* 70:57, 1987.

Scotti RJ, Ostergard DR, Guillaume AA, et al: Predictive value of urethroscopy as compared to urodynamics in the diagnosis of genuine stress incontinence, *J Reprod Med* 35:772, 1990.

Uehling DT: The normal caliber of the adult female urethra, *J Urol* 120:176, 1978.

Worth PH: Cystourethroscopy. In Stanton SL (ed): *Clinical gynecologic urology*, St Louis, 1984, Mosby–Year Book.

Pathology

Anderson MJ: The incidence of diverticula in the female urethra, *J Urol* 98:96, 1967.

Bergman A, Karram M, Bhatia NN: Urethral syndrome: a comparison of different treatment modalities, *J Reprod Med* 34:157, 1989.

Davis BL, Robinson DG: Diverticula of the female urethra: assay of 120 cases, *J Urol* 104:850, 1970.

Hunner GL: A rare type of bladder ulcer in women: report of cases, *Trans South Surg Gynecol Assoc* 27:247, 1914.

Lee RA: Diverticulum of the urethra. Clinical presentation, diagnosis and management, *Clin Obstet Gynecol* 27:490, 1984.

Lyon RP, Smith DR: Distal urethral stenosis, *J Urol* 89:414, 1963.

MacDermott JP, Charpied GC, Tesluk H, et al: Can histological assessment predict the outcome in interstitial cystitis? *Br J Urol* 67:44, 1991.

Marshall FC, Uson AC, Melicow MM: Neoplasms and caruncles of the female urethra, *Surg Gynecol Obstet* 110:723, 1960.

Messing EM, Stamey TA: Interstitial cystitis: early diagnosis, pathology, and treatment, *Urology* 12:381, 1978.

Numazaki Y, Kumasaka T, Yano N, et al: Further study on acute hemorrhagic cystitis due to adenovirus type II, *N Engl J Med* 289:344, 1973.

Mufson MA, Belshe RB, Horrigan TJ, et al: Cause of acute hemorrhagic cystitis in children, *Am J Dis Child* 126:605, 1973.

Richardson FH: External urethroplasty in women: technique and clinical evaluation, *J Urol* 101:719, 1969.

Scotti RJ, Ostergard DR: The urethral syndrome, *Clin Obstet Gynecol* 27:515, 1984.

Summary of the National Institute of Arthritis, Diabetes, Digestive and Kidney Diseases workshop on interstitial cystitis, National Institute of Health. Bethesda, Maryland, August 28-29, 1987, *J Urol* 140:203, 1988.

Walsh A: Interstitial cystitis. In Harrison JH, Gittes RF, Perlmutter AD, et al (eds): *Campbell's urology*, ed 4, Philadelphia, 1979, WB Saunders.

Complications and Postcystoscopy Care

Clark KR, Higgs MJ: Urinary infection following out-patient flexible cystoscopy, *Br J Urol* 66:503, 1990.

Denholm SW, Conn IG, Newsam JE, et al: Morbidity following cystoscopy: comparison of flexible and rigid techniques, *Br J Urol* 66:503, 1990.

Fozard JB, Green DF, Harrison GS, et al: Asepsis and out-patient cystoscopy, *Br J Urol* 55:680, 1983.

Manson AL: Is antibiotic administration indicated after out-patient cystoscopy? *J Urol* 140:316, 1988.

Marier R, Valenti AJ, Madri JA: Gram-negative endocarditis following cystoscopy, *J Urol* 119:134, 1978.

Richards B, Bastable JR: Bacteriuria after outpatient cystoscopy, *Br J Urol* 49:561, 1977.

CHAPTER 11

Radiologic Studies of the Lower Urinary Tract

Bruce A. Rosenzweig

Plain Films of the Abdomen
Intravenous Pyelogram
Cystourethrography
    Anteroposterior and lateral films
    Typical cystourographic findings
    Abnormal findings during cystourethrography
Positive Pressure Urethrography
Video-Cystourethrography
Ultrasound
MRI

Radiologic studies are an integral part of the evaluation of patients with dysfunction of the lower urinary tract. A variety of invasive and noninvasive techniques have evolved for this evaluation. The intravenous pyelogram was the first diagnostic radiographic test performed for urologic patients. In 1923, Osborne and associates noted that urine in the bladder was opaque on x-ray film in a group of patients treated for syphilis with large intravenous doses of sodium iodine.

In 1942, Barnes reported using chains of beads to radiographically determine urethral configuration. Later, Ball et al used a Foley catheter to evaluate urethral position radiographically. In 1949, Muellner used fluoroscopic techniques to demonstrate that de-scent of the bladder base during coughing resulted in funneling of the bladder neck. Jeffcoate and Roberts, in 1952, observed that patients with genuine stress urinary incontinence have loss of the posterior urethrovesical angle on cystourethrography. The technique of cine-roentgenography of the lower urinary tract was introduced in the 1950s to aid in the detection of normal and pathologic dynamic function of the bladder and urethra. Currently, ultrasound and magnetic resonance imaging (MRI) have become the focus of radiologic evaluation of the lower urinary tract. This chapter reviews both contrast and noncontrast techniques of lower urinary tract evaluation.

PLAIN FILMS OF THE ABDOMEN

The flat plate of the abdomen can be used as a scout film for intravenous pyelogram (IVP), or it can be used to screen for urinary stones. Because of the radiodensity of calcium found in the majority of stones, a significant number of them will be detected on a routine film.

INTRAVENOUS PYELOGRAM

IVP remains the most frequently performed contrast-agent-enhanced procedure in diagnostic radiology. IVP is the basic screening tool for many urologic and

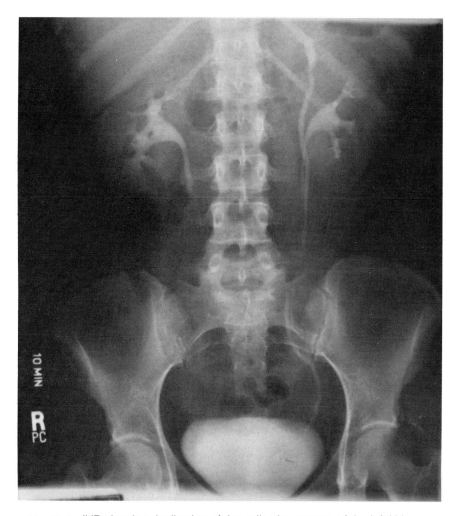

Fig. 11-1   IVP showing duplication of the collecting system of the left kidney.

urogynecologic abnormalities. It is part of the evaluation of women who have recurrent urinary tract infections to diagnose occult urinary tract stones or congenital abnormalities (such as duplication of the collecting system or ureters) (Fig. 11-1). An IVP is important in the initial assessment of hematuria. It also can be used to detect structural abnormalities such as bladder or suburethral diverticula (Fig. 11-2), particularly on the postvoid film.

Although the IVP is an integral part of the evaluation and staging of gynecologic malignancies, considerable debate has continued regarding routine IVPs before benign gynecologic surgery to avoid urologic injuries. Many clinicians use the IVP to trace the course of the pelvic ureters when evaluating patients with a large pelvic mass or myomatous uterus. Some believe that radiologic knowledge of the course of the ureters can facilitate intraoperative identification and avoid injury. Several studies, however, have failed to demonstrate a distinct advantage of IVPs in decreasing the rate of operative injury to the lower urinary tract. These studies noted that the most important information obtained from a preoperative IVP is the presence of a congenital anomaly of the urinary tract.

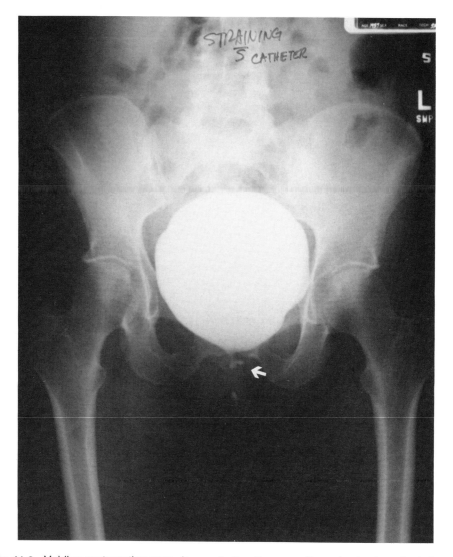

Fig. 11-2 Voiding cystourethrogram demonstrating three small proximal suburethral diverticula.

Postoperatively, however, IVP is an important element in the management of patients with a suspected ureteral injury (Fig. 11-3). These patients may present with (1) major operative complication, (2) development of unilateral or bilateral costovertebral angle tenderness, or (3) persistent fever despite appropriate antibiotic treatment for longer than 48 hours.

The three main risks and side effects of the IVP are: (1) exposure of the patient to ionizing radiation, (2) the possibility of allergic reaction to contrast agents, and (3) the potentially nephrotoxic effect of the contrast agents.

CYSTOURETHROGRAPHY

Cystourethrography is a useful imaging study for the evaluation of urogynecologic complaints. Cystourethrography determines the resting location of the urethrovesical junction in relation to the symphysis pubis as well as the amount of its downward and posterior

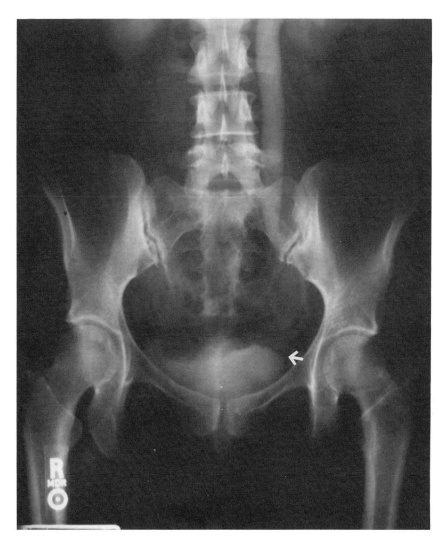

Fig. 11-3 IVP of a postoperative patient with left ureteral obstruction and hydroureter.

movement during strain. The main indications for this test include dysuria, irritative voiding symptoms, and urinary incontinence. It can also be helpful to detect suburethral diverticula and tumors and stones of both the upper and lower urinary tracts (Fig. 11-4). The main contraindication is acute urinary infection; indeed, the major complication associated with this procedure is infection to the lower urinary tract. This is why many advocate the use of prophylactic antibiotics for the procedure.

Typically a radiopaque solution containing either an organic iodine compound or a 10% to 20% solution of sodium iodine is used as the contrast agent. The selection of appropriate contrast material is of great importance. Some agents can irritate the bladder, leading to bladder or urethral spasm, mucosal irregularities, vesicoureteral reflux or uncontrolled urine loss. In a double-blind study evaluating the irritative properties of contrast agents, Shopfner found that diatrizoate meglumine and diatrizoate sodium (Hypaque)

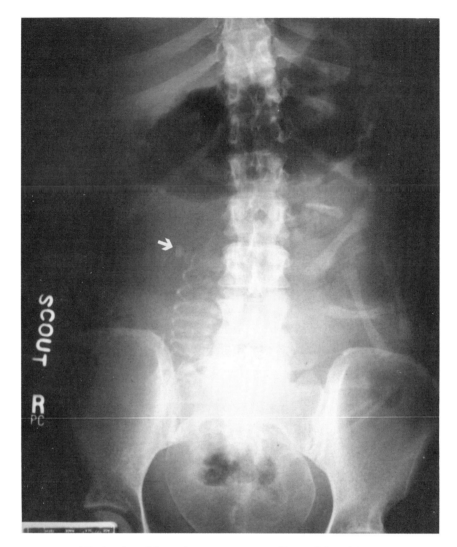

Fig. 11-4 AP view in a 32-week pregnancy revealing a right mid-ureteral stone.

is less noxious, whereas sodium acetrizoate (Cystokon) can be quite irritating.

The technique for performing standard cystourethrography is as follows. First, the patient is asked to empty her bladder and the postvoid residual urine volume is measured. The bladder is filled to capacity with contrast under low pressure. A catheter filled with contrast can be left in the urethra to help delineate the urethrovesical junction. Stanton has described the use of opaque materials of different viscosities as a

modification of this technique. A heavy barium paste is introduced into the urethra followed by a lighter radiopaque dye. The barium paste is used to highlight the urethrovesical junction and bladder base, whereas the more viscous dye outlines the remainder of the bladder. Anteroposterior (AP) and oblique views are obtained to provide visualization of vesicoureteral reflux and to determine the overall shape of the bladder. Next, the patient is placed in the standing position and AP and lateral films are obtained in both relaxed and straining positions. The patient is moved to the 30-degree oblique position, the catheter is removed, and the presence or absence of urinary incontinence is noted. The position of the bladder neck and the urethra in relation to the inferior border of the pubic symphysis is also noted. Films are then taken with the patient coughing to determine again if urine loss occurs. Finally, the patient is asked to void to obtain voiding and postvoid films.

Another technique advocated by Pochaczevsky and Grabstald is a double-contrast barium with carbon dioxide cystogram. This technique is particularly useful for evaluating bladder tumors. The bladder is first filled with sterile isotonic saline followed by 6 oz of barium sulfate. Films are then obtained. Next, 100 to 200 ml of carbon dioxide are added to the bladder and three additional films are taken. The carbon dioxide sits above the barium solution and gives a double-contrast image of the bladder.

Anteroposterior and Lateral Films

AP films are used mostly to study mobility and position of the bladder base. In the normal state during increased abdominal pressure, the bladder base should not descend below the level of the inferior border of the symphysis pubis. If a cystocele is present, however, the bladder base can descend below the inferior border of the symphysis pubis. It is difficult on an AP film to differentiate prolapse of the bladder base (distention cystocele) from prolapse of the urethrovesical junction or urethra (displacement cystocele) because these structures will be superimposed on one another, causing them to be obscured.

The lateral film assesses anatomic relationships of the lower urinary tract. It determines both the position of the bladder neck and urethra and also the degree of cystocele present. With a cystocele, the bladder base descends below the inferior ramus of the pubic symphysis. Straining films help to visualize the amount of descent and mobility of the bladder neck and urethra.

Oblique straining films in the upright position are also obtained during routine cystourethrography. These films can help verify if funneling of the bladder neck demonstrated on the lateral film is truly present. The cough film can demonstrate leakage of urine

through the entire length of the urethra in patients that have incompetence of the urethral sphincter mechanism. The last films obtained are the voiding and postvoiding films. These films are important to evaluate contractility of the bladder during voiding and the presence of significant postvoid residual urine volume.

Typical Cystourographic Findings

The bladder of the newborn is positioned high in the pelvis, but with advancing age, the bladder descends and in many cases lies at the level of the symphysis pubis. When filled with contrast material, the bladder distends upwards approximately symmetrically; when filled to maximum capacity, it assumes a round or oval shape. The base of the bladder is somewhat flat in the supine position, but on standing can assume a conical shape. Patients with acute or chronic cystitis may experience swelling of the mucosa, which causes irregularity of the borders of the bladder and prominent mucosal folds. These folds also can be seen when the bladder is actively contracting or when there is bladder outlet obstruction.

The urethra is a tubular structure running downward and forward from the bladder base. It can course in either a vertical or horizontal manner depending on the amount of descent of the bladder base with strain. There is a great deal of variability in the width of the urethra, and a number of shapes have been described including cylindrical fusiform, cone shaped, wineglass shaped, hourglass shaped, or string shaped. The distal urethra, because of its "nonelastic" collagen tissue composition, is nondistendable.

Abnormal Findings During Cystourethrography

The cystourethrogram was regarded previously as the most decisive study in the evaluation of stress urinary incontinence. Green thought that the cystourethrogram not only confirmed the anatomic defect responsible for stress incontinence, but also excluded incontinence of other causes. Green described two anatomic defects of stress incontinence based on cystourethrographic findings. Type I incontinence is associated with the loss of the posterior urethrovesical angle (greater than 115 degrees), with maintenance of the angle of in-

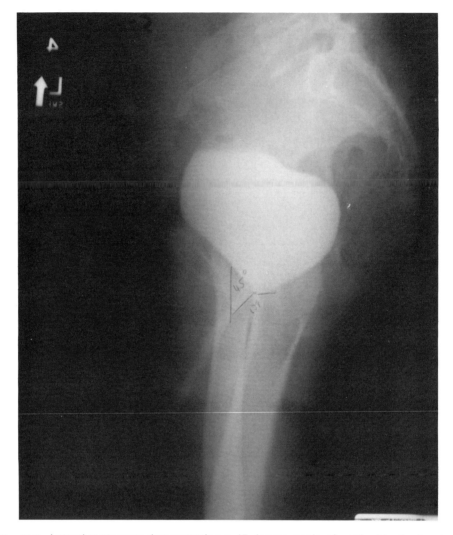

Fig. 11-5 Lateral cystogram demonstrating a 45-degree angle of urethral inclination in a woman with stress urinary incontinence and a posterior urethrovesical angle of 139 degrees.

clination of the urethral axis (less than 30 degrees). Type II incontinence is associated with loss of both angles (Fig. 11-5); however, Drutz et al found poor correlation between these radiographic findings and urodynamic results. Because of this and other studies, the preceding classification is no longer considered valid for women with stress incontinence.

Cystourethrography can be helpful in detecting neurologic conditions affecting bladder contractility.

An overactive bladder can appear as a pine tree shape or may be associated with urethral funneling. The bladder also can assume an hourglass appearance. A poorly contracting hypotonic bladder can appear as a large contrast-filled balloon, possibly containing bladder calculi.

The voiding cystourethrogram is particularly useful in documenting vesicoureteral reflux, which can be present in patients who have a history of frequent

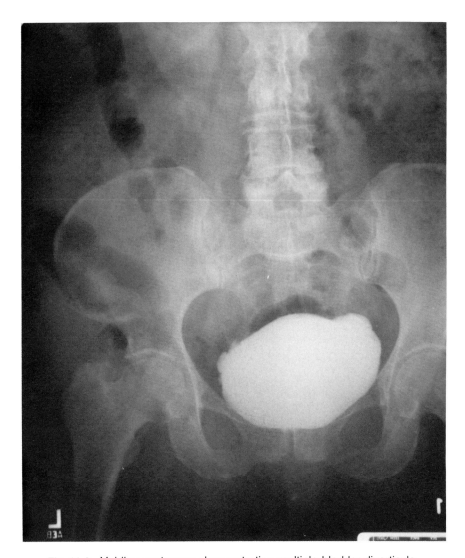

Fig. 11-6 Voiding cystogram demonstrating multiple bladder diverticula.

urinary tract infections and pyelonephritis. This finding is often associated with typical renal radiologic abnormalities.

Bladder diverticula (Fig. 11-6) are rarely found in women, accounting for only 3.4% of all bladder diverticula. They can be caused by congenital weak spots in the detrusor muscle, but are more frequently associated with bladder outlet obstruction, resulting in increased intravesical pressure. Other causes of acquired bladder diverticula are chronic inflammation,

bladder tumors, and stones. Patients with bladder diverticula usually present with frequency, urgency, dysuria, and hematuria. The most important film to demonstrate bladder diverticula is the oblique projection.

Bladder trabeculations are another sign of outlet obstruction or may be the result of chronic cystitis. Radiographically, trabeculations (Fig. 11-7) manifest as an increase in internal foldings of the bladder mucosa.

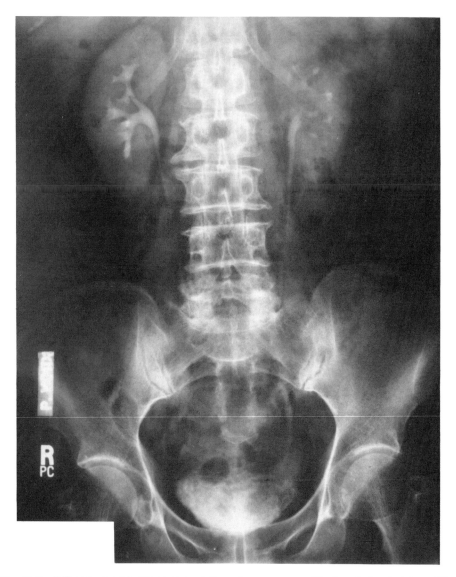

Fig. 11-7 IVP showing bladder trabeculations in a woman with chronic bacterial cystitis.

Tumors of the bladder can be detected with a cystourethrogram. They appear as a filling defect in the bladder, although carcinoma of the bladder is much less common in women than in men. Radiation cystitis presents as a small capacity bladder with irregular bladder folds caused by impaired circulation with inflammation, necrosis, ulceration, and scar formation.

Vesicovaginal or vesicouterine fistulas can be de-tected by noting spill of contrast material from the bladder into the vagina (Fig. 11-8). Small fistulas, which do not allow the passage of a significant amount of contrast, however, may not be seen radiographically. Urethral disorders that can be diagnosed using voiding cystourethrography include suburethral diverticula and urethrovaginal fistulas.

A metallic bead chain can be used in conjunction with cystography to describe the anatomic relation-

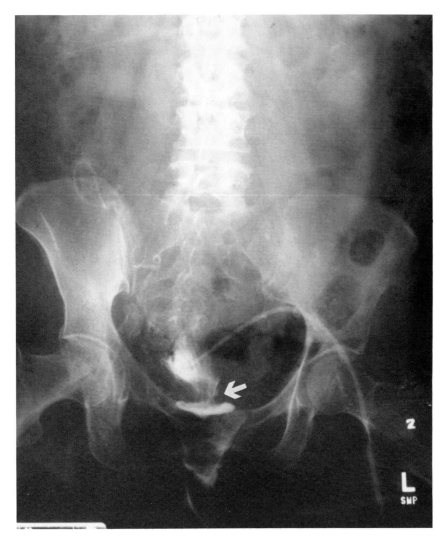

Fig. 11-8 Retrograde contrast installation into the bladder via a urethral catheter demonstrating a vesicovaginal fistula.

ships between the urethrovesical junction and the urethra. The bead chain is used to highlight the urethra and bladder neck. The technique entails placing the beaded chain measuring 25 cm long and 3 mm in diameter into the bladder through a soft bisected 18 French catheter. A contrast agent is then instilled to outline the bladder. Films are taken in the AP and lateral positions, with and without the patient straining. Various anatomic relationships, such as the presence of cystocele, the presence of stress urinary in-

continence, and the postoperative state, have been described and correlated with normal and abnormal findings. In studies by Kitzmiller et al and Greenwald et al, however, the utility of bead-chain studies were questioned. These studies found significant overlap in radiographic findings between women with stress urinary incontinence and continent parous women. Most investigators presently do not use bead-chain cystourethrography in the evaluation of genuine stress urinary incontinence.

POSITIVE PRESSURE URETHROGRAPHY

The use of positive pressure urethrography was first introduced by Davis and Cian in 1956 to evaluate the urethral anatomy. They described filling the female urethra with contrast using a double-balloon catheter to ensure a closed system. Before the advent of the double-balloon catheter, suburethral diverticula were rarely diagnosed. Since the introduction of this technique, suburethral diverticula have been found in approximately 3% of women.

Greenberg et al described six findings on positive pressure urethrography. Type I is considered normal. Type II, considered a normal variant, is a distal urethral ballooning, which is a symmetric dilation of the distal end of the urethra. Type III is proximal ballooning, which is thought to reflect the opening of the internal urethral sphincter by the pressure of the proximal balloon. Type IV is filling of the distal periurethral or Skene's glands. The majority of women with a type IV pattern remain asymptomatic; however, occasionally these patients require a surgical procedure to excise a mass near the external urethral meatus or to relieve symptoms of obstruction voiding. Type V is a localized outpouching of the urethral walls, and type VI is a definitive suburethral diverticulum.

Positive pressure urethrography is important in the diagnosis and management of suburethral diverticula because, on physical examination and cystoscopy, suburethral diverticula often are missed. This technique should be used in conjunction with a voiding cystourethrogram because the exact number and location of diverticula are not always determined with the double-balloon catheter.

VIDEO-CYSTOURETHROGRAPHY

Video-cystourethrography combines a fluoroscopic voiding cystourethrogram with simultaneous recording of intravesical and intraurethral pressures. This technique allows the visual assessment of urethral sphincter and bladder function while synchronously recording urodynamic data provided by pressure/flow studies. Bates et al evaluated over 200 patients using cine-pressure-flow cystourethrography and found that, although the investigation is complicated, it is not unduly difficult to perform and is undoubtedly valuable in select cases. Their data showed that video-cystourethrography can conclusively differentiate cough-induced stress incontinence from cough-induced urge incontinence. Their study also found that cinecystogram can evaluate both proximal and distal urethral sphincter incompetence. They believed that this method was the best approach available for the assessment of more complicated cases of urinary incontinence.

ULTRASOUND

The use of ultrasound for the evaluation of upper urinary tract function has evolved from merely using the bladder as a transparent window to scan pelvic structures. As opposed to conventional radiologic techniques, ultrasound is noninvasive, does not require contrast material, and does not expose the patient to ionizing radiation. Ultrasound is used to evaluate the upper urinary tract, particularly for the detection of hydronephrosis and renal stones, and to assess renal parenchyma. It also can be used to detect structural abnormalities of the lower tract, including bladder tumors and suburethral diverticula.

Recently, sonographic techniques have been used to evaluate stress urinary incontinence. Ultrasound has been used to detect anatomic alterations associated with genuine stress incontinence, to select the appropriate type of surgery, to assess surgical results (both intraoperatively and postoperatively), and to assess postoperative complications.

Transabdominal ultrasound of the lower urinary tract was the first method. The bladder neck can be seen on transabdominal ultrasound, but it is occasionally hidden behind the symphysis pubis. The bladder neck is especially difficult to locate in obese patients and in women with severe genitourinary prolapse. A urethral catheter may be needed to demonstrate the urethral axis. Transabdominal ultrasound can be used to determine the extent of mobility of the bladder and urethra and to detect detrusor instability in some patients. Finally, bladder and postvoid residual volumes can be determined with transabdominal scanning, although accuracy is not reliable for volumes less than 50 ml.

The bladder is scanned in two perpendicular planes

(transverse and sagittal) and three diameters (height, width, and depth) are measured. Height corresponds to the greatest superoinferior measurement; depth corresponds to the greatest AP measurement. Both are obtained in a sagittal plane scan. Width corresponds to the greatest transverse measurement obtained with a transverse plane scan. The simplest formula used to estimate volume is vol = $(H \times W \times D)(0.7)$. The correction factor of 0.7 is needed because the shape of the bladder is not circular until it is almost completely full. The same formula can be used for premicturition and postmicturition volume assessments. The error rate of this formula is approximately 21%.

Endosonography (vaginal and rectal procedures) involves probes of higher frequencies than transabdominal linear array scanners and, therefore, affords sharper, better focused pictures with high resolution. The endosonographic probes avoid interference from the symphysis pubis and subcutaneous fat. Transrectal sonography produces a good view of the bladder, urethra, and bladder neck, although the rectal probe can occasionally alter the alignment of the bladder neck. Patients find rectal sonography embarrassing and uncomfortable. Vaginal probes are better tolerated by patients, but they limit the degree of bladder neck movement during Valsalva maneuvers or coughing. They cannot be used in patients with significant pelvic relaxation.

Newer applications of sonography place the transducer on the perineum or just between the labia minora (introital sonography). These scanning techniques do not alter anatomic relationships, are not affected by patient straining, and can be used in patients with genitourinary prolapse.

Ultrasound evaluation of the bladder neck and urethra provides a wide range of information for the urogynecologist. The position of the bladder neck in the relaxed state and the degree of displacement with reference to the symphysis pubis can be measured. This information can be helpful in determining the type of surgical procedure. Surgical correction of the anatomic defect can be assessed intraoperatively or postoperatively. Detrusor contractions with concomitant funneling of the bladder neck are occasionally detected during scanning. Finally, postoperative voiding difficulties can be evaluated sonographically to determine the location of obstruction and the volume of residual urine.

MRI

MRI is rapidly becoming an important diagnostic tool in the assessment of pelvic pathology. It is noninvasive and does not require ionizing radiation. It also is more accurate than ultrasound in the detection of discrete structures, and its multiplanar imaging capabilities offer advantages over computerized tomography scanning.

MRI can be useful in detecting thickening of the bladder wall. The normal bladder is thin walled and cannot be identified as a discrete structure, but bladder tumors can be differentiated from both normal bladder wall and urine on MRI. MRI has been used to evaluate the pelvic floor musculature in an attempt to determine morphology and quality of the pelvic floor muscles. It has also been used for imaging the female urethra. Normal urethral structures imaged include the intrinsic urethral musculature, total urethral length, urethral wall thickness, intrinsic urethral function such as closure and coaptation, and periurethral musculature and connective tissue. MRI also can be used to detect various abnormalities of the urethra including scarring and diverticula. Finally, MRI has been applied in the evaluation and management of stress urinary incontinence. It may be beneficial in differentiating genuine stress incontinence resulting from malposition of the bladder neck from stress incontinence due to intrinsic urethral damage.

BIBLIOGRAPHY
X-ray Studies

Ball TL: Topographic urethrography. Part I, *Am J Obstet Gynecol* 59:1243, 1950.

Ball TL, Douglas RG, Fulkerson LL: Topographic urethrography: part II, *Am J Obstet Gynecol* 59:1252, 1950.

Barnes AC: The roentgenologic study of urethral sphincter strength in the female, *J Urol* 47:694, 1942.

Bates CP, Whiteside CG, Turner-Warwick R: Synchronous cine/pressure/flow/cysto-urethrography with special reference to stress and urge incontinence, *Br J Urol* 42:714, 1970.

Davis JH, Cian LG: Positive pressure urethrography: a new diagnostic method, *J Urol* 75:753, 1956.

Dawson P: Intravenous urography revisited, *Br J Urol* 66:561, 1990.

Drutz HP, Shapiro BJ, Mandel F: Do static cystourethrograms have a role in the investigation of female incontinence? *Am J Obstet Gynecol* 130:516, 1978.

Green TH: Development of a plan for the diagnosis and treatment of urinary stress incontinence, *Am J Obstet Gynecol* 83:632, 1962.

Greenberg M, Stone D, Cochran ST, et al: Female urethral diverticula: double-balloon catheter study. *Am J Roentgenol* 136:259, 1981.

Greenwald SW, Thronbury JR, Dunn LJ: Cystourethrography as a diagnostic aid in stress incontinence: an evaluation, *Obstet Gynecol* 29:324, 1967.

Hertz M: Cystourethrography. A radiographic atlas, *Excerpta Medica* 1973.

Hodgkinson CP: Relationships of the female urethra and bladder in urinary stress incontinence, *Am J Obstet Gynecol* 65:560, 1953.

Hodgkinson CP, Doub HP: Roentgen study of urethrovesical relationships in female urinary stress incontinence, *Radiology* 61:335, 1953.

Hodgkinson CP, Doub HP, Kelly WT: Urethrocystograms: metallic bead chain technique, *Clin Obstet Gynecol* 1:668, 1958.

Hutch JA, Shopfner CE: The lateral cystogram as an aid to urologic diagnosis, *J Urol* 99:292, 1968.

Jeffcoate TN, Roberts H: Observations on stress incontinence of urine, *Am J Obstet Gynecol* 64:721, 1952.

Kitzmiller JL, Manzer GA, Nebel WA, et al: Chain cystourethrogram and stress incontinence, *Obstet Gynecol* 39:333, 1972.

Lang EK, Davis HJ: Positive pressure urethrography: a roentgenographic diagnostic method for urethral diverticula in the female, *Radiology* 72:401, 1959.

Lund CJ, Fullerton RE, Tristan TA: Cinefluorographic studies of the bladder and urethra in women. II. Stress incontinence, *Am J Obstet Gynecol* 78:706, 1959.

Muellner SR: The etiology of stress incontinence, *Surg Gynecol Obstet* 88:237, 1949.

Ney C, Duff J: Cysto-urethrography: its role in diagnosis of neurogenic bladder, *J Urol* 63:640, 1950.

Osborne ED, Sutherland CG, Scholl AJ, et al: Roentgenography of urinary tract during excretion of sodium iodide, *JAMA* 80:368, 1923.

Piscitelli JT, Simel DL, Addison WA: Who should have intravenous pyelograms before hysterectomy for benign disease? *Obstet Gynecol* 69:541, 1987.

Pochaczevsky R, Grabstald H: Double contrast barium cystography utilizing carbon dioxide, *Am J Roentgenol* 92:365, 1964.

Rosenzweig BA, Seifer DB, Grant WD, et al: Urologic injury during vaginal hysterectomy: a case control study, *J Gynecol Surg* 6:27, 1990.

Sack RA: The value of intravenous urography prior to abdominal hysterectomy for gynecologic disease, *Am J Obstet Gynecol* 134:208, 1979.

Shopfner CE: Cystourethrography: methodology, normal anatomy and pathology, *J Urol* 103:92, 1970.

Shopfner CE: Cystourethrography: an evaluation of method, *Am J Roentgenol* 95:468, 1965.

Shopfner CE, Hutch JA: The normal urethrogram, *Radiol Clin North Am* 6:165, 1968.

Simel DL, Matchar DB, Piscitelli JT: Routine intravenous pyelograms before hysterectomy in cases of benign disease: possibly effective, definitely expensive, *Am J Obstet Gynecol* 159:1049, 1988.

Stanton SL: Radiological techniques for evaluation of bladder and urethra. In Ostergard DR: Gynecologic urology and urodynamics, ed 2, Baltimore, 1985, Williams and Wilkins.

Tanagho EA: Simplified cystography in stress urinary incontinence, *Br J Urol* 46:295, 1974.

van Nagel JR, Roddick JW: Vaginal hysterectomy, the ureter and excretory urography, *Obstet Gynecol* 39:784, 1972.

Ultrasound and MRI

Benson JT, Sumners JE: Ultrasound evaluation of female urinary incontinence, *Int Urogynecol J* 1:7, 1990.

Bhatia NN: Ultrasound in gynecologic urology. In Ostergard DR: Gynecologic urology and urodynamics, ed 2, Baltimore, 1985, Williams and Williams.

Bhatia NN, Ostergard DR: Use of ultrasound in management of stress incontinence. *Clin Diag Ultrasound* 15:73, 1984.

Bhatia NN, Ostergard DR, McQuown D: Ultrasonography in urinary incontinence, *Urology* 29:90, 1987.

Bryan PJ, Butler HE, LiPuma JP: Magnetic resonance imaging of the pelvis, *Radiol Clin North Am* 22:897, 1984.

Bryan PJ, Butler HE, LiPuma JP, et al: NMR scanning of the pelvis: initial experience with 0.3T system, *Am J Roentgenol* 141:1111, 1983.

Butler H, Bryan PJ, LiPuma JP, et al: Magnetic resonance imaging of the abnormal female pelvis, *Am J Roentgenol* 143:1259, 1984.

Chang HC, Chang SC, Kuo HC, et al: Transrectal sonographic cystourethrography: studies in stress urinary incontinence, *Urology* 36:488, 1990.

Clark AL, Creighton SM, Pearce JM, et al: Localization of the bladder neck by perineal ultrasound: methodology and applications (abstract), *Neurourol Urodyn* 9:56, 1990.

Creighton SM, Stanton SL: Ultrasound's role in urodynamics, *Contemp Obstet Gynecol* 36:60, 1991.

Debus-Thiede G, Hesse U, Mayr B, et al: NMRI of the pelvic floor—a preliminary report (abstract), *Neurourol Urodynam* 9:392, 1990.

Downing J, Mannion R, Sanchez J: Voiding cystourethrography under anesthesia, *J Urol* 103:357, 1970.

Ellenbogen PH, Scheible FW, Talner LB, et al: Sensitivity of Gray scale ultrasound in detecting urinary tract obstruction, *Am J Roentgenol* 130:731, 1978.

Griffiths CJ, Murray A, Ramsden PD: Accuracy and repeatability of bladder volume measurement using ultrasonic imaging, *J Urol* 136:808, 1986.

Hricak H, Alpers C, Crooks LE, et al: Magnetic resonance imaging of the female pelvis: initial experience, *Am J Roentgenol* 141:1119, 1983.

Jensen LP, Lynne CM: Sonographic diagnosis of a bladder polyp, *Am J Obstet Gynecol* 157:1168, 1987.

Klutkze C, Golomb J, Barbaric Z, et al: The anatomy of stress incontinence: magnetic resonance imaging of the female bladder neck and urethra, *J Urol* 143:563, 1990.

Koelbl H, Bernaschek G: A new method for sonographic urethrocystography and simultaneous pressure-flow measurements, *Obstet Gynecol* 74:417, 1989.

Koelbl H, Hanzal E, Bernaschek G: Sonographic urethrocystography—methods and application in patients with genuine stress incontinence, *Int Urogynecol J* 2:25, 1991.

Lee TG, Keller FS: Urethral diverticulum: diagnosis by ultrasound, *Am J Roentgenol* 128:690, 1977.

Mainprize TC, Drutz MP: Accuracy of total bladder volume and residual urine measurements: comparison between real-time ultrasonography and catheterization, *Am J Obstet Gynecol* 160:1013, 1989.

Orgaz RE, Gomez AZ, Ramirez CT, et al: Applications of bladder ultrasonography, I. Bladder content and residue, *J Urol* 125:174, 1981.

Poston GJ, Joseph AE, Riddle PR: The accuracy of ultrasound in the measurement of changes in bladder volume, *Br J Urol* 55:361, 1983.

Quinn MJ, Beynon J, Mortensen NN, et al: Vaginal endosonography in the postoperative assessment of colposuspension, *Br J Urol* 63:295, 1989.

Richmond DH, Sutherst JR: Burch colposuspension or sling for stress incontinence? A prospective study using transrectal ultrasound, *Br J Urol* 64:600, 1989.

Scheible W, Talner LB: Gray scale ultrasound and the genitourinary tract. A review of clinical applications, *Radiol Clin North Am* 17:281, 1979.

Shapiro RA, Raz S: Clinical applications of the radiologic evaluation of female incontinence. In Raz S: *Female urology,* Philadelphia, 1983, WB Saunders.

Shopfner CE: Clinical evaluation of cystourethrographic contrast media, *Radiology* 88:491, 1967.

Yang A, Mostwin J, Zerhouni E: Magnetic resonance imaging of the female urethra (abstract), *Neurourol Urodynam* 9:393, 1990.

PART THREE

Management of Genuine Stress Incontinence and Pelvic Organ Prolapse

CHAPTER **12**

Pathophysiology and Obstetrics Issues of Genuine Stress Incontinence

Mark D. Walters
Edward R. Newton

Mechanisms of Continence
   Bladder
   Urethra
Pathophysiology of Urethral Sphincteric Incompetence
Obstetric Delivery and Pelvic Floor Dysfunction
   Vaginal Delivery and Pelvic Floor Damage
   Vaginal Delivery and Perineal Damage
   Vaginal Delivery and Pudendal Nerve Damage
Conclusion

The female continence mechanism and factors contributing to its failure are not completely understood. Past theories of the mechanisms of stress urinary incontinence have tended to focus on single factors to explain bladder neck and urethral incompetence. The last decade has seen remarkable advances in our knowledge of the histology, biochemistry, and neurophysiology that control bladder neck and urethral support and function. We now believe that multiple physiologic factors make up the female continence mechanism. Defects in any of these factors can contribute to the presence and severity of stress incontinence in women.

This chapter reviews the anatomic and physiologic mechanisms of urinary continence and stress incontinence in women. The issues of urethral support defects and pelvic floor denervation are summarized to develop the current model of the mechanisms of urethral sphincteric incompetence. Finally, we discuss extensively obstetric factors as they affect pelvic floor and urethral function.

MECHANISMS OF CONTINENCE

The two functions of the lower urinary tract are the storage of urine within the bladder and the timely expulsion of urine from the urethra. The mechanisms that control urinary continence and voiding are complex. Normal function of the central and peripheral nervous systems, bladder wall, detrusor muscle, urethra, and pelvic floor musculature are required. Dysfunction can occur at any of these levels, resulting in various types of lower urinary tract dysfunction.

Bladder

During physiologic bladder filling, little or no increase in intravesical pressure is observed, despite large increases in urine volume. This process, called accommodation, is due primarily to passive elastic and viscoelastic properties of the smooth muscle and connective tissue of the bladder wall. As filling increases to a critical intravesical pressure, detrusor muscle contractility is probably inhibited by activation of a spinal sympathetic reflex, which results in inhibition of parasympathetic ganglionic transmission and stimulation of beta-adrenergic receptors in the bladder body. The net effect of these actions is filling and storage of urine within the bladder cavity, with little increase in intravesical pressure relative to volume. Abnormalities in the bladder wall, in the detrusor muscle, or in bladder innervation can result in incontinence—primarily detrusor instability or hyperreflexia—or voiding dysfunction.

Urethra
Resting Intraurethral Pressure

For a patient to remain continent, intraurethral pressure must be greater than intravesical pressure under both resting and stress conditions. At rest urethral resistance is generated by the interaction of urethral

smooth muscle, urethral wall elasticity and vascularity, and periurethral striated muscle. Each of these components contributes to about one third of overall intraurethral pressure. The smooth muscle and vascular-elastic tissue each provide a constant amount of tension along the urethra; the periurethral striated urogenital sphincter muscles function prominently in the distal one half of the urethra. Multiple clinical factors, such as age and obstetric history, can affect the function of these various urethral components (Fig. 12-1).

Urethral Support

On the basis of extensive work of Jeffcoate and Roberts, Hodgkinson, and others, it appears that intact support of the bladder neck and proximal urethra in a retropubic position is important for maintenance of urinary continence under stress. The proximal urethra and bladder base are supported in a slinglike fashion by the anterior vaginal wall, which is attached bilaterally to the pelvic diaphragm. The vagina provides

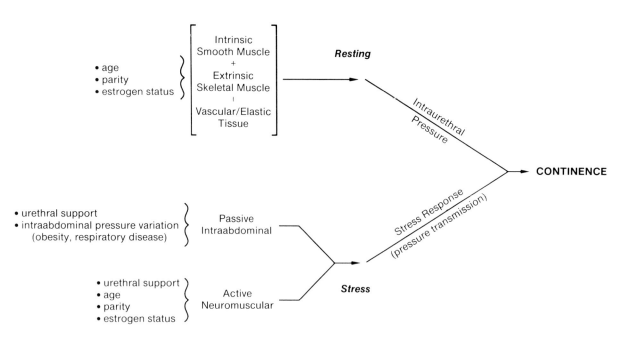

Fig. 12-1   Factors contributing to the female continence mechanism under resting and stress conditions. *(From Walters MD, Jackson GM: J Reprod Med 35:779, 1990.)*

a stable base onto which the urethra and bladder neck rest. With increases in intraabdominal pressure, as with coughing, pressure increases are transmitted equally to the bladder and urethra, maintaining urethral closure and thus continence (Fig. 12-2). In addition, intact bladder neck and urethral support also may allow for an efficient reflex pelvic muscle contraction with stress. Although this hypothesis is generally accepted, surprisingly little information is available comparing measures of urethral support and the urodynamic assessment of pressure transmission to the urethra in continent or stress incontinent women.

Urethral Innervation

Intact innervation of the urethra and periurethral muscles is also important in maintaining continence. With bladder filling, outlet resistance is increased by reflex stimulation of alpha-adrenergic receptors within the smooth muscle of the bladder neck and urethra. Voluntary and reflex stimulation of the muscles of the pelvic diaphragm and the striated urogenital sphincter also occurs, resulting from increased efferent pudendal nerve activity.

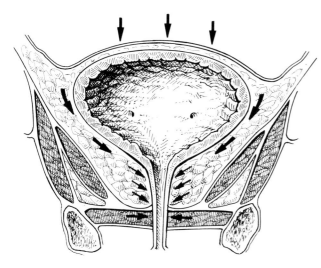

Fig. 12-2 Proposed mechanisms of urethral pressure augmentation with increases in intraabdominal pressure. *(Redrawn from Walters MD:* Obstet Gynecol Clin North Am *16:773, 1989.)*

Periurethral Musculature

The levator ani and periurethral striated muscles have a dual role in maintaining urinary continence: they provide resting urethral tone and assist in support (slow-twitch fibers), and they contract rapidly with increased intraabdominal pressure (fast-twitch fibers). The contributions to urethral resistance at rest were already disclosed.

Rapid voluntary and reflex periurethral striated muscle contraction, predominantly in the mid- and distal urethra, augments urethral pressure during rapid increases in intraabdominal pressure and interruption of urination. Using cine-fluorography, Lund et al observed two actions when a woman is asked to interrupt her urine stream. The first is a prompt constriction of the voluntary musculature, which immediately interrupts the urine stream in the mid-urethra. The urine distal to the constriction is voided but the contents of the proximal urethra are forced back into the bladder. Simultaneously, the base of the bladder is seen to rise and is drawn cephalad. Both of these actions are quick and decisive and are characteristic of voluntary fast-twitch muscle contraction. Rapid intraabdominal pressure rises reflexedly induce these same actions. Continence occurs primarily at the level of the bladder base; the mid-urethral periurethral muscles act as a backup mechanism by stopping and "milking back" urine that has entered the proximal urethra.

This concept was supported by Constantinou and Govan who showed that urethral pressure spikes precede, and are often greater than, intravesical pressure spikes during coughing in continent women. The area of greatest pressure increase was in the distal half of the urethra. Heidler et al noted that pressure increases in the distal urethra with sneezing in dogs decrease after transecting the pelvic muscles from the urethra. Koelbl et al showed that the diameter of fast-twitch levator ani muscles on biopsy correlated significantly with urethral closure pressure with stress.

Urethral Coaptation

The urethra is a pliable structure whose lumen must be completely sealed or coapted to maintain continence. The urethral wall must be sufficiently "soft" so that external forces can act on it to effect closure. Several studies by Zinner et al using mechanical models showed higher resistance to water flow when a softer lumen and a lubricating "filler" were used within the outflow tube. This finding makes clinical sense because a rigid urethra such as results from multiple surgeries or mucosal atrophy has poor closure properties. Because clinical scientific studies rarely address this issue, however, the actual importance of urethral softness and mucosal seal as they pertain to continence remains uncertain.

PATHOPHYSIOLOGY OF URETHRAL SPHINCTERIC INCOMPETENCE

Urethral sphincter incompetence (genuine stress incontinence) results when the bladder neck and urethra fail to maintain a watertight seal at rest and under conditions of increased intraabdominal pressure. By definition, the central nervous system and bladder wall function normally in this condition. Failure of urethral closure results when one or several of the factors that maintain continence become abnormal.

Adequate resting intraurethral resistance appears to be important for continence. Urethral pressure can be viewed as a threshold level, below which urine loss occurs in women with incomplete transmission of pressure to the urethra with stress. Compared to continent controls, mean resting urethral pressures are lower and vascular pulsations generally absent in women with genuine stress incontinence. In addition, maximum urethral pressure tends to be lower with increasing severity of incontinence.

Descent of the proximal urethra and bladder base to or below the level of perineal membrane with stress is generally regarded as the most important etiologic component of urethral sphincter incompetence. The basic anatomic defect appears to be the loss of integrity of the vaginal musculofascial attachments that support the bladder neck and urethra in a retropubic (intraabdominal) position. Hypermobility and descent of these structures with increased intraabdominal pressure lead to impaired pressure transmission to the urethra and possibly to an inefficient periurethral skeletal muscle response.

Damage to the nerves that control the pelvic floor and periurethral muscles probably contributes to the genesis of genuine stress incontinence. Damage to the pudendal nerve, as may occur during childbirth, can cause weakness and atrophy of the medial portions of the levator ani muscles as well as the voluntary muscles of the perineum. This damage can predispose to vaginal support defects and to decreased fast-twitch reflex pelvic muscle contraction—a factor that is believed to aid in continence during stress. Obstetric issues, as they relate to pelvic muscle denervation, are discussed more thoroughly later in the chapter.

Simultaneous measurement of urethral, bladder, and abdominal pressures, as with multichannel urethrocystometry, has provided a better understanding of the mechanisms of continence and stress incontinence. In a large, controlled study of urodynamic findings in women with genuine stress incontinence using microtransducer catheters to measure resting and stress urethral pressure profiles, Hilton and Stanton found that subjects with genuine stress incontinence had significantly decreased total urethral length, maximum urethral pressure, and pressure transmission ratios along the urethra as compared to continent controls. The total urethral length and maximum pressure decreased progressively with increasing severity of incontinence. Deficient pressure transmission ratios were noted in incontinent subjects, but not in continent controls, and did not correlate with severity. These investigators concluded that the main pathophysiologic event causing genuine stress incontinence is deficient pressure transmission to the urethra. The severity of incontinence is determined by the degree of abnormalities in resting maximum urethral pressure, urethral and intraabdominal pressure variations, and the urethral response to sustained stress. Because no attempt was made to correlate pressure transmission ratios with measures of urethral mobility, it is unknown whether deficient pressure transmission is from urethral hypermobility, abnormal reflex urethral muscle contraction, or other undefined factors.

As has been discussed, a continent woman with a well-supported bladder neck and urethra at rest and with straining has roughly equal transmission of pressures to the bladder and urethra during increased intraabdominal pressure. With anterior vaginal support defects, the bladder base descends and the urethra rotates during increases in intraabdominal pressure; resulting unequal pressure transmission sometimes

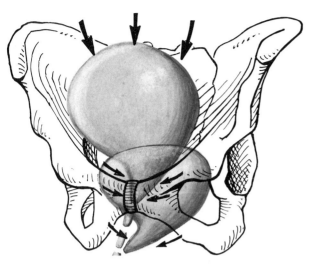

Fig. 12-3 Anatomic alterations in position of the bladder and urethra with genuine stress incontinence and an estimation of the relative transmission of intraabdominal pressure to the bladder and urethra. Worsening severity of anatomic displacement of the urethrovesical junction results in decreased pressure transmission of intraabdominal pressure to the urethra compared with the bladder.

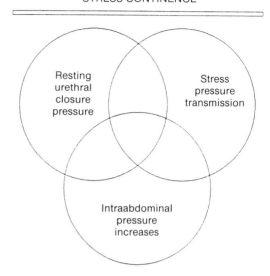

DETERMINANTS
OF
STRESS CONTINENCE

Resting urethral closure pressure

Stress pressure transmission

Intraabdominal pressure increases

Fig. 12-4 Determinants of stress incontinence. If the magnitude of the bladder pressure increase generated by the stress times the inefficiency of pressure transmission $[1 - (\Delta P_U / \Delta P_B)]$ exceeds the urethral closure pressure, genuine stress incontinence results. *(From Bump RC:* Obstet Gynecol Clin North Am *16:795, 1989.)*

leads to stress incontinence (Fig. 12-3). In these cases of "anatomic" stress incontinence, the bladder neck is always closed at rest in the absence of a detrusor contraction. During periods of rapid increased intraabdominal pressure, the proximal urethra opens and urine loss occurs. These patients are usually treated with simple elevation and stabilization of the bladder neck and urethra via a colposuspension or urethropexy procedure.

When the urethra no longer functions as a sphincter and cannot maintain a watertight seal even at rest, it is termed a type III urethra. The urethra is often well supported, but nonpliable and rigid; these cases are usually due to prior bladder neck surgery or pelvic radiation. This rigidity leads to failure of urethral coaptation and explains the radiologic finding of an open bladder neck at rest. These patients are often severely incontinent; leaking can occur with standing or with minimal exertion. Urodynamically, these patients tend to have lower maximal urethral closure pressures. Pressure transmission is usually incom-

plete, due not to anatomic disadvantage, as with urethral hypermobility, but to urethral wall rigidity. Cases of "low-pressure urethra" and "lead-pipe urethra" fit into this category.

The amplitude of rapid increases in intraabdominal pressure can influence the severity of stress incontinence. This relationship makes clinical sense because many women who are not incontinent normally still leak small amounts of urine with a full bladder during episodes of strong coughing or with aerobic exercise. Large amplitude rises can be seen with obesity, acute and chronic pulmonary problems, exercise, and occupational factors.

Thus three main factors determine the presence and severity of stress incontinence: resting urethral closure pressure, pressure transmission with stress, and the magnitude of intraabdominal pressure increases (Fig. 12-4). Mathematically, the three determinants can be combined in an equation. If the magnitude of the bladder pressure increase generated by a stress, multiplied by the inefficiency of pressure transmission $[1 - (\Delta P_U / \Delta P_B);$ see Fig. 8-3], is greater than the maximum urethral closure pressure, then bladder pressure will exceed urethral pressure and stress incontinence will result. In any given patient the relative importance of each of these three determinants varies, leading to the many clinical situations in which stress incontinence occurs.

OBSTETRIC DELIVERY AND PELVIC FLOOR DYSFUNCTION

For years circumstantial evidence has supported a relationship between obstetric trauma and stress incontinence. The evidence includes higher rates of incontinence among women of high parity than women of low parity and an association between anatomic pelvic floor abnormalities and stress incontinence. Unfortunately, obstetricians have introduced many interventions to prevent birth-related stress incontinence with neither an adequate evaluation of their efficacy nor an understanding of the pathologic mechanisms of stress incontinence. Examples of obstetric interventions include episiotomy, forceps operations, perineal massage, alternative birth positions, epidural anesthesia, and cesarean delivery.

A complete understanding of the problem requires review of the mechanism of birth, the onset of stress incontinence, the injuries associated with childbirth, and the efficacy of interventions designed to prevent perineal trauma.

Vaginal Delivery and Pelvic Floor Damage

In a classic review, Power described the mechanism by which the fetus negotiates the birth canal and is expelled through the pelvic diaphragm. In brief, as the flexed occiput anterior fetal head strikes the pelvic floor, the levator ani muscle segments are funneled from behind forward. The ischiococcygeus muscle is the first to receive the impact, but the head is often preceded by a dilating wedge of amniotic fluid and membranes that transfers most of the pressure onto the front of the pubococcygeus muscle. The anococcygeal raphe is pushed down until it becomes vertical.

The ischiococcygeus assumes a vertical plane and acts as a deflecting surface for the descending head, which is deflected downward and forward onto the iliococcygeus.

After the resistance of the ischiococcygeus is overcome, the head is shunted onto the pubococcygeus segment, which is stretched anteroposteriorly and peripherally. The perineal membrane is pulled upward as it is attached to the peripherally dilating vagina. The perineal body is pushed downward as the head is propelled along the axis of the pelvic outlet. The transverse perinei profundus muscle is flattened peripherally and stretched vertically. The rectovaginal septal fibers are stretched peripherally and longitudinally. As the sphincter group of muscles—the bulbocavernosus, ischiocavernosus, transverse perinei and periurethral muscles—are dilated, they are converted into a short muscular tube along the axis of the pelvic outlet.

As the biparietal diameter of the fetal head reaches the transverse diameter of the pelvic outlet, the uterovaginal canal is converted into one continuous hiatus. The lateral ligaments of the cervix uteri (endopelvic fascia) are flattened peripherally and stretched vertically. The vagina is dilated spherically and the pelvic diaphragm is changed from an oblique to a vertical plane. At this point—"crowning"—episiotomy and outlet forceps are often used to "prevent" pelvic injury; this moment is well after maximum stretching and possible injury has occurred to the levator ani muscles and endopelvic fascia supporting the uterus and vagina.

This sequence describes the process in an occiput anterior position. The shape of the pelvis, preexisting pelvic muscle mass and strength, strength of fascial supports, fetal presentation, position, and size all contribute to different strains, stresses, and locations of particular injuries to the pelvic floor and perineum. Childbirth injuries may involve disruption of anatomic relationships and subsequent loss of mechanical advantage, denervation of the pelvic floor muscles through injury to the pudendal nerve and/or its branches, or a combination of the two.

In a classic paper, Delee described the anatomic injuries as they occur. The fetal head advancing through the hiatus genitalis rips the vagina off its fascial anchorings, sliding it downward and outward.

Likewise, the rectum is torn from its attachments to the levator ani muscles and fascia. The head tears or overstretches the levator muscles causing their diastasis. Anteriorly, the fascia between the vagina and bladder is stretched in a radial and downward fashion. This motion may tear the vagina and bladder off their anchorage to the upper surface of the endopelvic fascia or the levator ani and posterior surface of the pubic symphysis.

Between 1945 and 1955, Gainey systematically evaluated 2000 patients for evidence of postpartum pelvic tissue damage. Table 12-1 describes the frequency of pelvic tissue damage. Episiotomy appeared to protect the patient from pelvic tissue damage; however, the data did not control for maternal/fetal size, socioeconomic status, fetal presentation, or maternal parity. A total of 92 (4.6%) patients complained of stress incontinence at postpartum evaluation. Examination of these patients with regard to pelvic tissue damage shows a statistically significant association between stress incontinence and both "levator atrophy" and urethral detachment.

The descriptions of Powers, Delee, Gainey, and others relied on personal observation of the birth process, as measured through serial rectal examinations or x-ray pelvimetry, and a superior knowledge of pelvic anatomy obtained through autopsy study. Most obstetric labors that they observed were heavily med-

icated. Current labor management and patient demographics are quite different. Vaginal examinations and ultrasound provide different, more objective measurements of soft tissue anatomy. The current use of epidural anesthesia paralyzes the voluntary pelvic muscle groups, radically changing their ability to resist and direct the position of the fetal head. Patients are having fewer children and many more are avoiding perineal trauma altogether by cesarean birth. Thus the classic descriptions need confirmation using modern methodology and obstetric management.

Vaginal Delivery and Perineal Damage

Recently, interest has renewed in perineal trauma through retrospective multivariate analyses and prospective randomized trials. The evaluations and outcome variables, however, usually relate to the severity of posterior perineal trauma, i.e., does the injury extend to or include the rectal sphincter and/or rectal mucosa? The average incidence of third-degree (anal sphincter only) or fourth-degree (anal sphincter and rectal mucosa) lacerations in the literature is 6.5% (0.4% to 23.9%) in patients with midline episiotomy, 1.3% (0.5% to 2.0%) in patients with mediolateral episiotomy, and 1.4% (0% to 6.4%) in patients without episiotomy.

Although posterior injury may be important for fecal incontinence, its relationship with urinary incontinence is not clear. Most recent studies have neither defined clearly nor ascertained systematically the frequency of anterior vaginal or periurethral injury. Labial, periclitoral, and periurethral injury usually are classified together and were reported in only two recent studies. The incidence was reported to be 12.7% and 21.9%.

Study of risk factors for perineal trauma has been limited to predictors of third- and fourth-degree lacerations. Table 12-2 describes the typical adjusted odds ratios for predictors of posterior vaginal trauma on multivariate analyses. Other risk factors for posterior trauma are reported in some, but not all, studies and include Asian race, black race, second stage of labor greater than 90 minutes, physician (versus midwife) delivery, and lithotomy position.

The positive association between episiotomy and posterior trauma has been supported by randomized,

TABLE 12-1   Incidence of postpartum pelvic injury

	Percent of patients	
Pelvic finding	No episiotomy (N = 1000)	Mediolateral (N = 1000)
Detached urethra	18	9
Vaginal relaxation	14	3
Levator atrophy	31	12
Cystocele	26	10
Rectocele	12	2
Detached rectovaginal septum	24	<1
Anal sphincter damage	<1	<1
Uterine descensus	1	3

From Gainey HL: *Am J Obstet Gynecol* 70:800, 1955.

TABLE 12-2 Predictors of posterior vaginal trauma after vaginal delivery

Risk factors	Adjusted odds ratios*
Midline episiotomy	4.9-16.5
Nulliparity	2.5-4.0
Operative delivery	2.5-3.5
Birthweight ≥4000 g	1.5-2.5
Occiput posterior	1.2-1.8

*Numbers represent the minimum and maximum adjusted odds ratios reported in the medical literature.

controlled trials. Harrison et al randomized 181 primigravid women to routine mediolateral episiotomy or to restricted use of mediolateral episiotomy. The episiotomy group sustained rectal injury in 5 of 89 cases (5.6%) compared to no cases of rectal injury in the restricted group. Sleep et al randomized 1000 women to liberal use of mediolateral episiotomy (51% of patients) or restricted mediolateral episiotomy (10% of patients). A liberal policy toward episiotomy resulted in significantly more maternal vaginal trauma and more suturing.

The association between operative delivery and perineal trauma has also been studied in a randomized fashion. Yancey et al randomly assigned uncomplicated, term gestations at 2+ station in occiput-anterior position to routine outlet forceps or to spontaneous delivery. Among patients delivered by outlet forceps, the incidence of third- or fourth-degree laceration was 30 of 165 (18%) versus 12 of 168 (7%) in women who delivered spontaneously. Midline episiotomy and outlet forceps were the only factors significantly associated with rectal trauma on multivariate analysis.

Sleep and Grant performed a postal questionnaire of the 1000 patients who participated in the randomized clinical trial 3 years earlier. No apparent differences were noted between nonresponders and responders in 674 subjects. Among women with no more children (n = 401), 129 (32%) described stress incontinence, 51 (12.7%) had urge incontinence and 53 (13.2%) had dyspareunia. Thirty-nine (9.7%) of the women had urinary incontinence severe enough to require a pad. These symptoms were reported with equal frequency in the episiotomy and no-episiotomy groups. These results were not correlated with the presence or absence of acute injuries in the original study. More important, they were not correlated with the presence or absence of levator injury or detached urethra at follow-up examination.

Vaginal Delivery and Pudendal Nerve Damage

More recently another theory has been developed to explain stress incontinence and pelvic organ prolapse. This theory states that primary obstetric injury occurs to the innervation of the pelvic floor muscles, especially the pudendal nerve. Damage to the pudendal nerve is thought to occur distal to the ischial spine in the pudendal canal and to the perineal branches of the pudendal nerve (Fig. 12-5). Nerve damage may occur by longitudinal stretching with perineal descent or by direct compression. This injury leads to abnormalities in neurologic control, resulting in pelvic muscle atrophy. The denervation and muscle atrophy exacerbates the mechanical disadvantages that result from childbirth-related perineal stretching trauma and subsequent repair.

Pudendal nerve terminal motor latency (PNTML) and single fiber electromyography (EMG) of the external anal sphincter muscle have been used to test this theory. An increase in the terminal motor latency implies (1) damage to, or loss of, a population of rapidly conducting, large myelinated motor fibers in the distal portion of the nerve or (2) conduction block representing damage to these motor fibers between the point of stimulation and the muscle itself. Single fiber EMG fiber density measurements can be used as a sensitive index of reinnervation (by collateral axial sprouting) after nerve damage has occurred.

Snooks et al studied 122 pregnant women antepartum, 24 to 72 hours after delivery, and 2 months after delivery. Thirty-four nulliparous women were controls. Pudendal nerve terminal motor latency and fiber density in the external anal sphincter muscle were increased significantly at 48 to 72 hours postpartum and at 2 months postpartum, respectively. These changes were associated with multiparity, forceps delivery, increased duration of second stage of labor, rectal sphincter tear, and high birthweight. Epidural

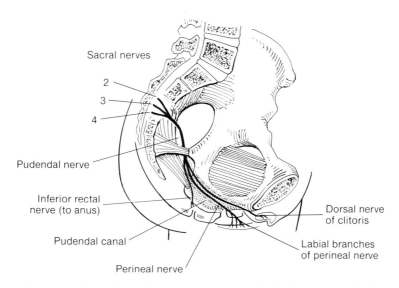

Sacral nerves

2

3

4

Pudendal nerve

Inferior rectal
nerve (to anus)

Pudendal canal

Perineal nerve

Dorsal nerve
of clitoris

Labial branches
of perineal nerve

Fig. 12-5   Course and branches of the pudendal nerve in the female pelvis. Shaded area represents section of nerve that is sometimes damaged with childbirth.

anesthesia and cesarean section did not increase the likelihood of abnormal results.

Using single-fiber EMG, Anderson demonstrated increased motor-unit fiber density of the external anal sphincter in women with genuine stress incontinence, compared to continent controls. The changes were independent of age, uterovaginal prolapse, or a history of previous surgery for incontinence. In a later study using similar methodology, Smith et al showed that partial denervation of pelvic floor muscles with subsequent reinnervation is a normal accompaniment of aging and is increased by childbirth. Women with stress incontinence and pelvic organ prolapse, or both, have significant increases in denervation of the pelvic floor compared with asymptomatic women. These studies suggest that peripheral denervation causes the periurethral and pelvic striated muscles to be mechanically less efficient. Abnormal function of these muscles could then result in lower resting urethral pressure, lower reflex striated muscle response with stress, and/or descent of the bladder base and urethra (with resulting decreased pressure transmission) with stress.

Recently, Snooks et al reported a 5-year follow-up in 14 of 24 multiparous women who participated in

the original study. All 14 women were delivered without the assistance of forceps. Five of 14 (38%) developed stress incontinence. Both fiber density and PNTML were increased in all five women who complained of stress incontinence.

Pudendal neuropathy may affect continence indirectly through a loss of muscle strength with neurogenic atrophy or directly by disruption of neurogenic control mechanisms. Decreased pelvic muscle tone secondary to denervation can lead to absent or weak fast-twitch skeletal muscle contractions with stress. Widening of the levator hiatus also results, which probably contributes to the development of pelvic organ prolapse.

A decrease in pelvic muscle strength after vaginal delivery is well documented using vaginal or anal pressure transducers or standardized digital measurement of pelvic muscle strength. Snooks et al measured maximum anal pressure in 14 multiparous women during pregnancy, 24 to 72 hours after delivery, and 2 months and 5 years postpartum. Twenty nulliparous women were controls. At 5 years, maximum anal canal pressure (50 cm H_2O) remained depressed from antepartum values in the same women (73.5 cm H_2O) and from nulliparous controls (104.7 cm H_2O). These results were similar to values found at 24 to 72 hours and 2 months postpartum.

Sampselle et al studied 20 nulliparous women at 32 to 36 weeks' gestation and at 6 weeks' postpartum. Measurements included digital muscle score, observed incontinence, and urine flow interruption time. Mean pelvic muscle strength scores were correlated inversely with observed standing stress incontinence and reported stress incontinence. Vaginal birth was associated with a highly significant loss in strength, whereas cesarean delivery was not. In another study, Gordon and Logue measured vaginal squeeze pressure with a pressure transducer. At 1 year postdelivery, neither perineal damage nor episiotomy influenced squeeze pressures, but when the data were stratified by no exercise, pelvic muscle exercises, and general exercise, highly significant improvement in pressures was noted in the exercise groups. This and other studies suggest that, when performed regularly and consistently, pelvic muscle exercises are effective in strengthening pelvic muscles.

The existence of an inherently weak urethral sphincter mechanism in women is apparent in epidemiologic studies of the onset of stress urinary incontinence. Five percent to 13% of young nulliparas suffer frequent stress incontinence. When pregnancy occurs, by 32 weeks' gestation, 30% to 53% of primiparas and 40% to 85% of multiparas experience occasional stress urinary incontinence. Postpartum, 6% to 11% of women will have stress incontinence. Retrospectively, Beck and Hsu noted that 65% of their patients with stress incontinence first complained of incontinence when pregnant and 14% developed incontinence in the puerperium. Theories that evoke anatomic or pudendal nerve injury at birth as a cause of urinary incontinence must incorporate and explain the common occurrence of incontinence before and during pregnancy.

CONCLUSION

Multiple physiologic factors, only one of which is urethral support, make up the female continence mechanism. Other important factors include resting intraurethral pressure, pressure transmission to the urethra with increases in intraabdominal pressure, and

the magnitude of rises in intraabdominal pressure. Abnormal urethral support and pelvic muscle denervation probably lead to deficient transmission of abdominal pressure to the urethra and to inefficient pelvic muscle contractions with stress. These factors result in genuine stress incontinence in some women.

The etiology of stress urinary incontinence is more complex than the simple theories that evoke anatomic or neurologic injury during childbirth. Most likely, maternal characteristics, fetal size and position, labor characteristics, and obstetric management define the likelihood of anatomic or nerve injury. These injuries unmask a susceptibility to stress incontinence, which is defined genetically (tissue strength, mechanical/anatomic relationships) and/or behaviorally (nutrition, smoking, and exercise).

For years obstetricians intervened at delivery to prevent perineal trauma and subsequent stress incontinence. The failure to systematically define and ascertain the frequency of perineal injuries at delivery and the failure to correlate those injuries with documented stress incontinence are surprisingly persistent deficiencies in the literature. Without the support of clinical trials with randomization of treatment, interventions such as midline episiotomy and outlet forceps have persisted for years. Recently, appropriately conducted trials not only have failed to show a benefit to episiotomy and outlet forceps, but have actually shown more posterior vaginal trauma with forceps and midline episiotomy. On the other hand, if urinary stress incontinence is the outcome variable of interest, then the incidence of posterior trauma may not be a proxy for that injury. Measures of postpartum urinary tract performance are a necessary part of future outcome analyses.

The massive social, medical, and financial impact of urinary incontinence in women warrants a major commitment to the understanding of the pathophysiology of the disease. The relationship between pregnancy, childbirth, and stress urinary incontinence will require longitudinal studies of the lower urinary tract before, during, and after pregnancy in a large, heterogenous group of primiparous women. Unbiased subject selection and standardized ascertainment of urogynecologic history, physical examination, and diagnostic testing (cystometrogram, urethral pressure profile, and studies of pudendal nerve function) are critical. Results then could be correlated in multivariate analyses with demographic, morphometric, and obstetric variables.

BIBLIOGRAPHY
Mechanisms of Urinary Continence

Awad SA, Downie JW: Relative contributions of smooth and striated muscles to the canine urethral pressure profile, *Br J Urol* 48:347, 1976.

Bazeed MA, Thuroff JW, Schmidt RA, et al: Histochemical study of urethral striated musculature in the dog, *J Urol* 128:406, 1982.

Constantinou CD, Govan DE: Spatial distribution and timing of transmitted and reflexly generated urethral pressures in healthy women, *J Urol* 127:964, 1982.

Enhorning G: Simultaneous recording of intravesical and intra-urethral pressure. *Acta Chir Scand* (suppl) 276:1, 1961.

Gosling JA, Dixon JS, Critchley HO: A comparative study of the human external sphincter and periurethral levator ani muscles, *Br J Urol* 53:35, 1981.

Heidler H, Casper F, Thuroff JW: Urethral closure under stress conditions: contribution and relative share of intraurethral and periurethral striated muscles, *Neurourol Urodyn* 6:151, 1987.

Hodgkinson CP: Relationships of the female urethra and bladder in urinary stress incontinence, *Am J Obstet Gynecol* 65:560, 1953.

Jeffcoate TN, Roberts H: Observations on stress incontinence of urine, *Am J Obstet Gynecol* 64:721, 1952.

Lund CJ, Fullerton RE, Tristan TA: Cinefluorographic studies of the bladder and urethra in women, *Am J Obstet Gynecol* 78:706, 1959.

Muellner SR: The physiology of micturition, *J Urol* 65:805, 1951.

Mundy AP: Clinical physiology of the bladder, urethra and pelvic floor. In Mundy AP, Stephenson TP, Wein AJ (eds): *Urodynamics: principles, practice and application,* New York, 1984, Churchill Livingstone.

Rud T, Andersson KE, Asmussen M, et al: Factors maintaining the intraurethral pressure in women, *Invest Urol* 17:343, 1980.

Walters MD: Mechanisms of continence and voiding, with International Continence Society classification of dysfunction, *Obstet Gynecol Clin North Am* 16:773, 1989.

Wein AJ, Barrett DM: *Voiding function and dysfunction,* Chicago, 1988, Year Book Medical Publishers.

Zinner NR, Sterling AM, Ritter RC: Evaluation of inner urethral softness, Urology 22:446, 1983.

Zinner NR, Sterling AM, Ritter RC: Role of inner urethral softness in urinary incontinence, *Urology* 16:115, 1980.

Pathophysiology of Urethral Sphincteric Incompetence

Blaivas JG, Olsson CA: Stress incontinence: classification and surgical approach, *J Urol* 139:727, 1988.

Blaivas JG: Classification of stress urinary incontinence, *Neurourol Urodyn* 2:103, 1983.

Bump RC: The urodynamic laboratory, *Obstet Gynecol Clin North Am* 16:795, 1989.

Bunne G, Obrink A: Urethral closure pressure with stress: a comparison between stress incontinent and continent women, *Urol Res* 6:127, 1978.

Hilton P, Stanton SL: Urethral pressure measurement by microtransducer: the results in symptom-free women and in those with genuine stress incontinence, *Br J Obstet Gynaecol* 90:919, 1983.

Koebl H, Strassegger H, Riss PA, et al: Morphologic and functional aspects of pelvic floor muscles in patients with pelvic relaxation and genuine stress incontinence, *Obstet Gynecol* 74:789, 1989.

McGuire EJ, Lytton B, Pepe V, et al: Stress urinary incontinence, *Am J Obstet Gynecol* 47:255, 1976.

Walters MD, Jackson GM: Urethral mobility and its relationship to stress incontinence in women, *J Reprod Med* 35:777, 1990.

Obstetric Issues

Anderson RS: A neurogenic element to urinary genuine stress incontinence, *Br J Obstet Gynaecol* 91:141, 1984.

Avery MD, Van Arsdale L: Perineal massage: effect on the incidence of episiotomy and laceration in a nulliparous population, J Nurse Midwifery 37:18, 1987.

Avery MD, Burket, BA: Effect of perineal massage on the incidence of episiotomy and perineal laceration in a nurse-midwifery service, *J Nurse Midwifery* 31:128, 1986.

Beck RP, Hsu N: Pregnancy, childbirth and the menopause related to the development of stress incontinence, *Am J Obstet Gynecol* 91:820, 1965.

Borgata L, Dieming SL, Cohen WR: Association of episiotomy and delivery position with deep perineal laceration during delivery in nulliparous women, *Am J Obstet Gynecol* 160:294, 1989.

Brendsel C, Peterson G, Mehl LE: Routine episiotomy and pelvic symptomatology, *Women Health* 5:49, 1980.

Delee JB: The prophylactic forceps operation, *Am J Obstet Gynecol* 1:34, 1920.

Dougherty MC, Bishop KR, Abrams RM, et al: The effect of exercise on the circumvaginal muscles in postpartum women, *J Nurse Midwifery* 34:8, 1989.

Ferguson KL, McKey PL, Bishop KR, et al: Stress urinary incontinence: effect of pelvic muscle exercise, *Obstet Gynecol* 75:671, 1990.

Fischer SR: Factors associated with the occurrence of perineal lacerations, *J Nurse Midwifery* 24:18, 1979.

Francis WJ: The onset of stress incontinence, *J Obstet Gynaecol Br Emp* 67:899, 1960.

Francis WJ: Disturbances in bladder function in relation to pregnancy, *J Obstet Gynaecol Br Emp* 67:353, 1960.

Gainey HL: Postpartum observation of pelvic tissue damage: further studies, *Am J Obstet Gynecol* 70:800, 1955.

Gordon H, Logue M: Perineal muscle function after childbirth, *Lancet* 2:123, 1985.

Green JR, Soohoo SL: Factors associated with rectal injury in spontaneous delivery, *Obstet Gynecol* 73:732, 1989.

Harrison RF, Brennan M, North PM, et al: Is routine episiotomy necessary? *Br Med J* 288:1971, 1984.

Nodine P, Roberts J: Factors associated with perineal outcome during childbirth, *J Nurse Midwifery* 32:123, 1987.

Power RM: The pelvic floor during parturition, *Surg Gynecol Obstet* 83:296, 1946.

Roberts JE, King D: Delivery positions and perineal outcome, *J Nurse Midwifery* 29:186, 1984.

Sampselle CM, Brink CA, Wells JJ: Digital measurement of pelvic muscle strength in childbearing women, *Nurs Res* 38:134, 1989.

Sampselle CM: Changes in pelvic muscle strength and stress urinary incontinence associated with childbirth, *J Obstet Gynecol Neonatal Nurs* 19:371, 1980.

Schuessler B, Hesse V, Dimpfel T, et al: Epidural anesthetic and avoidance of postpartum stress urinary incontinence, *Lancet* 1:762, 1988.

Scott JC: Stress incontinence in nulliparous women, *J Reprod Med* 2:96, 1969.

Shiono P, Klebanoff MA, Carey JC: Midline episiotomies: more harm than good? *Obstet Gynecol* 75:765, 1990.

Sleep J, Grant A, Garcia J, et al: West Berkshire perineal management trial, *Br Med J* 289:587, 1984.

Sleep J, Grant A: West Bershire perineal management trial: three year follow up, *Br Med J* 295:749, 1987.

Smith AR, Hosker GL, Warrell DW: The role of partial denervation of the pelvic floor in the aetiology of genitourinary prolapse and stress incontinence of urine. A neurophysiological study, *Br J Obstet Gynaecol* 96:24, 1989.

Snooks SJ, Swash M: Abnormalities of the innervation of the urethral striated sphincter musculature in incontinence, *Br J Urol* 56:401, 1984.

Snooks SJ, Swash M: Perineal nerve and transcutaneous spinal stimulation: new methods for investigation of the urethral striated sphincter musculature, *Br J Urol* 56:406, 1984.

Snooks SJ, Swash M, Henry MM, et al: Risk factors in childbirth causing damage to the pelvic floor innervation, *Int J Colorect Dis* 1:20, 1986.

Snooks SJ, Swash M, Mathers SE: The effect of vaginal delivery on the pelvic floor: a five year followup, *Br J Surg* 70:1358, 1990.

Stanton SL, Kerr-Wilson R, Harris VG: The incidence of urological symptoms in normal pregnancy, *Br J Obstet Gynaecol* 87:897, 1980.

Swash M, Snooks SJ, Henry MW: Unifying concept of pelvic floor disorders and incontinence, *J R Soc Med* 78:906, 1985.

Thorp JM, Bowes WA, Braune RG, et al: Selected use of midline episiotomy: effect on perineal trauma, *Obstet Gynecol* 70:260, 1987.

Thorp JM, Bowes WA: Episiotomy: can its routine use be defended? *Am J Obstet Gynecol* 160:1027, 1989.

Walker MP, Farine D, Rolbin SH, et al: Epidural anesthesia, episiotomy and obstetric laceration, *Obstet Gynecol* 77:668, 1991.

Wilcox LS, Strobino DM, Baruffi J, et al: Episiotomy and its role in the incidence of perineal laceration in a maternity center a tertiary hospital obstetric service, *Am J Obstet Gynecol* 160:1047, 1989.

Yancey MK, Herpolsheimer A, Jordan GD, et al: Maternal and neonatal affects of outlet forceps delivery compared with spontaneous vaginal delivery in term pregnancies, *Obstet Gynecol* 78:646, 1991.

Zacharin RF: "A Chinese anatomy": the pelvic supporting tissues of the Chinese and Occidental female compared and contrasted, *Aust NZ J Obstet Gynaecol* 17:1, 1977.

CHAPTER 13

Genuine Stress Incontinence: Nonsurgical Treatment

Molly C. Dougherty
Mark D. Walters

Behavioral Management
Preparation of the clinician
Key concepts in behavioral management of stress urinary incontinence
Assessment for behavioral management
Behavioral management techniques
Monitoring behavioral management at home
Implementing behavioral management
Pharmacologic Treatment
Estrogen
Alpha-adrenergic stimulating drugs
Estrogen combined with alpha-adrenergic stimulating drugs
Imipramine hydrochloride
Beta-adrenergic blocking agents
Functional Electrical Stimulation
Background
Mechanisms of action
Device characteristics
Clinical results
Mechanical Devices

Various forms of nonsurgical therapy effectively improve or cure stress urinary incontinence in some women. These patients may not desire surgery, are poor surgical candidates, or are not affected to a degree that justifies major surgery. In fact, some women with bothersome stress incontinence who traditionally would receive surgical treatment may obtain sufficient improvement with nonsurgical methods so that the remaining urine loss is no longer a social or hygienic problem. Thus we believe that women with genuine stress incontinence generally should have a trial of nonsurgical therapy before corrective surgery is offered.

Four types of conservative treatment are effective for some women with genuine stress incontinence: behavioral management (biofeedback, pelvic muscle exercises, and bladder training), pharmacologic therapy, functional electrical stimulation, and mechanical devices. In general, these treatments facilitate storage of urine by increasing bladder outlet resistance or by mechanically supporting the bladder neck. This chapter reviews these techniques.

BEHAVIORAL MANAGEMENT
Preparation of the Clinician

Behavioral management is carried out in an office/clinic setting with continued application of techniques by the woman in her home. The application of techniques discussed in this chapter is most readily learned by those who have a conceptual and clinical understanding of the anatomy and physiology of the pelvis. Instruction and monitoring of behavioral management require a positive, supportive relationship between the clinician and patient. Because behavioral management is time-consuming and intensive, the exchange between the clinician and the woman is critical for mastering behavioral techniques.

Key Concepts in the Behavioral Management of Stress Urinary Incontinence

Terminology in this area can be confusing. Currently, the term *pelvic muscles* (PM) is used for the meshwork of skeletal muscles that help support the bladder and urethra. Voluntary contractions of the PM directed toward strengthening and improving control are referred to as *pelvic muscle exercise* (PME). Biofeedback, defined as techniques that reveal to patients internal physical events by visual or auditory signals in order to teach them to manipulate these events, is used in this chapter to refer to PM biofeedback.

A complete description of the muscle groups and neural control of the bladder, urethra, and supportive musculature is beyond the scope of this chapter. Nevertheless, it is important to have a mental picture of the dynamic processes involved in micturition and in relaxation and contraction of the PM.

A series of studies by Snooks et al on pelvic muscle denervation posits concepts consistent with behavioral management. Denervation of the PM appears to progress over many years, and functional disorders usually appear in middle life. Partial denervation of the PM with subsequent reinnervation appears to be a normal process in aging and may be increased by childbirth. Delayed conduction to the striated periurethral and pelvic muscles, indicative of denervation injury, is present in women with stress urinary incontinence. Compared to normal continent women, these women have hypertrophy of type 2 (fast twitch) pelvic muscle fibers and an increase in the proportion of type 1 (slow twitch) fibers to all fibers. These results suggest localized partial denervation accompanied by reinnervation. Denervation may affect specific portions of the pelvic and periurethral striated muscles. The variable recuperative response of motor neurons to axonal injury and the process of denervation and regeneration may explain the value of behavioral management in stress incontinence. Taken together, these studies help to explain why some women become absolutely con-

tinent with behavioral management, whereas others report little benefit.

Assessment for Behavioral Management

A history of the woman's bladder control problem in her own words is a starting point for behavioral management. Important in this initial discussion is her goal(s) for treatment. An overview of the necessary physical and gynecologic examinations used with behavioral management is provided in Chapter 5. Direct physical assessment of the muscles palpated vaginally is essential. Clinical mapping of the underlying muscles is performed with the index finger while the woman relaxes and contracts the PM. Areas of the muscles that are absent or atrophied are noted. Tone is assessed by the degree of resistance provided to the finger during contraction. Two clinical rating scales have been published and have undergone clinical evaluation; these scales help ensure consistency during examinations and provide a numerical score on the results. Clinicians often rely on instrumentation to the neglect of clinical observation and assessment. Clinical assessment offers face validity that is not matched by complex technology and should always be included.

A bladder diary is used almost universally in the assessment of urinary incontinence and several versions are available. The bladder diary (Fig. 13-1) may be printed onto a card with instructions on the reverse side, which permits the woman to keep it with her and record events as they occur. This diary is used to document the severity of the problem (voids and leakage), discuss patterns of fluid intake, and help the woman develop insight into her daily behavior patterns. Usually, a record is kept for 7 days. The bladder diary may be used before initiating a behavioral technique; thereafter it is completed to quantitatively evaluate the results.

Behavioral Management Techniques
Education

Managing stress urinary incontinence requires the woman to change habitual behaviors. Rushing to the toilet tends to increase abdominal pressure and contribute to poor muscle coordination. When faced with possible urine loss, the woman should be taught to

7-Day Bladder Diary

This card is to help you keep a record of your voiding (urinating) pattern and leakage (incontinence) of urine. Please complete this record for 7 days according to the following instructions prior to your office/clinic visit. Start a new card for each day (use as many as you need for each day). We would like you to drink a minimum of 6 to 8 glasses of fluid each day you keep this record.

Example:

(1) Time	(2) Intake Type	 Amount	(3) Urge (X)	(4) Voided (X)	(5) Leak (X)	(6) Activity

A

(1) Record the time of all voiding and leakage of urine as well as the time of any liquid intake. (2) Describe the type of intake (coffee, water, etc) and the amount (1 cup, 12 oz., etc). Anything that is liquid at room temperature, for example, ice cream, is considered a liquid. (3) Make a mark anytime you note an "urge". (4) Make a mark each time you void (urinate). (5) Make a mark each time you note leaking. (6) Describe the activity you were performing at the time of leakage of urine. If you were not actively doing anything, record whether you were sitting, standing, or lying down.

REVERSE SIDE OF CARD

7-Day Bladder Diary

Name _____   Date _____

(1) Time	(2) Intake Type	 Amount	(3) Urge (X)	(4) Voided (X)	(5) Leak (X)	(6) Activity

B

Fig. 13-1 A, 7-day bladder diary: instructions may be copied on one side of card. **B,** 7-day bladder diary: the bladder record on the reverse.

Incontinence Organizations

The HIP Report
(Help for Incontinent People)
PO Box 544
Union, SC 29379

The Informer
(Helping People with Incontinence)
The Simon Foundation
Box 815
Wilmette, IL 60091

Write and enclose $15 donation to receive newsletters.

---

stop the activity she is engaged in, to sit down if possible until the urge passes, and to proceed slowly to the toilet.

Books and pamphlets often help women learn that they are not alone with their problem and reinforce information provided in the office/clinic setting. The clinician should review published materials carefully before use to avoid confusion resulting from discrepancies in various publications. Organizations dedicated to public education and self-help for urinary incontinence are an important source of information (see accompanying box) and may be helpful to women undertaking behavioral management. Several organizations for professionals also generate and disseminate information on urinary incontinence.

Dietary Modification

The bladder diary is useful to guide counseling for dietary change. When fluid intake is below average, documentation from the bladder diary may be used to urge adequate hydration, usually at least eight glasses of fluid daily. Limiting fluids as a way to manage incontinence is not recommended. Restricting fluids after 6 PM, however, often results in fewer nocturnal voids and may be particularly helpful to those with restricted mobility.

Review of the bladder diary provides an opportunity to discuss use of caffeinated foods and beverages and to recommend a reduction in their intake. Bowel habits should be scrutinized because constipation is often associated with urinary incontinence. Recommending high-fiber diets and enough fluid intake to control constipation is helpful. Although modification in diet based on education and self-monitoring probably does not result in significantly fewer leakage episodes, many women report symptomatic improvement after reducing caffeine in their diet and implementing other modifications.

Bladder Training

Scheduling regimens, including bladder training, are frequently used to manage urge and, more recently, stress incontinence. Several scheduling regimens are described in the literature. Becoming well acquainted with a specific approach may help the clinician use the method consistently.

Using an approach based on behavior modification that included patient education and scheduled voiding, Fantl et al reported a 57% reduction in incontinence episodes and a 54% reduction in amount of fluid lost. The effect was similar for both detrusor instability and genuine stress incontinence. The voiding schedule is based on the woman's daytime voiding interval, derived from the bladder diary. During the first week, the voiding interval is 30 or 60 minutes. The woman is encouraged to void on schedule, even if the desire to void is not present. Relaxation and distraction techniques are used to suppress urge sensations. When urgency cannot be suppressed and leakage is imminent, however, the woman may void to prevent leakage.

The woman meets with the clinician for 6 consecutive weeks. The bladder diary is reviewed and a decrease in the number of leak episodes and tolerance of the prescribed interval without interruptions signal readiness to increase the voiding interval by 30 minutes. During visits, the clinician provides positive reinforcement and optimism. The goal is to reach a 3- to 4-hour voiding interval. After 6 weeks, the woman is encouraged to assume a comfortable voiding schedule. Bladder training does not impose fluid modifications. It is designed to increase bladder volume in women who empty frequently to avoid leaks.

Biofeedback

Biofeedback is widely used to facilitate behavior change and to manage incontinence. Some investigators report good results with the use of a physiograph, which provides a visual recording of abdominal, bladder, and PM pressures. Others provide feedback on PM contractions and abdominal pressure. Stress incontinence not accompanied by an unstable bladder does not appear to require monitoring of detrusor pressure. Catheterization to obtain detrusor pressure was performed in some studies, but is not well accepted by many women.

Biofeedback is usually an intensive therapy, with sessions occurring weekly or more frequently. Gains from biofeedback are seen relatively quickly. Dougherty et al (unpublished) found that an average of 5.5 sessions scheduled two to three times per week was sufficient for women to develop control of abdominal pressure, attain characteristic PM pressure curves, and achieve improvement in leakage episodes and urine loss. Burgio et al (1989) report significant improvement in leak episodes, with one to eight sessions spaced 2 to 4 weeks apart.

Biofeedback requires equipment that (1) monitors signals representing relevant physiologic processes (i.e., from the abdomen and PM) and (2) provides the woman with auditory or visual information that varies with the signal produced. Ideally, a permanent record is obtained for review later. Sensors for monitoring may be surface electrodes or intravaginal or rectal probes. Many equipment systems dedicated to, or adaptable for, biofeedback are available. Systems may measure in units of pressure or electromyography or a combination thereof. Some systems are computer dependent and feature dedicated software; others rely on analog signals. The warranty and maintenance plans associated with the equipment are important, as is the company's reputation for service. Caution is recommended in selecting a system. At minimum, a clinician should use a system and become familiar with its features before purchase. One should read premarket research and talk with clinicians and investigators who use the equipment.

One advantage of biofeedback is that the procedures are individualized and focus on elements that contribute to incontinence. Although no single pattern for biofeedback has emerged in the literature, it may be organized around specific steps, as described in the accompanying box.

Controlling abdominal pressure is an early step in

Guidelines for Biofeedback

Guideline 1: Plan for approximately 20-minute sessions.

Guideline 2: Review woman's experience since last session.

Guideline 3: Review and record woman's progress toward goals at each session.

Biofeedback Routine—Progression of Activity

Step 1 Abdominal (ABD) pressure

Experiment with maneuvers to increase ABD pressure.

Cough, laugh. Head lift (hands on abdomen).

Head lift with inspiration and hold.

Head and shoulder lift.

Conscious tightening of abdomen.

Extend abdomen by voluntary extension of abdominal muscles.

OBJECTIVE: Learn and control increases in abdominal pressure.

Step 2 Quick, intense PM contraction of short duration

Contract quickly, briefly. Helps to get an initial "feel" for contraction. Relax to baseline. Work toward PM contractions without increasing ABD activity.

OBJECTIVE: PM contraction without ABD activity.

Step 3 10-second PM contraction

Contract firmly and quickly, hold. Relax to baseline. Work toward PM contractions without increasing ABD activity.

OBJECTIVE: PM contraction sustained for 10 seconds with ABD activity controlled.

Step 4 Slow deliberate PM contraction

Focus on slow, deliberate increases in PM activity and a controlled return to baseline.

Maintain stable, low ABD activity.

OBJECTIVE: To promote sensations associated with subtle changes in PM contraction and relaxation of PM.

Step 5 Individualized biofeedback sessions

Use sitting and standing positions. Perform PM biofeedback session with full bladder. Perform activities that provoke leakage at home—coughs, laughs—and practice control with PM contractions.

OBJECTIVE: Duplicate events in office/clinic that provoke leaks at home and practice control.

biofeedback. Many women make stress incontinence worse by increasing abdominal pressure instead of performing PM contractions. Biofeedback demonstrates changes during voluntary increases and decreases in abdominal pressure and helps the woman relate her habits to the leakage. For example, some women, on rising to a standing position, sense an imminent urine leak. They habitually inspire and contract the abdominal muscles, which increases abdominal pressure (and bladder pressure) and contributes to leakage. With biofeedback, the woman learns to control behaviors that increase abdominal pressure.

Abdominal contractions contribute to increases in PM activity in some women. Thus it is important to monitor abdominal activity during biofeedback. If only PM contractions are monitored, changes in abdominal pressure that produce changes in the PM may lead to imprecise and confusing signals to the woman.

A second step in biofeedback is mastering voluntary contractions of the PM. Women, both continent and incontinent, vary widely in the force with which they are able to contract the PM. A woman who cannot produce a palpable PM contraction on examination will benefit from biofeedback to help her produce PM contractions that she can monitor and enhance. The rehabilitation literature indicates that biofeedback for skeletal muscles should focus on slow and fast twitch fibers separately, but this level of specificity is not represented currently in the incontinence literature.

Mastering short (1 to 2 seconds), intense contractions seems to be easier for women with stress incontinence than sustaining a contraction (10 seconds). Each type of muscle contraction probably contributes to continence during increases in abdominal pressure. Gradually, increasing the intensity of a muscle contraction and then gradually relaxing is a technique used in biofeedback generally, and, when applied to the PM, also may play a role in continence.

The final step is to duplicate events in the office/clinic that reflect everyday activities that lead to leakage. In these sessions, the woman can practice relaxing her abdominal muscles and contracting the PM to overcome imminent leaks while monitoring the effect of her efforts with the biofeedback equipment. Having the woman drink 250 to 500 ml fluid an hour before the session so that her bladder is full helps produce realistic practice. The woman may sit and/or stand as she duplicates behavior that provokes leaks (coughs, laughs) while monitoring her behavior on the biofeedback equipment. These steps help her link activities that produce incontinence to techniques she is learning and provide practice. During her daily activities, she can use the techniques. The biofeedback steps may be modified depending on the woman's preferences and her goals for management.

Most research on biofeedback includes PME. Burns et al studied PME alone, PME in combination with biofeedback, and a control group. Results showed that biofeedback increased the effect of PME. Because of the time commitment required by biofeedback, however, some women select PME before or instead of biofeedback.

Pelvic Muscle Exercise

Women who are able to effectively contract the PM and do not contract the abdominal or auxiliary muscles during PM contractions may use PME alone. The quality of PM contractions may be assessed with a digital examination or with biofeedback equipment (discussed earlier). One session may be devoted to assessing the woman's ability to identify the PM and control abdominal pressure. If any coordination or control deficits are observed, implementing biofeedback in the office/clinic setting is recommended before PME at home is undertaken.

PME is best approached like other physical conditioning programs. The program should be graded and regular. Repeated, sustained contractions with rest intervals between each contraction and periodic clinical assessments should be used. The exercise program should begin with three sessions per week requiring 15 repetitions of a 10-second PM contraction. Ten repetitions should be added every 4 weeks, so that 35 repetitions are completed during the last interval of training (see accompanying box).

In a study of 130 women, including 65 with stress incontinence, PME as described earlier resulted in significant improvement in pelvic muscle variables, episodes of incontinence, and urine loss. Bo et al, who based PME on principles of exercise physiology and used intensive training in the research institution, achieved similar results. However, exercise with an

Pelvic Muscle Exercise Instructions

The muscles that surround the vagina, the pelvic muscles, help support the pelvic organs. Pelvic muscle exercise (PME) was popularized by Dr. Arnold Kegel and often is called Kegel exercises. Most health professionals agree that PME is beneficial to women. Weakened PM often result in loss of urine during an increase in abdominal pressure, which can occur when laughing, coughing, jogging, etc.

Begin by emptying your bladder. Adjust your clothing so that you can be comfortable and relaxed. Lie down with your head slightly elevated (at a 20-degree angle), your knees bent and comfortable.

Try tensing your fist into a tight ball, to a count of five. Now completely relax your fist. Can you feel the difference between the two states? It is important that you are able to do so. When you contract or tighten your PM, it is important but often difficult to keep your abdominal, buttock, and thigh muscles relaxed. Should you note a problem with tightening too many muscles, take a deep breath, and focus on relaxing your whole body before proceeding.

Isolating and tightening a specific muscle, as you did with your fist, may help you learn to concentrate and focus on the PM. Try to think about the area around your vagina. Draw the muscles together quickly as though you are trying to stop urinating or a bowel movement. When you have pulled the muscles together quickly and deliberately, actively hold the contraction for 10 seconds. Relax completely after the contraction subsides. Relax approximately 15 seconds before beginning another PM contraction.

When you begin to exercise these muscles, you may note that your muscles tire easily or that you are not able to hold the contraction for 10 seconds. As you continue to exercise, this problem will develop less frequently. In addition, a short 30-second break at these points may be helpful. If you think that you are no longer tightening or contracting your muscles, it is important not to tighten them during the remainder of the 10-second count. What you are trying to do is gain control and strength in the muscles. By retightening, or "flicking" the muscle, you will not be as successful in gaining control and strength.

Directions for a PM Exercise Contraction

To the count of 10 seconds:
1. Contract deliberately, quickly, and hard.
2. Actively hold the contraction, hard and firm.
3. Hold it, hard and firm.
4. Hold it, hard and firm.
5. Hold it, hard and firm.
6. Hold it, hard and firm.
7. Hold it, hard and firm.
8. Hold it, hard and firm.
9. Hold it, hard and firm.
10. Relax completely.

Begin by doing 15 of these contractions each session (day) three times a week every other day. Add 10 contractions at the end of each month until you build up to 35 contractions in a session. Good luck!

Adapted from Dougherty M, Bishop K: *Circumvaginal muscle (CVM) exercise instructions*, 1987.

---

intravaginal device to provide resistance did not improve results obtained with PME alone in two clinical trials.

Characteristics of the PME prescription that are important to communicate to women are the following:
1. Isolate the pelvic muscles during exercise. Avoid tightening the abdomen, buttocks, or thighs during PME. Generally, the woman should assume a recumbent position because maintaining upright posture involves muscles in the legs and abdomen.
2. Relax completely between contractions. If relaxation is not attained, a generalized muscular tonus in the pelvis may occur, making it more difficult for the woman to sense the intensity of her efforts.
3. Concentrate on each contraction. The woman may be counseled to set aside a time during the day that she can devote to PME.
4. Rest for 1 to 3 minutes, or as needed, between each set of 10 contractions to maintain general relaxation.

5. Give a strong, maximum effort with each contraction.
6. Hold each contraction firmly and steadily. Retightening during a contraction contributes to general muscle tension. Instead, if concentration and focus are lost, relax completely and begin another contraction.

Some women find that keeping a record of their PME is motivating and useful as a reminder. An audiocassette tape recording to guide the exercise sessions is also well accepted. Similarly, periodic assessments in the office reinforce home PME and allow for monitoring PME technique.

Little is known about the level of PME needed to maintain gains attained during the PME protocol. PME is not effective in about 25% of healthy aging women. Older women respond more slowly to PME and achieve less improvement on PM variables. If denervation partially explains stress urinary incontinence, those who do not identify and control the PM initially may benefit from biofeedback followed by PME. Because the reasons for failure to improve are not entirely clear, clinicians should base their statements about expected improvement on the research literature and not offer false assurance about outcomes.

Monitoring Behavioral Management at Home
Self-examination and Biofeedback Devices

It is relatively easy for women who are comfortable with their bodies to learn to monitor their PM contractions. Tact and urging are needed with others. Nevertheless, self-monitoring techniques have a place in behavioral management and provide women with a way to feel independent in tracking their progress. By encouraging improved compliance, these techniques may contribute to the success of behavioral management.

To monitor one's own progress, the woman places her index finger intravaginally and contracts the PM while standing (with one foot elevated and supported) or recumbent. The pressure of the PM contraction against her finger provides some information about the quality of her contraction. The clinician may discuss this technique during the PM assessment. The second self-monitoring technique using the PM con-

traction is to stop the urine stream. This technique demonstrates the relationship between effective PM contraction and continence and reinforces the importance of PME. It is not recommended for the performance of PME, however, because it may contribute to urine retention. Many women cannot stop their urine stream with a PM contraction, but may attain continence with behavioral management. For many women, returning to the clinic/office is an opportunity to monitor PME progress and may provide other benefits as well.

A number of devices are designed to be used at home to promote PME or biofeedback. The caveats discussed earlier for biofeedback equipment also apply to take-home devices.

Weighted Vaginal Cones

A relatively new approach to PME is a set of five cones with graduated weights (Fig. 13-2). The woman inserts the cone with the least weight into her vagina as she would a tampon. As she goes about her activities, the weight of the cone causes it to slip out unless she contracts the PM firmly and consistently to keep the cone in place. She is instructed to retain the cone for 15 minutes twice a day. When successful with a specific cone on two successive occasions, she graduates to the next heavier cone. Preliminary studies

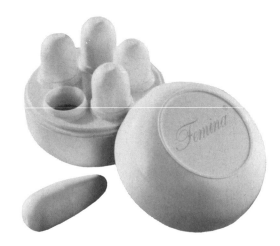

Fig. 13-2 Vaginal cones of graduated weights (Femina, Dacomed Corp, Minneapolis, Minn).

with relatively small samples show promising results in women with stress incontinence. With wide use, more information will be available regarding women for whom the technique is not suitable, as well as on clinical and PM changes associated with the use of cones.

Implementing Behavioral Management

This chapter separates assessment procedures from management strategies. Yet the bladder diary is used to monitor the effect of management techniques. The behavioral management techniques of dietary modification, scheduled voiding, biofeedback, and PME are presented as discrete techniques. It is possible to combine strategies, such as biofeedback and PME or dietary modification and scheduled voiding. For the clinician new to behavioral management, it may be beneficial to implement one technique at a time to minimize confusion.

Behavioral management has limitations. It is time-consuming and requires considerable commitment from the woman. Not all women benefit from behavioral management of genuine stress incontinence. In fact, across studies of all behavioral interventions for multiple problems, approximately 12% of patients drop out and 30% fail to improve. Little is known about what characteristics of the woman or of her situation predict "cure" versus minimal to moderate improvement. Keeping abreast of the literature permits the clinician to use research-based statements to place the potential outcomes of behavioral management in perspective for women.

PHARMACOLOGIC TREATMENT

See Table 13-1 for a review of pharmacologic therapy available to treat stress incontinence.

Estrogen

In the vagina, estrogen treatment results in an increased karyopyknotic index, increased vaginal blood flow, increased quantity of vaginal fluid, and de-

TABLE 13-1   Pharmacologic therapy for genuine stress incontinence

Classification of drug	Name of drug	Minimum/maximum dosage	Potential side effects
Hormone	Conjugated estrogen (or comparable estrogen preparation)	Oral: 0.3 mg QD/1.25 mg QD cyclically or continuously Vaginal: 2 g QD/4 g QD then weekly for maintenance	Increased risk of endometrial carcinoma (unless opposed with cyclic progestin), irregular vaginal bleeding
Alpha-sympathomimetic	Pseudoephedrine hydrochloride	15 mg BID/30 mg QID	Drowsiness, dry mouth, hypertension
	Phenylpropanolamine hydrochloride	50 mg QD/75 mg BID	Drowsiness, dry mouth, hypertension
Tricyclic antidepressant	Imipramine hydrochloride	25 mg QD/75 mg BID	Anticholinergic effects, orthostatic hypotension, hepatic dysfunction, mania, cardiovascular effects (especially in the elderly); MAO inhibitors prohibited
Beta-sympathetic blocker	Propranolol hydrochloride	10 mg BID/40 mg TID	Fatigue, lethargy, cardiovascular effects

creased vaginal pH. Clinically, improvement in vulvovaginal pain, itching, vaginal lubrication, and dyspareunia often result. The proportion of vaginal lactobacilli increases relative to enteric bacteria, thus protecting against periurethral colonization by pathogenic bacteria. This protective effect has been shown to reduce the incidence of urinary tract infection in postmenopausal women.

In the urethra, estrogen treatment results in mucosal cytologic changes similar to those of the vagina, with changes toward more intermediate and superficial cells, and fewer transitional cells. Bergman et al showed that cytologic changes in the mid-urethra correlated well with clinical response.

Using castrated female baboons to measure the effects of hormonal manipulation on urethral function, Bump and Friedman showed that estrogen replacement enhances measures of urethral sphincter function. Estrogen treatment resulted in significantly increased urethral length, as well as total urethral pressure profile area in paralyzed animals. The increased area reflects increases in both functional urethral length and mean urethral pressure. The addition of testosterone had no significant effect on the urethral pressure profile measurements.

The mechanisms by which estrogen therapy may improve urethral sphincteric function are unknown. The cytologic changes of urethral mucosa that occur in response to estrogen may lead to an improved mucosal seal effect, thereby increasing urethral resistance and lessening symptoms of urgency and frequency. Alternatively, or perhaps additionally, intrinsic urethral function may be improved, both at rest and with increases in intraabdominal pressure. This improvement may be achieved by augmentation of periurethral vascularity, by improved efficiency of smooth and striated periurethral muscles, or by both mechanisms. These physiologic changes probably cause the urodynamic improvements frequently observed with estrogen therapy: increased maximum urethral closure pressure and increased pressure transmission to the urethra with cough.

Numerous studies have addressed the efficacy of estrogen in treating lower urinary tract symptoms in postmenopausal women. Subjective improvement or cure of stress incontinence has been reported in 20%

to 71% of women. Similar results have been found using various estrogen preparations, whether orally or vaginally, although Hilton et al showed greater improvement after vaginal estrogen. Fewer symptoms of urgency, frequency (diurnal and nocturnal), and voiding difficulties also have been observed after estrogen therapy. No improvement in urinary symptoms occurs after treatment with progestin.

Urodynamic changes after estrogen therapy have been inconsistent among studies. Augmentation of maximum urethral pressure and functional urethral length has been noted by some, but not by others. Improvement in pressure transmission ratio, a measure of the urethra's response to increased intraabdominal pressure, has been demonstrated, but poor correlation was found between symptom and urodynamic improvements.

Clinical results have been less encouraging in the few placebo-controlled or long-term studies addressing estrogen treatment for urinary incontinence. In a double-blind, placebo-controlled study of the effect of estrogen on urge incontinence in postmenopausal women, Walter et al (1978) described significant improvement in sensory and motor urgency after estrogen treatment compared to placebo. Nevertheless, there were no statistically significant changes in the maximal urethral closure pressure or functional urethral length between estrogen- and placebo-treated groups.

In another prospective, double-blind study by Wilson et al, oral piperazine estrone sulfate or placebo was given to 36 postmenopausal women with genuine stress incontinence for 3 months. There was no statistical difference in the subjective response to treatment between the two groups. Although vaginal cytology and hormone profiles were significantly affected by estrogen, there were no differences between the groups with respect to urethral pressure profile or pad test measurements.

In a more recent randomized, double-blind, placebo-controlled study, Walter et al (1990) noted cure or improvement in incontinence complaints in 43% of women given estriol, compared to no improvement in the placebo group. Significant improvement was noted in 1-hour pad test results, but not in the number of leakage episodes per 24 hours.

Regarding the long-term effects of estriol implants on urinary tract symptoms in postmenopausal women, Versi et al studied 12 climacteric women for 1 year in an open, noncontrolled study. No improvement in symptoms of stress incontinence or urgency was noted after treatment. Although improvement in nocturnal frequency occurred, it may have been due to the known sleep-enhancing effects of estrogen treatment. Slight but statistically significant decreases in residual urine volume and cystometric capacity were observed after treatment. Increases in total functional area under the urethral pressure profile at rest, but not with stress, were found. The authors concluded that estrogen replacement therapy has little benefit for treatment of lower urinary tract dysfunction during the climacteric.

It is clear from this summary that the data regarding treatment effects of estrogen on lower urinary tract dysfunction are inconsistent and confusing. Most studies agree that estrogen replacement alleviates sensory urgency, urge incontinence, frequency, nocturia, and dysuria. However, no evidence from controlled clinical trials indicate that estrogen improves or cures genuine stress incontinence.

Whether a postmenopausal woman should use hormone replacement therapy is a complex issue. A considerable body of literature supports substantial long-term health benefits with the use of hormone replacement therapy, especially related to cardiovascular disease and osteoporosis. Therefore, in the absence of contraindications and after considering the risks and benefits, we believe that most eligible incontinent women should be offered hormone replacement therapy.

Alpha-Adrenergic Stimulating Drugs

The bladder neck and proximal urethra in women contain predominantly alpha-adrenoreceptors. Stimulation of these receptors produces smooth muscle contraction, which results in increased bladder outlet resistance.

Treatment of patients with stress incontinence with alpha-adrenergic stimulating drugs improves symptoms in some patients. Drugs that have been studied include ephedrine, phenylephrine, midodrine, norfenefrine, and phenylpropanolamine (PPA). Ephedrine is a noncatecholamine sympathomimetic agent that owes part of its peripheral action to the release of noradrenalin, which also directly stimulates alpha- and beta-adrenergic receptors.

Studies using norephedrine chloride have shown an increase in maximal urethral closure pressure, but not functional urethral length. In a 14-week, double-blind, cross-over study that compared the effects of norephedrine chloride with placebo, Ek et al showed reduction of urinary leakage with the drug in 12 of 22 patients. Diokno and Taub reported good to excellent results in 27 of 38 patients with genuine stress incontinence treated with ephedrine sulfate. In general, effects are most notable in patients with mild to moderate symptoms, but do not sufficiently improve severe symptoms of stress incontinence to offer an alternative to surgical treatment.

Lose et al and others have reported improvement of stress incontinence with norfenefrine, a sustained release alpha-agonist agent. In one study, 32% of patients awaiting surgical correction for genuine stress incontinence claimed to be continent or so much improved that further treatment was considered unnecessary. Of the patients who still had stress incontinence with treatment, an additional 25% preferred to resume the pharmacologic treatment rather than undergo surgery. Thus over half of women in this study avoided surgery after pharmacologic treatment.

PPA shares the pharmacologic properties of ephedrine and is approximately equal in peripheral potency, while causing less central stimulation. Several placebo-controlled studies have evaluated PPA in the treatment of women with genuine stress incontinence. Using the dose of 50 mg twice daily, improvement is noted in 60% to 70% of patients, mainly in those with less severe disease. Although modest increases in maximum urethral pressure were noted, these did not correlate with either serum concentration or subjective urinary symptom response.

PPA is a component of numerous prescription and over-the-counter medications that are marketed for the treatment of nasal and sinus congestion and appetite suppression. Pharmacologic studies of PPA in these doses revealed few clinically significant adverse effects. Nevertheless, reports of serious complications, including seizures, stroke, and death, with over-the-counter preparations containing PPA suggest that these drugs be used with care. Alpha-adrenergic stimulating drugs are usually used for the temporary, intermittent, or seasonal relief of stress incontinence symptoms. If long-term cure is desired, other treatments are probably more appropriate.

Estrogen Combined With Alpha-Adrenergic Stimulating Drugs

Estrogen appears to modify the responses of the urethra and bladder to alpha-adrenergic stimulation. Hodgson et al demonstrated that urethral segments of estrous rabbits were more sensitive to phenylephrine than were bladder segments. This difference was abolished by castration and restored with estrogen treatment. The estrogen-induced increased sensitivity of urethral smooth muscle is due, at least in part, to an increase in the number of postjunctional alpha-2 adrenoreceptors. In the rabbit bladder body, estrogen induces a significant increase in alpha-adrenergic and muscarinic, but not beta-adrenergic, receptors. This mechanism and others (Fig. 13-3) have been proposed

to explain the clinically observed estrogen-induced enhancement to alpha-adrenergic stimulation.

Schreiter et al demonstrated that primary treatment with estrogen augments the effect of subsequent alpha-adrenoreceptor stimulants on maximal urethral pressure, suggesting that estrogen has a tonicizing effect on urethral smooth musculature. Several other studies verified that the use of estrogen plus PPA is more efficacious than either agent alone. Walter et al (1990), however, found only marginal improvement after pretreatment with estrogen. The effects seem to be additive, but not synergistic.

Imipramine Hydrochloride

Imipramine hydrochloride, an antidepressant with alpha-adrenergic agonist and anticholinergic effects, appears to improve symptoms in some women with stress urinary incontinence. Gilja et al reported a 71% cure rate in 21 women after treatment with imipramine. These investigators documented an increase in functional urethral length and maximum urethral pres-

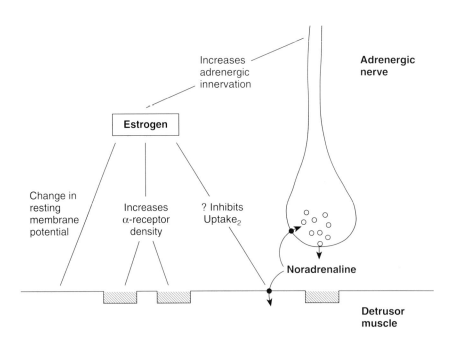

Fig. 13-3 Mechanisms by which estrogen may alter adrenergic responses *(From Miodrag A, Castleden CM, Vallance TR:* Drugs *36:491, 1988.)*

sure after a daily dose of 75 mg of imipramine hydrochloride.

Beta-Adrenergic Blocking Agents

Theoretically, beta-adrenergic blocking agents might be expected to potentiate an alpha-adrenergic effect, thereby increasing resistance in the urethra. Gleason et al reported success in treating stress incontinent patients with the beta-adrenergic blocking agent propranolol, in oral doses of 10 mg, four times daily. Although such treatment has been suggested as alternative drug therapy in patients with sphincteric incompetence and hypertension, no reports of such efficacy have appeared. Other reports have noted no significant changes in urethral pressure profile measurements in normal women after beta-adrenergic blockade.

FUNCTIONAL ELECTRICAL STIMULATION

Background

In 1963, Caldwell first introduced electrical stimulation for the correction of urinary incontinence. A surgically implantable, radio-linked electrical stimulator with electrodes placed adjacent to the urethral musculature was used. Various types of incontinence were treated with an overall success rate of about 50%. Because of the risks of surgical implantation and various technical failures requiring reoperation, implantable electrical devices generally were replaced by removable external devices. However, implantable sacral anterior root nerve stimulators still are available for detrusor hyperreflexia and neuropathic voiding disorders.

Automatic integrated functional electrical stimulation (FES) systems in the form of anal and vaginal plugs (independent or connected to a portable battery-operated stimulator) were then developed. Different designs and sizes of electrodes have been used, such as the vaginal ring pessary, the elliptical Hodge's pessary, and cylindrical anal and vaginal plug electrodes.

Mechanisms of Action

Intravaginal FES has been shown both to augment urethral sphincteric function and to inhibit bladder contractility. Pelvic muscle stimulation probably is achieved by direct electrical stimulation of afferent fibers in the pudendal nerve, which results in polysynaptic reflex responses. This mechanism activates a number of muscles from a single stimulation site. The electrical impulse runs along the afferent limb of the pudendal nerve to the sacral nerve roots and by efferent pathways to the pelvic floor muscles. Pelvic muscle contraction occurs and results in increased urethral closure pressure. Erlandson and Fall determined that a frequency of between 20 and 50 Hz with a pulse duration of 1 to 5 msec was most effective for augmenting urethral closure.

Intravaginal electrical stimulation also causes bladder inhibition. At low intravesical volumes, the hypogastric (sympathetic) nerves mediate bladder inhibition. At higher volumes, inhibition of the pelvic nerve (parasympathetic) completes the reflexogenic bladder inhibition. Both reflex arcs (pudendal-to-hypogastric and pudendal-to-pelvic) are activated by stimulation of pudendal nerve afferents. Both mechanisms can operate without supraspinal control. Bladder inhibition is optimal when alternating pulses at a frequency of about 10 Hz are used.

FES is indicated for the treatment of most storage and filling disorders in adult women. Based on their observations, Godec and Kralj predicted favorable results from the application of FES for urinary incontinence when (1) the morphology of the urinary tract is preserved, (2) the spinal center for micturition is preserved, (3) there is a low degree of peripheral denervation of the muscles of the pelvic floor, (4) urodynamic and neurophysiologic responses·to FES are positive, and (5) any lesion of the medulla spinalis is between T_6 and T_{12}. The clinical indications and contraindications of FES are presented in the box on p. 176.

Device Characteristics

Intravaginal electrodes are available as independent systems or attached to external stimulating devices. Complete independent systems consist of a battery and electronic circuit placed in a waterproof housing made of plexiglass with electrodes made of stainless steel. This system is automatically turned on when the electrodes come in contact with the walls of the vagina and turned off when the contact is broken by their

---

Indications and Contraindications of Functional Electrical Stimulation

Indications

Genuine stress incontinence
Detrusor instability
Mixed genuine stress incontinence and detrusor instability
Sensory urgency
Detrusor hyperreflexia
Neuropathic voiding dysfunction

Contraindications

Extraurinary

Severe vaginal prolapse
Pregnancy
Vaginal infections
Heavy menstruation or other vaginal bleeding
History of cardiac arrhythmia
Demand cardiac pacemaker

Urinary

Urinary retention, elevated residual urinary volumes due to incomplete bladder emptying
Extraurethral incontinence
Urinary infection
Vesicoureteral reflex

---

removal. The device contains a microvibrator, from which a continuous train of monophasic rectangular pulses of different frequencies and pulse widths is delivered.

Intravaginal electrodes that are used with an external stimulator can be connected to office stimulators for periodic acute maximal FES or to home stimulators for daily FES. The stimulators have switches to adjust device characteristics, including current intensity, character of stimulation (continuous or intermittent), and frequency. Several devices that are available for use in the United States and Canada are shown in Figs. 13-4 and 13-5.

In clinical use, a maximal response with minimal energy consumption is desired. This response requires two types of electrical characteristics: alternating pulses and intermittent stimulation. Intermittent, rather than constant, stimulation circumvents the problem of muscle fatigue without sacrificing effectiveness. As has been stated, a stimulation frequency of 20 to 50 Hz and a pulse duration of 1 to 5 msec is most effective for urethral closure; a stimulation frequency of 10 Hz is most effective for bladder inhibition.

Response also varies with current intensity. At lower currents (<35 mA), only pelvic floor muscles are affected. Stronger currents (>65 mA vaginally or >40 mA rectally) achieve both contraction of pelvic floor muscles and inhibition of bladder activity. Various stimulus amplitudes ranging from 4 to 12 volts have been used in clinical studies.

Clinical Results

Because of the various devices that have been used and the many variations in their electrical characteristics, clinical results are difficult to compare among studies. In addition, no prospective, placebo-controlled clinical trial has been performed with FES for the treatment of urinary incontinence in women. Despite these methodologic flaws, FES seems to be effective for some women with stress and/or urge incontinence.

Eriksen et al reported on the treatment of 121 women with stress and motor urge incontinence with an integrated, automatic electrical anal stimulator. Twenty-three patients discontinued treatment because of various side effects, most notably anal discomfort and pain. The remaining 98 women were treated with anal stimulation for an average of 9 months. Continence was achieved in 64% of the patients with stress incontinence, in 65% of those with motor urge incontinence, and in 53% of the patients with mixed stress and motor urge incontinence. Continence was more difficult to achieve in patients who had undergone previous unsuccessful incontinence operations.

Urodynamic changes after FES include increased bladder volume measured at first desire to void, increased maximum cystometric capacity, and fewer detrusor contractions. In 45% of patients with detrusor instability, a stable bladder with normal sensation and capacity was found after therapy. In patients with stress incontinence, a significant increase was observed in functional urethral length. The slight

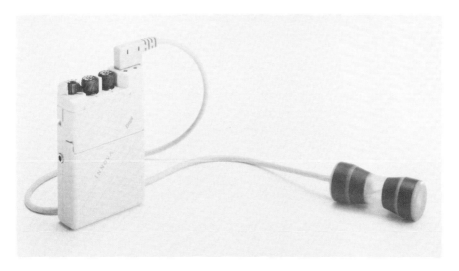

Fig. 13-4   Innova intravaginal functional electrical stimulator *(Empi Inc, St. Paul, Minn).*

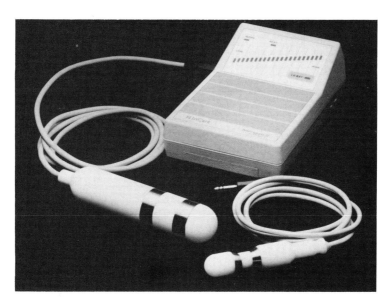

Fig. 13-5   Microgyn II stimulation device: vaginal and anal electrodes are shown with home unit *(InCare Medical Products, Libertyville, Ill).*

increase in maximum urethral closure pressure after therapy was not significant. In patients reporting cure of stress incontinence, 94% had a positive urethral closure pressure during stress provocation after therapy.

In a prospective study of 55 women with stress incontinence awaiting surgical repair, Eriksen and Mjølnerød prescribed FES for at least 2 months. Surgical treatment was avoided in 56% of these patients. A cost-benefit analysis showed that the total cost of stress incontinence therapy could be reduced by 40% with long-term FES use.

MECHANICAL DEVICES

Traditionally, mechanical devices such as pessaries have been used to alleviate symptoms of pelvic relaxation and for patients with urinary incontinence who have not responded to other therapies or for those who are medically unfit for surgical treatment. These devices may also be appropriate for women with intermittent urinary incontinence, such as during upper respiratory infections or with exercise.

A number of inflatable and noninflatable devices have been developed and marketed in various countries. The mechanical device designed by Bonnar and marketed in England is made of soft latex with an inflatable balloon on its upper surface. When inflated, it elevates the urethrovesical junction and proximal urethra. For voiding, the balloon is deflated without extraction by reversing the pump. Cardozo and Stanton found that 9 of 20 patients who used the device for 1 month showed subjective improvement in urinary leaking. Urodynamically, the investigators noted an increase in urethral pressure when the device was inflated. Eight of the 20 patients reported problems with the size of the device and only two chose to keep the device after the trial. Other vaginal devices that have been developed include the Edwards pubovaginal spring, the Suarez Continence Ring (Cook Urological, Inc, Spencer, IN), and the Cook Continence Ring (Cook Urological, Inc, Spencer, IN).

Bhatia et al, noted that placement of a Smith-Hodge vaginal pessary resulted in consistent and significant increases in functional urethral length and urethral closure pressure under stressful conditions, when compared with prepessary studies. Clinically, 10 of 12 patients became continent, probably by stabilizing the urethra and urethrovesical junction to assure adequate pressure transmission during increases in intraabdominal pressure. Simultaneous voiding urethrocystometry and instrumented uroflowmetry demonstrated absence of outflow obstruction when voiding with the pessary in place.

Realini and Walters reported that vaginal diaphragm rings may be used to treat stress incontinence. Four of ten women with genuine stress incontinence experienced clinically significant improvement in the amount of urine lost during pad tests, number of leaking episodes per week, and overall assessment of response. Urodynamic findings were essentially unchanged by wearing the diaphragm rings, although mild restrictions in urethral mobility were noted as measured by the Q-tip test. In another study, Suarez et al reported complete resolution of stress incontinence in 11 of 12 patients, although two of the patients who improved withdrew from the study because of vaginal discomfort. Augmented maximal urethral pressures were noted in this study, possibly suggesting that a large, obstructive, diaphragm ring size may have been used.

SUMMARY

Although surgery is usually curative for genuine stress incontinence, it is invasive and costly. All of the various types of nonsurgical treatments improve or cure stress urinary incontinence in selected women. Although time-consuming for the patient and caregiver, behavioral treatments are safe and effective therapy for stress incontinence. Ideally, behavioral therapy should be tried on every patient with stress incontinence before more invasive interventions are considered. Similarly, we believe that most eligible postmenopausal women with incontinence should be offered estrogen replacement therapy, both for the enhanced urogenital effects and for other long-term health benefits.

The other nonsurgical treatments of stress incontinence—alpha-adrenergic stimulating drugs, functional electrical stimulation, and mechanical devices—should be used more selectively. Alpha-adrenergic agonists and mechanical devices probably are most appropriate for temporary relief of stress incontinence symptoms while more definitive therapy is being considered. Intravaginal functional electrical stimulation is a promising treatment option for incontinent women and has been shown in many studies to improve or cure a substantial proportion of these patients. The long-term outcomes of patients treated with functional electrical stimulation are still unknown and await further study.

BIBLIOGRAPHY
Behavioral Management

Basmajian JV (ed): *Biofeedback principles and practice for clinicians,* Baltimore, 1989, Williams & Wilkins.

Bo K, Hagen RH, Kvarstein B, et al: Pelvic floor muscle exercise for the treatment of female stress urinary incontinence, *Neurourol Urodyn* 9:489, 1990.

Burgio KL, Pearce KL, Lucco AJ: *Staying dry. A practical guide to bladder control,* Baltimore, 1989, Johns Hopkins.

Burgio KL, Whitehead WE, Engel BT: Urinary incontinence in the elderly, *Ann Intern Med* 103:507, 1985.

Burns PA, Pranikoff K, Nochajski T, et al: Treatment of stress incontinence with pelvic floor exercises and biofeedback, *J Am Geriatr Soc* 38:341, 1990.

Cardozo LD, Stanton SL, Hefner J, et al: Idiopathic bladder instability treated by biofeedback, *Br J Urol* 50:250, 1978.

Chalker R, Whitmore KE: *Overcoming bladder disorders,* New York, 1990, Harper & Row.

Diokno AC, Brown MB, Brock BM, et al: Prevalence and outcome of surgery for female incontinence, *Urology* 33:285, 1989.

Dougherty MC, Bishop KR, Mooney RA, et al: The effect of circumvaginal muscle exercise, *Nurs Res* 38:331, 1989.

Dougherty MC, Bishop KR, Mooney RA, et al: Graded exercise: effect on pressures developed by the pelvic muscles. In Funk SG, Tornquist EM, Champagne MT, et al (eds): New York, 1992, Springer.

Fantl JA, Wyman JF, McClish DK, et al: Efficacy of bladder training in older women with urinary incontinence, *JAMA* 265:609, 1991.

Ferguson KL, McKey PL, Bishop KR, et al: Stress urinary incontinence: effect of pelvic muscle exercise, *Obstet Gynecol* 75:671, 1990.

Graber B, Kline-Graber G, Golden CJ: A circumvaginal muscle nomogram: a new diagnostic tool for evaluation of female sexual dysfunction, *J Clin Psychiatry* 43:157, 1981.

Hadley EC: Bladder training and related therapies for urinary incontinence in older people, *JAMA* 256:372, 1986.

Peattie AB, Plevnik S, Stanton SL: Vaginal cones: a conservative method of treating genuine stress incontinence, *Br J Obstet Gynaecol* 95:1049, 1988.

Sampselle CM, Brink CA, Wells TJ: Digital measurement of pelvic muscle strength in childbearing women, *Nurs Res* 38:134, 1990.

Smith ARB, Hosker GL, Warrell DW: The role of pudendal nerve damage in the aetiology of genuine stress incontinence in women, *Br J Obstet Gynaecol* 96:29, 1989.

Snooks SJ, Badenoch DF, Tiptaft RC, et al: Perineal nerve damage in genuine stress urinary incontinence: an electrophysiological study, *Br J Urol* 57:422, 1985.

Snooks SJ, Swash M: Abnormalities of the innervation of the urethral striated sphincter musculature in incontinence, *Br J Urol* 56:401, 1984.

Tries J: Kegel exercises enhanced by biofeedback, *J Enterostomal Ther* 17:67, 1990.

Wells TJ: Pelvic (floor) muscle exercise, *J Am Geriatr Soc* 38:333, 1990.

Worth AM, Dougherty MC, McKey PL: Development and testing the circumvaginal muscles (CVM) rating scale, *Nurs Res* 35:166, 1986.

Wyman JF, Choi SC, Harkins SW, et al: The urinary diary in evaluation of incontinent women: a test-retest analysis, *Obstet Gynecol* 71:812, 1988.

Wyman JF, Fantl JA: Bladder training in ambulatory care management of urinary incontinence, *Urol Nurs* 11:11, 1991.

Pharmacologic Treatment—Hormonal

Abrams R, Stanley H, Carter R, et al: Effect of conjugated estrogens on vaginal blood flow in surgically menopausal women, *Am J Obstet Gynecol* 143: 375, 1982.

Bergman A, Karram M, Bhatia N: Changes in urethral cytology following estrogen administration, *Gynecol Obstet Invest* 29:211, 1990.

Beisland HO, Fossberg E, Moer A, et al: Urethral sphincteric insufficiency in postmenopausal females: treatment with phenylpropanolamine and estriol separately and in combination, *Urol Int* 39:211, 1984.

Bhatia NN, Bergman A, Karram MM: Effects of estrogen on urethral function in women with urinary incontinence, *Am J Obstet Gynecol* 160:176, 1989.

Bump RC, Friedman CI: Intraluminal urethral pressure measurements in the female baboon: effects of hormonal manipulation, *J Urol* 136:508, 1986.

Cardozo L: Role of estrogens in the treatment of female urinary incontinence, *J Am Geriatr Soc* 38:326, 1990.

Faber P, Heidenreich J: Treatment of stress incontinence with estrogen in postmenopausal women, *Urol Int* 32:221, 1977.

Hilton P, Stanton SL: The use of intravaginal oestrogen cream in genuine stress incontinence, *Br J Obstet Gynaecol* 90:940, 1983.

Hilton P, Tweddell AL, Mayne C: Oral and intravaginal estrogens alone and in combination with alpha-adrenergic stimulation in genuine stress incontinence, *Int Urogynecol* J 1:80, 1990.

Hodgson BJ, Dumas S, Bolling DR, et al: Effect of estrogen on sensitivity of rabbit bladder and urethra to phenylephrine, *Invest Urol* 16:67, 1978.

Kinn AC, Lindskog M: Estrogens and phenylpropanolamine in combination for stress urinary incontinence in postmenopausal women, *Urology* 32:273, 1988.

Larsson B, Andersson KE, Batra S, et al: Effects of estradiol on norepinephrine-induced contraction, alpha adrenoreceptor number and norepinephrine content in the female rabbit urethra, *J Pharmacol Exper Ther* 229:557, 1984.

Levin RM, Shofer FS, Wein AJ: Estrogen-induced alterations in the autonomic responses of the rabbit urinary bladder, *J Pharmacol Exper Ther* 215:614, 1980.

Miodrag A, Castleden CM, Vallance TR: Sex hormones and the female urinary tract, *Drugs* 36:491, 1988.

Molander U, Milsom I, Ekelund P, et al: Effect of oral oestriol on vaginal flora and cytology and urogenital symptoms in postmenopause, *Maturitas* 12:113, 1990.

Onuoro CO, Ardoin JA, Dunnihoo DR, et al: Vaginal estrogen therapy in the treatment of urinary tract symptoms in postmenopausal women, *Int Urogynecol J* 2:3, 1991.

Rud T: The effects of estrogens and gestagens on the urethral pressure profile in urinary continent and stress incontinent women, *Acta Obstet Gynecol Scand* 59:265, 1980.

Schreiter F, Fuchs P, Stockamp K: Estrogenic sensitivity of α-receptors in the urethra musculature, *Urol Int* 31:13, 1976.

Semmens JP, Wagner G: Estrogen deprivation and vaginal function in postmenopausal women, *JAMA* 248:445, 1982.

Solomon C, Panagotopoulos P, Oppenheim A: The use of urinary sediment as an aid in endocrinological disorders in the female, *Am J Obstet Gynecol* 76:56, 1958.

Ulmsten U, Stormby N: Evaluation of the urethral mucosa before and after oestrogen treatment in postmenopausal women with a new sampling technique, *Gynecol Obstet Invest* 24:208, 1987.

Versi E, Cardozo L, Studd J: Long-term effects of estradiol implants on the female urinary tract during the climacteric, *Int Urogynecol J* 1:87, 1990.

Walter S, Kjaergaard B, Lose G, et al: Stress urinary incontinence in postmenopausal women treated with oral estrogen (estriol) and alpha-adrenoreceptor-stimulating agent (phenylpropanolamine): a randomized double blind placebo-controlled study, *Int Urogynecol J* 1:74, 1990.

Walter S, Wolf H, Barlebo H, et al: Urinary incontinence in postmenopausal women treated with estrogens, *Urol Int* 33:135, 1978.

Wilson PD, Faragher B, Butler B, et al: Treatment with oral piperazine oestrone sulphate for genuine stress incontinence in postmenopausal women, *Br J Obstet Gynaecol* 94:568, 1987.

Pharmacologic Treatment—Nonhormonal

Awad SA, Downie JW, Kiruluta HG: Alpha-adrenergic agents in urinary disorders of the proximal urethra. I. Sphincteric incontinence, *Br J Urol* 50:332, 1978.

Bernstein E, Diskant BM: Phenylpropanolamine: a potentially hazardous drug, *Ann Emerg Med* 11:311, 1982.

Collste L, Lindskog M: Phenylpropanolamine in treatment of female stress urinary incontinence, *Urology* 30:398, 1987.

Diokno A, Taub M: Ephedrine in treatment of urinary incontinence, *Urology* 5:624, 1975.

Donker P, van der Sluis C: Action of beta adrenergic blocking agents on the urethral pressure profile, *Urol Int* 31:6, 1976.

Ek A, Andersson KE, Gullberg B, et al: The effects of long-term treatment with norephedrine on stress incontinence and urethral closure pressure profile, *Scand J Urol Nephrol* 12:105, 1978.

Fossberg E, Beisland HO, Lundgren RA: Stress incontinence in females: treatment with phenylpropanolamine, *Urol Int* 38:293, 1983.

Gilja I, Radej M, Kovacic M, et al: Conservative treatment of female stress incontinence with imipramine, *J Urol* 132:909, 1984.

Gleason D, Reilly R, Bottaccini M, et al: The urethral continence zone and its relation to stress incontinence, *J Urol* 112:81, 1974.

Lehtonen T, Rannikko S, Lindell O, et al: The effect of phenylpropanolamine on female stress urinary incontinence, *Ann Chir Gynaecol* 75:236, 1986.

Liebson I, Bigelow G, Griffiths R, et al: Phenylpropanolamine effects on subjective and cardiovascular variables at recommended over-the-counter dose levels, *J Clin Pharmacol* 27:685, 1987.

Lose G, Diernæs E, Rix P: Does medical therapy cure female stress incontinence? *Urol Int* 44:25, 1989.

Montague DK, Stewart BH: Urethral pressure profiles before and after Ornade administration in patients with stress urinary incontinence, *J Urol* 122:198, 1979.

Öbrink A, Bunne G: The effect of alpha-adrenergic stimulation in stress incontinence, *Scand J Urol Nephrol* 12:205, 1978.

Stewart BH, Banowsky LHW, Montague DK: Stress incontinence: conservative therapy with sympathomimetic drugs, *J Urol* 115:558, 1976.

Wein AJ: Pharmacologic treatment of incontinence, *J Am Geriatr Soc* 38:317, 1990.

Functional Electrical Stimulation

Alexander S, Rowan D: An electric pessary for stress incontinence, *Lancet* 1:728, 1968.

Caldwell KP: The electrical control of sphincter incompetence, *Lancet* 2:174, 1963.

Eriksen BC: Electrostimulation of the pelvic floor in female urinary incontinence, *Acta Obstet Gynecol Scand* 69:359, 1990.

Eriksen BC, Bergmann S, Mjølnerød OK: Effect of anal electrostimulation with the 'Incontan' device in women with urinary incontinence, *Br J Obstet Gynaecol* 94:147, 1987.

Eriksen BC, Eik-Nes SH: Long-term electrostimulation of the pelvic floor: primary therapy in female stress incontinence? *Urol Int* 44:90, 1989.

Eriksen BC, Mjølnerød OK: Changes in urodynamic measurements after successful anal electrostimulation in female urinary incontinence, *Br J Urol* 59:45, 1987.

Erlandson BE, Fall M: Intravaginal electrical stimulation in urinary incontinence. An experimental and clinical study, *Scand J Urol Nephrol* 44 (suppl):1, 1977.

Fall F, Erlandson C, Carlsson A, et al: Effects of electrical intravaginal stimulation on bladder volume. An experimental and clinical study, *Urol Int* 33:440, 1978.

Fall M, Ahlstrom K, Carlsson CA, et al: Contelle: pelvic floor stimulator for female stress-urge incontinence, *Urology* 27:282, 1986.

Fossberg E, Sørensen S, Ruutu M, et al: Maximal electrical stimulation in the treatment of unstable detrusor and urge incontinence, *Eur Urol* 18;120, 1990.

Godec C, Fravel R, Cass AS: Optimal parameters of electrical stimulation in the treatment of urinary incontinence, *Invest Urol* 18:239, 1981.

Godec C, Kralj B: Selection of patients with urinary incontinence for application of functional electrical stimulation, *Urol Int* 31:124, 1976.

Kralj B: The treatment of female urinary incontinence by functional electrical stimulation. In Ostergard DR, Bent AE (eds): *Urogynecology and urodynamics,* ed 3, Baltimore, 1991, Williams & Wilkins.

Lindstrom S, Fall M, Carlsson CA, et al: The neurophysiological basis of bladder inhibition in response to intravaginal electrical stimulation, *J Urol* 129:405, 1983.

Plevnik S: Electrical therapy. In Stanton SL (ed): *Clinical gynecologic urology,* St Louis, 1984, Mosby–Year Book.

Plevnik S, Suhel P, Rakovec S: Effects of functional electrical stimulation on the urethral closing muscles, *Med Biol Eng Comput* 15:155, 1977.

Sundin T, Carlsson CA: Reconstruction of several dorsal roots innervating the urinary bladder: an experimental study in cats.I. Studies on the normal afferent pathways in the pelvic and pudendal nerves, *Scand J Urol Nephrol* 6:176, 1972.

Sundin T, Carlsson CA, Kock NG: Detrusor inhibition induced from mechanical stimulation of the anal region and from electrical stimulation of the pudendal nerve afferents, *Invest Urol* 11:374, 1974.

Tanagho EA, Schmidt RA, Orvis BR: Neural stimulation for control of voiding dysfunction: a preliminary report in 22 patients with serious neuropathic voiding disorders, *J Urol* 142:340, 1989.

Trontelj JV, Janko M, Godec C, et al: Electrical stimulation for urinary incontinence, *Urol Int* 29:213, 1974.

Mechanical Devices

Bhatia N, Bergman A, Gunning J: Urodynamic effects of a vaginal pessary in women with stress urinary incontinence, *Am J Obstet Gynecol* 147:876, 1983.

Bonnar J: Silicone vaginal appliance for control of stress incontinence, *Lancet* 2:8049, 1977.

Cardozo LD, Stanton SL: Evaluation of female urinary incontinence device, *Urology* 13:398, 1979.

Edwards L: Control of incontinence of urine in women with a pubovaginal spring device: objective and subjective results, *Br J Urol* 43:211, 1971.

Realini JP, Walters MD: Vaginal diaphragm rings in the treatment of stress urinary incontinence, *J Am Board Fam Pract* 3:99, 1990.

Suarez GM, Baum NH, Jacobs J: Use of standard contraceptive diaphragm in management of stress urinary incontinence, *Urology* 37:119, 1991.

CHAPTER 14

Transvaginal Needle Suspension Procedures for Genuine Stress Incontinence

Mickey M. Karram

Surgical Anatomy and Terminology
Indications
Surgical Procedures
    Pereyra
    Stamey
    Raz
    Gittes
    Vaginal Colposuspension (Muzsnai)
Results
Complications
    Infection
    Hemorrhage
    Voiding Dysfunction
    Detrusor Instability
    Lower Urinary Tract Injury
    Nerve Damage
    Immediate Postoperative Urinary Incontinence

In 1959, Pereyra described the first transvaginal bladder neck suspension for stress incontinence using a long needle to suspend sutures from the vagina to the anterior abdominal fascia. The aim of the procedure was to combine a high cure rate with a low operative morbidity. When compared to retropubic procedures, these procedures were quicker, did not require splitting of the anterior abdominal fascia, and had reduced perioperative and postoperative morbidity. The transvaginal approach also permitted the simultaneous correction of other vaginal pathology such as cystocele, rectocele, and enterocele. Over 30 years later, at least 15 modifications of the original Pereyra procedure have been described; inferring efficient treatment of stress incontinence with these operations is an unresolved issue. Increasing popularity of these various modifications has led to confusion among gynecologists and urologists with regard to nomenclature and procedural details. This chapter traces these procedures from their origin, stresses important clinically relevant milestones as they evolved, and discusses current indications, techniques, results, and complications.

SURGICAL ANATOMY AND TERMINOLOGY

In the numerous modifications described, many different supportive tissues are used as anchoring tissue to elevate the bladder neck. Lack of a clear understanding of anatomic relations as well as inconsistency in the terminology used to describe these various tissues have contributed to the confusion surrounding these procedures. The anatomy of the urethra, bladder neck, and their supporting structures is both controversial and confusing. Only a few recent studies discuss periurethral and perivesical anatomy relative to function. Tissues that have been used to anchor vaginally placed sutures have included vaginal wall, pubocervical fascia, pubourethral ligaments, and the periurethral attachment to the inferior ramus of the pubic bone.

The bladder rests on the pubocervical fascia, which incorporates the entire vagina whose anterior lateral sulci is attached to the pelvic fascia's tendinous arch (white line). The integrity of these tissues may be affected by the plane of dissection of the vaginal wall off the proximal urethra and bladder neck. The pubocervical fascia is the anchoring tissue for sutures or vaginal buffers in the Stamey modification.

The periurethral attachment to the pubic bone is referred to as endopelvic fascia. To obtain this tissue, there must be either blunt or sharp dissection into the retropubic space to free this attachment from the pubic bone. When the retropubic space is entered sharply, the scissor tips are most likely to enter the space of Retzius medial to the arcus tendineus fasciae pelvis and lateral to the vaginal veins. The medial aspect of this incision is the desired location for placement of transvaginal sutures for the modified Pereyra procedure. This tissue is the medial condensation of endopelvic fascia that is densely adherent to the urogenital diaphragm lying immediately beneath it.

The pubourethral ligaments are composed of an anterior and posterior band. The posterior pubourethral ligament is thought to be an important structure with regard to urethral support and thus the development of stress incontinence. It is a dense band of connective tissue, which can be seen beside the urethra arising primarily from the vagina and periurethral tissue to attach laterally to the pelvic wall. There are two parts of this lateral attachment: the fascial attachment to the arcus tendineus fasciae pelvis and a muscular attachment to the medial edge of the levator ani. In his final modification, Pereyra included these structures in his helical suture of endopelvic fascia and claimed that when elevated retropubically, it held the posterior ligament firmly against the pubic bone.

Finally, some modifications have included the use of the vaginal wall either in its full thickness or excluding the epithelium.

INDICATIONS

As with retropubic procedures, needle suspensions are aimed at correcting anatomic genuine stress incontinence. The intent of these procedures is to elevate and support the bladder neck, which achieves continence by maintaining the bladder neck inside the sphere of abdominal pressure transmission during increased intraabdominal pressure.

Although various modifications of needle suspension procedures have been advocated for the correction of what has been termed a type III urethra (poorly functioning urethral sphincteric mechanism at rest with or without urethral mobility), other procedures such as suburethral slings, artificial sphincters, or periurethral injections will yield better results.

Whether one should perform a needle suspension or a retropubic procedure depends on numerous factors such as associated pathology, age, and physical well-being of the patient and skill and training of the surgeon. Results of recent prospective studies (see Results) comparing the two types of procedures also should be considered.

SURGICAL PROCEDURES
Pereyra

The original technique described bilateral passage of a special needle carrier through an abdominal stab incision without prior dissection. The needle carrier passed retropubically and penetrated the unopened vaginal mucosa. Extension of a stylet resulted in a Y-shaped, double, unilateral vaginal penetration. Subsequent placement of a suture, followed by needle carrier withdrawal, resulted in vaginal wall elevation. The original suture material described was No. 30 steel wire, which later penetrated the epithelium into the fibrous tissue of the vaginal wall. Thus the original description was a no incision needle suspension procedure almost identical to a recently popularized procedure (the Gittes procedure), which will be discussed later.

Because the wire loops left in the vaginal wall eventually cut through the anterior vaginal wall resulting in recurrent anatomic defects, Pereyra and Lebherz, working independently in 1967, reported their first modification. This report summarized their experience using a technique for suprapubic urethro-vesical angulation and suspension in conjunction with vesical neck plication to create a suburethral shelf. Theoretically, the plication sutures helped relieve some of the strain placed on the suspensory sutures.

Because longer follow-up of the 1967 modification revealed recurrences due to cutting through and pulling out of catgut sutures from the periurethral tissue, Pereyra and Lebherz described their second modification in 1978. They believed that to minimize the incidence of bladder injury, the space of Retzius had to be exposed completely per vagina so that each step of the operation could be performed under direct vision. In this modification, the authors first described entering the retropubic space through the vagina (Figs. 14-1 and 14-2). The anterolateral attachments of the periurethral tissue to the inferior pubic ramus were released by blunt dissection from the level of the

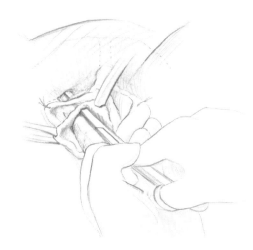

Fig. 14-2 Technique of vaginal entrance using Metzenbaum scissors. Endopelvic fascia is perforated at inferior margin of pubic bone as guided by surgeon's index finger. Blades of scissors are separated and dissection is completed by inserting a finger into space created as in Fig. 14-1. *(From Karram MM: In Hurt WG (ed): Urogynecologic surgery, Gaithersburg, Md, 1992, Aspen.)*

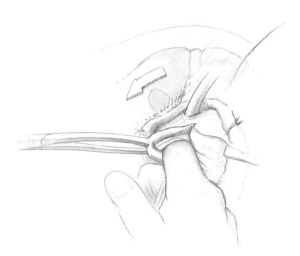

Fig. 14-1 Technique of blunt dissection into retropubic space. With tip of index finger flexed anteriorly against posterior symphysis, paraurethral attachment to pubic bone is perforated downward toward ischial spine, completely detaching endopelvic fascia. *(From Karram MM: In Hurt WG (ed): Urogynecologic surgery, Gaithersburg, Md, 1992, Aspen.)*

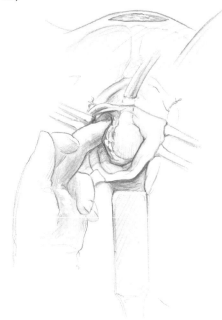

Fig. 14-3 Finger is placed behind detached endopelvic fascia, mobilizing it into vaginal field, to facilitate placement of helical suture. *(From Karram MM: In Hurt WG (ed): Urogynecologic surgery, Gaithersburg, Md, 1992, Aspen.)*

urethrovesical junction, up to but not including the attachments of the urethral meatus (Fig. 14-1). The endopelvic fascia was then brought down into the vaginal field (Fig. 14-3), and a permanent suture was passed in a helical fashion several times through this detached endopelvic fascia. Traction on both suture ends resulted in ruffling and thickening of the periurethral tissues producing multiple pleats to impede the sutures from pulling through. This revised procedure was safer because a vaginal finger could be inserted to the rectus muscle to provide direct guidance of the Pereyra ligature carrier (Fig.14-4) through the retropubic space (Fig.14-5). Using an aneurysm needle, the suspensory sutures were then anchored into the anterior rectus fascia. This revision included patients operated on between 1974 and 1977. In the latter portion of 1978, Pereyra believed that the revised procedure was incomplete because it did not include the posterior pubourethral ligaments in the suspensory sutures even though the procedure laid open to view laterally the posterior pillars of the pubourethral ligaments. He believed that inclusion of the posterior pubourethral pillars in the helical suture with the detached endopelvic fascia would provide maximal resistance to suspensory suture penetration. This modification is referred to as the modified Pereyra procedure (Fig. 14-6).

Stamey

Once Pereyra demonstrated the feasibility of suspending the pubocervical fascia by the passage of a suture through a special needle from the abdominal wall to the vagina, other investigators began to modify his techniques. Stamey believed that an appealing way to restore the posterior urethrovesical angle with great

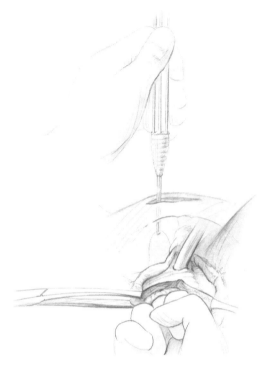

Fig. 14-5 Passage of needle is under direct finger guidance. Vaginal finger is inserted to posterior aspect of rectus muscle. *(From Karram MM: In Hurt WG (ed): Urogynecologic surgery, Gaithersburg, Md, 1992, Aspen.)*

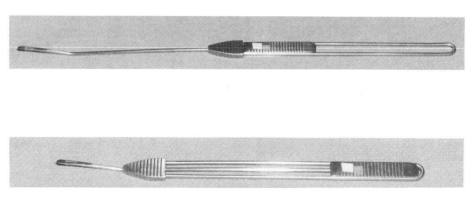

Fig. 14-4 Pereyra Ligature carrier *(El Ney Industries, Inc, Upland, Calif).*

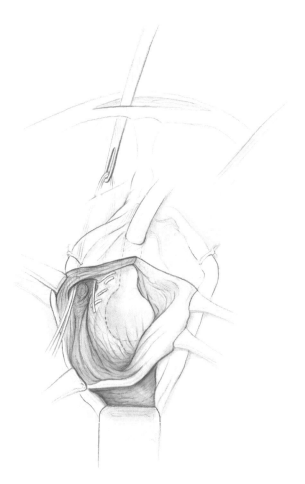

Fig. 14-6 Modified Pereyra procedure. Permanent suture is anchored in pubourethral ligament; then numerous passes are taken through detached endopelvic fascia. *(From Karram MM: In Hurt WG (ed):* Urogynecologic surgery, *Gaithersburg, Md, 1992, Aspen.)*

accuracy was to visualize the urethrovesical junction directly through the cystoscope while placing heavy monofilament suture on each side of the vesical neck. The theory was to raise a broad band of tissue on each side of the vesical neck extending from the pubocervical fascia to the anterior rectus fascia. In this procedure, bilateral transverse skin incisions are made, 2 to 4 cm long, about two finger breaths above the upper border of the symphysis pubis. A T-shaped vaginal incision is then made and the vaginal wall is

separated from the overlying urethra and trigone. One of three special long needles of different degrees of angulation is passed vertically alongside the vesical neck (Fig. 14-7). A cystoscope is then inserted to ensure that the lateral motion of the needle produces an indentation on the bladder wall at the vesical neck. Once proper placement of the needle is assured, the tip is passed into the vagina and is threaded with a No. 2 monofilament nylon suture and then withdrawn suprapubically. The needle is again passed through the same incision about 1 to 2 cm lateral to the original entry. It should exit in the vagina about 1 cm distal to the nylon suture. The vaginal end of the nylon suture is threaded through the eye of the needle and pulled out suprapubically. A broad band of tissue along one side of the vesical neck is within the nylon loop. If the pubocervical tissue is poor and unlikely to hold, the nylon suture can be passed through a 1 cm long 5 mm Dacron arteriograph to buttress the vaginal loop (Fig. 14-8).

Raz

The Raz modification differs from the 1978 modification of Pereyra in that an inverted U-shaped vaginal incision is used to allow dissection to be lateral to the urethra and bladder neck. The suspension sutures are anchored not only in the detached endopelvic fascia, but also through the full thickness of the vaginal wall excluding the epithelium (Fig. 14-9). Sutures are passed suprapubically under direct finger guidance. Cystoscopy is performed to inspect for any injury to the urethra, bladder, or ureters and to verify adequate bladder neck elevation. The claimed advantage over the modified Pereyra procedure is that anchoring the suspension sutures in the vaginal wall lateral to the urethra precludes the possibility of permanent urinary retention caused by overzealous traction on the sutures.

Gittes

In this modification, a small puncture is made in the suprapubic subcutaneous tissue, 2 cm superior to the pubic bone and 5 cm lateral to the midline on each side. A special long mattress-type needle or a Stamey needle with a 30-degree deflection is passed through the subcutaneous tissue and rectus fascia. The tip is

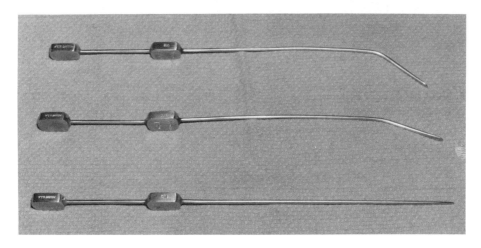

Fig. 14-7 A series of Stamey needles, a straight needle, a 15-degree angled needle, and a 30-degree angled needle *(Pilling Company, Fort Washington, Pa)*.

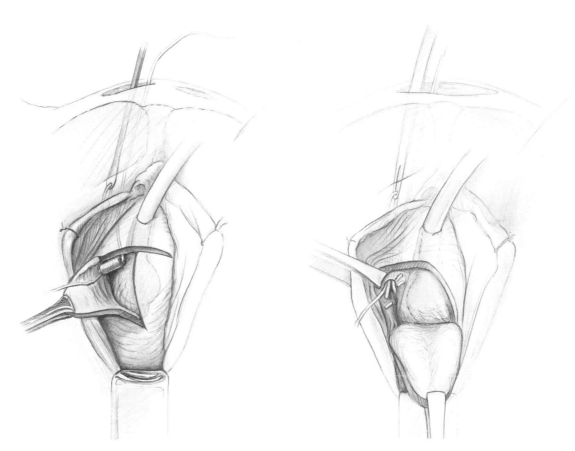

Fig. 14-8 Stamey procedure. Dacron loops are placed in pubovesico-cervical fascia on each side of bladder neck. These loops are suspended to anterior rectus fascia with nylon sutures. *(From Karram MM: In Hurt WG (ed): Urogynecologic surgery, Gaithersburg, Md, 1992, Aspen.)*

Fig. 14-9 Raz procedure. Helical suture is taken through detached endopelvic fascia and anchored in full-thickness vaginal wall excluding epithelium. *(From Karram MM: In Hurt WG (ed): Urogynecologic surgery, Gaithersburg, Md, 1992, Aspen.)*

advanced carefully down the posterior aspect of the pubic bone. A second hand elevates the anterior vaginal wall lateral to the bladder neck as palpated from the Foley balloon. The tip is then pierced through the vaginal wall. No vaginal incision is made in this procedure. A No. 2 nylon suture is threaded into the needle eyelet and withdrawn to the suprapubic area. A second pass of the needle is then made taking care to pass it through a different spot on the rectus fascia. The second perforation site on the vaginal wall is selected tactilly and visually to be 1.5 to 2 cm cephalad or caudad to the first puncture site with the suture in it. A free needle is used to take a full-thickness bite

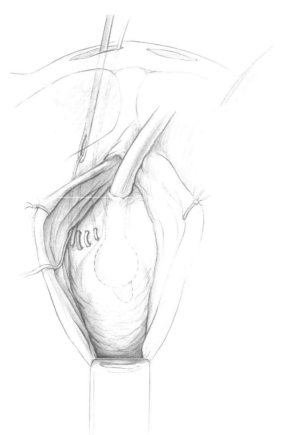

Fig. 14-10 Gittes Procedure. Stitches are taken through full thickness of vaginal wall and transferred suprapubically. No vaginal incision is made. *(From Karram MM: In Hurt WG (ed): Urogynecologic surgery, Gaithersburg, Md, 1992, Aspen.)*

through the portion of the anterior vaginal wall between the first and second vaginal perforations. The mattress suture is threaded and passed forward (Fig.14-10).

Cystourethroscopy is performed during passage of these sutures to detect any bladder damage or penetration by suture material. The sutures are tied tightly into the stab incision resulting in elevation of the anterior vaginal wall. The tied sutures are pulled upward and trimmed just above the knot, which then retracts below the skin. The tension on these tissues has been noted to relax slightly after 1 to 2 days.

Vaginal Colposuspension (Muzsnai)

In 1981, Muzsnai et al reported results on a new needle suspension procedure that used full-thickness vaginal wall excluding the epithelium as anchoring tissue, thus performing a vaginal colposuspension. A Foley catheter with a 30 ml balloon is used for easy identification of the bladder neck. Before beginning the surgery, the level of the bladder neck (as palpated by the Foley balloon) is marked on each side of the anterior vaginal wall. A midline anterior vaginal wall incision is used extending to approximately 2 cm proximal to the external urethral meatus. The incision should be carried through the full thickness of the vaginal wall, including the loose connective tissue. Sharp dissection is used to separate the vaginal wall from the bladder anterior and lateral to the pubic rami. Thus two vaginal flaps are created leaving the urethra and vesical wall denuded. At the level of the bladder neck, the anterolateral attachment of the periurethral tissue to the inferior ramus of the pubic bone is bluntly (Fig. 14-1) or sharply (Fig. 14-2) separated, allowing access into the retropubic space. The endopelvic fascia is completely detached and freed from the pubic bone, thus completely mobilizing the bladder neck. Nonabsorbable suture is then placed through the inner surface of the vaginal wall. One helical suture is taken from the level of the mid-urethra to the bladder neck and a second suture is placed from the bladder neck down to the level of the bladder base. A finger is placed on the outside of the vagina to ensure that the sutures do not penetrate through the vaginal epithelium. These sutures are taken approximately 1.5 to 2 cm inside the edge of each vaginal flap (Fig. 14-11).

In patients with severe anterior vaginal wall relaxation in which the surgeon anticipates trimming some vaginal wall, the sutures should be 2 cm inside the trimmed edge. In instances in which the vaginal wall is very thin, the sutures can be passed through the detached endopelvic fascia, either in conjunction or separate from the vaginal wall. A Pereyra needle (Fig. 14-2) is then used to transfer these sutures to the suprapubic area under direct finger guidance. If necessary, an anterior colporrhaphy is performed at this time. Cystourethroscopy is performed to assure no

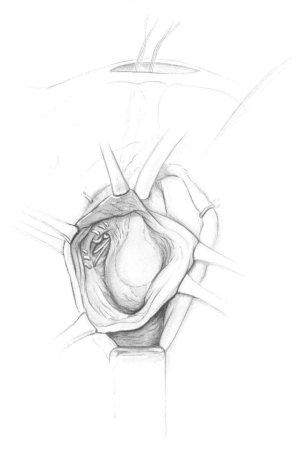

Fig. 14-11 Vaginal colposuspension (Muzsnai). Permanent sutures are taken through full thickness of vaginal wall (excluding epithelium). Two stitches are placed on each side and transferred suprapubically under direct finger guidance. *(From Karram MM: In Hurt WG (ed):* Urogynecologic surgery, *Gaithersburg, Md, 1992, Aspen.)*

bladder injury or stitch penetration. Five milliliters of indigo-carmine is given intravenously to help visualize and assure patency of the ureters.

The anterior vaginal wall is closed with continuous or interrupted No. 3-0 sutures. With a hand in the vagina elevating the anterior vaginal wall, the suprapubic stitches are tied down so that there is a small amount of dimpling in the lateral vaginal fornix on each side, thus simulating the abdominal colposuspension (modified Burch procedure).

Fig. 14-12 and Table 14-1 compare commonly performed needle suspension procedures.

RESULTS

The evaluation of any surgery for the correction of stress incontinence is hampered by several factors. First, the diagnostic criteria, including the need for urodynamic testing, is controversial. Second, variations in patient populations including prior pelvic surgery, age, weight, childbearing history, associated medical conditions, and coexistent detrusor instability influence the surgical success rates. Variations in surgical technique, including modifications of a so-called standard procedure, may be significant. Finally, and most important, is the length and method of followup for these patients. How long must a patient remain continent and what constitutes a cure or failure?

Many studies have reported clinical experiences with needle suspension procedures. The major problem with most studies is that objective parameters were not used preoperatively and postoperatively to establish diagnosis and outcome of surgery. A recent review of published results of needle suspension procedures noted a cure rate of 85% for over 1950 procedures. Most of these studies, however, were based on subjective criteria for cure and had relatively short follow-up periods. This review also noted that only three studies, with a total of 60 patients, used objective urodynamic criteria preoperatively and postoperatively.

Several studies have reported objective results with much lower cure rates. Probably the best published data to date are two prospective randomized studies by Bergman et al. They compared Burch urethropexy to modified Pereyra to anterior colporrhaphy in pa-

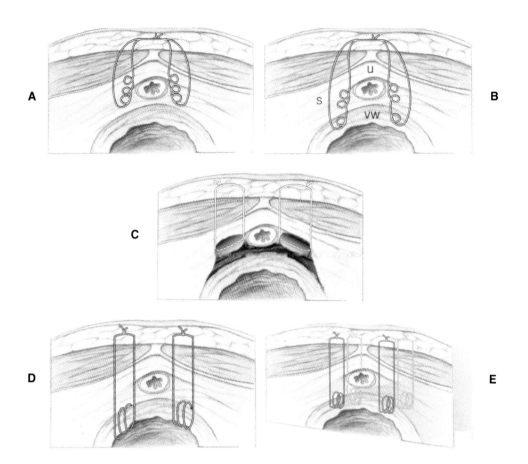

Fig. 14-12 Cross-section of various anchoring sutures used in needle procedures. **A**, Modified Pereyra: helical stitch through paraurethral ligament and detached endopelvic fascia. **B**, Raz procedure: helical stitch through detached endopelvic fascia and anchored in vaginal wall. **C**, Stamey procedure: buttresses are placed in the pubocervicovesical fascia on each side of the bladder neck. **D**, Gittes Procedure: stitches through the full thickness of the vaginal wall. **E**, Muzsnai: two stitches on each side through vaginal wall excluding epithelium. *(From Karram MM: In Hurt WG (ed): Clinical urogynecology, Gaithersburg, Md, 1992, Aspen.)*

TABLE 14-1 Differences among various needle suspension produres

Procedure	Vaginal incision	Needle passage	Anchoring tissue	Cystoscopy
Modified Pereyra	Midline	Under direct finger guidance	Pubourethral ligament and endopelvic fascia	To assure no injury
Stamey	T-shaped	Blindly	Pubocervical fascia	For proper needle and suture placement
Raz	Inverted-U	Under direct finger guidance	Endopelvic fascia and vaginal wall	To assure no injury
No incision urethropexy (Gittes)	None	Blindly	Full-thickness vaginal wall	For proper needle and suture placement
Vaginal colposuspension (Muzsnai)	Midline	Under direct finger guidance	Vaginal wall excluding epithelium	To assure no injury

tients with associated pelvic relaxation defects (289 patients) and also in patients with the isolated finding of genuine stress incontinence (107 patients). The studies were randomized for the procedure as well as for the surgeon. All patients had preoperative and postoperative urodynamic studies with a minimum follow-up of 1 year. The cure rate for the Burch procedure (88%) was significantly higher than the anterior repair (67%) and modified Pereyra (68%). Weil et al studied 86 patients clinically and urodynamically at least 6 months after either Burch procedure, modified Pereyra, or anterior repair and noted similar results (Table 14-2). Recent reports on the Stamey procedure have also noted objective cure rates approximating 65%, 3 to 6 months after surgery. Peattie and Stanton noted only a 40% success rate after a Stamey procedure in women over the age of 65. Mundy also noted an objective cure rate of only 40% in patients 12 months after a Stamey procedure.

No data with objective follow-up have been published regarding the results of the noincision urethropexy (Gittes). The only study of vaginal colposuspension by Muzsnai et al involved 98 patients. All patients were followed for a minimum of 6 months with a 95% cure rate. Cure was defined as no subjective complaints of incontinence and no visual loss of urine during coughing at the time of follow-up.

Table 14-2 lists all published studies on needle suspension procedures in which preoperative and postoperative urodynamics were performed.

COMPLICATIONS

Complications of these procedures can be classified broadly into those complications mutual to all needle suspension procedures and complications associated with specific modifications.

Infection

Infection can occur after any of these procedures but is probably more common in Stamey-type procedures in which Dacron or silicon buttresses are used. Because most surgeons use permanent suture when performing these procedures, stitch abscesses can occur and point transvaginally or suprapubically. These complications rarely occur in the immediate postop-

TABLE 14-2   Published studies on needle procedures in which preoperative and postoperative urodynamic studies were perfomred

Author	Patients (No.)	Time of follow-up	Cure rate (%)				
			Stamey	Pereyra	Burch	AR	Sling
Bergman et al	289	1 year		70	87	69	
Bergman et al	107	1 year		65	89	67	
Weil et al	86	6 months		50	91	57	
Griffith-Jones and Abrams	17	9 months	76				
English and Fowler	45	6 months	58				
Peattie and Stanton	44	3 months	40				
Mundy	51	1 year	40		73		
Hilton	21	6 months	80				90
Karram et al	103	1 year		60			
Bhatia and Bergman	64	1 year		85	98		
Leach et al	20	14 months		90			

AR, Anterior repair.

erative period, but can present months and even years postoperatively. We routinely use prophylactic antibiotics at surgery; however, there is no published data showing the efficacy of this practice.

Hemorrhage

Hemorrhage is more common after modifications in which the retropubic space is entered. While doing this, a significant amount of venous bleeding may occur, which is usually from perforating vessels at the medial edge of the periurethral attachment to the pubic bone. Surprisingly, bleeding from the retropubic space is almost always self-limited even though it can appear to be severe at the time of surgery. We recently reported on 103 modified Pereyra procedures of which 7% of patients required blood transfusion, with no patient requiring reexploration to control active bleeding or evacuate a hematoma. When excessive, uncontrollable bleeding occurs from the retropubic space, transvaginal tamponade can be achieved with a Foley catheter, described by Katske and Raz. Gauze packing is inserted around the catheter; the Foley balloon is inflated until adequate tamponade is achieved.

Voiding Dysfunction

Voiding dysfunction is a potential complication of any antiincontinence procedure. In our experience, needle procedures have been more obstructive than retropubic procedures in the immediate postoperative period. Nevertheless, numerous studies have noted a low incidence of long term voiding dysfunction. Patients with more severe anterior vaginal wall relaxation, those with high preoperative postvoid residual urine volumes, and those with underactive or areflexic detrusor muscles on pressure-flow studies are at higher risk for prolonged voiding dysfunction and probably should be taught intermittent self-catheterization preoperatively.

Detrusor Instability

Detrusor instability is a common cause of either persistence or recurrence of incontinence after antiincontinence surgery. Detrusor instability should be aggressively looked for when antiincontinence surgery is being contemplated because it has been shown to coexist in 5% to 30% of patients with genuine stress incontinence. The postoperative course of detrusor instability is unpredictable, as it may persist, worsen, improve, or develop de novo. All patients should be warned preoperatively that they may require anticholinergic medications postoperatively. When instability develops postoperatively, it is usually self-limited and responds quite well to therapy.

Lower Urinary Tract Injury

Cystotomy can occur during any of the steps of vaginal dissection and is probably more common during secondary procedures. In the modified Pereyra procedure, dissection directly on the medial aspect of the ischial pubic ramus during mobilization of the bladder neck and entrance of the retropubic space, minimizes bladder injury. In addition, the modified Pereyra procedure permits fingertip control of needle passage through the retropubic space to the vagina, minimizing the risk of injury to the bladder and urethra. This advantage is not offered by the Stamey or Gittes procedures. Routine use of intraoperative cystoscopy should recognize this complication. If a suture is noted in the anterolateral bladder wall, it should be removed and repassed under fingertip guidance. Nonrecognition of a penetrating suture or intravesical migration of a permanent suture can lead to chronic infection and stone formation. Any patient with recurrent urinary tract infection or irritative symptoms who has undergone a suspension should have a radiographic and endoscopic evaluation to rule out this complication.

Urethral injuries are rare; immediate closure with long-term catheter drainage is recommended.

Nerve Damage

Neural injury can occur, because the patient is in a dorsal lithotomy position during these procedures. This complication is most commonly due to direct compression of the nerve against various structures and results in a first degree injury (neuropraxia) resolving in 1 to 6 weeks. Rarely a second-degree injury (axonotmesis) will occur, which takes 2 to 6 months to resolve. The most frequent nerve involved is the common peroneal but injury to the obturator, sciatic, tibial, femoral, or saphenous nerves can occur (Table 14-3). Neurologic and physical medicine consultations are recommended after early recognition.

Another category of nerve injury is nerve entrapment of the ilioinguinal nerve, which can occur when

TABLE 14-3   Various nerves that can be injured during needle suspension procedures

Nerve	Mechanism of injury	Clinical presentation
Common peroneal	Direct compression between fibular neck and leg brace	Foot drop
Sciatic	Pressure against sciatic notch or stretching of the nerve during hip flexion	Weakness during knee flexion, or variable loss of common peroneal or tibial nerve function
Obturator	Compression of nerve at undersurface of pubic ramus	Weakness of ipsilateral thigh adduction
Femoral	Hyperflexion of hips compressing femoral nerve against inguinal ligament	Quadriceps weakness, gait impairment, decreased sensation over anterior thigh and medial calf
Saphenous	Hyperflexion of hips creating undue stretch of nerve against medial aspect of knee	Buring or aching pain in medial calf
Ilioinguinal	Entrapment of nerve by suture when needle passed lateral to pubic tubercle	Pain in medial groin, labia, or inner thigh

the bladder neck suspension sutures are anchored to the anterior rectus fascia. These patients will complain of localized pain in the medial groin, labia, or inner thigh. The character of the pain varies from a severe constant burning pain to sharp shooting pains. The pain is uniformly aggravated by Valsalva maneuver and by lifting the ipsilateral leg. This type of nerve injury has been reported in as many as 16% of patients undergoing transvaginal needle suspensions. The nerve is most vulnerable to entrapment near its exit from the superficial inguinal ring which lies almost directly above the pubic tubercle. Thus to avert injury to this nerve, sutures should always be passed medial to the pubic tubercle. When injury is suspected, the diagnosis is confirmed by a local nerve block in the inguinal canal with 10 to 15 ml of 1% lidocaine (Xylocaine). Initial management of this type of pain should include analgesic and antiinflammatory agents. The decision to remove and reposition the offending sutures depends on the severity and duration of pain.

Immediate Postoperative Urinary Incontinence

The immediate demonstration of urinary incontinence after surgery for stress incontinence is a very distressing finding to both patient and physician. The surgeon must differentiate among persistent stress incontinence, detrusor instability, lower urinary tract fistula, overflow incontinence, urinary tract infection, or a watery vaginal discharge simulating urinary incontinence.

Persistent stress incontinence will most commonly be secondary to failure of the surgical procedure to stabilize and support the bladder neck (anatomic stress incontinence). Rarely, it will be due to persistence or development of a type III or poorly functioning urethra.

Overflow incontinence is a manifestation of iatrogenic retention, and it can be managed with a combination of fluid restriction and self-catheterization.

As previously mentioned, detrusor instability can develop de novo after bladder neck suspension. This type of detrusor instability usually responds to anticholinergic therapy and is usually self-limited, undergoing spontaneous resolution within 3 months of surgery.

SUMMARY

Based on recently published objective studies, we believe that the procedure of choice for primary anatomic stress incontinence is a retropubic urethropexy. We reserve needle suspension procedures for elderly patients with medical disabilities in which anesthetic and operative time is best kept to a minimum, continent patients with marked anterior vaginal wall relaxation who are at high risk for developing stress urinary incontinence, and patients with severe pelvic prolapse as a primary complaint who also have coexistent mild stress incontinence as a secondary complaint.

Our needle procedure of choice is a vaginal colposuspension similar to that described by Muzsnai et al. The advantages of this modification are the following: (1) use of strong anchoring tissue in full thickness vaginal wall, (2) complete mobilization of bladder neck; (3) needle passage under direct finger guidance; and (4) facilitation of anterior vaginal wall support. These potential advantages await confirmation via controlled randomized trials.

These operations are still evolving and many procedural details remain controversial. Many of the currently held beliefs have been advocated empirically with little supportive data. There is a definite advantage, in certain patients, to correcting stress incontinence via a vaginal route. It is hoped that continued experience with these procedures will lead to modifications, resulting in better long-term cure rates.

BIBLIOGRAPHY

Surgical Anatomy and Terminology

Delancy JO: Correlative study of paraurethral anatomy, *Obstet Gynecol* 68:91, 1986.

Delancy JO: Pubovesical ligament: a separate structure from the urethral supports ("pubo-urethral ligaments"), *Neurourol Urodyn* 8:53, 1989.

Delancy JO: Structural aspects of the extrinsic continence mechanism, *Obstet Gynecol* 72:296, 1988.

Mostwin JL: Current concepts of female pelvic anatomy and physiology, *Urol Clin North Am* 18:175, 1991.

Richardson AC, Lyon JB, Williams NL: A new look at pelvic relaxation, *Am J Obstet Gynecol* 126:568, 1976.

Surgical Procedures

Karram MM, Bhatia NN: Transvaginal needle bladder neck suspension procedures for stress urinary incontinence: a comprehensive review, *Obstet Gynecol* 73:906, 1989.

Muzsnai D, Carrillo E, Dubin C, Silverman I: Retropubic vaginopexy for correction of urinary stress incontinence, *Obstet Gynecol* 59:113, 1982.

Pereyra AJ: A simplified surgical procedure for the correction of stress incontinence in women, *West J Surg* 1959; 67:223, 1959.

Pereyra AJ: Revised Pereyra procedure using colligated pubourethral supports. In Slate WG (ed): *Disorders of the female urethra and urinary incontinence*, Baltimore, 1978, Williams & Wilkins.

Pereyra AJ, Lebherz TB: Combined urethral vesical suspension vaginal urethroplasty for correction of urinary stress incontinence, *Obstet Gynecol* 30:537, 1967.

Pereyra AJ, Lebherz TB: The revised Pereyra procedure. In Buchsbaum H, Schmidt JD (eds): *Gynecologic and obstetric urology*, ed 1, Philadelphia, 1978, WB Saunders.

Raz S: Modified bladder neck suspension for female stress incontinence, *Urology* 17:82, 1981.

Stamey TA: Endoscopic suspension of the vesical neck for urinary incontinence in females, *Ann Surg* 192:465, 1980.

Stamey TA: Endoscopic suspension of vesical neck for urinary incontinence, *Surg Gynecol Obstet* 136:547, 1973.

Stamey TA, Schaffer AJ, Condy M: Clinical and roentgenographic evaluation of endoscopic suspension of the vesical neck for urinary incontinence, *Surg Gynecol Obstet* 140:355, 1975.

Results

Bergman A, Ballard CA, Koonings PP: Comparison of three different surgical procedures for genuine stress incontinence: prospective randomized study, *Am J Obstet Gynecol* 160:1102, 1989.

Bergman A, Kooning PP, Ballard CA: Primary stress urinary incontinence and pelvic relaxation: prospective randomized comparison of three different operations, *Am J Obstet Gynecol* 161:91, 1989.

Bhatia NN, Bergman A: Modified Burch versus Pereyra retropubic urethropexy for stress urinary incontinence, *Obstet Gynecol* 66:255, 1985.

English PJ, Fowler JW: Videourodynamic assessment of the Stamey procedure for stress incontinence, *Br J Urol* 62:550, 1988.

Griffith-Jones MD, Abrams PH: The Stamey endoscopic bladder neck in the elderly, *Br J Obstet Gynecol* 65:170, 1990.

Hilton P: A clinical and urodynamic study comparing the Stamey bladder neck suspension and suburethral sling procedures in the treatment of genuine stress incontinence, *Br J Obstet Gynecol* 96:213, 1989.

Karram MM, Angel O, Koonings P, et al: The modified Pereyra procedure. A clinical and urodynamic review, *Br J Obstet Gynecol* 99:655, 1992.

Leach GE, Yip CM, Donovan BJ: Mechanism of continence after modified Pereyra bladder neck suspension, *Urology* 29:328, 1987.

Mundy AR: A trial comparing the Stamey bladder neck suspension procedure with colposuspension for the treatment of stress incontinence, *Br J Urol* 55:687, 1983.

Peattie AB, Stanton SL: The Stamey operation for correction of genuine stress incontinence in the elderly woman, *Br J Obstet Gynecol* 96:983, 1989.

Weil A, Reyes H, Bischoff P, et al, Modification of the urethral rest and stress profile after different types of surgery for stress incontinence, *Br J Obstet Gynecol* 91:46, 1984.

Complications

Ashken MH, Abrams PH, Lawrence WT: Stamey endoscopic bladder neck suspension for stress incontinence, *Br J Urol* 56:629, 1984.

Bhatia NN, Bergman A: Use of preoperative uroflowmetry and simultaneous urethrocystometry for predicting risk of prolonged postoperative bladder drainage, *Urology* 28:440, 1986.

Cardozo LD, Stanton SL, Williams JE: Detrusor instability following surgery for genuine stress incontinence, *Br J Urol* 51:204, 1979.

Diaz DL, Fox BM, Walzak MP, et al: Endoscopic vesicourethropexy, *Urology* 24:321, 1984.

Karram MM, Bhatia NN: Management of coexistent stress and urge urinary incontinence, *Obstet Gynecol* 73:4, 1989.

Katske FA, Raz S. Use of Foley catheter to obtain transvaginal tamponade, *Urol Urotech*, May 1987, p 8.

Kelly MJ, Knielsen K, Bruskewitz R, et al: Symptom analysis of patients undergoing modified Pereyra bladder neck suspension for stress urinary incontinence. Preoperative and postoperative findings, *Urology*, 28:213, 1991.

Kelly MJ, Zimmern PE, Leach GE: Complications of bladder neck suspension procedures, *Urol Clin North Am* 18:342, 1991.

McGuire EJ, Savastano JA: Stress incontinence and detrusor instability/urge incontinence, *Neurourol Urodyn* 1985;4:313, 1985.

Zimmern PE, Schmidbauer CP, Leach GE, et al: Vesicovaginal and urethrovaginal fistulae, *Semin Urol* 424, 1986.

CHAPTER 15

Genuine Stress Incontinence: Retropubic Surgical Procedures

Mark D. Walters

Indications for Retropubic Procedures
Surgical Techniques
    Operative set-up and general entry into the retropubic
      space
    Burch colposuspension
    Marshal-Marchetti-Krantz procedure
    Paravaginal and VOS procedures
    Laparoscopic retropubic bladder neck surgery
    General intraoperative and postoperative procedures
Clinical Results
Mechanisms of Cure
Complications
    Short-term postoperative
    Postoperative voiding difficulties
    Detrusor instability
    Osteitis pubis
    Enterocele
Role of Hysterectomy in the Treatment of
    Incontinence
Pregnancy After Retropubic Surgery

Since 1949, when Marshall et al first described retropubic urethrovesical suspension for the treatment of stress urinary incontinence, retropubic procedures have emerged as consistently curative. Although numerous terminologies and variations of retropubic repairs have been described, the basic concept remains the same: to suspend and to stabilize the bladder neck and proximal urethra in a retropubic position to prevent their descent outside the sphere of abdominal pressure transmission during stress. Selection of a retropubic approach (versus a vaginal approach) depends on many factors, such as the need for laparotomy for other pelvic disease, the amount of pelvic relaxation, the age and health status of the patient, and the preference and expertise of the surgeon.

Few data differentiate one retropubic procedure from another, although all have advantages and disadvantages. This chapter describes the surgical techniques for the three most studied and popular retropubic procedures: the Marshall-Marchetti-Krantz (MMK) procedure, the Burch colposuspension, and the paravaginal and vaginal obturator shelf (VOS) repairs. The surgical techniques described herein are contemporary modifications of the original operations: Krantz in 1986 described the MMK technique and Tanagho in 1976 described the modified Burch colposuspension. The paravaginal and VOS repairs are similar procedures; the techniques have been described by Richardson et al and Shull and Baden (paravaginal repair) and by Turner-Warwick and Webster and Kreder (VOS repair). Although less critically studied, these techniques are regionally popular and widely performed in the United States and Great Britain. The operations described do not represent one correct technique, but a commonly used and proven method.

INDICATIONS FOR RETROPUBIC PROCEDURES

Retropubic urethrovesical suspension procedures are indicated for women with the diagnosis of genuine stress incontinence and a hypermobile proximal urethra and bladder neck. These procedures yield the best results when the urethral sphincter is capable of maintaining a watertight seal at rest, but cannot withstand the unequal transmission of abdominal pressure to the proximal urethra, relative to the bladder, with straining. This situation corresponds to types I and II genuine stress incontinence as described by McGuire. Although retropubic procedures can be used for type III genuine stress incontinence (poorly functioning urethral sphincteric mechanism at rest, with or without urethral mobility), other more obstructive operations probably yield better long-term results (see Chapter 16).

To diagnose genuine stress incontinence, clinical and urodynamic (simple or complex) tests must be performed to evaluate bladder filling, storage, and emptying. Clinically, the urethra is shown to be incompetent by visually observing loss of urine simultaneous with increases in intraabdominal pressure. Urodynamic or radiologic methods may also be used for diagnosis. Abnormalities of bladder-filling function, such as detrusor instability, can coexist with urethral sphincter incompetence, but may be associated with a lower cure rates after retropubic surgery.

Women with genuine stress incontinence should generally have a trial of conservative therapy before corrective surgery is offered. Conservative treatment comes in the form of pelvic muscle exercises, bladder retraining, pharmacologic therapy, functional electrical stimulation, and mechanical devices, such as pessaries. Eligible postmenopausal patients with atrophic urogenital changes should be prescribed estrogen before surgery is considered.

SURGICAL TECHNIQUES

Operative Setup and General Entry into the Retropubic Space

The patient is supine, with the legs supported in a slightly abducted position, allowing the surgeon to operate with one hand in the vagina and the other in the retropubic space. The vagina, perineum, and abdomen are sterilely prepped and draped in a fashion that permits easy access to the lower abdomen and vagina. A three-way 16 or 20 French Foley catheter with a 20 to 30 ml balloon is inserted sterilely into the bladder and kept in the sterile field. The drainage port of the catheter is left to gravity drainage and the irrigation port is connected to a dilute methylene blue solution. One to three perioperative intravenous doses of an appropriate antibiotic should be given as prophylaxis against infection.

A Pfannenstiel or Cherney incision is made. During intraperitoneal surgery, the peritoneum is opened, the surgery is completed, and the cul-de-sac is plicated. The retropubic space is then exposed. Staying close to the back of the pubic bone, the surgeon's hand is introduced into the retropubic space and the bladder and urethra gently moved downward. Sharp dissection is not usually necessary in primary cases. To aid visualization of the bladder, 100 ml of sterile water with methylene blue dye may be instilled into the bladder after the catheter drainage port is clamped.

If previous retropubic (especially MMK) procedures have been performed, dense adhesions from the anterior bladder wall and urethra to the symphysis pubis are frequently present. These adhesions should be dissected sharply from the pubic bone until the anterior bladder wall, urethra, and vagina are free of adhesions and are mobile. If identification of the urethra or lower border of the bladder is difficult, one may perform a cystotomy, which, with a finger inside the bladder, helps to define the bladder's lower limits for easier dissection, mobilization, and elevation.

Burch Colposuspension

Once the retropubic space is entered, the urethra and anterior vaginal wall are depressed downward. No dissection should be performed in the midline over the urethra or at the urethrovesical junction, thus protecting the delicate musculature of the urethra from surgical trauma. Attention is directed to the tissue on either side of the urethra. Most of the overlying fat should be cleared away, using a swab mounted on a curved forceps. This dissection is accomplished with forceful elevation of the surgeon's vaginal finger (or a Deaver retractor in the vagina) until glistening white

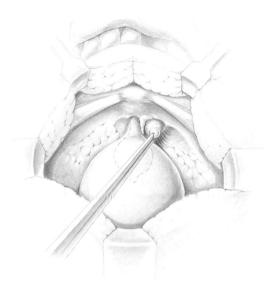

Fig. 15-1 Dissection of the lateral retropubic space. After forceful elevation of the surgeon's vaginal finger, the fat overlying the glistening white periurethral fascia is cleared in preparation for suture placement.

periurethral fascia and vaginal wall are seen (Fig. 15-1). This area is extremely vascular, with a rich, thin-walled venous plexus that should be avoided, if possible. The position of the urethra and the lower edge of the bladder should be determined by palpating the Foley balloon and by partially distending the bladder to define the rounded lower margin of the bladder as it meets the anterior vaginal wall.

Once dissection lateral to the urethra is completed and vaginal mobility is judged to be adequate by using the vaginal fingers to lift the anterior vaginal wall upward and forward, sutures should be placed. Number 0 or 1 delayed absorbable or nonabsorbable sutures are placed as far laterally in the anterior vaginal wall as is technically possible. We apply two sutures bilaterally, using double bites for each suture. The distal suture is placed approximately 2 cm lateral to the midurethra. The proximal suture is placed approximately 2 cm lateral to the reflection of the anterior bladder wall at, or slightly proximal to, the level of the urethrovesical junction.

In placing the sutures, one should take a full thickness of vaginal wall, excluding the epithelium, with

the needle parallel to the urethra (Fig. 15-2, *inset*). This maneuver is best accomplished by suturing over the vaginal finger at the appropriate selected sites. On each side, after the two sutures are placed, they are then passed through the pectineal (Cooper's) ligament, so that all four suture ends exit above the ligament (Fig. 15-2). Before tying the sutures, a 1 × 4 cm strip of Gelfoam may be placed between the vagina and obturator fascia below Cooper's ligament to aid adherence and hemostasis.

As noted previously, this area is extremely vascular, and visible vessels should be avoided if at all possible. When excessive bleeding occurs, it can be controlled by direct pressure, sutures, or vascular clips. Less severe bleeding usually stops once the fixation sutures are tied.

After all four sutures are placed in the vagina and through the Cooper's ligaments, the assistant ties first the distal sutures and then the proximal ones, while the surgeon elevates the vagina with the vaginal hand. In tying the sutures, one does not have to be concerned about whether the vaginal wall meets Cooper's ligament, so one should not place too much tension on the vaginal wall. A suture bridge may be placed between the two points without causing complications. After the sutures are tied, one can easily insert two fingers between the pubic bone and the urethra, thus avoiding compression of the urethra against the pubic bone. Continued vaginal fixation and urethral support depend more on fibrosis and scarring of periurethral and vaginal tissues over the obturator internus fascia than on the suture material itself.

Marshall-Marchetti-Krantz Procedure

The retropubic space is exposed and the urethra and bladder base palpated with the Foley catheter in place. The surgeon's left hand is placed into the vagina and the index and middle fingers are placed at the urethrovesical neck on either side of the urethra. Gentle dissection of periurethral fat is made at the urethrovesical junction on each side over the vaginal fingers. This area is extremely vascular, having a rich, thin-walled venous plexus that should be avoided, if possible.

Delayed absorbable sutures are usually used and are placed at right angles to the urethra and parallel

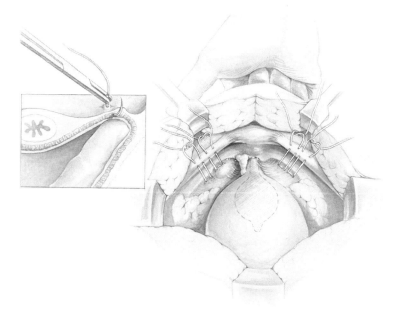

Fig. 15-2 Technique of Burch colposuspension. After the two sutures are placed on each side, they are passed through the pectineal (Cooper's) ligament, so that all four suture ends exit above the ligament to facilitate knot tying. *Inset,* In placing the sutures, one should take a full thickness of vaginal wall, excluding the epithelium, with the needle parallel to the urethra. This maneuver is best achieved by suturing over the vaginal finger.

to the vesical neck. A single suture is placed bilaterally at the urethrovesical junction. A double bite is taken over the surgeon's finger, incorporating full thickness of the vaginal wall, but excluding the vaginal epithelium. After placement of the sutures, the point of fixation of the urethra to the symphysis pubis can be determined by elevating the two vaginal fingers to the point where the vesical neck comes in contact with the pubic symphysis and noting the position at which the sutures will be placed into the pubic periosteum. The needle is placed medially to laterally against the periosteum, and turned with a simple wrist action. It may involve the cartilage in the midline, depending on the width, thickness, and availability of the periosteum. The sutures on each side are placed accordingly and tied, with the vaginal finger elevating the urethrovesical junction (Fig. 15-3). Venous bleeding is usually controlled after tying the sutures or with direct pressure.

Paravaginal and VOS Procedures

The object of the paravaginal and VOS repairs is to reattach, bilaterally, the anterolateral vaginal sulcus with its overlying pubocervical fascia to the pubococcygeus and obturator internus muscles and fascia at the level of the arcus tendineus fasciae pelvis. The retropubic space is entered and the bladder and vagina are depressed and pulled medially to allow visualization of the lateral retropubic space, including the obturator internus muscle, and the fossa containing the obturator neurovascular bundle. Blunt dissection can be carried dorsally from this point until the ischial spine is palpated. The arcus tendineus fasciae pelvis is frequently visualized as a white band of tissue running over the pubococcygeus and obturator internus muscles from the back of the lower edge of the symphysis pubis toward the ischial spine. A lateral paravaginal defect representing avulsion of the vagina off the arcus tendineus fasciae pelvis or of the arcus ten-

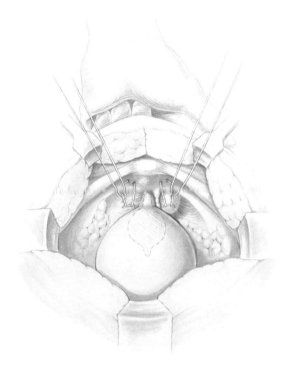

Fig. 15-3 Marshall-Marchetti-Krantz procedure. One suture is placed bilaterally at the level of the bladder neck and then into the periosteum of the pubic symphysis.

dineus fasciae pelvis off the obturator internus muscle may be visualized (Fig. 15-4).

The surgeon's left hand is inserted into the vagina. While gently retracting the vagina and bladder medially, the surgeon elevates the anterolateral vaginal sulcus. Starting near the vaginal apex, a suture is placed, first through the full thickness of the vagina (excluding the vaginal epithelium), and then into the obturator internus fascia or arcus tendineus fasciae pelvis, 3 to 4 cm below the obturator fossa. After this first stitch is tied, additional (five or six) sutures are placed through the vaginal wall and overlying fascia and then into the obturator internus at about 1-cm intervals toward the pubic ramus (Fig. 15-4, *inset*). The most distal suture should be placed as close as possible to the pubic ramus, into the pubourethral ligament. No. 3-0 nonabsorbable suture on a medium-sized, tapered needle is usually used for the paravaginal repair.

The VOS repair enters the retropubic space as noted previously, but does not continue dissection to the ischial spine. Three interrupted No. 0 or 1 nonabsorbable or delayed absorbable sutures are placed bilaterally at 1-cm intervals through the paravaginal fascia and vaginal wall (excluding the vaginal epithelium), beginning at the urethrovesical junction

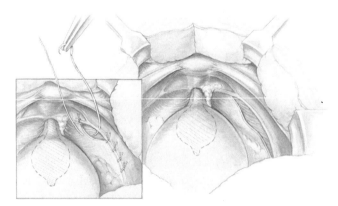

Fig. 15-4 Lateral paravaginal defect and technique of paravaginal repair. Five or six sutures are placed, first through the full thickness of the vagina (excluding the vaginal epithelium), and then into the obturator internus fascia or arcus tendineus fasciae pelvis, 3 to 4 cm below the obturator fossa.

and continuing proximally toward the bladder base. These sutures are then passed horizontally through the adjacent obturator fascia and underlying muscle and tied. To fill the retropubic dead space, the peritoneum is opened and an omental pedicle is brought down into the retropubic space.

Both procedures leave free space between the symphysis pubis and the proximal urethra, but secure support so that rotational descent of the proximal urethra and bladder base is prevented with sudden increases in intraabdominal pressure. According to Turner-Warwick, these procedures avoid overcorrection and fixation of the paraurethral fascia, which might compromise the functional movements of the urethra and bladder base and lead to obstruction and voiding difficulty. This principle may explain why the paravaginal repair and VOS procedure usually result in spontaneous voiding on the first or second postoperative day. In fact, the VOS repair has been used to correct patients with dysfunctional voiding symptoms after previous retropubic surgery.

Laparoscopic Retropubic Bladder Neck Surgery

Due to improved surgical technique and technology, many operative procedures traditionally performed by laparotomy can be accomplished endoscopically. A recent case report of nine laparoscopic MMK procedures undoubtedly heralds the use of the endoscopic approach for selected cases of retropubic surgery. Although surgical access is quite different, the principles of elevation and stabilization of the bladder neck and proximal urethra are not altered. Any retropubic procedure theoretically can be performed laparoscopically. Further research is needed to determine whether laparoscopic urethral suspension procedures can be performed technically and whether their long-term cure rates are comparable to those performed by laparotomy.

The procedure is accomplished with the patient positioned in modified lithotomy. The main modification is that the legs are positioned so that they lie in the same plane as the upper body. The knees are abducted and flexed, the heels are turned inward, and the thighs are kept in the same plane as the trunk. This position allows access to the perineum.

Laparoscopy is preceded by intubation and placement of gastric and Foley catheters. A small incision is made within the hollow of the umbilicus. A Verres needle, which is fitted with a retractable blunt obturator, is pierced through fascia and peritoneum. CO_2 gas is insufflated at a rate of 1 to 6 L/min. After abdominal distention, the main trocar, which is 11 mm in diameter, is inserted through the umbilical incision. The pelvic cavity is visualized with the aid of a video screen monitor. The important landmarks are the umbilical ligaments, which actually delineate the lateral borders of the bladder. The urachus can usually also be seen. Although transection of the urachus improves access to the space of Retzius, this practice probably should be avoided so that accidental damage to the bladder is less likely to occur.

Three more incisions are made. One is placed in the midline, approximately half way between the pubic bone and the umbilicus, and an 11-mm trocar is introduced. The two other trocars are 5 mm in diameter and placed lateral to the rectus muscle, approximately half way between the anterior iliac spine and the umbilicus. The surgeon (if right handed) uses the left lateral and medial ports; the assistant uses the remaining port.

The initial peritoneal incision is made along the medial border of the patient's left umbilical ligament. It is made long enough to reach well above the level of the upper border of the pubic bone. Once the peritoneum has been incised, the surgeon's immediate focus is to reach the pubic bone. Because of the angle of approach, there is a tendency to slip away from the medial aspect of the umbilical ligament, with the inherent risk of injury to the bladder. After the posterior aspect of the pubic bone is identified, the assistant can retract the bladder toward the right side, away from the field, which lowers the risk of vesical injury while providing access to the space of Retzius. The surgeon enters the retropubic space and dissects the pubic arch, either with scissors or with dissecting spatula. The fat within the space generally is removed to expose the anatomy of the region. One can examine in excellent detail the bladder neck, urethra, and surrounding anatomy.

Blood vessels, mainly capillaries and veins, are easily distinguished because of the magnification inherent to all fixed focused optical systems. Meticulous hemostasis is mandatory because fluids tend to pool in the space of Retzius and because blood tinges the tissues, which interferes with visual identification of critical landmarks.

With the anatomy clearly identified, the operator inserts a suture through the suprapubic trocar. A long, nonabsorbable, No. 0 or 2-0 suture is preferred. Suturing and knotting is technically the most difficult part of the procedure. Vancaillie and Schuessler use a slip knot outside the abdominal cavity, which is then pushed into place with a special extracorporeal knot-tying instrument. The type of knot has been described in detail by Weston. The main advantage of this knot, besides the fact that it is a slip knot that can be made on the outside, is that it can be fixed at any point during insertion. Thus the surgeon has available an extremely precise mechanism, which allows elevation of the bladder neck under direct visual control to the optimal level.

The right side suture is placed first and tied. The needle is placed into the anterior vaginal wall while the surgeon has the left hand in the patient's vagina, permitting displacement of the urethra to the left, so as to increase the available space. During actual placement of the needle, mobility of the needle and needle holder is greater if the obturator displaces the vagina to the left, rather than toward the pubic bone. The needle is then pushed through the symphysis pubis (if an MMK procedure is chosen). Further steps of the procedure are not hampered by tying the first knot.

This maneuver is repeated on the left side. The number of sutures placed on each side varies according to the technique preferred. The peritoneal defect can be closed, but this maneuver probably is not necessary. At the end of the procedure, the four abdominal incisions are closed with subcutaneous sutures or adhesive strips. A suprapubic or Foley catheter is used to drain the bladder postoperatively and can be removed according to the surgeon's usual protocol. Early ambulation and hospital discharge are encouraged.

General Intraoperative and Postoperative Procedures

If the surgeon is concerned that intravesical suture placement or ureteral obstruction may have occurred, cystoscopy—either transurethrally or through the dome of the bladder—or cystotomy may be performed to document ureteral patency and absence of intravesical sutures after retropubic procedures.

Closed suction drains of the retropubic space are used only as necessary when hemostasis is incomplete and there is concern about postoperative hematoma. The bladder is routinely drained with a suprapubic or transurethral catheter for 2 to 3 days. After that time, the patient is allowed to begin voiding trials, and postvoid residual urine volumes are checked.

CLINICAL RESULTS

Many studies have reported clinical experiences with retropubic urethral suspension procedures for stress urinary incontinence. Unfortunately, most of these studies are methodologically flawed by modern standards. Most did not use objective parameters preoperatively and postoperatively to establish diagnosis and outcome. Few prospective studies are available comparing the results of the various procedures for genuine stress incontinence, and those that do compare retropubic procedures with vaginal procedures.

Mainprize and Drutz summarized 56 articles reporting results of MMK procedures. Few of these articles used preoperative diagnostic urodynamic tests and only Milani et al reported postoperative urodynamic data after 1 year. Of 2712 cases, 2334 (86.1%) succeeded, 73 (2.7%) improved, and 305 (11.2%) failed. The success rate of primary MMK procedures was 92.1%; the success rate was 84.5% when the MMK procedure was used for recurrent incontinence.

In the study by Milani et al, the rate of continence confirmed by urodynamic studies was 71% after 1 year. After MMK procedures, the recurrence of stress incontinence increases over time: the longer the observation period, the more cases of recurrence may be seen. Using a self-reported interview, Park and Miller showed that 86% of patients treated with primary MMK procedures were cured during the first 3 years after surgery and only 66% were still continent after 3 to 10 years.

The Burch colposuspension is the best studied of the retropubic procedures. From 1980 to 1990, 18 studies have reported using the Burch colposuspension in women with urodynamically proved genuine stress incontinence and with objective measures of cure. Follow-up times range from 3 months to 7 years. A summary of the outcomes is presented in Tables 15-1 and 15-2. At 3 to 24 months after surgery, 59% to 100% of patients became continent, for an overall average cure rate of 84.0%. At 3 to 7 years, continence rates range from 63% to 89%, for an average rate of 76.9%. Although objectively incontinent, a small percentage of additional patients were judged to be im-

proved and satisfied with their surgical results. The overall reported absolute failure rate is 13.6% at 3 to 24 months and 14.0% at 5 to 7 years.

In one of the best long-term studies to date, Eriksen et al reported 91 women with urodynamically proved genuine stress incontinence, with or without bladder stability, who had undergone Burch colposuspension. Urodynamic evaluation was accepted by 76 patients after 5 years. Stress incontinence was cured in 71%

TABLE 15-1   Summary of Burch procedure studies to treat genuine stress incontinence (1980-1990)

Author, year	Number of patients	Number (%) cured	Follow-up time (months)
Milani et al, 1985	44	35 (79.5)	12
Bhatia and Ostergard, 1981	12	10 (83.3)	4-12
Walter et al, 1982	38	27 (71.0)	12-30
Kujansuu, 1983	29	17 (58.6)	15 (mean)
Hilton and Stanton, 1983	25	22 (88.0)	3
Mundy, 1983	26	22 (84.6)	12
Weil et al, 1984	34	31 (91.2)	6
Bhatia and Bergman, 1985	44	43 (97.7)	12
van Geelen et al, 1988	34	29 (85.3)	12-24
Bergman et al, 1989	38	34 (89.5)	12
Bergman et al, 1989	101	88 (87.1)	12
Penttinen et al, 1989a	29	29 (100)	8-12
Thunedborg et al, 1990	17	15 (88.2)	6
Langer et al, 1990	122	96 (78.7)	3-6
TOTAL	593	498 (84)	

Objective urodynamic outcomes were available after 3 to 24 months.

TABLE 15-2   Summary of studies reporting long-term follow-up of Burch procedures to treat genuine stress incontinence (1980-1990)

Author, year	Number of patients	Number (%) cured	Follow-up time (years)
van Geelen et al, 1988	33	25* (75.8)	5-7
Thunedborg et al, 1990	14	11† (78.6)	6
Eriksen et al, 1990	76	48 (63.1)	5
Rydhström and Iosif, 1988	30	26 (86.7)	3 (mean)
Galloway et al, 1987	50	42 (84.0)	1-6
Gillon and Stanton, 1984	35	31† (88.6)	3-5
Total	238	183 (76.9)	

Objective urodynamic outcomes were available after 3 to 7 years.
*determined by questionnaire only.
†determined by pad test, urolog only.

of the patients with stable bladders preoperatively and in 57% of those with stress incontinence and detrusor instability, a nonsignificant difference. After 5 years, only 52% of the study group was completely dry and free of complications; about 30% needed further incontinence therapy.

Demographic conditions that increase the risk of surgical failure for retropubic urethropexy are shown in the accompanying box. They include menopause, prior hysterectomy, and prior antiincontinence procedures. Advanced age does not appear to be associated with lower rates of cure after colposuspension, although one study described a somewhat higher mean age in patients who failed incontinence surgery. Clinical and urodynamic findings that increase the risk of surgical failure include maximum urethral closure pressure less than 20 cm H_2O, abnormal perineal electromyography, and concurrent detrusor instability. The first condition may identify women who are at higher risk of having type III genuine stress incontinence. These patients are probably better treated with a more obstructive operation, such as a sling.

Women with mixed detrusor instability and genuine stress incontinence who undergo surgical correction have lower postoperative continence rates than do women with pure genuine stress incontinence. Although in 60% to 70% of patients with mixed incontinence detrusor instability resolves after urethropexy, residual urgency and incontinence often persist and may be interpreted by the patient as surgical failure. Although not all authors agree, patients with mixed incontinence should probably receive medical therapy first; surgery is then suggested for those who have continued stress incontinence.

MECHANISMS OF CURE

Early work by Lapides stated that urethral suspension restores continence by applying longitudinal tension (stretching) to the urethra, thereby increasing intraluminal resistance. This theory was based on the principle that the resistance of a tubular structure varies directly with the length of the tube. Nevertheless, most urodynamic reports have failed to verify this alleged urethral-lengthening effect of retropubic procedures.

Retropubic suspension procedures elevate and stabilize the bladder neck and proximal urethra in a high retropubic position. The principal urodynamic change in urethrovesical function postoperatively is increased pressure transmission to the urethra, relative to the bladder, during elevations in intraabdominal pressure. Resting urethral pressure and functional urethral length are unchanged, suggesting that the intrinsic function of the urethra is not altered appreciably by this type of surgery.

The greater the difference in preoperative and postoperative pressure transmission ratios, the more likely the patient will be continent after Burch colposuspension. If the retropubic procedure fails to elevate and stabilize the urethra and postoperative pressure transmission ratios remain less than 100%, the patient may continue to have sphincteric incompetence postoperatively. Appropriate elevation of the bladder neck and urethra, accompanied by pressure transmission ratios near 100%, result in continence in most patients. This concept is supported by a study by Penttinen et al (1989b), who noted a significant negative correlation between postoperative bladder neck mobility and pressure transmission ratios, indicating that correction of the urethrovesical anatomic disorder eliminates the functional disorder and restores continence.

Mechanical compression of the urethra against the posterosuperior aspect of the symphysis pubis may result during episodes of increased abdominal pressure after retropubic procedures. Hertogs and Stanton

---

Conditions That Decrease the Chance of Cure After Retropubic Urethropexy

Demographic

Advanced age (?)
Postmenopausal
Prior hysterectomy
Prior procedures to correct genuine stress incontinence

Urodynamic

Concurrent detrusor instability
Urethral closure pressure less than 20 cm H_2O
Abnormal perineal electromyography

showed that colposuspension restores urinary continence by placing the proximal urethra against the posterior surface of the symphysis pubis and exposing the urethra to direct compression against the bone during stress. These authors noted that compared to unsuccessful operation, successful operation repositioned the bladder neck significantly closer to the posterosuperior surface of the symphysis pubis, although not significantly higher. Thus continence after retropubic suspension may depend on compression of the urethra by the bladder base during exertion.

Both MMK and Burch procedures probably tend to overelevate and fix the urethra in a retropubic position. Hilton and Stanton found that pressure transmission profiles after successful Burch colposuspensions differed from those of continent control subjects, with pressure transmission ratios in the proximal half of the urethra significantly higher than 100% (Fig. 15-5). This observation suggests that an additional mechanism, probably partial outflow obstruction, results. Bump et al determined that patients with postoperative voiding abnormalities and detrusor insta-

bility had pressure transmission ratios significantly greater than 100%, supporting the hypothesis that obstruction may play a role in postcontinence-surgery voiding dysfunction and detrusor instability.

COMPLICATIONS
Short-term Postoperative

Of the retropubic procedures, the MMK procedure is the most extensively studied with regard to complications. In a thorough review of the literature, Mainprize and Drutz summarized the postoperative complications (excluding urinary retention) of MMK procedures (Table 15-3). Wound complications and urinary infections are the most common surgical complications. Direct surgical injury to the urinary tract occurs relatively infrequently. Bladder lacerations occurred in 0.7% of patients; sutures through the bladder and urethra and catheters sewn into the urethra occurred in 0.3% of patients. Ureteral obstruction occurred in 0.1% of patients. Accidental placement of sutures into the bladder during the Burch or paravaginal repair, resulting in vesical stone formation, recurrent cystitis, or fistula, has not been reported.

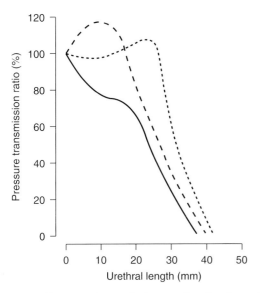

Fig. 15-5 Pressure transmission profiles in stress incontinent women before (—) and after (---) successful colposuspensions, compared with a group of 20 symptom-free women (. . . .). *(From Hilton P, Stanton SL: Br J Obstet Gynaecol 90:934, 1983.)*

TABLE 15-3   Postoperative complications in 2712 Marshall-Marchetti-Krantz procedures

Type of Complication	Percent
Wound, total	5.5
infection or hematoma	3.4
hernia or dehiscence	1.8
other	0.3
Urinary tract infection	3.9
Osteitis pubis	2.5
Direct surgical injury to the urinary tract	1.6
bladder tears	0.7
urethral obstruction	0.5
sutures through bladder or urethra with/ without catheter sewn in	0.3
Ureteral obstruction or hydronephrosis	0.1
Fistula	0.3
Death	0.2

Modified from Mainprize TC, Drutz HP: *Obstet Gynecol Surv* 43:724, 1988.

Ureteral obstruction occurs rarely after Burch colposuspension and results from ureteral kinking after elevation of the vagina and bladder base. One study reported three unilateral ureteral obstructions and three bilateral ureteral obstructions in 483 Burch colposuspensions (1.2%). All patients were treated successfully with removal of sutures and ureteral stenting. No cases of transected ureters have been reported. Ericksen et al found that 1 of 75 patients (1.3%) followed for 5 years after Burch procedures had absent unilateral renal function due to presumed complete ureteral obstruction. This patient had developed only transient postoperative fever.

Lower urinary tract fistulae are uncommon after retropubic procedures, with various types occurring after 0.3% of MMK procedures. Fistulae are probably less common after Burch and paravaginal repairs because the sutures are placed several centimeters lateral to the urethra.

Postoperative Voiding Difficulties

The incidence of voiding difficulties after colposuspension varies widely, although patients rarely have difficulty voiding after 30 days. Eriksen et al found that only 2 of 91 patients had delayed spontaneous micturition after Burch colposuspension when the catheter was removed the third day postoperatively. Fifteen percent of these patients had residual urine volumes of 100 to 300 ml the fifth day after surgery. In contrast, Korda et al had a mean postoperative catheter drainage of 10 days (range 5 to 60 days) for 174 patients after colposuspension. Twenty-five percent of these patients required catheter drainage for more than 10 days.

Lose et al found that colposuspension may change the original micturition pattern and introduce an element of obstruction that can disturb the balance between voiding forces and outflow resistance, resulting in immediate postoperative as well as late voiding difficulties. Urodynamic findings that may occur after colposuspension include decreased flow rate, increased micturition pressure, and increased urethral resistance.

Urodynamic tests may be used to predict early postoperative voiding difficulties. Bhatia and Bergman found that all patients with adequate detrusor con-

traction and flow rates preoperatively were able to resume spontaneous voiding by the seventh postoperative day after Burch colposuspension. One third of patients who voided without detrusor contraction required bladder drainage for 7 days or longer. No patients with decreased flow rates and absent detrusor contraction during voiding were able to void in less than 7 days postoperatively. The use of a Valsalva maneuver during voiding may further lead to postoperative voiding difficulties, perhaps by intensifying obstruction at the bladder neck. In another study, these authors found that preoperative uroflowmetry and postvoid residual urine volumes were not predictive of postoperative voiding difficulties after Burch procedures.

Detrusor Instability

Detrusor instability is a recognized postoperative complication of retropubic procedures. Unstable bladders as demonstrated on cystometrogram have been reported in 7% to 27% of patients with genuine stress incontinence and stable bladders preoperatively, with follow-up up to 5 years after Burch colposuspension. Postoperative detrusor instability is more common in patients with previous bladder neck surgery and in those with mixed detrusor instability and sphincteric incompetence preoperatively. In a study of 148 patients with genuine stress incontinence and stable bladders preoperatively, Steel et al reported that 24 (16.2%) patients had postoperative detrusor instability on cystometrogram 6 months after surgery. Ten of the 24 patients with detrusor instability were completely asymptomatic. Of the 14 symptomatic patients, four were improved with drugs aimed at correcting the instability. The remaining 10 patients (6.8%) remained symptomatic with detrusor instability 3 to 5 years after surgery.

The mechanism for this phenomenon is unknown. Cardozo et al suggested that postoperative onset of detrusor instability may be due to disruption of the autonomic innervation of the bladder, although this relationship has not been proved. As noted previously, excessive urethral elevation or compression may lead to partial outflow obstruction and resulting detrusor instability. Whatever the mechanism, postoperative detrusor instability predictably occurs in a small, but significant number of patients. Patients undergoing retropubic urethropexy should understand that the operation may cause urinary incontinence due to detrusor instability, even if it cures their sphincteric incontinence.

Osteitis Pubis

Osteitis pubis is a painful inflammation of the periosteum, bone, cartilage, and ligament of structures of the anterior pelvic girdle. It is a recognized postoperative complication of urologic and radical gynecologic procedures involving the prostate gland or urinary bladder. In urogynecology, osteitis pubis occurs after 2.5% of Marshall-Marchetti-Krantz procedures. It also can occur, although rarely, after placement of artificial urinary sphincters and after radical pelvic surgery for gynecologic malignancies.

The cause of osteitis pubis is unclear. In noninfectious cases, it may result from trauma to the periosteum or from impaired circulation in the vessels around the symphysis pubis. Krantz has suggested that osteitis pubis after MMK procedures is caused by using cutting rather than tapered needles. The onset of the disease occurs 2 to 12 weeks postoperatively. Typically, osteitis pubis is characterized by suprapubic pain radiating to the thighs and exacerbated by walking or abduction of the lower extremities, marked tenderness and swelling over the symphysis pubis, and radiographic evidence of bone destruction with separation of the symphysis pubis. The clinical course varies from prolonged, progressive debilitation over several months to spontaneous resolution after several weeks. Suggested treatments include rest, physical therapy, steroids, nonsteroidal antiinflammatory agents, and wedge resection of the symphysis pubis for recalcitrant cases. Whatever the therapy, however, noninfectious osteitis pubis tends to be self-limiting.

Osteomyelitis of the symphysis pubis has been documented in a small number of cases. Diagnosis is made by bone biopsy and bacterial culture. Treatments are antibiotics and incision and drainage if abscess formation occurs.

Enterocele

Burch first reported that enteroceles occurred in 7.6% of cases as a late complication after the Burch procedure, but only two thirds of these patients required surgical correction. Langer et al (1989) reported that 13.6% of patients who had undergone Burch procedures, but no hysterectomy or cul-de-sac obliteration, developed an enterocele 1 to 2 years postoperatively. Whenever possible, a cul-de-sac obliteration in the form of uterosacral plication, Moschcowitz procedure, or McCall culdoplasty should be performed at the time of retropubic suspension to prevent enterocele formation.

ROLE OF HYSTERECTOMY IN THE TREATMENT OF INCONTINENCE

Gynecologists frequently perform hysterectomies at the time of retropubic or vaginal surgery for genuine stress incontinence. Although it was generally believed that the presence of a uterus somehow contributed to the genesis of sphincteric incompetence, few data support this theory. Langer et al (1989) assessed the effect of concomitant hysterectomy during Burch colposuspension on the cure rate of genuine stress incontinence. Forty-five patients were randomly assigned to receive colposuspension only or colposuspension plus abdominal hysterectomy and cul-de-sac obliteration. Using urodynamic investigations 6 months after surgery, the rate of cure for stress incontinence between the two groups did not differ statistically (95.5% and 95.7% for the no-hysterectomy and the hysterectomy groups, respectively). This study clearly suggests that hysterectomy adds little to the efficacy of Burch colposuspension in curing genuine stress incontinence. In general, hysterectomies should be performed only for specific uterine pathology or for the treatment of uterovaginal prolapse.

PREGNANCY AFTER RETROPUBIC SURGERY

Most physicians suggest that the patient finish her childbearing before surgical correction of stress incontinence is attempted. Few data demonstrate the continence status when pregnancy or vaginal delivery occurs after a retropubic repair. Only eight pregnancies have been reported after MMK procedures. Seven patients delivered vaginally and one delivered by cesarean section because she also had undergone a vesicovaginal fistula repair. All of the patients were reportedly continent after delivery, although no long-term follow-up is available. Although in general surgical treatment for stress incontinence should be reserved for those women who have finished their child-bearing, no data demonstrate that a pregnancy and vaginal delivery would not be satisfactory for women after retropubic surgery.

BIBLIOGRAPHY

Surgical Technique

Bhatia NN, Karram MM, Bergman A: Role of antibiotic prophylaxis in retropubic surgery for stress urinary incontinence, *Obstet Gynecol* 74:637, 1989.

Blaivas JG, Olsson CA: Stress incontinence: classification and surgical approach, *J Urol* 139:727, 1988.

Burch JC: Urethrovaginal fixation to Cooper's ligament for correction of stress incontinence, cystocele, and prolapse, *Am J Obstet Gynecol* 81:281, 1961.

Gleason DM, Reilly RJ, Pierce JA: Vesical neck suspension under vision with cystotomy enhances treatment of female incontinence, *J Urol* 115:555, 1976.

Haylen BT, Frazer MI, Golovsky D, et al: Elevation of the vagina during colposuspension: the use of a Deaver retractor, *Br J Urol* 63:220, 1989.

Korda A, Ferry J, Hunter P: Colposuspension for the treatment of female urinary incontinence, *Aust NZ J Obstet Gynaecol* 29:146, 1989.

Krantz KE: The Marshall-Marchetti-Krantz procedure. In Stanton SL, Tanagho EA (eds): *Surgery of female incontinence*, ed 2, New York, 1986, Springer-Verlag.

Linder A, Golomb J, Korczak D: Endoscopic control during colposuspension procedure for the treatment of stress urinary incontinence, *Eur Urol* 16:372, 1989.

McGuire EM: Urodynamic findings in patients after failure of stress incontinence operations. In Zinner NR, Sterling AM (eds): *Female incontinence*, New York, 1981, Alan R Liss.

McGuire EJ, Lytton B, Pepe V, et al: Stress urinary incontinence, *Obstet Gynecol* 47:255, 1976.

Marshall VF, Marchetti AA, Krantz KE: The correction of stress incontinence by simple vesicourethral suspension, *Surg Gynecol Obstet* 88:509, 1949.

Richardson AC, Edmonds PB, Williams NL: Treatment of stress urinary incontinence due to paravaginal fascial defect, *Obstet Gynecol* 57:357, 1981.

Shull BL, Baden WF: A six-year experience with paravaginal defect repair for stress urinary incontinence, *Am J Obstet Gynecol* 160:1432, 1989.

Tanagho EA: Colpocystourethropexy: the way we do it, *J Urol* 116:751, 1976.

Timmons MC, Addison WA: Suprapubic teloscopy: extraperitoneal intraoperative technique to demonstrate ureteral patency, *Obstet Gynecol* 75:137, 1990.

Turner-Warwick R: Turner-Warwick vagino-obtruator shelf urethral repositioning procedure. In Debruyne FMJ, van Kerrebroeck EVA (eds): *Practical aspects of urinary incontinence*, Dordrecht, 1986, Martinus Nejhoff.

Vancaillie TG, Schuessler W: Laparoscopic bladderneck suspension, *J Laparoendo Surg* 1:169, 1991.

Webster GD, Kreder KJ: Voiding dysfunction following cystourethropexy: its evaluation and management, *J Urol* 144:670, 1990.

Weston PV: A new clinch knot, *Obstet Gynecol* 78:144, 1991.

Results and Mechanism of Cure

Bergman A, Koonings PP, Ballard CA: Primary stress urinary incontinence and pelvic relaxation: prospective randomized comparison of three different operations, *Am J Obstet Gynecol* 161:97, 1989.

Bergman A, Ballard CA, Koonings PP: Comparison of three different surgical procedures for genuine stress incontinence: prospective randomized study, *Am J Obstet Gynecol* 160:1102, 1989.

Bhatia NN, Bergman A: Modified Burch versus Pereyra retropubic urethropexy for stress urinary incontinence, *Obstet Gynecol* 66:255, 1985.

Bhatia NN, Ostergard DR: Urodynamic effects of retropubic urethropexy in genuine stress incontinence, *Am J Obstet Gynecol* 140:936, 1981.

Bump RC, Fantl JA, Hurt WG: Dynamic urethral pressure profilometry pressure transmission ratio determinations after continence surgery: understanding the mechanism of success, failure, and complications, *Obstet Gynecol* 72:870, 1988.

Enhorning G: Simultaneous recording of intravesical and intraurethral pressure, *Acta Chir Scand* (suppl) 276:1, 1961.

Eriksen BC, Hagen B, Eik-Nes SH, et al: Long-term effectiveness of the Burch colposuspension in female urinary stress incontinence, *Acta Obstet Gynecol Scand* 69:45, 1990.

Gillon G, Stanton SL: Long-term follow-up of surgery for urinary incontinence in elderly women, *Br J Urol* 56:478, 1984.

Henriksson L, Ulmsten U: A urodynamic evaluation of the effects of abdominal urethrocystopexy and vaginal sling urethroplasty in women with stress incontinence, *Am J Obstet Gynecol* 131:77, 1978.

Hertogs K, Stanton SL: Mechanism of urinary continence after colposuspension: barrier studies, *Br J Obstet Gynaecol* 92:1184, 1985.

Hilton P, Stanton SL: A clinical and urodynamic assessment of the Burch colposuspension for genuine stress incontinence, *Br J Obstet Gynaecol* 90:934, 1983.

Karram MM, Bhatia NN: Management of coexistent stress and urge urinary incontinence, *Obstet Gynecol* 73:4, 1989.

Koonings PP, Bergman A, Ballard CA: Low urethral pressure and stress urinary incontinence in women: risk factor for failed retropubic surgical procedure, *Urology* 36:245, 1990.

Kujansuu E: Urodynamic analysis of successful and failed incontinence surgery, *Int J Gynaecol Obstet* 21:353, 1983.

Langer R, Ron-El R, Neuman N, et al: The value of simultaneous hysterectomy during Burch colposuspension for urinary stress incontinence, *Obstet Gynecol* 72:866, 1988.

Langer R, Golan A, Ron-El R, et al: Colposuspension for urinary stress incontinence in premenopausal and postmenopausal women, *Surg Gynecol Obstet* 171:13, 1990.

Lapides J: Structure and function of the internal vesical sphincter, *J Urol* 80:341, 1958.

Mainprize TC, Drutz HP: The Marshall-Marchetti-Krantz procedure: a critical review, *Obstet Gynecol Surv* 43:724, 1988.

Milani R, Scalambrino S, Quadri G, et al: Marshall-Marchetti-Krantz procedure and Burch colposuspension in the surgical treatment of female urinary incontinence, *Br J Obstet Gynaecol* 92:1050, 1985.

Mundy AR: A trial comparing the Stamey bladder neck suspension procedure with colposuspension for the treatment of stress incontinence, *Br J Urol* 55:687, 1983.

Park GS, Miller EJ: Surgical treatment of stress urinary incontinence: a comparison of the Kelly plication, Marshall-Marchetti-Krantz, and Pereyra procedures, *Obstet Gynecol* 71:575, 1988.

Penttinen J, Käär K, Kauppila K: Colposuspension and transvaginal bladder neck suspension in the treatment of stress incontinence, *Gynecol Obstet Invest* 28:101, 1989a.

Penttinen J, Lindholm EL, Käär K, et al: Successful colposuspension in stress urinary incontinence reduces bladder neck mobility and increases pressure transmission to the urethra, *Arch Gynecol Obstet* 244:233, 1989b.

Rosenzweig BA, Bhatia NN, Nelson AL: Dynamic urethral pressure profilometry pressure transmission ratio: what do the numbers really mean? *Obstet Gynecol* 77:586, 1991.

Rydhström H, Iosif CS: Urodynamic studies before and after retropubic colpourethrocystopexy in fertile women with stress urinary incontinence, *Arch Gynecol Obstet* 241:201, 1988.

Sand PK, Bowen LW, Ostergard DR, et al: Hysterectomy and prior surgery as risk factors for failed retropubic cystourethropexy, *J Reprod Med* 33:171, 1988.

Sand PK, Bowen LW, Panganiban R, et al: The low pressue urethra as a factor in failed retropubic urethropexy, *Obstet Gynecol* 69:399, 1987.

Stanton SL, Cardozo L, Williams JE, et al: Clinical and urodynamic features of failed incontinence surgery in the female, *Obstet Gynecol* 51:515, 1978.

Thunedborg P, Fischer-Rasmussen W, Jensen SB: Stress urinary incontinence and posterior bladder suspension defects, *Acta Obstet Gynecol Scand* 69:55, 1990.

van Geelen JM, Theeuwes AGM, Eskes TKAB, et al: The clinical and urodynamic effects of anterior vaginal repair and Burch colposuspension, *Am J Obstet Gynecol* 159:137, 1988.

Walter S, Olesen KP, Hald T, et al: Urodynamic evaluation after vaginal repair and colposuspension, *Br J Urol* 54:377, 1982.

Weil A, Reyes H, Bischoff P, et al: Modifications of the urethral rest and stress profiles after different types of surgery for urinary stress incontinence, *Br J Obstet Gynaecol* 91:46, 1984.

Wheelan JB: Long-term results of colposuspension, *Br J Urol* 65:329, 1990.

Complications

Applegate GB, Bass KM, Kubik CJ: Ureteral obstruction as a complication of the Burch colposuspension procedure: case report, *Am J Obstet Gynecol* 156:445, 1987.

Bergman A, Bhatia N: Uroflowmetry for predicting postoperative voiding difficulties in women with stress urinary incontinence, *Br J Obstet Gynaecol* 92:835, 1985.

Bhatia NN, Bergman A: Urodynamic predictability of voiding following incontinence surgery, *Obstet Gynecol* 63:85, 1984.

Bhatia NN, Bergman A: Use of preoperative uroflowmetry and simultaneous urethrocystometry for predicting risk of prolonged postoperative bladder drainage, *Urology* 28:440, 1986.

Bouza E, Winston DJ, Hewitt WL: Infectious osteitis pubis, *Urology* 12:663, 1978.

Burch JC: Cooper's ligament urethrovesical suspension for stress incontinence, *Am J Obstet Gynecol* 100:764, 1968.

Burns JR, Gregory JG: Osteomyelitis of the pubic symphysis after urologic surgery, *J Urol* 118:803, 1977.

Cardozo LD, Stanton SL, Williams JE: Detrusor instability following surgery for genuine stress incontinence, *Br J Urol* 51:204, 1979.

Ferriani RA, Silva de Sá MF, de Moura MD, et al: Ureteral blockage as a complication of Burch colposuspension: report of 6 cases, *Gynecol Obstet Invest* 29:239, 1990.

Galloway NTM, Davies N, Stephenson TP: The complications of colposuspension, *Br J Urol* 60:122, 1987.

Hoyme OB, Tamimi HK, Eschenbach DA, et al: Osteomyelitis pubis after radical gynecologic operations, *Obstet Gynecol* 63:47S, 1984.

Langer R, Ron-El R, Newman M, et al: Detrusor instability following colposuspension for urinary stress incontinence, *Br J Obstet Gynaecol* 95:607, 1988.

Lose G, Jørgensen L, Mortensen SO, et al: Voiding difficulties after colposuspension, *Obstet Gynecol* 69:33, 1987.

Maulik TG: Kinked ureter with unilateral obstructive uropathy complicating Burch colposuspension, *J Urol* 130:135, 1983.

Muschat M: Osteitis pubis following prostatectomy, *J Urol* 54:447, 1945.

Rebenack P, Thompson RJ, Wilf LH: Osteomyelitis pubis following a Burch retropubic urethropexy, *J Gynecol Surg* 6:205, 1990.

Rosenthal RE, Spickard WA, Markham RD, et al: Osteomyelitis of the symphysis pubis: a separate disease from osteitis pubis, *J Bone Joint Surg* 64:123, 1982.

Sand PK, Bowen LW, Ostergard DR, et al: The effect of retropubic urethropexy on detrusor stability, *Obstet Gynecol* 71:818, 1988.

Sjöberg B: Hydrodynamics of micturition following Marshall-Marchetti-Krantz procedure for stress urinary incontinence, *Scand J Urol Nephrol* 16:11, 1982.

Steel SA, Cox C, Stanton SL: Long-term follow-up of detrusor instability following the colposuspension operation, *Br J Urol* 58:138, 1986.

Turner-Warwick RT: The pathogenesis and treatment of osteitis pubis, *Br J Urol* 32:464, 1960.

Wiskind AK, Creighton SM, Stanton SL: The incidence of genital prolapse after the Burch colposuspension, *Am J Obstet Gynecol* 167:399, 1992.

CHAPTER 16

Surgical Correction of Genuine Stress Incontinence Secondary to Intrinsic Urethral Sphincter Dysfunction

Mickey M. Karram

Suburethral Sling Procedures
  History
  Indications
  Preoperative evaluation
  Operative technique
  Results
  Complications
Periurethral Injection of Bulk-Enhancing Agents
  Indications
  Bulk-enhancing agents
  Technique
  Postoperative management and complications
  Efficacy and safety of bulk-enhancing agents
Implantation of Artificial Urinary Sphincters
  Description of the AMS 800 prosthesis
  Indications and preoperative preparation
  Surgical techniques
  Results and complications
Summary

In the vast majority of patients, genuine stress incontinence is due to loss of support of the urethro-vesical junction. The mechanism of incontinence in such cases is believed to be poor abdominal pressure transmission to the proximal urethra, relative to the bladder, during rises in intraabdominal pressure. The internal sphincter is closed at rest, which can be confirmed by radiographic and endoscopic tests. Standard bladder neck suspension procedures that have been discussed previously are generally successful in correcting this form of incontinence. Urethral closure pressure is not changed by successful repositioning and elevation of the bladder neck, which is required for continence in these patients. In others words, cure of the condition does not depend on compression of the urethra to engineer a better closure mechanism. Rather, it depends on suspension of the urethra so that it no longer descends with increases in intraabdominal pressure.

A smaller group of women demonstrate severe stress incontinence, with little or no urethral mobility during changes in intraabdominal pressure. Most commonly, these patients have had previous operations to correct stress incontinence, radiation therapy, neurologic insult, or pelvic trauma and have developed poor urethral resistance. They lose urine with minimal exertion and usually have very low urethral closure pressure. These women demonstrate endoscopically and radiographically a partially or totally open internal sphincter (type III stress incontinence).

This chapter discusses various surgical techniques that can be used to improve or cure patients with stress incontinence secondary to urethral damage. Discussions on suburetheal sling procedures, periurethral injections of bulk-enhancing agents, and placement of artificial urinary sphincters are presented.

SUBURETHRAL SLING PROCEDURES

History

In 1907, von Giordano was the first to describe a suburethral sling procedure using a gracilis muscle flap. Numerous modifications of this procedure have been described subsequently. Many of the early modifications used various other muscle tissues. Eventually, however, muscular slings were abandoned due to the difficulty in maintaining the muscle's blood supply and to the mechanical problems associated with incorporating bulky tissue beneath the urethra. Over the years, numerous other autologous tissues have been used, including rectus fascia, fascia lata, round ligament, strips of external oblique fascia, and palmaris longus tendon. In the early 1950s, Bracht was the first to use synthetic nylon material that was strapped underneath the urethra. Since then Mersiline, Marlex, silicone, Vicryl, and Gore-tex have all been used successfully to sling the urethra.

Indications

Unfortunately, a clear exposition of the indications for sling procedure as opposed to a less complicated urethropexy is not apparent in the literature. A suburethral sling procedure should be considered whenever it is believed that simple elevation and stabilization of the urethrovesical junction will not produce continence.

These patients have genuine stress incontinence secondary to a poorly-functioning or nonfunctional internal urethral sphincteric mechanism (type III). They usually have had previous bladder neck suspension or anterior colporrhaphy. They often have de-

creased urethral mobility and decreased vaginal pliability. Urodynamic studies usually reveal low resting urethral closure pressure and low leak point pressures. Endoscopic or radiographic studies will commonly reveal an open bladder neck at rest.

Whether a suburethral sling procedure is ever indicated as primary treatment in neurologically intact, nonradiated women with anatomic stress incontinence is controversial. Some investigators have advocated the placement of a suburethral sling in any patient with stress incontinence who has a resting urethral closure pressure of less than 20 cm H_2O regardless of the presence or absence of urethral mobility.

Other situations in which a sling may be considered as a primary procedure include patients with chronic pulmonary disease, obesity, athleticism, and congenital tissue weakness.

Preoperative Evaluation

All patients should have a complete history, general physical and neurologic examinations, and urodynamic and endoscopic evaluations to assure the proper diagnosis and to exclude any contraindications to sling procedures. Due to the procedure's obstructive nature, all patients should be taught intermittent self-catheterization and be warned of the need for prolonged postoperative bladder drainage. Patients who void on preoperative evaluation with a Valsalva maneuver and have minimal or no bladder contraction must understand that spontaneous voiding may never resume and that they may need to remain permanently on intermittent self-catheterization.

Patients with mixed stress incontinence and detrusor instability must also be warned that the course of detrusor instability after sling procedures is unpredictable. Many times the obstructive nature of the sling procedure will cause the instability to worsen. The rate of de novo detrusor instability developing after suburethral sling procedures ranges from 5% to 20%.

Operative Technique

Prophylactic antibodies are routinely given preoperatively, and an antibiotic solution is used liberally throughout the procedure. Before performing a suburethral sling procedure, one must determine the material to be used for the sling. The ideal material is easily accessible and provides adequate tensile strength. It should be associated with minimal risk of infection, graft rejection, or excessive scarring. Intuitively, one would think that synthetic material, when compared to autologous material, would have a higher infection and erosion rate. One small comparative study in the literature (Ogundipe et al) noted no significant differences between Gore-tex and fascia lata, there was a trend for the synthetic Gore-tex to be more obstructive with regard to resumption of normal voiding after surgery.

Most surgeons perform sling procedures via a combined abdominal-vaginal route, with the major portion of the dissection performed vaginally. The procedure also can be performed entirely via an abdominal approach with tunneling of the sling between the urethra and vagina; however, this approach increases the likelihood of urethral trauma. A separate vaginal incision does not seem to increase the infectious morbidity of the operation or increase the incidence of sling erosion.

Most reports on sling procedures describe fixing the sling to the anterior rectus fascia. One can also fix it to other structures, such as the pectineal ligament.

Sling procedures generally have been performed with a continuous band of tissue that is fixed to the undersurface of the urethra and each end tied above the anterior rectus fascia. More recently, some investigators (Hadley et al; McGuire; Karram and Bhatia) have advocated the use of a patch of synthetic or autologous tissue fixed to the suburethra. Sutures are placed along the longitudinal axis of the patch and transferred via a needle suspension ligature carrier to above the anterior rectus fascia over which they are tied. Currently, no published data compare these two different methods of performing sling procedures.

The following is a description of our current technique for suburethral sling placement.

1. A patch of fascia lata is used for the sling and is obtained by making a 3 to 4 cm transverse skin incision approximately four finger-breadths above the midpatella, lateral to the knee in the lower thigh. A 4 × 6 cm piece of

fascia lata is removed (Fig. 16-1, *B*). Subcutaneous tissue is approximated, the skin is closed, and a pressure bandage is placed. If a full sling is preferred, a long strip of fascia lata can be obtained using a Wilson fascial stripper or a vein stripper (Fig. 16-1, *A*). Another commonly obtained fascia for this procedure is the anterior rectus abdominal fascia; a patch or full strip of fascia can be obtained using a low transverse abdominal incision, followed by closure of the defect.

2. The patient is placed in stirrups in a dorsal lithotomy position. The vaginal and lower abdominal area are appropriately prepped and draped. Injectable saline or a dilute Neo-Synephrine solution is used to inject beneath the epithelium of the anterior vaginal wall. A midline anterior vaginal wall incision is made from just above the apex of the vagina to approximately 1 cm proximal to the external urethral meatus. The epithelium is carefully dissected off the underlying periurethral and paravesical fascia. Because many of these patients have undergone previous surgery, the dissection is usually performed sharply. A plane between the vaginal wall and periurethral fascia, which is white and glistening, should be followed laterally to underneath the pubic bone; this is the proper plane in which the retropubic space is bluntly or sharply entered (see Chapter 14).

3. Once this space is entered, it is important to completely mobilize the bladder and urethrovesical junction. This procedure is usually performed bluntly with a sweeping motion of the finger along the backside of the pubic bone.

4. The patch of fascia is now brought into the field and fixed to the posterior aspect of the urethra with numerous delayed absorbable sutures.

5. Permanent sutures are placed at the lateral surfaces of the patch, as noted in Fig. 16-2, and these sutures are also fixed to the periurethral endopelvic fascia. The sutures are transferred with a needle ligature carrier under direct finger guidance to above the anterior rectus fascia. If

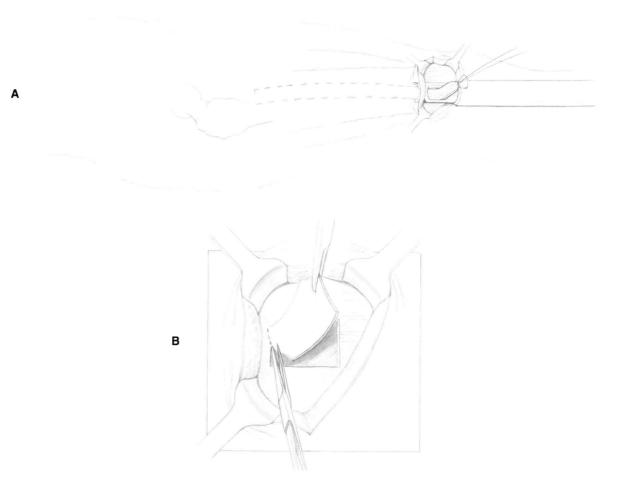

Fig. 16-1 A, Technique of obtaining strip of fascia lata using vein stripper. **B**, Technique of obtaining patch of fascia lata.

a full sling is being performed, dressing forceps are used to transfer the ends of the sling above the anterior rectus fascia after making a small fascial incision (Fig. 16-3).

6. Cystourethroscopy is performed to assure that no inadvertent bladder or urethral injury has occurred. The ureteral orifices can be visualized and the urethrovesical junction observed with and without tension on the sling.

7. The anterior vaginal wall incision is then closed with running absorbable suture. The sutures or

the sling material itself are fixed above the anterior rectus fascia. Some surgeons advocate tying the sling under direct endoscopic vision with a urethroscope in place. Others believe that the sling should be tied so that the urethral axis is horizontal. Unfortunately, the proper amount of tension placed on these sutures or the sling remains a matter of experience. In most situations the sling should be tied under relatively little tension.

8. A suprapubic catheter is placed and we usually

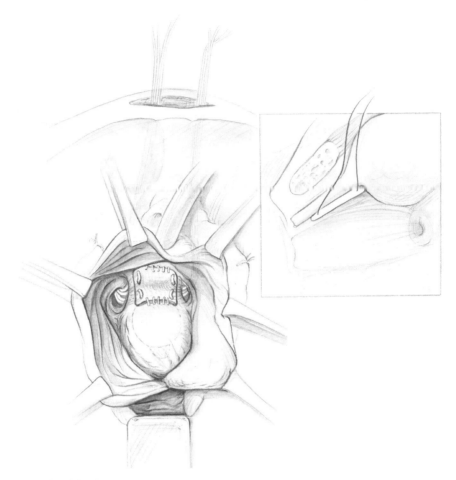

Fig. 16-2 Combined needle suspension sling procedure in which suburethral patch of fascia is suspended with permanent sutures to the anterior rectus fascia.

place a packing in the vagina for at least 24 hours.

Results

As with any antiincontinence surgery, it is difficult to assess outcome because the definition of cure in the literature is inconsistent. Most authors report subjective cure rates; few studies report any objective follow-up. In addition, the length of follow-up in most series is small. In general, sling procedures appear to be successful in curing most patients with stress incontinence. Two objective studies by Low and Parker et al using fascia lata reported cure rates of 95% and

84%, respectively. There does not seem to be any significant difference in cure rates between sling procedures performed with autologous tissue versus synthetic tissue. Horbach et al and Stanton et al have reported objective cure rates of 85% and 83%, respectively, using Gore-tex and silastic. Furthermore, results do not seem to differ significantly regardless of whether a full sling or a patch type of sling is used.

Complications

Because sling procedures significantly increase urethral outlet resistance, most of the complications that occur relate to the obstruction produced resulting in

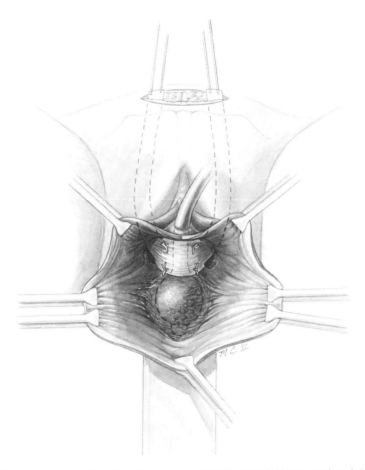

Fig. 16-3   Suburethral sling in which fascia or synthetic material is passed and tied above the anterior rectus fascia.

various forms of voiding difficulty. Sudden nonpainful urgency and urge incontinence can occur immediately after surgery because many of these patients did not have normal bladder capacity preoperatively due to defunctionalization after long-term severe incontinence. This form of incontinence usually is transient and responds well to anticholinergic therapy; it must be remembered, however, that these agents will cause a delay of normal voiding.

We begin suprapubic catheter clamping on the second postoperative day. If the patient is not voiding spontaneously by approximately 1 week postoperatively, the catheter is removed and the patient, if able, begins intermittent self-catheterization. If complete

urinary retention continues, one must decide whether it would be in the patient's best interest to undergo a second operation to loosen the sling to allow for spontaneous voiding. If the patient demonstrated a bladder contraction on pressure-flow study preoperatively, then such an operation is much more likely to be successful. On the other hand, if the patient voided preoperatively with excessive straining and no detrusor contraction, loosening the sling may not be adequate to allow for spontaneous voiding.

If it is decided to loosen the sling, we prefer a vaginal approach. A midline anterior vaginal wall incision is made and sharp dissection is performed along the pathway of the sling as it passes into the retropubic space. A vaginal urethrolysis is performed until some urethral mobility is achieved. This mobility can best be measured by downward traction on a Foley catheter. If possible, one should not undo the sling completely because of the possibility of recurrent incontinence.

Pain related to nerve injury that can occur after transvaginal needle suspension procedures can also occur after suburethral sling procedures. This complication is described extensively in Chapter 14.

Detrusor instability can persist or develop in a small group of patients, especially those who had an overactive detrusor before surgery.

A number of complications are related more to the use of synthetic rather than autologous tissue. When erosion of the sling occurs, either through the vagina or into the urethra, the sling material must be removed by the easiest method. Other complications such as wound infection, persistent urinary tract infections, sinus formation, and persistent urgency and frequency can also occur in a small group of

patients. Table 16-1 is a compilation of complications that have been previously reported in the literature and is broken down into those complications occurring with synthetic material versus those with autologous tissue.

PERIURETHRAL INJECTION OF BULK-ENHANCING AGENTS

The use of periurethral bulk-enhancing agents for urinary incontinence in women was described initially in 1938 by Murless who injected a sclerosing solution (moorhuate sodium) into the anterior vaginal wall in 20 patients. Berg, in 1973, first described the use of polytetrafluoroethylene (PTFE) injections around the urethra. This therapy has since been used extensively in certain centers in the United States and Europe. Reports of asymptomatic polytef granulomas at distant sites in laboratory animals, however, have led to a search for potentially safer injectable materials. Glutaraldehyde cross-linked collagen has recently been investigated and appears effective as a bulk-enhancing agent.

Indications

As with suburethral sling procedures, bulk-enhancing agents are best used for patients with urinary incontinence secondary to a poorly functioning urethral sphincter (type III). Because these procedures can be performed on an outpatient basis in an office setting, they are attractive for patients in which a major operative procedure is an unacceptable risk. The procedure is also attractive for patients who have had previous pelvic or vaginal radiation; these patients are at high risk for infection or erosion after placement of artificial sphincter or suburethral sling.

As with complex and severe forms of incontinence, complete urodynamic and endoscopic evaluations should be performed before the injection. Best results occur if the patient has a compliant bladder with a bladder capacity of at least 125 ml. An overactive detrusor, whether hyperreflexic or unstable, should be controlled before periurethral injections. The only absolute contraindications to injectables are uncontrollable detrusor overactivity and known hypersensitivity to the injectable agents.

TABLE 16-1   Review of literature noting prevalence of complications after suburethral sling operations

Complications	Autologous sling (N = 493)	Synthetic sling (N = 616)	Total (N = 1109)
Urinary retention	3.8%	10.2%	7.4%
Detrusor instability	7.9%	1.5%	4.3%
Urgency/frequency	3.6%	2.9%	3.2%
Wound infection	2.4%	1.8%	3.0%
Urinary tract infection	4.4%	1.6%	2.9%
Urethral/bladder injury	3.8%	1.3%	2.4%
Sling revision/removal	1.6%	2.4%	2.1%
Fistula	0.8%	0.8%	0.8%
Poor vaginal healing	—	1.5%	0.8%
Sling erosion	—	1.0%	0.5%
Wound abscess	—	0.6%	0.4%
Sinus tract formation	—	0.8%	0.4%
Other	1.8%	—	0.8%

From Horbach NS: Suburethral sling procedures. In Ostegard D, Bent A, editors: *Urogynecology and urodynamics, theory and practice,* ed 3, Baltimore, 1991, Williams & Wilkins.

Bulk-Enhancing Agents

Two materials have been popularized for periurethral use. The first, polytetrafluoroethylene (PTFE), is a paste consisting of a sterile colloidal suspension of PTFE micropolymer particles that range from 4 to 100 μm and are formed in irregular shapes. The paste is thick and requires special instrumentation for its injection under pressure.

The second, Contigen, is a sterile nonpyrogenic material composed of a highly purified bovine dermal collagen that is cross-linked with glutaraldehyde and dispersed in phosphate buffered physiologic saline. Both of these agents can be injected either transurethrally or transvaginally. It should be mentioned, however, neither of these substances has been approved by the United States FDA for use in women.

Technique of Periurethral Injection

Most investigators prefer a transvaginal periurethral approach. The periurethral area is covered with a 2% lidocaine jelly. At 5 and 7 o'clock positions, 1% lidocaine is injected periurethrally up to a total of 2 ml on each side of the urethra. A 0 or 30-degree endoscope is then placed into the urethra. If polytef paste is to be used, an Arnold-Breuning intercordal injection

set is necessary, which is readily available from the otolaryngology department because polytef has FDA approval for use in certain vocal cord dysfunction. The technique requires an assistant to pull the trigger of the device while the surgeon holds the cystoscope in one hand and stabilizes the needle periurethrally with the other hand.

If Contigen is used, the delivery system consists of a beveled 20-gauge needle, approximately 1.2 cm long, attached to a thermal plastic catheter. Contigen is provided in a 3 ml luer-lock syringe, which attaches easily to the long needle. Each syringe contains 2.5 ml of Contigen.

The needle is slowly advanced periurethrally under direct vision through the urethra. The surgeon looks for any bulging of the tip of the needle against the lining of the urethra to determine proper positioning of the needle. Injection is initiated when the needle is at the level of the bladder neck. The surgeon visualizes the material layering up outside the urethra, gradually pressing the lumen closed (Fig. 16-4). When approximately 50% of the lumen is closed the needle is removed and placed in the 8 o'clock position on the opposite side, and the exact same procedure is repeated. The needle is then removed and the patient

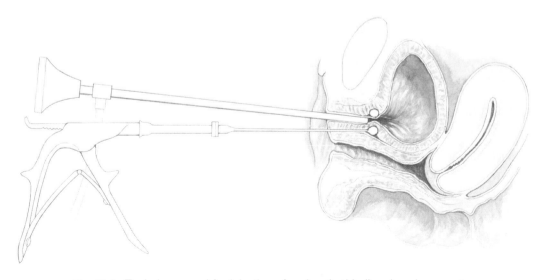

Fig. 16-4 Technique used for injection of periurethral bulk-enhancing agents.

is asked to stand and undergo various provocative maneuvers to assure that urinary continence has been obtained.

Postoperative Management and Complications

Before surgery patients should be instructed in the use of intermittent self-catheterization. The use of an indwelling urethral catheter should be avoided to prevent molding of the bulk-enhancing agent around the catheter. The patient is instructed to perform intermittent self-catheterization if necessary and is given a short course of oral antibiotic therapy. The patient should be seen approximately 24 to 48 hours after the injection to determine a postvoid residual urine volume, as well as to assess subjectively the success of the procedure. If continence is not restored completely, further injections can be performed approximately 7 to 14 days apart.

Efficacy and Safety of Bulk-Enhancing Agents

Bulk-enhancing agents have been reported to improve or cure 50% to 100% of patients with urinary incontinence secondary to sphincteric damage. Table 16-2 reviews published results of PTFE injections. These procedures offer the obvious advantage of being performed as an outpatient under local anesthesia when

TABLE 16-2   Published results of the effectiveness of periurethral PTFE injections for genuine stress incontinence

Investigation	Number of patients	Improvement or cure	No improvement
Politano et al	43	30 (70%)	13 (30%)
Politano	51	36 (71%)	15 (29%)
Lim et al	28	15 (53%)	13 (47%)
Deane et al	28	17 (61%)	11 (39%)
Lockhart et al	20	18 (90%)	2 (10%)
Schulman et al	56	48 (86%)	8 (14%)
Osther and Rohe	36	13 (50%)	13 (50%)
Vesey et al	36	24 (67%)	12 (33%)
Smart	24	15 (63%)	9 (37%)

compared to more invasive inpatient procedures. The major issue with use of bulk-enhancing agents for urinary incontinence is safety, which has delayed approval by the FDA.

The concerns regarding the safety of PTFE relate to particle migration and granuloma formation. Granuloma formation signifies a chronic foreign body reaction, resulting in long-term fibrosis and possibly carcinogenesis. More relevant is the fact that related polymers of PTFE have been shown to be carcinogenic in rats. Despite these data and three decades of use of PTFE in the discipline of otolaryngology and at certain centers in the United States and in Europe for urinary incontinence, there have been no reports of such complications in human subjects. Because the material is approved for use in men with postprostatectomy incontinence, it should certainly be available for elderly women as well.

Contigen, on the other hand, does not migrate or produce granuloma formation because it begins to degrade in 12 weeks and is completely degraded in 9 to 19 months. The primary safety concern with contigen is with respect to immunogenicity. Some persons undergoing collagen injections for soft tissue augmentation have developed collagen vascular disorders such as dermatomyositis. Despite these claims, there is no evidence to link injection of bovine collagen with these disorders. In fact, Lyon et al noted a lower incidence of such disorders in these women when compared to the incidence expected in the general population. In addition, none of the patients in the multicentered studies assessing the efficacy of contigen have had adverse events related to immunogenicity.

IMPLANTATION OF ARTIFICIAL URINARY SPHINCTERS

The third method of therapy for the female patient with severe stress incontinence secondary to urethral damage is implantation of an artificial urinary sphincter. Theoretically, this is an attractive mode of therapy because it can be considered a controlled obstruction. Only implantation of an artificial sphincter allows for urethral obstruction to be voluntarily relieved at the time of voiding. The use of this mode of therapy has not gained wide acceptance, probably because of lack of experience among urogynecologic surgeons, technical difficulties encountered during placement of the cuff, and fear of mechanical difficulties with the device.

The first artificial sphincter implanted in a woman was in 1972 by Brantly Scott. This model (AS721) consisted of a set of valves that controlled the direction of fluid flow within the system, as well as the pressure of the urethra and bladder neck by means of a cuff placed around it. Since then, numerous modifications of the original device have been made. Currently, the most sophisticated artificial sphincter available is the AMS 800.

Description of the AMS 800 Prosthesis

The AMS 800 artificial urinary sphincter consists of a cuff, a pressure-regulating balloon, a control pump, and tubing (Fig. 16-5). The control pump assembly is placed subcutaneously in the labia majora (Fig. 16-6). It contains one-way valves, resistors, and a poppet valve. The poppet valve controls the flow of fluid from the balloon to the cuff. The position of the poppet valve is easily palpated through the skin because of a nipple that has been incorporated in the plastic of the pump control assembly. Pressure on the nipple prevents the cuff from filling, thus deactivating the device. Activation of the device requires a firm squeeze over the pump, which allows for primary deactivation and delayed activation without a second operation.

The cuff is placed around the bladder neck and consists of an inner pliable leaflet attached to a firm Dacron backing. The cuff is available in various sizes. The smallest having a diameter of 4 to 5 cm with increments of 0.5 cm up to 8 cm, and then 1 cm increments up to 11 cm.

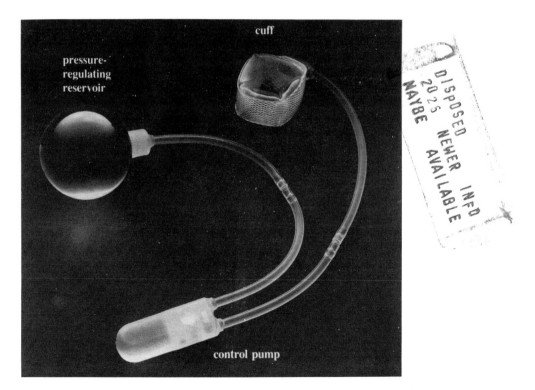

Fig. 16-5 AMS 800 artificial urinary sphincter. Note small button on control pump for activation and deactivation of the device. *(Courtesy of American Medical Systems, Minnetonka, MN.)*

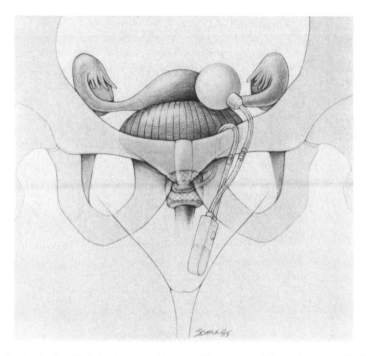

Fig. 16-6   Implanted artificial urinary sphincter. *(Courtesy of American Medical Systems, Minnetonka, MN.)*

The balloon is placed in the retropubic space where it is subjected to the effects of changes in intraabdominal pressure. Balloon pressures range from 51 to 60 cm H_2O to 71 to 80 cm H_2O in 10 cm H_2O increments.

Unlike earlier models, the tubing is now all "resistant" and color coded for easy intraoperative identification. The balloon-pump tubing is black, and the cuff-pump tubing is white.

When the patient feels the urge to urinate, she squeezes the pump through the labia, which transfers fluid to the balloon. On releasing the pump, fluid is sucked from the cuff into the pump. The process is repeated until the pump goes flat signifying the cuff is deflated. The patient is then able to void. The balloon automatically beings repressurization. About 3 minutes are required for the cuff to refill, thus allowing adequate time to complete urination.

Indications and Preoperative Preparation

The artificial urinary sphincter has been implanted in both men and women for various types of incontinence including postprostatectomy incontinence, stress incontinence, epispadias, and neuropathic bladder dysfunction secondary to meningomyelocele, spinal cord injury, multiple sclerosis, sacral agenesis, and spinal cord tumors.

Specifically with regard to incontinence in women, the AMS 800 is most suitable for patients with stress incontinence secondary to poor urethral sphincteric function. The preoperative evaluation of potential candidates is aimed at excluding patients who have underlying disease that would result in a high risk of device failure or who would be at risk for upper urinary tract injury once the device was implanted. This evaluation should include urine culture and sensitivity, intravenous urography, voiding cystourethrography, cystourethroscopy, and urodynamic evaluation.

Patients with urinary tract infections must be treated before implantation to reduce the risk of device contamination. Patients with an overactive detrusor should be controlled medically before implantation. Patients with poor urinary flow and excessive postvoid residual urine can still undergo implantation if they accept the possibility that permanent intermittent self-catheterization will be required. Previous surgery, radiation, or trauma in the region of the urethrovaginal septum can make cuff placement difficult and increase the possibility of cuff erosion, and urethral damage.

Patient motivation is the foremost consideration when selecting patients for artificial sphincter implantation. They must have adequate manual dexterity, mental capacity, and motivation to manipulate the pump mechanism each time they need to urinate. The only two absolute contraindications for implanting an artificial sphincter are uncontrollable detrusor instability or hyperreflexia and high-grade vericoureteral reflux.

Because this is a synthetic device inserted into a closed space, excessive precautions must be taken preoperatively to reduce the chance of infection. Thus the device and instruments are soaked in antimicrobial solutions and proper antibiotic levels are achieved in all tissues before implantation.

Surgical Techniques for Implantation

Implantation of the artificial urinary sphincter has historically been via an abdominal approach to minimize infection and contamination. More recently, however, a transvaginal approach has also been described. Regardless of the route of cuff placement, certain precautions must always be taken. Excessive handling of the device should be avoided. All components of the device except the control assembly are composed of silicone rubber and are thus vulnerable to puncture from needles or sharp instruments. Silicone-shod hemostats to clamp the tubing are used to avoid injury to the device. Blood must not enter the tubing because it will block the one-way valves in the pump assembly and result in device malfunction.

If an abdominal approach is elected, a low transverse muscle cutting incision allows for the best exposure of the retropubic space. A urethral catheter with a 30 ml balloon is placed for easy identification of the bladder neck. The retropubic space is entered and dissection is carried down to the level of the bladder neck. If the patient has undergone previous retropubic surgery, excessive scar tissue may be encountered and one should not hesitate to open the bladder to facilitate the dissection. A small incision is made

in the endopelvic fascia on each side of the bladder neck. Dissection proceeds between the urethra and the vagina with care, as there is no anatomic plane between these two structures.

Caution must be taken to make sure that the plane of dissection is distal to the ureteral orifices. A cutter clamp or right angle scissors is helpful for this dissection. The placing of a finger in the vagina and the elevation of the urethra with a babcock clamp will help delineate the correct plane. Once created, the suburethral tunnel is gently dilated with a right-angle clamp so that it will accept a 2 cm cuff.

A cuff sizer is then passed to measure the circumference of the bladder neck. The adult female bladder neck generally requires a 7 to 9 cm cuff. With the use of a right angle clamp, the appropriately sized cuff is slid into position. The tubing is routed through the layers of the anterior abdominal wall to emerge in the subcutaneous position near the left side of the incision. The pressure-regulating balloon is placed in the prevesical space and its tubing routed in a manner similar to that described for the cuff.

A Hegar dilator is bluntly dissected into one labium majorum to create a space for the pump. The pump is then placed in the dissected space so that it rests immediately beneath the skin to allow for easy palpation and manipulation. All tubing from the three components are passed to the subcutaneous space and filling of the system and connections are made according to the published instructions from the manufacturers.

The device is then left in a deactivated mode for approximately 6 weeks to allow adequate tissue healing. A Foley catheter is left in place for 24 to 48 hours. If the bladder or urethra was opened, drainage should be continued for 7 to 10 days.

More recently, Appell advocated a transvaginal approach for insertion of the cuff. The premise is to decrease the chance of injury to the proximal urethra and bladder neck, which can easily occur with the abdominal route. An inverted u-shaped incision is made in the anterior vaginal wall, and the vaginal mucosa is dissected away from the posterior urethra and bladder neck. At the level of the bladder neck, the dissection is extended laterally and the retropubic space is sharply or bluntly entered between the pubic bone and the endopelvic fascia. Sharp and blunt dissection is used to completely mobilize the proximal urethra and bladder neck. The catheter is removed and the cuff sizer is passed circumferentially around the bladder neck. The appropriate sized cuff is inserted and snapped in place.

A 6 cm transverse skin incision is then made approximately one finger-breadth above the symphysis pubis. The rectus muscle on one side is transected to allow access to the retropubic space. Using a tubing passer, the tubing from the cuff is passed superiorly to exit through the lower abdominal incision. The vaginal incision is then closed with a 2-0 absorbable suture and a vaginal packing is placed.

If there is concern about the integrity of the vaginal wall, interposition of a Martius fat pad from the labium not containing the pump may be considered. A space is bluntly created in the retropubic space to accommodate the pressure-regulating balloon. The remainder of the connections and implantation of the pump are performed as previously described.

Results and Complications

The artificial urinary sphincter has been shown to be effective in restoring continence in appropriately selected female patients. Diokno et al reported a 91% success rate in 32 women who had the device implanted abdominally. Mechanical complications requiring surgical repair occurred in 21% of these patients. These complications included two loose cuffs, two cuff leaks, two tubing kinks, and one connector leak. All of these complications were successfully corrected. Two nonmechanical complications were reported: One pelvic abscess occurred, which required removal of the device, and one superficial wound dehiscence developed. These results are in agreement with a previous study by Light and Scott. More recently, Appell reported 34 women who underwent implantation via a combined vaginal and abdominal approach; he achieved a 100% cure rate for incontinence with no case of erosion or infection. Other studies by Scott, Donovan et al, Mundy and Stephenson, and Stanton have also reported good results.

SUMMARY

Three procedures have been discussed to manage female patients with genuine stress incontinence sec-

ondary to intrinsic urethral dysfunction (type III). Although periurethral injections of bulk-enhancing agents are currently not approved for use in the United States, if and when this approval occurs, this mode of therapy will be suitable for elderly patients as well as postradiation patients. Currently, suburethral sling procedures remain the most commonly used of the three procedures, as most urogynecologic surgeons are familiar with this operation. With further experience and follow-up, the artificial sphincter will probably become more popular and may be a more feasible option in the patient at high risk for complete retention after suburethral sling procedures.

REFERENCES

Suburethral Slings

Aldridge AH: Transplantation of fascia for relief of urinary stress incontinence, *Am J Obstet Gynecol* 44:398, 1942.

Barns HH: Round ligament sling operation for stress incontinence, *J Obstet Gynaecol Br Emp* 57:404, 1950.

Beck RP: The sling operation. In Buchsbaum HJ, Schmidt JD, editors: *Gynecologic and obstetric urology*, ed 2, Philadelphia, 1982, WB Saunders.

Beck RP, McCormick RN, Nordstrom L: The fascia lata sling procedure for treating recurrent genuine stress incontinence of urine, *Obstet Gynecol* 72:699, 1988.

Bryans FE: Marlex gauze hammock sling operation with Cooper's ligament attachment in the management of recurrent urinary incontinence, *Am J Obstet Gynecol* 133:292, 1979.

Goebell R: Zur operativen Beseitigung der Angeborenen, *Incontinentia Vesicae Z Gynakol Urol* 2:187, 1910.

Hadley RH, Zimmern PE, Staskin DR, et al: Transvaginal needle bladder neck suspension, *Urol Clin North Am* 12:299, 1985.

Hilton P: A clinical and urodynamic study comparing the Stamey bladder neck suspension and suburethral sling procedures in the treatment of genuine stress incontinence, *Br J Obstet Gynaecol* 96:213, 1989.

Hilton P, Stanton SL: Clinical and urodynamic evaluation of the polypropylene (Marlex) sling for genuine stress incontinence, *Neurol Urodyn* 2:145, 1983.

Hodgkinson CP, Kelly W: Urinary incontinence in the female. III. Round ligament technique for retropubic suspension of the urethra, *Obstet Gynecol* 10:493, 1957.

Horbach NS, Blanco JS, Ostergard DR, et al: A suburethral sling procedure with polytetrafluoroethylene for the treatment of genuine stress incontinence in patients with low urethral closure pressure, *Obstet Gynecol* 71:648, 1988.

Horbach NS: Suburethral sling procedures. In Ostegard D, Bent A, editors: *Urogynecology and urodynamics, theory and practice*, ed 3, Baltimore, 1991, Williams & Wilkins.

Jarvis GJ, Fowlie A: Clinical and urodynamic assessment of the porcine dermis bladder sling in the treatment of genuine stress incontinence, *Br J Obstet Gynaecol* 92:1189, 1985.

Karram MM, Bhatia NN: Patch procedure: modified transvaginal fascia lata sling for recurrent or severe stress urinary incontinence, *Obtet Gynecol* 75:461, 1990.

Kersey J: The gauze hammock sling operation in the treatment of stress incontinence, *Br J Obstet Gynaecol* 90:945, 1983.

Low JA: Management of severe anatomic deficiencies of urethral sphincter function by a combined procedure with a fascia lata sling, *Am J Obstet Gynecol* 105:149, 1969.

McGuire EJ, Bennett CJ, Konnak JA, et al: Experience with pubovaginal slings for urinary incontinence at University of Michigan, *J Urol* 138:525, 1987.

McGuire EJ, Lytton B: Pubovaginal sling procedure for stress incontinence, *J Urol* 119:82, 1978.

McGuire EJ: Urodynamic findings in patients after failure of stress incontinence operations, *Prog Clin Biol Res* 78:351, 1981.

McGuire EJ: Abdominal procedures for stress incontinence, *Urol Clin North Am* 12:285, 1985.

McGuire EJ, Wang CC, Usitalo H, et al: Modified pubovaginal sling in girls with myelodysplasia, *J Urol* 135:94, 1986.

McLaren HC: Late results from sling operations, *J Gynecol* 75:10, 1968.

McLaren HC: Fascial slings for stress incontinence, *J Obstet Gynaecol Br Emp* 64:673, 1957.

Millin T, Read C: Stress incontinence of urine in the female: Millin's sling operation for stress incontinence, *Postgrad Med J* 24:51, 1948.

Morgan JE: A sling operation using Marlex polypropylene mesh for treatment of recurrent stress incontinence, *Am J Obstet Gynecol* 106:369, 1970.

Morgan JE, Farrow GA, Steward FE: The Marlex sling operation for the treatment of recurrent stress urinary incontinence. A 16-year review, *Am J Obstet Gynecol* 151:224, 1985.

Nichols DH: The mersilene mesh gauze hammock for severe urinary stress incontinence, *Obstet Gynecol* 41:88, 1973.

Obrink A, Bunne G: The margin of incontinence after three types of operation for stress incontinence, *Scand J Urol Nephrol* 12:209, 1978.

Ogundipe A, Rosenzweig BA, Karram MM, et al: Modified suburethral sling procedures for treatment of recurrent or severe stress urinary incontinence, *Surg Obstet Gynecol* 175:173, 1992.

Parker RT, Addison WA, Wilson CJ: Fascia lata urethrovesical suspension for recurrent stress urinary incontinence, *Am J Obstet Gynecol* 135:843, 1979.

Poliak A, Daniller AI, Liebling RW: Sling operation for recurrent stress incontinence using the tendon of the palmaris longus. *Obstet Gynecol* 63:850, 1984.

Ridley JG: Appraisal of the Goebell-Frankenheim-Stoekel sling procedure, *Am J Obstet Gynecol* 95:714, 1966.

Stanton SL, Brindley GS, Holmes DM: Silastic sling for urethral sphincter incompetence in women, *Br J Obstet Gynaecol* 92:747, 1985.

Stoeckel W: Uber die Verwendung der Musculi Pyridimale beider operativen Behandlung der Incontinentia Urinae, *Gynakologe* 41:11, 1917.

Williams TJ, TeLinde RW: The sling operation for urinary incontinence using mersilene ribbon, *Obstet Gynecol* 19:241, 1962.

Periurethral Injections

Appell RA: New developments: injectables for urethral incompetence in women, *Int Urogynecol J* 1:117, 1990.

Appell RA: Injectables for urethral incompetence, *World J Urol* 8:208, 1990.

Arnold GE: Alleviation of aphonia or dysphonia through intrachordal injection of Teflon paste, *Ann Otol Rhinol Laryngol* 72:384, 1963.

Berg S: Polytef augmentation urethroplasty, *Arch Surg* 379:1973.

Boykin W, Rodriguez FR, Brizzolara JP, et al: Complete urinary obstruction following periurethral polytetrafluoroethylene injection for urinary incontinence, *J Urol* 141:1199, 1989.

Claes H, Stroobants D, Van Meerbeek J, et al: Pulmonary migration following periurethral injection for urinary incontinence, *J Urol* 142:821, 1989.

Deane AM, English P, Hehir M, et al: Teflon injection in stress incontinence, *Br J Urol* 140:1101, 1985.

Ford CN, Martin DW, Warren TF: Injectable collagen in laryngeal rehabilitation, *Laryngoscope* 95:513, 1988.

Leonard MP, Canning DA, Epstein JI, et al: Local tissue reaction to the subureteric injection of glutaraldehyde cross-linked bovine collagen in humans, *J Urol* 143:1209, 1990.

Lim KB, Ball AJ, Feneley RCL: Periurethral teflon injection: a simple treatment for urinary incontinence, *Br J Urol* 55:208, 1983.

Lockhart JL, Walker RD, Vorstam B, et al: Periurethral polytetrafluoroethylene injection following urethral reconstruction in female patients with urinary incontinence, *J Urol* 140:51, 1988.

Malizia AA, Reiman MM, Myers RP, et al: Migration and granulation after periurethral injection of Polytef (Teflon), *JAMA* 251:3277, 1984.

Mittleman RE, Marraccini JV: Pulmonary Teflon granulomas following periurethral Teflon injection for urinary incontinence (letter), *Arch Pathol Lab Med* 107:611, 1983.

Oppenheimer BS, Oppenheimer ET, Stout AP: The latent period in carcinogenesis by plastic in rats and its relation to the presarcomatous stage, *Cancer* 11:204, 1958.

Osther PJ, Rohe HF: Female urinary stress incontinence treated with Teflon injections, *Acta Obstet Gynecol Scand* 66:333, 1987.

Politano VA: Periurethral Teflon injection for urinary incontinence, *Urol Clin North Am* 5:451, 1978.

Politano VA, Small MP, Harper JM, et al: Periurethral teflon injection: a simple treatment for urinary incontinence, *J Urol* 111:180, 1974.

Politano VA: Periurethral polytetrafluorethylene injection for urinary urethral incontinence, *J Urol* 172:439, 1982.

Politano VA: Migration of polytetrafluoroethylene polytef (letter), *JAMA* 254:1903, 1985.

Schulman CC, Simon J, Wespes E, et al: Endoscopic injection for Teflon for female urinary incontinence, *Eur Urol* 9:246, 1982.

Shortliffe LMD, Freiha FS, Kessler R, et al: Treatment of urinary incontinence by the periurethral implantation of glutaraldehyde cross-linked collagen, *J Urol* 141:538, 1989.

Smart RF: Polytef paste for urinary incontinence, *Aust NZ J Surg* 61:663, 1991.

Vesey SG, Rivett A, O'Boyle PJ: Teflon injection in female stress incontinence. Effect on urethral pressure profile and flow rate, *Br J Urol* 62:39, 1988.

Artificial Urinary Sphincter

Appell RA: Techniques and results in the implantation of the artificial urinary sphincter in women with type III stress urinary incontinence by vaginal approach, *Neurourol Urodyn* 7:613, 1988.

Diokno AC, Hollander JB, Alderson TP: Artificial urinary sphincter for recurrent female urinary incontinence: indications and results, *J Urol* 137:778, 1987.

Diokno AC, Sonda LP: Compatibility of genitourinary prostheses and intermittent self-catheterization, *J Urol* 125:659, 1981.

Donovan MG, Barrett DM, Furlow WL: Use of the artificial urinary sphincter in the management of severe incontinence in females, *Surg Gynecol Obstet* 161:17, 1985.

Furlow WL: Implantation of a new semiautomatic artificial genitourinary sphincter: experience with primary activation and deactivation in 47 patients, *J Urol* 126:741, 1981.

Hadley HR: The artificial sphincter in the female, *Prob Urology* 5:123, 1991.

Light JK: Abdominal approach for implantation of the AS800 artificial urinary sphincter in females, *Neurourol Urodyn* 7:603, 1988.

Mundy AR, Stephenson TP: Selection of patients for implantation of the Brantley Scott artificial urinary sphincter, *Br J Urol* 56:717, 1984.

Perulkar BC, Barrett DM: Application of the AS-800 artificial sphincter for intractable urinary incontinence in females, *Surg Gyncol Obstet* 171:131, 1990.

Scott FB: The use of the artificial sphincter in the treatment of urinary incontinence in the female patient, *Urol Clin North Am* 12:305, 1985.

Scott FB, Bradley WE, Timm GW: Treatment of urinary incontinence by an implantable prosthetic urinary sphincter, *Urology* 1:252, 1973.

Scott FB, Bradley WE, Timm GW: Treatment of urinary incontinence by an implantable prosthetic urinary sphincter, *J Urol* 112:75, 1974.

Stanton SL: Artificial urinary sphincters (letter), *Br Med J* 291:413, 1985.

Webster GD, Sihelnik SA: Trouble-shooting the malfunctioning Scott artificial urinary sphincter, *J Urol* 131:269, 1985.

CHAPTER **17**

Pelvic Organ Prolapse: Cystocele and Rectocele

Mark D. Walters

Anatomy and Pathology
    Cystocele
    Rectocele
Evaluation
    History
    Physical examination
    Diagnostic tests
Surgical Repair Techniques—Cystocele
    Anterior colporrhaphy with vesical neck plication
    Abdominal cystocele repair
Surgical Repair Techniques—Perineal Relaxation and Rectocele
Results
Complications

Defects of anterior and posterior vaginal wall support are common problems in women that may coexist with disorders of micturition and defecation. Mild cystoceles and rectoceles frequently occur in parous women, but usually present few problems for the patient. As pelvic support defects progress and symptoms develop and worsen, treatment may be indicated. This chapter reviews the anatomy and pathology of anterior and posterior vaginal wall descent and describes methods of their surgical repair.

ANATOMY AND PATHOLOGY

Cystocele

Cystocele is defined as pathologic descent of the anterior vaginal wall and overlying bladder base. According to Nichols, cystoceles are classified as distention cystoceles or as displacement cystoceles. *Distention cystocele* results from overstretching and attenuation of the anterior vaginal wall. It is mainly due to overdistention of the vagina associated with vaginal delivery or to atrophic changes associated with aging and menopause. Rugal folds of the anterior vaginal epithelium are usually diminished or absent due to thinning or loss of midline vaginal fascia. *Displacement cystocele* results from pathologic detachment or elongation of the anterolateral vaginal supports to the arcus tendineus fasciae pelvis. It may occur unilaterally or bilaterally and frequently coexists with some degree of distention cystocele and with descent of the proximal urethra. Although a true cystocele is usually associated only with symptoms of pelvic prolapse, descent of the proximal urethra and bladder base may be associated with urinary incontinence or voiding difficulty.

Rectocele

Rectocele may be defined as herniation or bulging of the posterior vaginal wall and underlying rectum anteriorly, into the vaginal lumen. Rectocele is fundamentally a defect of the vagina and its support, not of the rectum. It is predominantly due to stretching and dehiscence of the rectovaginal septum and the adjacent vaginal fascial envelope during childbirth.

Within the rectovaginal septum is a thin, membranelike connective tissue called the *fascia of Denonvilliers*, which is fused to the underside of the posterior vaginal wall. This tissue extends downward from the bottom of the cul-de-sac of Douglas to its attachment to the upper margin of the perineal body. When this caudal attachment is avulsed, as during childbirth, defects occur in the rectovaginal fascia and the perineum is destabilized. Such weakness leads to rectocele and perineal descent.

Failure of peritoneal fusion of the obliterated extension of the pelvic cavity in the rectovaginal septum can result in congenital deepness of the cul-de-sac and congenital weakness of the posterior vaginal wall in adults. These anatomic variations account in part for the frequent coexistence of high rectocele with enterocele. So frequent is this association that, when one condition is found, the other must be routinely sought and repaired at the same time.

Rectocele and enterocele appear to be disorders confined to parous women. One or both were seen in 39% of asymptomatic women who underwent laparoscopy for other indications. Parturition is associated with a significant increase in the length of the dorsal vaginal wall. This increase in dorsal vaginal length was ascribed to the increase in length of the rectovaginal septum alone, as there was no change in the depth of the cul-de-sac between parous and nulliparous women.

EVALUATION

History

When evaluating women with urogenital prolapse or stress incontinence, attention should be paid to all potential pelvic support defects, including the anterior vaginal wall and overlying urethra and bladder base; the uterus (if present) and vaginal apex; and the posterior vaginal wall, rectum, and perineum. Careful assessment of the rectovaginal space should be made to detect enterocele, which frequently coexists with,

and mimics, rectocele. The reconstructive surgeon must determine the specific sites and causes of damage for each patient, with the ultimate goal of restoring both anatomy and function.

Patients with vaginal prolapse complain either of symptoms related directly to the herniated tissue in the vagina or of associated symptoms, such as urinary incontinence or voiding difficulty. Symptoms directly related to genital prolapse include the sensation of a mass or bulge in the vagina, pelvic pressure and pain, low back pain, and sexual difficulty. Stress urinary incontinence may be related to anterior vaginal wall prolapse. Voiding difficulty may result from large pelvic support defects, especially cystocele and uterovaginal prolapse. Postevacuation rectal discomfort or the inability to completely empty the bowel, requiring manual vaginal or perineal expression to evacuate, sometimes are related to rectocele. Constipation per se is not a symptom of rectocele, although it may coexist. Finally, fecal incontinence frequently coexists with pelvic prolapse.

Physical Examination

The physical examination should be conducted with the patient in lithotomy position as for a routine pelvic examination. The examination is first performed with the patient in the supine position, then, if symptoms do not correspond to physical findings, the woman is reexamined in the standing position. The standing rectovaginal examination is the most reliable position for examining for enterocele.

The genitalia are inspected, and if no displacement is apparent, the labia are gently spread to expose the vestibule and introitus. The integrity of the perineal body is evaluated and the approximate size of all prolapsed parts is assessed. After the resting examination, the patient is instructed to strain down forcefully or to cough vigorously. During this maneuver, the order of descent of the pelvic organs is noted, as is the relationship of the pelvic organs at the peak of straining. Anterior vaginal wall descent usually represents a cystocele with or without rotational descent of the urethra. Less commonly, an anterior enterocele can mimic a cystocele on physical examination. The position of the cervix and uterus or, if absent, the vaginal apex, should be assessed. Digital depression of the perineal body while the patient strains enlarges the genital hiatus and may be helpful to visualize the anatomy. Visualization can be facilitated by displacement of the posterior vaginal wall with a speculum.

Posterior vaginal wall prolapse represents a rectocele, an enterocele, or both. The rectovaginal area is examined to differentiate between these conditions (Fig. 17-1). The rectal finger is elevated into the va-gina to assess for anterior displacement of the rectal wall (rectocele) and for the integrity and thickness of the perineal body. An enterocele is diagnosed on rectovaginal examination by noting a sac of tissue, which may or may not contain small bowel, in the rectovaginal space. When a standing rectovaginal examination is performed, small bowel can frequently herniate into this space between the fingers.

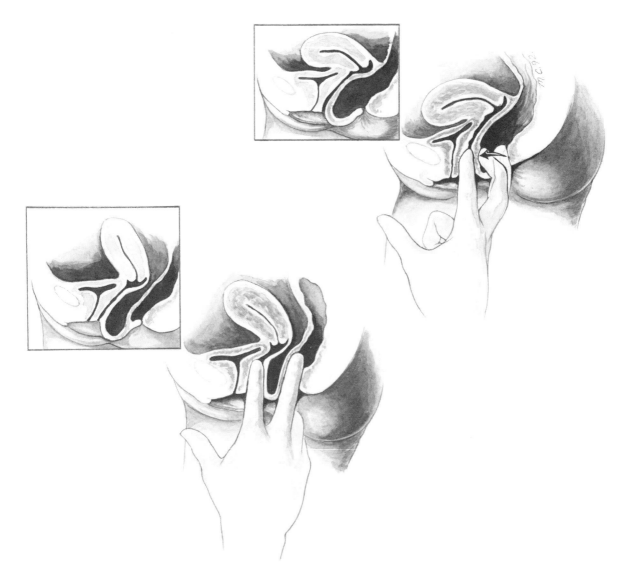

Fig. 17-1 Posterior vaginal wall prolapse, with findings on standing rectovaginal examination for rectocele (*top*) and enterocele (*bottom*).

The severity of vaginal relaxation can be classified using criteria modified from Beecham and Baden et al (see accompanying box). It is helpful to use this classification of position of the pelvic organs during both resting and straining. Classification of rectoceles is aided by performing a rectovaginal examination.

Despite the development of many classification systems, no objective standards have been universally agreed upon. Thus although the system presented here

may be useful, the examining physician also should describe the anatomy of the pelvic findings, with careful reference to each quadrant of the vagina. This approach will facilitate communication among examiners and minimize confusion.

Diagnostic Tests

After careful history and physical examination, few diagnostic tests are needed to evaluate patients with genital prolapse. A urinalysis should be performed to rule out urinary infection if the patient complains of any lower urinary tract dysfunction. If the patient's estrogen status is unclear, vaginal cytologic smears can be obtained to assess maturation index. For third-degree uterovaginal prolapse, a pyelogram or renal ultrasound should be performed to evaluate for ureteral patency and hydronephrosis, which frequently result.

If coexistent urinary incontinence is present, further diagnostic testing may be indicated to differentiate detrusor instability from genuine stress incontinence. Urodynamic, endoscopic, or radiologic assessments of filling and voiding function are probably necessary only when symptoms of incontinence or voiding dysfunction are present. Even if no urologic symptoms are noted, voiding function should be assessed to evaluate for completeness of bladder emptying. This procedure usually involves only a timed, measured micturition or electronic uroflowmetry, followed by urethral catheterization to measure residual urine volume.

Although mild to moderate prolapse is often associated with stress urinary incontinence, patients with severe genitourinary prolapse and cystocele extending beyond the vaginal introitus rarely develop urinary incontinence. Furthermore, stress incontinence may occur after prolapse surgery. Severe genital prolapse is a risk factor for recurrence of stress incontinence after surgery, perhaps because severe uterovaginal prolapse results in urethral kinking, which generates increased urethral resistance. In addition direct compression on the urethra may occur by descending parts of the genital tract. Urethrovesical angulation or extrinsic compression could explain the very high pressure transmission ratios observed when urethral pressure profiles are performed in women with uterovaginal prolapse.

Classification of the Severity of Pelvic Relaxation

Rectocele

First degree—The saccular protrusion of the rectovaginal wall descends half way to the introitus.
Second degree—The sacculation descends to the introitus.
Third degree—The sacculation protrudes or extends outside the introitus.

Cystocele

First degree—The anterior vaginal wall, from the urethral meatus to the anterior fornix, descends half way to the introitus.
Second degree—The inferior bladder wall and its attached vaginal wall extend to the introitus.
Third degree—The entire urethra and bladder are outside the vagina. This cystocele usually is part of a third-degree uterine or posthysterectomy vaginal vault prolapse.

Uterine or vaginal vault prolapse

First degree—The cervix or vaginal apex descends half way to the introitus.
Second degree—The cervix or vaginal apex extends to the introitus or over the perineal body.
Third degree—The cervix and corpus uteri extend totally outside the introitus or the vaginal vault is totally everted.

Enterocele

The presence and depth of the enterocele sac, relative to the hymen, should be described anatomically, with the patient in the supine and standing positions during Valsalva maneuver.

It is important to check urethral function after the prolapse is repositioned in women with severe uterovaginal prolapse and large cystoceles. A pessary can be used to reduce the prolapse before clinical or electronic urodynamic testing. If urinary leaking occurs with stress and/or the urethral closure pressure profile becomes positive after reduction of the prolapse, the urethral sphincter is probably incompetent, even if the patient is normally continent. In this situation, the surgeon can choose an antiincontinence procedure in conjunction with anterior colporrhaphy. If sphincteric incompetence is not present even after reduction with a pessary, an anterior colporrhaphy with vesical neck plication is appropriate.

SURGICAL REPAIR TECHNIQUES—CYSTOCELE

Anterior Colporrhaphy with Vesical Neck Plication

The patient is supine, with the legs elevated and abducted and the buttocks placed just past the edge of the operating table. The vagina and perineum are sterilely prepped and draped, and a 16 French Foley catheter with a 10 ml balloon is inserted for easy identification of the bladder neck. One to three perioperative intravenous doses of an appropriate antibiotic may be given as prophylaxis against infection. If indicated, a suprapubic catheter is placed into the bladder.

A weighted speculum is placed into the vagina. Hemostatic solutions or saline may be injected submucosally, along the midline of the anterior vaginal wall, to decrease bleeding and to aid in dissection of the vesicovaginal space. If a vaginal hysterectomy has been performed, the incised apex of the anterior vaginal wall is grasped transversely with two Allis clamps and elevated. A third Allis clamp is placed about 1 cm below the posterior margin of the urethral meatus and pulled up. The points of a pair of curved Mayo scissors are inserted between the vaginal epithelium and the bladder wall and gently forced upward while partially opening and closing the scissors. Countertraction during the maneuver is important to minimize the likelihood of perforation of the bladder wall.

After development of the vesicovaginal space, the vaginal epithelium is incised in the midline to the level of the midurethra. When the entire vaginal wall has

been cut, the edges are grasped with Allis or T-clamps and drawn laterally for further mobilization. Dissection of the vaginal flaps and mobilization of the cystocele are then accomplished by turning the clamps back across the forefinger and incising the vaginal fascia with a scalpel or Metzenbaum scissors, while the assistant maintains constant traction on the bladder superiorly and medially. This procedure is performed bilaterally until the entire bladder base has been dissected free. The spaces lateral to the urethrovesical junction are sharply and bluntly dissected towards the inferior pubic ramus. When a vaginal hysterectomy has been performed previously, the bladder base often will be firmly adherent to the apex of the vagina. The bladder base should be carefully mobilized from the vaginal apex using sharp dissection with Metzenbaum scissors (Fig. 17-2).

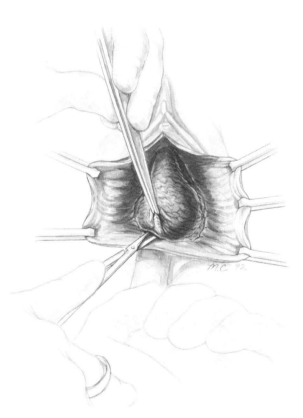

Fig. 17-2 Sharp dissection is used to mobilize the bladder base from the vaginal apex during anterior colporrhaphy.

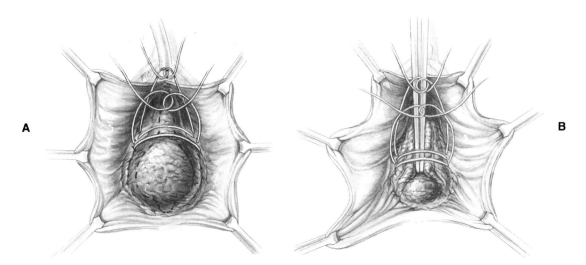

Fig. 17-3   Technique of anterior colporrhaphy. **A**, After dissection of vaginal wall from the bladder and urethra, 1 to 3 plication sutures are placed into the periurethral endopelvic fascia at the urethrovesical junction. **B**, The plication sutures at the vesical neck are tied.

When the vaginal flaps have been developed and the cystocele delineated, the urethrovesical junction can be identified visually or by pulling the Foley catheter downward until the bulb obstructs the vesical neck. Repair should begin at the urethrovesical junction. In most cases, regardless of whether the patient suffers from urinary incontinence, plicating sutures at the urethrovesical junction should be placed to preserve the posterior urethral support and to ensure that stress incontinence, if not present at the time of operation, does not develop postoperatively.

The vesical neck and cystocele are repaired by turning in the remains of the submucosal fascia and bladder adventitia with vertically placed Lembert sutures, using No. 2-0 or 0 delayed absorbable suture. The first plicating suture is placed into the periurethral endopelvic fascia at the urethrovesical junction and tied (Fig. 17-3, *A,B*). After the urethrovesical junction is supported with two or three sutures, the remaining cystocele is repaired with several additional plication sutures, so that each successive stitch incorporates some of the previous stitch. Depending on the size of the cystocele, one or two rows of plication sutures or a purse-string suture followed by plication sutures is placed (Fig. 17-3, *C,D*). After the entire cystocele

has been repaired, vaginal epithelium is trimmed bilaterally and the anterior vaginal wall is closed with a running or interrupted No. 3-0 subcuticular suture.

Needle urethropexy procedures effectively treat small cystoceles associated with descent of the urethra and bladder base. Larger cystoceles usually involve bulging of the posterior bladder wall above the interureteric ridge and will not be treated adequately with needle urethropexies. In these cases, a cystocele repair should be accomplished using the procedure of anterior colporrhaphy described previously. If the cystocele is very large, a purse string suture may be placed to partially reduce the cystocele. This maneuver is followed by standard plication sutures of the bladder muscularis, trimming of the anterior vaginal wall, and closure. If this procedure is combined with a needle urethropexy, the cystocele should be repaired before the urethropexy sutures are tied.

Abdominal Cystocele Repair

Retropubic surgical procedures are effective for treating small cystoceles, although they are generally not used for that purpose. Both the Burch colposuspension and the vaginal obturator shelf and paravaginal repairs suspend the anterior vaginal wall for the treatment of

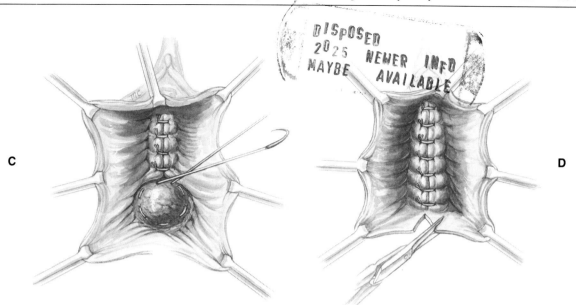

C

D

Fig. 17-3, cont'd.   C, A purse-string suture can be placed in the bladder muscularis to reduce large cystoceles. **D,** The entire cystocele has been repaired with plication sutures and the vaginal epithelium is trimmed before closure.

genuine stress incontinence. These operations effectively treat displacement cystoceles, although the Burch colposuspension may leave a high cystocele located above the trigone.

Abdominal repair of a posterior distention cystocele can be accomplished after abdominal hysterectomy. After the cervix has been amputated from the vagina, the bladder is dissected off the anterior vaginal wall, nearly to the level of the ureters. A full-thickness midline wedge of anterior vaginal wall is excised, and the vagina is closed with running delayed absorbable suture. The vaginal cuff then is repaired according to the surgeon's preference. This procedure will have no effect on bladder neck or urethral support, and care should be taken not to unmask latent stress incontinence by treating a high cystocele without simultaneous urethral suspension.

SURGICAL REPAIR TECHNIQUES—PERINEAL RELAXATION AND RECTOCELE

The repair of a relaxed perineum and rectocele are two distinct operative procedures, although they are usually performed together. Before beginning the repair, the surgeon should estimate the severity of the rectocele and the perineal defect, as well as the desired postoperative caliber of the vagina and introitus. The ultimate size of the vaginal orifice is determined by placing Allis clamps on the inner aspect of the labia minora bilaterally and approximating them in the midline. The final vaginal opening should admit three fingers easily, taking into account that the levator ani and perineal muscles are completely relaxed from the general anesthesia and that the vagina may further constrict postoperatively.

To begin the posterior colporrhaphy, Allis clamps are placed bilaterally on the posterior perineum. A triangular-shaped incision is made in the perineal body and the overlying perineal skin is removed. A subepithelial tunnel is made in the rectovaginal space using Mayo scissors. The dissection is extended to the apex of the vagina and bilaterally in the rectovaginal space using blunt and sharp dissection. The surgeon removes a triangular strip of full-thickness vaginal wall, wide enough to repair the rectocele but leaving an appropriate caliber vagina (Fig. 17-4, *A*).

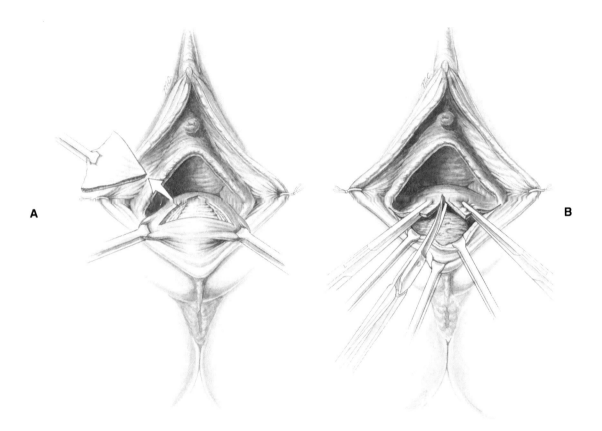

Fig. 17-4 Repair of moderate-sized rectocele. **A,** After a transverse perineal incision and dissection of the vagina from rectum, a triangular strip of full-thickness vaginal wall, sufficiently wide to repair the rectocele while leaving an appropriate caliber vagina, is removed. **B,** Alternatively, the posterior vaginal wall is incised in the midline to the vaginal apex before bilateral rectovaginal dissection.

Alternatively, the posterior vaginal wall is incised in the midline along its entire length (Fig. 17-4, *B*). In a manner similar to the anterior colporrhaphy, lateral traction is placed on each vaginal flap and the underlying rectum and rectovaginal fascia are dissected bluntly and sharply from the vaginal epithelium. The dissection should be extended laterally as far as possible to mobilize perirectal fascia and to expose the medial margins of the puborectalis muscles. The terminal ends of the bulbocavernosus and transverse perineal muscles are also freed from the adherent epithelium in the lower vagina.

The rectovaginal fascia is identified and any defects or lacerations are repaired with No. 2-0 or 0 delayed absorbable suture. Identification of rectovaginal defects is aided by rectal examination with the surgeon's finger elevated toward the vagina. Vertical mattress sutures then are used to plicate the pararectal and rectovaginal fascia over the rectal wall. Repair and plication of this fascia may be sufficient to treat small rectoceles. If the rectocele and levator hiatus are large, however, additional No. 0 delayed absorbable sutures are placed deeply into the medial portions of the puborectalis muscles, and the muscles are brought together in the rectovaginal space (Fig. 17-4, *C*). Although levator plication effectively treats rectocele, it also tends to decrease the caliber of the vaginal lumen and to create a transverse ridge in the posterior vaginal

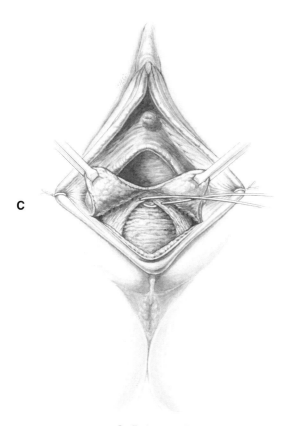

C

Fig. 17-4, cont'd. C, Puborectalis muscle and fascia are approximated in the midline with deep sutures of No. 0 or 1 delayed absorbable material.

wall, both of which may lead to dyspareunia. After the pararectal fascia and levator muscles are plicated, as appropriate, redundant vaginal epithelium is trimmed bilaterally and the posterior vaginal wall and epithelium are closed with No. 3-0 delayed absorbable running suture. A perineoplasty is then performed by placing deep sutures into the perineal muscles and fascia to build up the perineal body. The overlying vulvar skin is closed with No. 3-0 running subcuticular suture.

For anterior and posterior colporrhaphy, a vaginal pack is placed and removed the first postoperative day. Ambulation and diet are advanced rapidly as tolerated by the patient. The bladder is routinely drained after anterior colporrhaphy for 2 or 3 days, after which trials of voiding are begun.

Results

The main indication for anterior colporrhaphy with vesical neck plication is for repair of cystocele. This procedure also may be effective for treatment of mild stress incontinence associated with urethral hypermobility. Several subjective studies have described continence rates as high as 90% after 1 year, although recurrences frequently occur with longer follow-up. In a prospective, randomized study, Bergman et al showed that continence was restored in 69% of women with genuine stress incontinence and pelvic relaxation 1 year after anterior colporrhaphy. This study demonstrated similar cure rates between anterior colporrhaphy and needle urethropexy.

Van Geelen et al treated 90 women with genuine stress incontinence with either anterior colporrhaphy or Burch colposuspension. The choice of surgical procedure was not randomized and was based on the degree of genital prolapse and mobility of the anterior vaginal wall. Urodynamic testing was performed preoperatively and 1 to 2 years postoperatively, with clinical follow-up at 5 to 7 years. At 1 to 2 years after surgery, 45% of women treated with anterior colporrhaphy were cured and 36% were improved. With the Burch colposuspension, 85% of women were cured and 12% were improved 1 to 2 years after surgery. Five years after surgery, 38% of the women who had undergone anterior colporrhaphy were incontinent, compared with 11% of those who had undergone Burch colposuspension. These differences were highly statistically significant for both periods of follow-up, suggesting that the Burch colposuspension is more effective than the anterior colporrhaphy for correcting genuine stress incontinence.

Women with large cystoceles, with or without stress incontinence, frequently have other abnormal bladder symptoms such as urgency, urge incontinence, and voiding difficulty. In a study of surgical repair of large cystoceles by Gardy et al, stress incontinence resolved in 94%, urge incontinence in 87%, and significant residual urine (greater than 80 ml) in 92% of patients 3 months after needle suspension procedures and anterior colporrhaphy. Approximately 5% of patients developed a recurrent cystocele and 8% a recurrent enterocele after an average of 2 years of follow-up.

Few studies have addressed the long-term success of vaginal plastic procedures for treating cystocele and rectocele. Vaginal prolapse recurs with increasing age, but the actual frequency is unknown. Early recurrence is usually due to failure to identify and individually repair all support defects, including the anterior vaginal wall, vaginal apex, rectovaginal septum, posterior vaginal wall, and perineum. Late recurrence is probably due to weakening of the patient's own supporting tissue, which occurs with advancing age and after menopause. Other characteristics that may increase chances of recurrence are pregnancy, heavy lifting, chronic pulmonary disease, smoking, obesity, absence of estrogen replacement after menopause, and genetic predisposition.

COMPLICATIONS

The intraoperative complications of anterior and posterior colporrhaphy include blood loss requiring a blood transfusion and damage to the lumina of the bladder and rectum. Accidental cystotomy or proctotomy should be repaired in layers at the time of the injury. After repair of cystotomy, the bladder is generally drained for 7 to 14 days to allow for adequate healing. After repair of proctotomy, oral feedings should not begin postoperatively until after approximately 48 hours, during which time intravenous fluid replacement is maintained, and bowel function is gradually restored. Patients can then advance to clear liquids and to a soft, low-residue diet for an additional 48 hours. Patients may resume a regular diet after they pass flatus or after the first soft bowel movement. The use of laxatives should be avoided for 4 or 5 days to keep the terminal rectum and anal canal free of fecal material for as long as possible postoperatively, until the mucosal suture line is healing adequately. Failure of healing can result in formation of rectovaginal fistula.

Voiding difficulty can occur after anterior colporrhaphy. This problem occurs primarily in women with subclinical preoperative voiding dysfunction, especially those with low micturition flow rates and absent detrusor contractions with voiding. Treatment is bladder drainage or intermittent self-catheterization until

spontaneous voiding resumes, usually within 6 weeks. Other rare complications include ureteral damage, intravesical or urethral suture placement (and associated urologic problems), and fistula, either urethrovaginal or vesicovaginal. These complications occur rarely; their actual incidence is unknown.

Sexual function may be positively or negatively affected by the vaginal operations for genital prolapse and urinary incontinence. Francis and Jeffcoate found that about one half of sexually active women had some sexual problems after anterior and posterior colpoperineorrhaphy, with or without hysterectomy. Fifty-five percent of these patients reported loss of sexual desire or impotence (male or female) which frequently predated the vaginal surgery. The remaining women reported sexual difficulties due to shortened or stenotic vaginas, dyspareunia, or fear of injury.

Haase and Skibsted studied 55 sexually active women who underwent a variety of operations for stress incontinence or genital prolapse. Postoperatively, 24% of the patients experienced improvement in their sexual satisfaction, 67% experienced no change, and 9% experienced deterioration. Improvement often resulted from cessation of urinary incontinence. Deterioration was always due to dyspareunia after posterior colporrhaphy. These authors concluded that the prognosis for an improved sexual life is good after surgery for stress incontinence, but that posterior colpoperineorrhaphy causes dyspareunia in some patients.

BIBLIOGRAPHY
Anatomy and Pathology

Harrison JE, McDonagh JE: Hernia of Douglas' pouch and high rectocele, *Am J Obstet Gynecol* 60:83, 1950.

Kuhn RJP, Hollyock MD: Observations on the anatomy of the rectovaginal pouch and septum, *Obstet Gynecol* 59:445, 1982.

Milley PS, Nichols DH: A correlative investigation of the human rectovaginal septum, *Anat Rec* 163:443, 1969.

Nichols DH: Posterior colporrhaphy and perineorrhaphy: separate and distinct operations, *Am J Obstet Gynecol* 164:714, 1991.

Nichols DH, Randall CL: Vaginal surgery, ed 3, Baltimore, 1989, Williams & Wilkins.

Richardson AC, Lyon JB, Williams NL. A new look at pelvic relaxation, *Am J Obstet Gynecol* 126:568, 1976.

Evaluation

Addison WA, Livengood CH, Parker RT: Post hysterectomy vaginal vault prolapse with emphasis on management by transabdominal sacral colpopexy, *Postgrad Obstet Gynecol* 8:1, 1988.

Arnold EP, Webster JR, Loose H, et al: Urodynamics of female incontinence: factors influencing the results of surgery, *Am J Obstet Gynecol* 117:805, 1973.

Baden WF, Walker T, Lindsey JH: The vaginal profile, *Tex Med* 64:56, 1968.

Beecham CT: Classification of vaginal relaxation, *Am J Obstet Gynecol* 136:957, 1980.

Bhatia NN, Bergman A: Pessary test in women with urinary incontinence, *Obstet Gynecol* 65:220, 1985.

Bump RC, Fantl JA, Hurt WG: The mechanism of urinary continence in women with severe uterovaginal prolapse: results of barrier studies, *Obstet Gynecol* 72:291, 1988.

deGregorio G, Hillemanns HG: Urethral closure function in women with prolapse, *Int Urogynecol J* 1:143, 1990.

Hadar H, Meiraz D: Total uterine prolapse causing hydroureteronephrosis, *Surg Gynecol Obstet* 150:711, 1980.

Porges RF: A practical system of diagnosis and classification of pelvic relaxations, *Surg Gynecol Obstet* 117:769, 1963.

Richardson DA, Bent AE, Ostergard DR: The effect of uterovaginal prolapse on urethrovesical pressure dynamics, *Am J Obstet Gynecol* 146:901, 1983.

Stabler J: Uterine prolapse and urinary tract obstruction, *Br J Radiol* 50:493, 1977.

Surgical Repair Techniques and Complications-Cystocele and Rectocele

Beck RP, McCormick S: Treatment of urinary stress incontinence with anterior colporrhaphy, *Obstet Gynecol* 59:269, 1982.

Bergman A, Koonings PP, Ballard CA: Primary stress urinary incontinence and pelvic relaxation: prospective randomized comparison of three different operations, *Am J Obstet Gynecol* 161:97, 1989.

Bhatia NN, Bergman A: Use of preoperative uroflowmetry and simultaneous urethrocystometry for predicting risk of prolonged postoperative bladder drainage, *Urology* 28:440, 1986.

Francis WJA, Jeffcoate TNA: Dyspareunia following vaginal operations, *Br J Obstet Gynaecol* 68:1, 1961.

Gardy M, Kozminski M, DeLancey J, et al: Stress incontinence and cystoceles, *J Urol* 145:1211, 1991.

Haase P, Skibsted L: Influence of operations for stress incontinence and/or genital descensus on sexual life, *Acta Obstet Gynecol Scand* 67:659, 1988.

Macer GA: Transabdominal repair of cystocele, a 20-year experience, compared with the traditional vaginal approach, *Am J Obstet Gynecol* 131:203, 1978.

Mitchell GW: Vaginal hysterectomy: anterior and posterior colporrhaphy; repair of enterocele; and prolapse of vaginal vault. In Ridley JH (ed): *Gynecologic surgery; errors, safeguards, salvage*, ed 2, Baltimore, 1981, Williams & Wilkins.

Pelusi G, Bacchi P, Demaria F, et al: The use of Kelly plication for the prevention and treatment of genuine stress urinary incontinence in patients undergoing surgery for genital prolapse, *Int Urogynecol J* 1:196, 1990.

Stanton SL, Norton C, Cardozo L: Clinical and urodynamic effects of anterior colporrhaphy and vaginal hysterectomy for prolapse with and without incontinence, *Br J Obstet Gynaecol* 89:459, 1982.

Symmonds RE, Jordan LT: Iatrogenic stress incontinence of urine, *Am J Obstet Gynecol* 82:1231, 1961.

Mattingly RF, Thompson JD: Relaxed vaginal outlet, rectocele, and enterocele. In *Operative gynecology*, ed 6, Philadelphia, 1985, JB Lippincott.

van Geelen JM, Theeuwes AG, Eskes TK, et al: The clinical and urodynamic effects of anterior vaginal repair and Burch colposuspension, *Am J Obstet Gynecol* 159:137, 1988.

CHAPTER 18

Pelvic Organ Prolapse: Enterocele and Vaginal Vault Prolapse

Mickey M. Karram
Mark D. Walters

Pathology of Pelvic Organ Prolapse
Enterocele
    Definition and types
    Surgical repair of enterocele
Vaginal Vault Prolapse: General Concepts
Vaginal Surgical Approaches
    Fixation of the vaginal vault to the sacrospinous
      ligament
    LeFort partial colpocleisis
    Colpectomy
Abdominal Sacral Colpopexy
Nonsurgical Treatment of Uteropelvic and Vaginal
    Prolapse

In the last several years, the problem of pelvic organ prolapse has been given much more attention. Many women are living longer and there is more interest in maintaining self-image of femininity and the capacity of sexual activity beyond the menopause. Although few data on the incidence or prevalence of various forms of pelvic organ prolapse exist, the incidence appears to be rising based on increased longevity of women.

The management of pelvic organ prolapse can at times be difficult; several support defects often coexist and simple anatomic correction of the various defects does not always result in normal function of the vagina and surrounding organs. To accomplish the goals of pelvic reconstruction, the surgeon must thoroughly understand normal anatomic support and physiologic function of the vagina, bladder, and rectum. These goals are to restore anatomy, maintain or restore normal bowel and bladder function, and maintain vaginal capacity for sexual intercourse.

This chapter discusses the pathology and surgical correction of enterocele and vaginal vault prolapse. Normal anatomy of the pelvic diaphragm is discussed in detail in Chapter 1. The evaluation of patients with pelvic organ prolapse, especially regarding their symptomatology, physical examination, and diagnostic tests, is discussed in Chapter 17.

PATHOLOGY OF PELVIC ORGAN PROLAPSE

Pelvic organ prolapse can result when normal pelvic organ supports are subjected chronically to increases in intraabdominal pressure, or when defective genital support responds to normal intraabdominal pressure. Individual organs that pass through the pelvic floor can lose support singly or in combination, resulting in various degrees and combinations of pelvic organ prolapse. This loss of support occurs as a result of damage to any one or more of the pelvic supportive systems. These systems include the bony pelvis, to which the soft tissues ultimately attach; the subperitoneal retinaculum and smooth muscle component of the endopelvic fascia (the cardinal and uterosacral ligament complex); the pelvic diaphragm, with the levator ani muscles and their fibromuscular attachments to the pelvic organs; and the perineal membrane. The perineal body and the walls of the vagina can lose tone and weaken from pathologic stretching from childbirth and attenuating changes of aging and menopause.

Loss of support or integrity of anterior and posterior vaginal walls results in cystocele and enterorectocele, respectively. Uterovaginal prolapse occurs with damage or attenuation of endopelvic fascia that supports the uterus and upper vagina over the pelvic diaphragm. Furthermore, when the muscles within the pelvic diaphragm weaken as a result of congenital weakness, childbirth injury, pelvic neuropathy, or aging, the levator ani lose resting tone and fail to contract quickly and strongly with increases in the intraabdominal pressure. Muscle atrophy and a wider levator hiatus result; weaker and less rapid muscle contractions with intraabdominal pressure rises contribute to related symptoms of urinary and fecal incontinence.

The normal vaginal axis in a standing woman is nearly horizontal in the upper half of the vagina, with the uterus and upper 3 or 4 cm of the vagina lying over the levator plate in the hollow of the sacrum (Fig. 18-1). Funt et al found that the vagina is directed toward the S3 and S4 vertebrae and extends approximately 3 cm past the ischial spines in most nulliparous women. Increases in intraabdominal pressure compress the vagina anteriorly to posteriorly over the contracted levator muscles in the midline (levator plate). Laxity of the muscles results in loss of stability of the levator plate and widening of the levator hiatus. This provides less of a base to support the upper vagina and uterus in the midpelvis.

Genetically or hormonally determined connective tissue defects have been found in women with uterine prolapse and stress incontinence. In several studies, Mäkinen and co-workers found abnormal histologic changes in the pelvic connective tissue in 70% of women with uterine descent, as compared to 20% of normal controls. The observed changes were decreased cellularity (fibroblasts) and an increase in collagen fibers. Ulmsten et al reported 40% less total

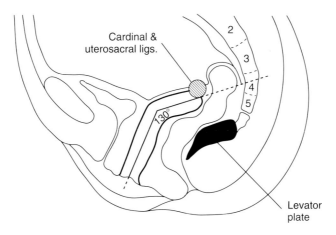

Fig. 18-1 Normal vaginal axis of nulliparous woman in the standing position. Note that the upper third of the vagina is nearhorizontal and is directed toward the S3 and S4 sacral vertebrae. *(From Funt MI, Thompson JD, Birch H:* South Med J *71:1534, 1978.)*

collagen in the skin and round ligaments in women with stress incontinence, compared with continent women. These studies suggest that deteriorated connective tissue may be associated with pelvic organ prolapse and stress incontinence in women.

ENTEROCELE

Definition and Types

Enterocele is defined as herniation of peritoneum, with or without portions of intraperitoneal contents, in areas of the pelvic floor where they are not normally found. The location typically involves the posterior cul-de-sac (pouch of Douglas). This herniation may or may not involve the uterus or vaginal apex. Enteroceles occurring anterior as well as lateral to the vaginal apex have been described, but are exceedingly rare.

Enteroceles are divided into four types: congenital, traction, pulsion, and iatrogenic. **Congenital enteroceles** are rare and are thought to occur secondary to incomplete fusion of anterior and posterior peritoneum in the rectovaginal septum. Other congenital factors that may predispose to the development of enterocele or vaginal prolapse include neurologic disorders, as with spina bifida, and connective tissue disorders. **Traction enterocele** occurs secondary to uterovaginal descent, while **pulsion enterocele** occurs from prolonged increased intraabdominal pressure. Both of these types of enterocele may be associated with various degrees of vaginal vault prolapse, cystocele, and rectocele. **Iatrogenic enterocele** occurs after surgical procedures that change the normally near horizontal vaginal axis toward vertical. This change commonly occurs after colposuspension operations for stress incontinence.

Enteroceles occur frequently in association with rectocele. When these conditions coexist, rectovaginal examination demonstrates the rectocele as distinct from the bulging sac that arises from a higher point in the vagina. Inspection of the posterior vaginal wall also normally reveals a transverse furrow between the two hernias. If the pathology is not evident in the supine position, patients should be examined in the standing position because smaller enteroceles can remain completely reduced in the supine position.

Surgical Repair of Enterocele

Surgical repair of enterocele can be performed vaginally or abdominally. No data exist comparing the various types of repairs; the type of procedure performed depends on the surgeon's preference and whether there is coexistent vaginal or abdominal pathology. Vaginal surgical techniques described herein are the vaginal enterocele repair and McCall culdoplasty; other types of vaginal excision of a deep cul-de-sac have been described by Torpin and by Waters. Abdominal approaches include the Moschcowitz procedure, Halban procedure, and uterosacral ligament plication.

Vaginal Enterocele Repair

The vaginal enterocele repair is usually used for enteroceles that develop after a hysterectomy. Concurrent vaginal vault suspension and/or rectocele repair are frequently necessary. The technique is as follows:

1. The patient is positioned as for posterior colporrhaphy. A midline posterior vaginal wall incision is made over the enterocele sac up to the vaginal apex and extended to the perineum if a rectocele is also present. Sharp and blunt dissection is used to dissect the posterior vaginal wall from the enterocele sac and the anterior rectal wall. The dissection should extend laterally to the medial margins of the levator ani muscles.

2. The enterocele sac should be mobilized completely from the vagina and rectum. Sometimes the enterocele sac is difficult to distinguish from the rectum. This differentiation is aided by a rectal examination with simultaneous dissection of the enterocele sac from the rectal wall. At times it may also be difficult to distinguish the enterocele sac from a large cystocele. In this situation placement of a probe into the bladder or transillumination with a cystoscope may be helpful.

3. After the enterocele sac has been separated from the vagina and rectum, traction is placed on it with two Allis clamps and the sac is entered with Metzenbaum scissors (Fig. 18-2, *A*). The enterocele sac is digitally explored to ensure that no small bowel or omental adhesions are

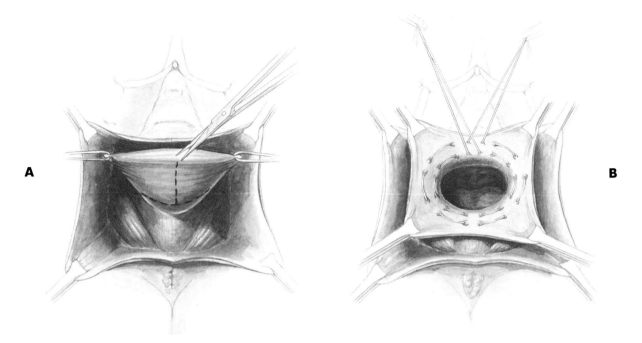

Fig. 18-2 Vaginal enterocele repair. **A,** Isolation and entry of the enterocele sac in the rectovaginal space. **B,** Purse-string sutures are placed close to the enterocele sac.

within the sac. The sac is widely opened and dissected circumferentially up to the level of its neck.

4. Under direct visualization, circumferential purse-string sutures of No. 2-0 or 0 silk (or other nonabsorbable suture) are used to close the enterocele sac (Fig. 18-2, *B*). Usually three purse-string sutures are placed before tying and then they are all tied in sequence. The peritoneum distal to the neck is excised. If the uterosacral-cardinal ligament complex can be indentified, it should be incorporated into the purse-string sutures. Care should be taken to avoid kinking the ureter with the purse-string sutures.

5. The surgeon then can proceed with posterior colporrhaphy and vaginal vault suspension, as indicated.

McCall Culdoplasty

McCall described the technique of surgical correction of enterocele and deep cul-de-sac immediately after vaginal hysterectomy. The advantage of the McCall's culdoplasty is that it closes the redundant cul-de-sac and associated enterocele, while bringing the uterosacral ligaments together in the midline. The posterior vaginal wall is sutured to the uterosacral ligaments providing apical support, as well as lengthening of the vagina. This procedure should be applied as part of every vaginal hysterectomy, even when an enterocele is not present, to help prevent future enterocele formation and vaginal vault prolapse.

The technique is as follows (Fig. 18-3):

1. After the vaginal hysterectomy has been accomplished and a running, locking suture has been placed on the posterior vaginal edge, the surgeon puts a finger into the posterior cul-de-sac to evaluate its depth. Lateral traction is placed on the previously tagged uterosacral ligaments.

2. With the patient in Trendelenburg position, a small packing is placed intraperitoneally to prevent descent of omentum or bowel into the operator's field. Using silk or other permanent

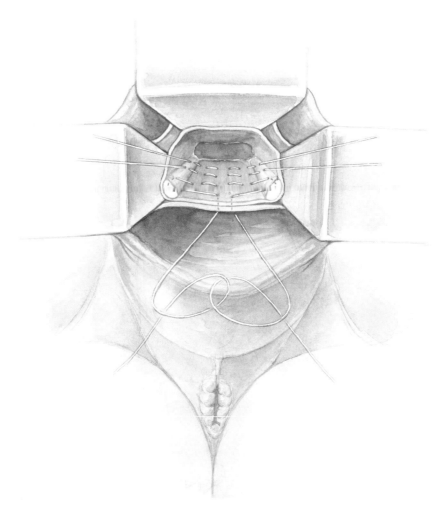

Fig. 18-3 McCall culdoplasty technique. Note that the lowest suture incorporates the posterior vaginal wall thus providing additional support.

suture, the needle is initially passed through one uterosacral ligament as high as possible. Successive bites are then taken at 1 to 2 cm intervals through the anterior serosa of the sigmoid colon until the opposite uterosacral ligament is reached. This suture is held and one to three more identical sutures are placed, progressing toward the posterior vaginal cuff. The number of internal sutures placed depends on the size and depth of the enterocele. In this way, the entire dependent portion of the cul-de-sac is obliterated.

3. After all the internal silk sutures have been placed and their ends held laterally without tying, one or two sutures of delayed absorbable, No. 0 suture are placed. These are inserted from the vaginal lumen just below the middle of the cut edge of the posterior vaginal cuff. With an Allis clamp pulling the posterior vaginal incision upward, the needle is passed through both the vagina and peritoneum. The needle is then picked up within the lower peritoneal cavity and passed through the right uterosacral ligament. Successive bites are taken across the cul-de-sac

as before, and into the left uterosacral ligament. This suture is then passed through the peritoneum and into the vagina next to where the suture originated.

4. The silk sutures are then tied in sequence. The final suture that is tied is the one that exits out through the posterior vaginal wall. During tying of this knot, care is taken to push the posterior vagina onto the uterosacral ligaments while securing the knot.

Few studies have reported long-term results after vaginal repair of enterocele. In a study of 48 women who had McCall culdoplasties for large enterocele, complete procidentia, or complete vaginal vault prolapse, only two enteroceles (4%) recurred 2 to 22 years (average follow-up, 7 years) postoperatively.

Complications that have been reported after McCall culdoplasty are shown in Table 18-1. Care must be taken to not place sutures too deep into the uterosacral ligaments so that the ureters are not damaged or kinked. Given reported this complication in one of 48 McCall culdoplasty procedures. Stanhope et al found that culdoplasty sutures were implicated in a significant proportion of ureteral obstructions after vaginal surgery, although this complication occurred rarely.

Abdominal Enterocele Repairs

Moschcowitz Procedure. The Moschcowitz procedure is performed by placing concentric, purse-string sutures around the cul-de-sac (Fig. 18-4, *A*). The initial suture is placed at the base of the cul-de-sac. Peritoneal sutures should be placed over the posterior vaginal wall, the right pelvic side wall, the serosa of the sigmoid, and the left pelvic side wall. The number of sutures used depends on the depth of the cul-de-sac. Usually, three or four sutures will completely obliterate the enterocele. The purse-string sutures are tied so that no small defects remain that could entrap small bowel or lead to enterocele recurrence. Care should be taken not to include the ureter in the purse-string sutures or to allow the ureter to be kinked medially when tying the sutures.

Halban Procedure. Halban described a similar technique to obliterate the cul-de-sac except that he used interrupted sagittally placed sutures. Sutures are placed in a longitudinal fashion through the serosa of

TABLE 18-1   Complications after McCall culdoplasty*

Complication	Percent of patients (N = 48)
Removal of silk suture	10
Postoperative cuff infection	4
High rectocele	4
Partial prolapse of vaginal vault	4
Shortened vagina	4
Introital stenosis	2
Pulmonary emboli	2
Nerve palsy	2
Ureteral obstruction	2

From Given FT: *Am J Obstet Gynecol* 153:135, 1985.
*Follow-up was 2 to 22 (average 7) years.

the sigmoid, then into the deep peritoneum of the cul-de-sac, and then up the posterior vaginal wall (Fig. 18-4, *B*). Four or five sutures are placed across the pelvis. Sutures are not placed into the lateral pelvic peritoneum or adjacent to the ureters. After all sutures are placed, they are tied in sequence to obliterate the cul-de-sac.

Uterosacral Ligament Plication. If the uterus is present, or if identifiable uterosacral ligaments are found, a uterosacral ligament plication can be performed (Fig. 18-4, *C*). Sutures are placed into the medial portion of one uterosacral ligament, then into the back wall of the vagina, then into the medial portion of the other uterosacral ligament. Three to five sutures are placed from the upper portion of the vagina down toward the rectum. The lowest suture incorporates the anterior rectal serosa to bring the rectum adjacent to the uterosacral ligaments and vagina. After all sutures are tied, the entire lengths of the uterosacral ligaments are brought together in the midline and the cul-de-sac below is closed. Again, care should be taken to avoid entrapment or kinking of the ureter.

VAGINAL VAULT PROLAPSE: GENERAL CONCEPTS

The true incidence and prevalence of vaginal vault prolapse are unknown. Eversion of the vagina prob-

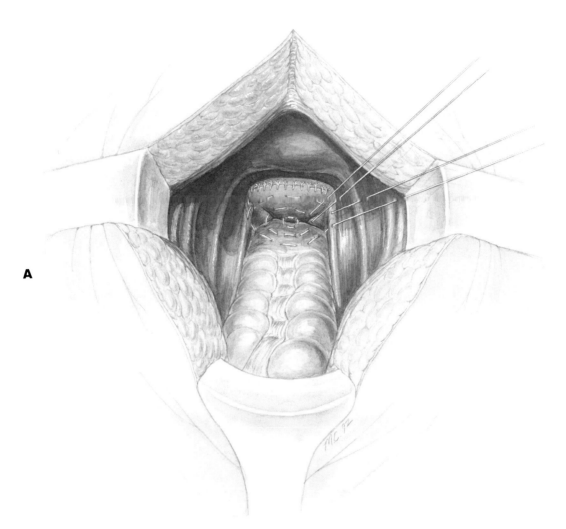

Fig. 18-4 Techniques of enterocele repair via the abdominal route. **A,** Moschcowitz procedure.

ably occurs in about 0.5% of patients who have undergone vaginal or abdominal hysterectomy. Prophylactic measures performed at the time of hysterectomy (vaginal or abdominal) probably decrease the incidence of vaginal vault prolapse. These measures include routine reattachment of endopelvic fascia—cardinal and uterosacral ligaments—to the vaginal vault, and routine use of culdoplasty sutures, cul-de-sac obliteration, or enterocele excision after removal of the uterus.

When mild to moderate forms of either isolated vault prolapse or uterovaginal prolapse (descent of the vaginal vault not beyond the midportion of the vagina) present, vaginal hysterectomy and culdoplasty with anterior and posterior colporrhaphy are usually sufficient operations to relieve the patient's symptoms and restore normal vaginal function. When the vault descends beyond this point, however, simple hysterectomy with repair often will not result in acceptable vaginal depth or prevent vaginal prolapse recurrences. In these cases, one must look to procedures aimed at suspending the apex of the vagina, or in rare circum-

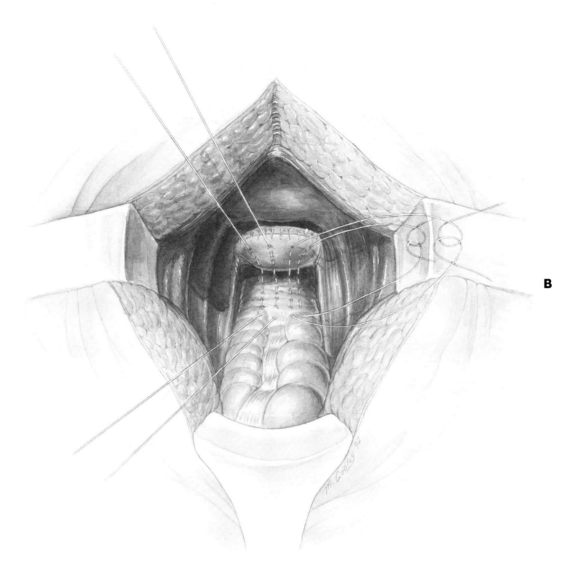

Fig. 18-4, cont'd. B, Halban procedure.

Continued.

stances, completely obliterating the vagina. When this has been decided, certain other decisions must be made:

1. If the uterus is still present, should hysterectomy be part of the surgical correction? The majority of patients require removal of the uterus. The techniques of vaginal and abdominal hysterectomy are sufficiently discussed in other texts and will not be mentioned further.

If hysterectomy is not desired, then pessary use or LeForte partial colpocleisis should be considered. If surgical correction is needed and the patient desires fertility potential, then an abdominal approach with uterosacral ligament plication and perhaps modified sacral colpopexy can be performed. Few studies have addressed this issue; a review of the subject was recently published by Nichols.

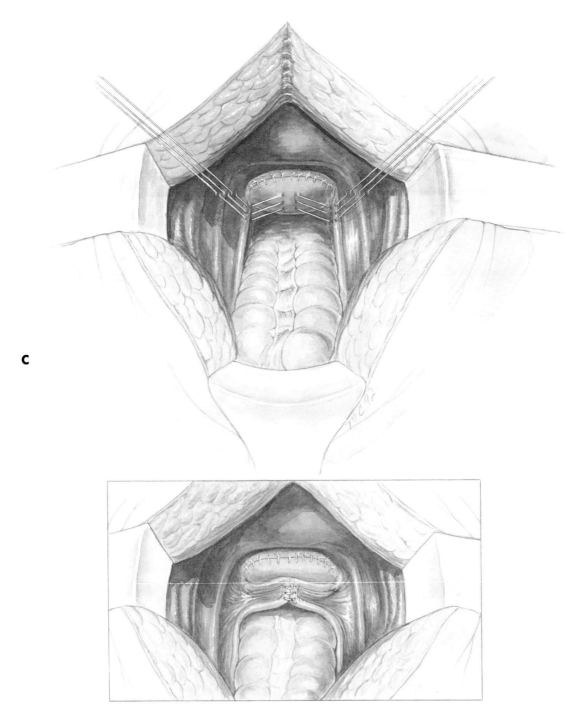

C

Fig. 18-4, cont'd. C, Uterosacral ligament plication.

2. Is the surgical correction intended to preserve a functional vagina? Most of the operations discussed in this chapter will be aimed at preservation of vaginal and coital function. For patients in whom future sexual function is not a goal or operative time and morbidity are best kept at a minimum, partial or complete colpocleisis and colpectomy operations are indicated.

3. Should the surgical correction be approached via a vaginal or abdominal route? Factors such as the patient's general medical condition and weight, the need for concurrent surgical procedures, and the preference and expertise of the surgeon influence this decision. Studies have not addressed the comparison of efficacy between the various operations.

4. Does the patient have real or potential stress urinary or fecal incontinence? When deciding the route of surgical correction, the surgeon must always consider the correction of lower urinary tract and lower gastrointestinal dysfunction. Preoperative reduction of the prolapse followed by urodynamic and/or rectal manometric tests will help to answer this question and to decide which operations are required.

Any reconstructive surgery should return the upper vagina to the normal near-horizontal axis. Ventral (abdominal wall) vaginal suspensions change the axis of the vagina anteriorly and predispose to recurrent posterior vaginal wall prolapse. Failure to recognize an enterocele or failure to reconstruct a widened levator hiatus also may predispose to postoperative vaginal prolapse. Finally, the length of the vagina may be an important factor for surgical success. The upper 3 to 4 cm of the vagina lies horizontally over the levator plate. Operations that shorten the vagina, such as partial vaginectomy, do not allow the upper vagina to lie over the levator plate and may predispose to recurrent vaginal prolapse.

Although many different techniques have been described to suspend or to obliterate the vagina, only the most popular techniques will be discussed. These techniques include sacrospinous ligament fixation, abdominal sacral colpopexy, LeFort partial colpocleisis, and colpectomy.

VAGINAL SURGICAL APPROACHES
Fixation of the Vaginal Vault to the Sacrospinous Ligament
Surgical Anatomy

To perform this procedure correctly and safely, the surgeon must be familiar with pararectal anatomy as well as the anatomy of the sacrospinous ligament and its surrounding structures (Fig. 18-5).

The sacrospinous ligaments extend from the ischial spines on each side to the lower portion of the sacrum and coccyx. Nichols and Randall described the sacrospinous ligament as a cordlike structure lying within the substance of the coccygeus muscle. However, the fibromuscular coccygeus muscle and sacrospinous ligament are basically the same structure and will thus be referred to as the coccygeus-sacrospinous ligament (C-SSL). The coccygeus muscle has a large fibrous component that is present throughout the body of the muscle and on the anterior surface where it appears as white ridges. The C-SSL can be identified when one palpates the ischial spine initially and traces the flat triangular thickening posteriorly to the sacrum. The fibromuscular coccygeus is attached directly to the underlying sacrotuberous ligament.

Posterior to the C-SSL and sacrotuberous ligament are the gluteus maximus muscle and the fat of the ischiorectal fossa. The pudendal nerves and vessels lie directly posterior to the ischial spine. The sciatic nerve lies superior and lateral to the C-SSL. Also superiorly lies an abundant vascular supply that includes inferior gluteal vessels and a hypogastric venous plexus.

Surgical Technique

Before this operation is initiated, one should have preoperatively recognized the ischial spine and C-SSL on pelvic examination. The patient should have been evaluated for stress incontinence after reducing the prolapse and the decision about whether to perform simultaneous bladder neck suspension should have been made. Estrogen replacement therapy should be liberally given preoperatively, if appropriate. We prefer to use a vaginal estrogen cream for 4 to 6 weeks preoperatively.

The performance of this operation almost always

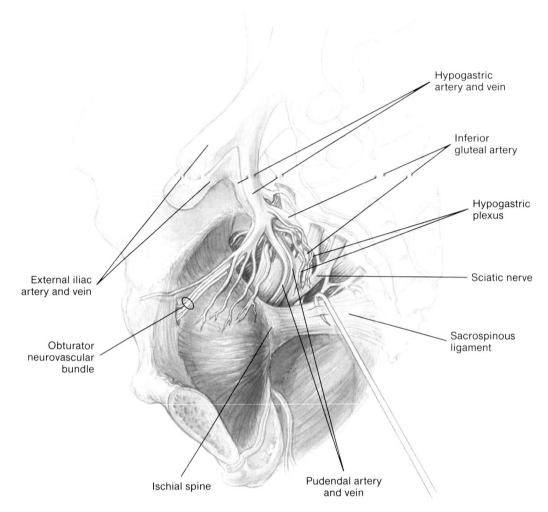

Fig. 18-5 Anatomy of the coccygeus-sacrospinous ligament (C-SSL) complex and surrounding structures. Note close proximity of pudendal vessels, hypogastric plexus, inferior gluteal vessels, and sciatic nerve to C-SSL.

requires simultaneous correction of the anterior and posterior vaginal walls and enterocele repair. Displacing the prolapsed vaginal apex to the sacrospinous ligament to see if the anterior and posterior vaginal wall prolapse disappears with a Valsalva maneuver helps to determine whether cystocele and rectocele repairs are needed. The patient should be routinely consented for these repairs as many times it is difficult to discern the extent of the various defects preoperatively.

The technique of sacrospinous fixation is as follows:

1. With patient in dorsal lithotomy position, vaginal area is prepped and draped. Prophylactic perioperative antibiotics are given routinely.
2. The apex of the vagina is grasped with two Allis clamps, and downward traction is used to determine the extent of the vaginal prolapse and associated pelvic support defects. The vaginal apex is then reduced to the sacrospinous ligament intended to be used. Although bilateral sacrospinous fixations have been described, most surgeons prefer unilateral fixa-

tion of the vaginal vault. At times the apex of the vagina is foreshortened and will not reach the intended area of fixation. We recommend in these circumstances that a new apex be created from a more prominent area of vaginal prolapse. This process usually entails moving the apex to a portion of the vaginal wall over an enterocele or a cystocele. The intended apex is then tagged with two sutures for its later identification.

3. If the patient has complete eversion of the vagina and requires anterior vaginal wall repair and bladder neck suspension, we prefer doing this portion of the operation first. During this procedure, one can separate the bladder base away from the vaginal apex, thus lowering the risk of cystotomy. After the anterior colporrhaphy and urethropexy, if indicated, are finished, the anterior vaginal wall is closed with a continuous running suture.

4. The posterior vaginal wall is then incised. After a transverse perineal incision, a midline posterior vaginal wall incision is made just short of the apex of the vagina leaving a small vaginal bridge of approximately 3 or 4 cm wide. In the majority of cases, an enterocele sac is present. This sac should be dissected off the posterior vaginal wall as described under the section on vaginal enterocele repair. Once the enterocele has been incised and ligated, one is ready to begin the sacrospinous fixation.

5. The first step is entry into the perirectal space. The right rectal pillar separates the rectovaginal space from the right perirectal space. The rectal pillar is areolar tissue that extends from the rectum to the arcus tendineous and overlies the levator muscle. It has two layers and may contain a few small muscle fibers and blood vessels. In the majority of cases, entry into the perirectal space is best achieved by breaking through the fibroareolar tissue just lateral to the enterocele sac at the level of the ischeal spine. This maneuver can usually be accomplished bluntly by mobilizing the rectum medially. At times, however, the use of gauze on the index finger or a tonsil clamp is necessary to break through into this space.

6. Once the perirectal space is entered, the ischial spine is identified and, with dorsal and medial movement of the fingers, the C-SSL is palpated.

7. Blunt dissection is used to further remove tissue from this area. The surgeon should take great care to assure that the rectum is adequately retracted medially. At this time, we recommend performing a rectal examination to assure that no inadvertent rectal injury has occurred.

8. Two techniques have been popularized for the actual passage of sutures through the ligament (Fig. 18-6, *A* and *B*). The first is the technique of Randall and Nichols using a long-handled Deschamps ligature carrier and nerve hook (Fig. 18-7, *A*). Long straight retractors are used to expose the coccygeus muscle. Heaney retractors or Briesky-Navratil retractors (Fig. 18-7, *B*) are preferred. One must take great care not to let the tip of the retractor be pushed across the anterior surface of the sacrum risking potential damage to vessels and nerves. If the right sacrospinous ligament is to be used, the middle and index fingers on the left hand are placed on the medial surface of the ischial spine and, under direct vision, the tip of the ligature carrier penetrates the C-SSL at a point two finger breadths medial to the ischial spine. When pushing the ligature carrier through the body of the C-SSL, considerable resistance should be encountered; this must be overcome by forceful, yet controlled, rotation of the handle of the ligature carrier. If visualization of the C-SSL is difficult, the muscle and ligament can be grasped in the tip of a long Babcock or Allis clamp, which helps to isolate the tissue to be sutured from underlying vessels and nerves. After suture passage, the fingers of the left hand are withdrawn. The retractor is suitably repositioned and the tip of the ligature carrier is visualized. The suture is then grasped with a nerve hook (see Fig. 18-6, *A*). A second suture is similarly placed 1 cm medial to the first. If one wishes to avoid a second passage

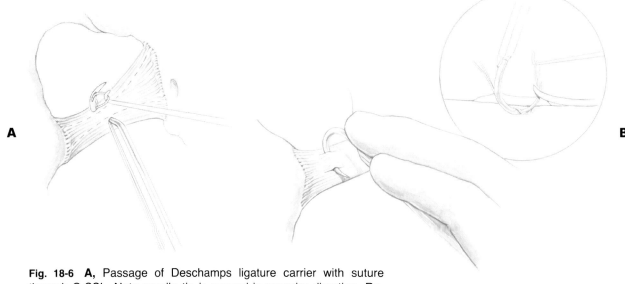

Fig. 18-6 **A,** Passage of Deschamps ligature carrier with suture through C-SSL. Note needle tip is passed in superior direction. Retrieval of suture is with nerve hook. **B,** Passage of Miya hook through C-SSL. Note needle tip is passed inferiorly. Retrieval of suture is facilitated by using notched speculum.

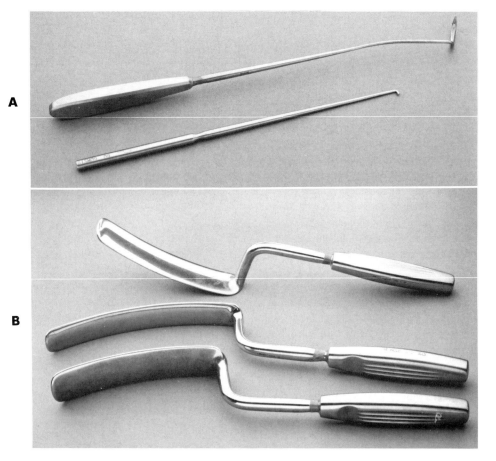

Fig. 18-7 **A,** Long-handled Deschamps ligature carrier and nerve hook. Note slight bend near the tip to facilitate suture placement into the C-SSL. **B,** Briesky-Navratil retractors: various sizes.

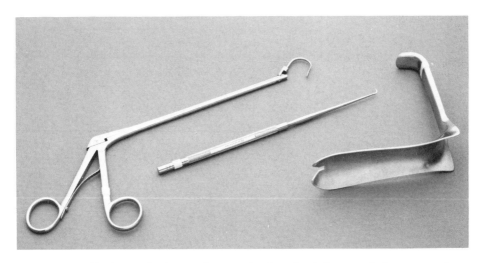

Fig. 18-8 Miya Hook, notched speculum, and suture hook for use during sacrospinous ligament fixation.

of the ligature carrier, the original long suture can be cut in the center and each end of the cut loop paired with its respective free suture. This obtains two sutures through the ligament with only one penetration of the ligature carrier. To assure that an appropriate bite of tissue has been obtained, one should be able to gently move the patient with traction of the sutures.

A second technique that has been recently popularized for passing the sutures through the C-SSL is the technique of Miyazaki using a Miya hook ligature carrier (Fig. 18-8). The proposed advantage of this technique is that it is safer and easier, as the ligature carrier enters the C-SLL under direct palpation of distinct landmarks and is then pulled down into the safe perirectal space below.

To perform this modification, the right middle finger tip is placed on the C-SSL just below its superior margin, approximately two finger breadths medial to the ischial spine. With the Miya hook in the left hand in a closed position, it is slid along the palmar surface of the right hand. The hook point should come to rest just beneath the previously positioned tip of the right middle finger. The handles are then opened and lowered to a near horizontal position. This points the hook into the C-SSL at about a 45-degree angle. If a high perineum prevents lowering the handle, then an episiotomy should be performed. With the tip of the middle finger, the hook point is placed two finger breadths medial to the ischial spine, approximately 0.5 cm below the superior edge. With experience, the hook point can actually be passed above the superior edge. With the middle and index fingers, apply firm pressure downward just behind the hook hump so the hook point penetrates the C-SSL (see Fig. 18-6, *B*). Downward pressure with two fingers on the top, plus traction with the back of the thumb on the back handle, produces enough force to penetrate the ligament. Close and elevate the handles of the Miya hook, and with the index and middle fingers, push the tissue from the hook point so as to make the suture clearly visible. If too much tissue is in the hook, simply back the hook out a little and take a smaller bite. An assistant should hold the elevated handles in a closed position. A long retractor is then placed to mobilize the rectum medially and a notched speculum is inserted by palpation underneath the hook point. A nerve hook is then used to retrieve the suture (see Fig. 18-6, *B, inset*).

9. Now the surgeon is ready to bring the stitches

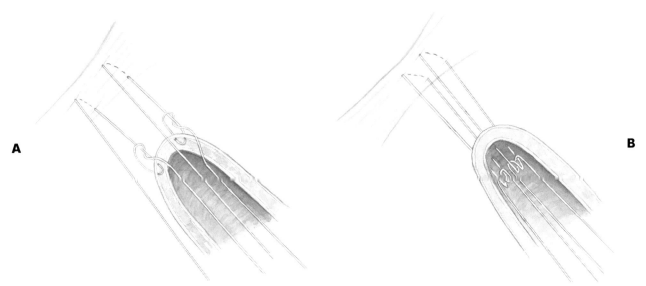

Fig. 18-9 Technique of fixing vaginal apex to C-SSL. **A,** "Pulley" stitch. Permanent sutures should be used. **B,** Stitches are placed through the vaginal epithelium and tied in the vaginal lumen. Delayed absorbable sutures should be used.

out to the apex of the vagina. Again, two methods have been popularized for this maneuver (Fig. 18-9, *A* and *B*). The first involves bringing the vaginal apex to the surface of the C-SSL with the use of a "pulley stitch." After the stitch has been placed in the ligament, one end of the suture is rethreaded on a free needle, sewn into the full thickness of the fibromuscular layer of the undersurface of the vaginal apex, and tied by a single half hitch, while the free end of the suture is held long (see Fig. 18-9, *A*). Traction of the free end of the suture pulls the vagina directly onto the muscle and ligament. A square knot will then fix it in place. With this type of fixation, a permanent suture should be used as the suture is not exposed through the epithelium of the vagina.

The second technique is used if the vaginal wall is thin, or if greater vaginal length is desired or, simply by surgeon's preference. This method inserts each end of the suture through the vaginal epithelium (see Fig. 18-9, *B*). When this method is used, a delayed absorbable suture should be used because the

knot remains in the vagina. We recommend a No. 2 delayed absorbable suture. After the sutures have been brought out through the vagina, the anterior and upper portion of the posterior vaginal walls are closed with interrupted or continuous 3-0 sutures. The vaginal vault suspension stitches are then tied, thus elevating the apex of the vagina to the C-SSL (Fig. 18-10). It is important that the vagina comes into contact with the coccygeus muscle and no suture bridge exists, especially if delayed absorbable sutures are being used. While tying these sutures, it may be useful to perform a rectal examination to detect any suture bridges.

10. After these sutures are tied, the posterior colpoperineorrhaphy is completed, as needed, and the vagina is packed with a moist gauze for 24 hours.

Results and Complications

The results of sacrospinous fixation are difficult to evaluate, as few studies report long-term follow-up. The largest published series to date is by Nichols who performed the operation on 163 patients and followed

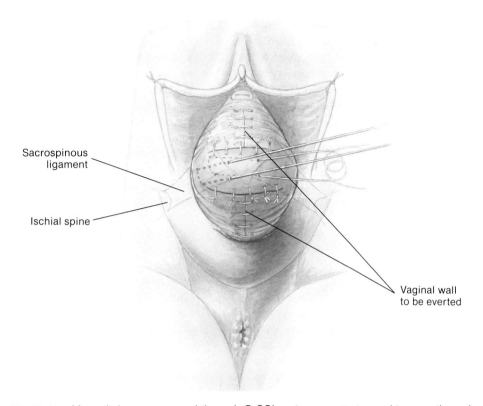

Fig. 18-10   After stitches are passed through C-SSL, a free needle is used to pass through entire thickness of the vaginal wall at the level of the vaginal apex. Tying of suture inverts vagina by fixing vaginal apex to C-SSL.

them for at least 2 years. He reports only a 3% incidence of recurrent vaginal eversion and did not specify whether other pelvic support defects recurred. More recently, Morley and DeLancey reported on 100 patients who underwent sacrospinous fixation with or without anterior and posterior vaginal wall repairs. Subjective 1-year follow-up was available on 71 patients; only three had recurrent vaginal vault prolapse. These authors did note, however, that 22 patients had recurrent or persistent mild to moderate anterior vaginal wall relaxation or symptomatic cystoceles.

Shull et al has reported on the results of 81 patients treated with sacrospinous ligament fixation, as well as other pelvic reconstructive surgery. The authors performed site-specific analysis of pelvic support defects preoperatively and at consecutive postoperative visits. The findings at 6 weeks postoperatively and at subsequent visits were noted for each of five sites:

urethra, bladder, vaginal cuff, cul-de-sac, and rectum. The most common site for recurrent prolapse was the anterior vaginal wall.

Miyazaki has reported on 74 cases of sacrospinous fixation using the Miya hook. Results with regard to treatment of the prolapse were not discussed; but the safety of the technique was documented as no patients had injuries to the bladder, rectum, nerves, or blood vessels and no blood transfusions were performed. Average blood loss was approximately 75 ml.

Although infrequently reported, serious intraoperative complications can occur with sacrospinous fixation. Potential complications of the procedure are:

1. **Hemorrhage.** Severe hemorrhage can occur from overzealous dissection superior to the coccygeus muscle or lateral to the ischial spine. This can result in hemorrhage from the inferior gluteal vessels, hypogastric venous plexus, or

internal pudendal vessels. Hemorrhage from these vessels can be difficult to control. For this reason, we prefer the technique described by Miyazaki in which the needle tip is passed into the safe ischiorectal space, compared to the technique using the Deschamps ligature carrier in which the needle tip is passed superiorly toward an abundant vasculature. If severe bleeding should occur in the area around the coccygeus muscle, we recommend initially packing the area. If this does not control the bleeding then visualization and attempted ligation with clips or sutures should be performed. This area is difficult to approach transabdominally, so bleeding should be controlled vaginally, if at all possible.

2. **Buttock pain.** It has been our experience that approximately 10% to 15% of patients experience moderate to severe buttock pain on the side that the sacrospinous suspension was performed. This is probably due to injury of a small nerve that runs through the C-SSL. This nerve injury is always self-limiting and should resolve completely by 6 weeks postoperatively. Reassurance and antiinflammatory agents usually are all that are necessary.

3. **Nerve injury.** Due to the close proximity of the sciatic nerve to the C-SSL, the potential for its injury is present. Although rarely reported, if this injury were to occur, reoperation with removal of suture material may be necessary.

4. **Rectal injury.** Rectal examinations should be performed frequently during this operation due to the close proximity of the rectum to the C-SSL. Rectal injury can occur during entering of the perirectal space as well as during mobilization of tissue off of the C-SSL. If a rectal injury is identified, it can usually be repaired primarily transvaginally by conventional techniques.

5. **Stress urinary incontinence.** This may occur after vaginal vault suspension procedures and is probably secondary to straightening of the vesicourethral junction coincident with restoration of vaginal length and depth. Stress incontinence should be tested for preoperatively by performing a stress test in the standing position with reduction of the vaginal prolapse. We believe that any patient with a poorly supported bladder neck who is undergoing a vaginal vault suspension should undergo concomitant bladder neck suspension.

6. **Vaginal stenosis.** Although this is not a common complication, it can be distressing to the patient who desires future coital function. Stenosis may occur if too much anterior and posterior vaginal wall tissue is trimmed or if too tight a posterior colporrhaphy is performed. We recommend postoperative use of estrogen vaginal cream in these patients in the hope of preventing or decreasing the incidence of this problem.

7. **Recurrent anterior vaginal wall prolapse.** As mentioned earlier, the pelvic support defect that recurs with the highest incidence is the anterior vaginal wall. We concur with others that approximately 20% of patients will return with a moderate anterior vaginal wall prolapse within a year after surgery.

LeFort Partial Colpocleisis

The LeFort partial colpocleisis reduces the uterovaginal prolapse and apposes the anterior and posterior vaginal walls. This operation should be used only as a last resort to cure prolapse because the procedure does not leave a functional vagina. It is useful because it can be performed quickly, has minimal risk of blood loss, and can be performed safely under regional or even local anesthesia. The procedure is commonly used in elderly patients of relatively poor surgical risk who otherwise would have no other treatment options except indefinite pessary use. The patient must understand that the procedure involves complete closure of the vagina and thus will terminate any potential for vaginal intercourse.

Other potential problems are associated with this procedure. A postoperative urinary stress incontinence rate has been reported as high as 30% in some studies. This high rate is probably due to the fusion of the anterior rectal wall to the base of the bladder, thus causing descent and flattening of the bladder neck and proximal urethra. Simultaneous bladder neck plication or needle urethropexy should be performed with the LeFort procedure if stress incontinence or the potential for postoperative stress incontinence exists.

Because the uterus is not removed, any bleeding that the patient has in the future will be difficult to evaluate because the vaginal canal is obstructed. An endometrial biopsy or dilation and curettage and Pap smear with cervical biopsies, if necessary, should always be performed preoperatively to assure that no cervical or endometrial pathology is present.

The LeFort procedure is as follows:

1. Traction is placed on the cervix to evert the vagina completely. A 0.5% lidocaine in 1:200,000 epinephrine solution is used to inject the vaginal tissue below the epithelium. A pudendal nerve block can be used if the procedure is to be performed under local anesthesia. A Foley catheter with a 30 ml balloon is placed for easy identification of the bladder neck.
2. A dilation and curettage should be performed, if it was not performed preoperatively.
3. The areas to be denuded anteriorly and posteriorly are marked out with a scalpel as indicated in Fig. 18-11, *A* and *B*. The rectangular piece of anterior vaginal wall should extend from 2 cm away from the tip of the cervix to approx-

imately 5 cm from the external urethral meatus.

4. Sharp and blunt dissection is used to remove the vaginal epithelium. These flaps should be thin, leaving a maximum amount of underlying fascia on the bladder and rectum. Sufficient vagina should be left bilaterally to form canals for draining cervical secretions or blood. Posteriorly, the cul-de-sac peritoneum may be encountered when vaginal mucosa is excised, but it should not be entered, if possible. Bleeding is controlled with fulguration. Absolute hemostasis is necessary to avoid a postoperative hematoma in the vaginal canal.
5. The cut edge of the anterior vaginal wall is sewn to the cut edge of the posterior vaginal wall with interrupted, delayed absorbable sutures. This is achieved in such a way that the knot is turned into, and remains in, the epithelium-lined tunnels that are created bilaterally. Suturing in this way will gradually push the uterus and vaginal apex inward (Fig. 18-11, *C*). When the entire vagina has been inverted, the superior and inferior margins of the rectangle can be sutured horizontally.
6. We almost routinely perform a plication of the bladder neck (see Fig. 18-11, *A*) during a LeFort

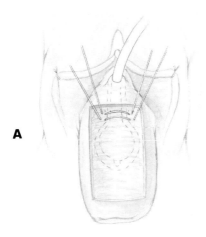

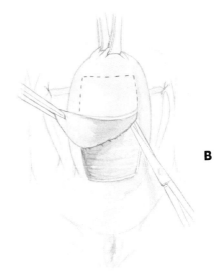

Fig. 18-11 Technique of LeFort partial colpocleisis. **A,** Anterior vaginal flap is removed and plication stitch is placed at the bladder neck. **B,** Posterior vaginal wall is removed.

Continued.

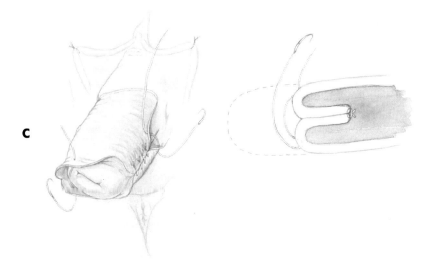

Fig. 18-11, cont'd. **C,** Cut edge of anterior vaginal wall is sewn to cut edge of posterior vaginal wall in such a way that the uterus and vagina are inverted.

LeFort operation and drain the bladder with a suprapubic catheter. A perineorrhaphy is usually performed to increase posterior pelvic muscle support and to narrow the introitus.

7. Postoperatively, the patient is mobilized early. Heavy lifting should be avoided for at least 2 months to avoid recurrence of the prolapse secondary to breakdown of repair. Voiding trials are begun several days postoperatively.

Early complications include hematoma, infection, or nonhealing (with acute herniation) of the prolapse. Urinary urgency, retention, and infection can also occur, especially if a urethral plication is completed. Since most patients are elderly and may be debilitated the risk of thromboembolic complications is significant. Pressure stockings and early ambulation should be used.

Late postoperative complications and results of a modified LeFort operation as reported by Goldman et al are shown in Table 18-2. In this report, anterior colporrhaphy or other urethropexies were not performed; this may explain the 10.2% rate of postoperative urinary incontinence. In general, total relief of uterine prolapse symptoms with good anatomic results can be expected in over 90% of patients. Complete breakdown with recurrent prolapse occurs in about 2% to 5% of patients.

TABLE 18-2 Late postoperative complications and results of modified LeFort operation

Outcome and complications	No. of patients
Good anatomic results	107 (90.7%)
Relief of symptoms	101 (85.6%)
Recurrence of prolapse complete breakdown (1 patient) partial recurrence (2 patients)	3 (2.5%)
Urinary tract symptoms, incontinence (minor degrees or worsened by operation)	12 (10.2%)
Occurrence of late vaginal bleeding	2 (1.8%)

From Goldman J, Ovadia J, Feldberg D: *Eur J Obstet Gynecol Reprod Biol* 12:31, 1985.

Colpectomy

Another operation that can be used for severe post-hysterectomy vaginal vault prolapse is colpectomy. This operation is performed in cases of vault prolapse in which operating time is kept at a minimum, and future vaginal intercourse is not anticipated by the patient. It can be performed under regional or local anesthesia.

The operation is performed by completely excising

the vaginal mucosa from the underlying vaginal or endopelvic fascia. Any coexistent enterocele should be identified and excised using the technique described earlier. A series of purse-string, delayed absorbable sutures is placed, slowly inverting the vaginal fascia and remaining cul-de-sac. A posterior colporrhaphy with high levator plication is usually performed, followed by vaginal closure. As with the LeFort procedure, anterior colporrhaphy and perineorrhaphy are often performed with a colpectomy.

ABDOMINAL SACRAL COLPOPEXY

Suspension of the vagina to the sacral promontory via the abdominal approach is an effective treatment for uterovaginal prolapse and vaginal eversion, and offers several advantages over vaginal surgical approaches. It is the procedure of choice for those patients that have other indications for abdominal surgery, such as ovarian masses. The laparotomy incision offers the advantage of performing a simultaneous retropubic suspension of the anterior vaginal wall and bladder neck, if necessary. For patients with genuine stress incontinence, the Burch procedure is the procedure of choice for many urogynecologists. A step-by-step comparison of the authors' recommendations for surgically correcting uterovaginal prolapse by vaginal and abdominal routes is shown in Table 18-3.

Many different materials, both autologous and synthetic, have been used for the graft in the sacral colpopexy. Natural materials that have been used include fascia lata, rectus fascia, and dura mater. Synthetic materials include polypropylene mesh, polyester fiber mesh, polytetrafluoroethylene mesh, Dacron mesh, and Silastic silicone rubber. No studies have compared the efficacy of the various graft materials and individual reports of long-term rates of cure are consistently good. Therefore, we believe that, as with the sling procedure, no important differences exist between the materials regarding efficacy and safety.

As was noted earlier, the normal vaginal axis directs toward sacral segments S3 and S4 in the nulliparous woman. Although some authors have advocated connecting the graft material at this level, Sutton et al encountered life-threatening hemorrhage from presacral vessels at this low level on the sacrum. As

TABLE 18-3 Surgical management of complete eversion of the vagina: abdominal and vaginal approaches (authors' recommendations)

Abdominal	Vaginal
1. Perform abdominal hysterectomy, close vaginal apex	1. Perform vaginal hysterectomy
2. Place graft on vaginal apex and posterior vaginal wall	2. Perform anterior colporrhaphy and/or needle urethropexy
3. Obliterate cul-de-sac	3. Repair enterocele vaginally
4. Fix graft to sacral promontory and reperitonize	4. Place sutures in sacrospinous ligament and suture to vagina (don't tie)
5. Perform retropubic urethropexy or paravaginal repair, if indicated	5. Perform posterior colporrhaphy, if rectocele present
6. Perform posterior colporrhaphy, if rectocele present	6. Close upper portion of posterior vaginal wall
	7. Tie sacrospinous ligament sutures
	8. Tie needle urethropexy sutures, if placed

these authors suggest, we recommend fixing the graft to the upper one third of the sacrum, near the sacral promontory, thus improving safety without sacrificing outcome or future vaginal function.

The technique of abdominal sacral colpopexy using graft placement is described as follows (Fig. 18-12):

1. The patient should be placed in Allen stirrups or in frogleg position so that the surgeon has digital access to the vagina during the operation. A sponge stick can be placed in the vagina for manipulation of the apex, if desired. A Foley catheter is placed into the bladder for drainage. Prophylactic perioperative antibiotics are generally used during this procedure.

2. A laparotomy is performed through a low transverse or midline incision. Small bowel is packed into the upper abdomen and the sigmoid colon is packed into the left pelvis as much as possible. The ureters are identified bilaterally for their entire course into the blad-

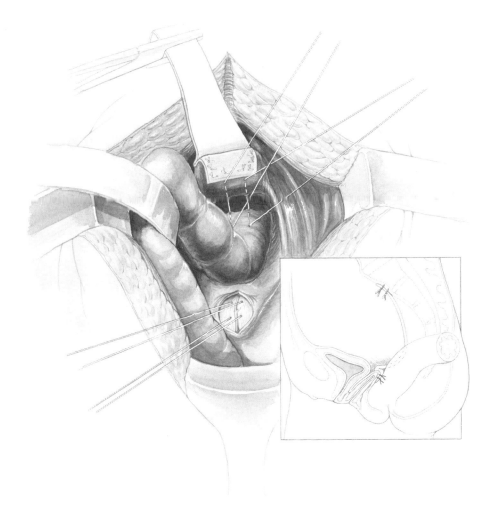

Fig. 18-12 Abdominal sacral colpopexy. Note Halban technique is used to obliterate cul-de-sac below graft. *Inset,* Graft connects vagina to sacrum and lies without tension in the deep pelvis.

der. If the uterus is present, a hysterectomy should be performed and the vaginal cuff closed. The depth of the cul-de-sac and the length of the vagina when completely elevated are estimated.

3. While the vagina is elevated cephalad using the sponge stick, the peritoneum over the vaginal apex is incised transversely and the bladder dissected from the anterior vaginal wall (this may have already been done if the uterus was removed). The peritoneum over the posterior vaginal wall into the cul-de-sac is incised

longitudinally and dissected for several centimeters bilaterally. The vaginal apex is elevated bilaterally with clamps or guide sutures.

4. Three to five pairs of nonabsorbable, No. 0 sutures are placed in the posterior vaginal wall, transversely, 1 to 2 cm apart. Sutures are placed through the full fibromuscular thickness of the vagina, but not into the vaginal epithelium. The vaginal pack is removed to assure that no sutures have perforated the pack. Sutures are then fed through the graft in pairs and tied. The graft should extend approxi-

mately half way down the length of the posterior vaginal wall.

5. A Moschcowitz or Halban procedure is then performed to obliterate the cul-de-sac. These procedures were described under the section of surgical treatment of enterocele.

6. A longitudinal incision, approximately 6 cm long, is made in the peritoneum over the sacral promontory. At this point the surgeon should carefully palpate the aortic bifurcation, common and internal iliac vessels, sigmoid colon, and right ureter so that these structures can be avoided during the procedure. The left common iliac vein is medial to the left common iliac artery and is particularly vulnerable to damage during this procedure. The middle sacral artery and vein should be identified and, at times, may need to be ligated to perform the graft placement.

7. Blunt and sharp dissection caudally may be used to create a subperitoneal tunnel into the full depth of the cul-de-sac so that the graft can be extraperitonized. The graft can then be tunneled retroperitoneally, or placed above the previous Halban or Moschcowitz cul-de-sac closure.

8. The bony sacral promontory and anterior longitudinal ligaments are directly visualized for approximately 4 cm using blunt and sharp dissection through the subperitoneal fat. Special care should be taken to avoid the delicate plexus of presacral veins that is frequently present, especially as one dissects more caudally.

9. Using a stiff but small half-curved tapered needle with permanent, No. 0 suture, two to four pairs of sutures are placed through the anterior sacral longitudinal ligament, over the sacral promontory. The graft should be trimmed to the appropriate length and passed, if desired, through the subperitoneal tunnel. The sutures are then fed through the graft in pairs and tied. The appropriate amount of vaginal elevation should provide gentle tension without undue traction on the vagina.

10. The peritoneum over the presacral space is closed with a running, absorbable suture. The bladder flap peritoneum is also closed transversely over the graft.

11. When appropriate, retropubic urethropexy or paravaginal repair should be accomplished at this time, followed by placement of a suprapubic catheter, if desired, and closure of the abdomen.

12. Posterior colporrhaphy and perineoplasty are generally performed to treat the remaining rectocele and perineal defect.

If attention has been paid to repairing all the support defects of the vagina at the time of sacral colpopexy, then recurrences of vaginal vault prolapse are quite uncommon. Addison et al (1989) reported three cases of recurrent vaginal prolapse after the sacral colpopexy with Mersiline mesh. In two patients, the mesh separated from the vaginal apex. In the remaining patient, the posterior vaginal wall ruptured distal to the attachment of the mesh to the vagina. These authors and others believe that failures of this procedure can be minimized by suturing the suspensory mesh to the posterior vagina and vaginal apex over as extended an area as possible. This is the justification for suturing the graft to the posterior vagina with four to six pairs of permanent sutures.

Intraoperative complications are uncommon but can be life-threatening. When there is bleeding from presacral vessels, hemostasis can be difficult to achieve because of the complex interlacing of the venous network, both beneath and on the surface of the sacral periosteum. When these veins have been damaged, they can retract beneath the bony surface of the anterior sacrum and recede into the underlying channels of cancellous bone. Communications with adjacent pelvic veins, especially the left common iliac vein, can be particularly troublesome. Packing of the presacral space may control bleeding temporarily, but often recurs when the pack is removed, and may further lacerate delicate veins. Sutures, metalic chips, cautery, and bone wax should be used initially. If these measures are not successful, sterilized stainless steel thumb tacks can be placed on the retracted bleeding presacral vein to treat life-threatening hemorrhage that has not responded to other measures.

Other complications that have been reported after

abdominal sacral colpopexy tend to be similar to procedures that require laparotomy, retropubic surgery, and extensive pelvic dissection. The complications include enterotomy, ureteral damage, cystotomy, proctotomy, extrafascial wound infections, and persistent granulation tissue in the vaginal vault. Remarkably, graft rejections are exceedingly rare. Lansman reported a small bowel obstruction after colpopexy that was due to a loop of ileum adherent to a hole in the posterior peritoneum, near the side wall of the pelvis. This problem underscores the importance of reperitonization over the hollow of the sacrum to avoid the potential for small bowel getting trapped in the cul-de-sac or behind the graft.

NONSURGICAL TREATMENT OF UTEROPELVIC AND VAGINAL PROLAPSE

Patients who do not desire surgical repair of vaginal prolapse, or who are not surgical candidates because of medical problems, have few treatment options, vaginal pessary being the main alternative. Successful pessary use can allow the patient to eliminate the morbidity associated with severe pelvic organ prolapse without undergoing the cost and risk of surgical repair. Vaginal pessary can be used as a permanent treatment of pelvic relaxation or as a temporary treatment while the patient is awaiting surgery. As has been mentioned in Chapter 17, the vaginal pessary can be used in the diagnostic evaluation of women with uterovaginal prolapse to determine if they have incompetent urethral sphincteric function after the vagina has been reduced. Finally, the pessary has been used successfully in several studies to treat genuine stress incontinence.

Many styles of pessaries are available in the United States. Smith, Hodge, and Risser pessaries are designed to be used in cases of uterine retroversion and small cystocele. The Smith pessary has a rounded top and is designed for use in women with a well-defined pubic notch. The Hodge pessary has a squared anterior surface, which prevents pressure on the urethra, yet aids pessary retention.

The ring, donut, inflatable ball, cube, and Gellhorn pessaries are useful in cases of uterine prolapse. The ring and donut pessaries are designed for patients with uterine prolapse associated with cystocele. The Gell-

horn pessary is supplied in a rigid, acrylic form and a flexible form; it is indicated for treatment of severe uterovaginal prolapse. The cube pessary is generally considered a pessary of last resort, i.e., when there is markedly decreased vaginal tone or an extremely relaxed perineal body.

The Gehrung pessary is an archlike pessary designed to raise the bladder floor in cases of large cystocele. It is also designed to thin out a rectocele and support apical prolapse.

After the pessary has been properly fitted, the patient should be reexamined in 1 week to ensure that no vaginal skin erosion has developed. The physician can also examine for fit and satisfaction of the patient and determine if any urinary symptoms developed. Vaginal estrogen therapy is usually given several times a week to ensure an estrogenized vaginal epithelium. If no contraindications exist, oral estrogen replacement therapy also should be considered.

The patient can be taught to remove the pessary periodically for cleaning and to allow for sexual intercourse. If the patient is unable to remove the pessary, she should be seen at 2- to 3-month intervals for vaginal examination, changing, and cleaning of the pessary.

The main complications to pessary use are vaginal skin erosion and vaginal infections. These problems can generally be managed easily by removing the pessary until the abrasions heal. Vaginal infections respond well to douching or to a course of antibiotic therapy. If patients with pessaries are not seen at regular intervals, or if the pessary is forgotten by the patient, pessary impaction or chronic vaginal infection can occur leading to more severe ulceration and ultimately damage to the bladder or rectum.

SUMMARY

The prevalence of enterocele and vaginal prolapse appears to be increasing, undoubtedly due to the increased longevity of women, but also as a result of inadequate recognition and repair of pelvic organ support defects when pelvic surgery has previously been performed. A heightened awareness of this problem and careful attention at pelvic examination should improve the recognition of enterocele. The standard use of cul-de-sac plication at every hysterectomy and ure-thropexy would probably decrease the likelihood of iatrogenic enterocele. Finally, improved education of the principles of pelvic and vaginal reconstructive surgery is needed to improve care to all affected women.

REFERENCES

Enterocele

Dicke J: Small bowel obstruction secondary to a prior Moschcowitz procedure, *Am J Obstet Gynecol* 152:887, 1985.

Given FT: "Posterior culdeplasty": revisited, *Am J Obstet Gynecol* 153:135, 1985.

Kuhn RJ, Hollyock VE: Observations on the anatomy of the rec-tovaginal pouch and septum, *Obstet Gynecol* 59:445, 1982.

McCall ML: Posterior culdeplasty, *Obstet Gynecol* 10:595, 1957.

Milley PS, Nichols DH: A correlative investigation of the human rectovaginal septum, *Anat Rec* 163:443, 1968.

Moschcowitz AV: The pathogenesis, anatomy, and cure of prolapse of the rectum, *Surg Gynecol Obstet* 15:7, 1912.

Nichols DH, Randall CL: *Vaginal surgery,* ed 3, Baltimore, 1989, Williams & Wilkins.

Stanhope CR, Wilson TO, Utz WJ, et al: Suture entrapment and secondary ureteral obstruction, *Am J Obstet Gynecol* 164:1513, 1991.

Symmonds RE, Williams TJ, Lee RA, et al: Posthysterectomy enterocele and vaginal vault prolapse, *Am J Obstet Gynecol* 140:852, 1981.

Thompson JD, Rock JA, editors: *TeLinde's operative gynecology,* ed 7, Philadelphia, 1992, JB Lippincott.

Torpin R: Excision of the cul-de-sac of Douglas for the surgical care of hernias through the female caudal wall, including prolapse of the uterus, *J Int Coll Surg* 24:322, 1955.

Waters EG: Vaginal prolapse: technique for correction and prevention at hysterectomy, *Obstet Gynecol* 8:432, 1956.

Zacharin RF: Pulsion enterocele: review of functional anatomy of the pelvic floor, *Obstet Gynecol* 55:135, 1980.

Zacharin RF: *Pelvic floor anatomy and the surgery of pulsion enterocele,* New York, 1985, Springer-Verlag/Wein.

Vaginal Vault Prolapse

Addison WA, Livengood CH, Sutton GP, et al: Abdominal sacral colpopexy with Mersilene mesh in the retroperitoneal position in the management of posthysterectomy vaginal vault prolapse and enterocele, *Am J Obstet Gynecol* 153:140, 1985.

Addison WA, Timmons CM, Wall LL, et al: Failed abdominal sacral colpopexy: observations and recommendations, *Obstet Gynecol* 74:480, 1989.

Addison WA, Livengood CH, Parker RT: Posthysterectomy vaginal vault prolapse with emphasis on management by transabdominal sacral colpopexy, *Postgrad Obstet Gynecol* 8:1, 1988.

Baker KR, Beresford JM, Campbell C: Colposacropexy with Pro-lene® mesh, *Surg Gynecol Obstet* 171:51, 1990.

DeLancey JO: Anatomic aspects of vaginal eversion after hyster-ectomy, *Am J Obstet Gynecol* 166:1717, 1992.

Funt MI, Thompson JD, Birch H: Normal vaginal axis, *South Med J* 71:1534, 1978.

Given FT: "Posterior culdeplasty": revisited, *Am J Obstet Gynecol* 153:135, 1985.

Goldman J, Ovadia J, Feldberg D: The Neugebauer-LeFort operation: a review of 118 partial colpocleises, *Eur J Obstet Gynecol Reprod Biol* 12:31, 1985.

Harris TA, Bent AE: Genital prolapse with and without urinary incontinence, *J Reprod Med* 35:792, 1990.

Keetel LM, Hebertson RM: An anatomic evaluation of the sacro-spinous ligament colpopexy, *Surg Gynecol Obstet* 168:318, 1989.

Langmade CF, Oliver JA: Partial colpocleisis, *Am J Obstet Gynecol* 154:1200, 1986.

Lansman HH: Posthysterectomy vault prolapse: sacral colpopexy with dura mater graft, *Obstet Gynecol* 63:577, 1984.

Mäkinen J, Kähäri V, Söderström K, et al: Collagen synthesis in the vaginal connective tissue of patients with and without uterine prolapse, *Eur J Obstet Gynecol Reprod Biol* 24:319, 1987.

Mäkinen J, Söderström K, Kiilholma P, et al: Histologic changes in the vaginal connective tissue of patients with and without uterine prolapse, *Arch Gynecol* 239:17, 1986.

Miyazaki FS: Miya hook ligature carrier for sacrospinous ligament suspension, *Obstet Gynecol* 70:286, 1987.

Morley G, DeLancey JO: Sacrospinous ligament fixation for eversion of the vagina, *Am J Obstet Gynecol* 158:872, 1988.

Nagata I, Kato K: Sacrospinous ligament fixation of vaginal apex for repair operation of uterine prolapse—operative procedure and postoperative outcome evaluated with score system and x-ray subtraction colpography, *Acta Obstet Gynaecol Jpn* 38:29, 1986.

Nichols DH: Sacrospinous fixation for massive eversion of the vagina, *Am J Obstet Gynecol* 142:901, 1982.

Nichols DH: Fertility retention in the patient with genital prolapse, *Am J Obstet Gynecol* 164:1155, 1991.

Richter K, Albrich W: Long-term results following fixation of the vagina on the sacrospinal ligament by the vaginal route, *Am J Obstet Gynecol* 151:811, 1981.

Ridley JG: Evaluation of the colpocleisis: a report of fifty-eight cases, *Am J Obstet Gynecol* 113:1114, 1972.

Shull BL, Capen CV, Riggs MW, et al: Preoperative analysis of site-specific pelvic support defects in 81 women treated with sacrospinous ligament suspension and pelvic reconstruction, *Am J Obstet Gynecol* 166:1764, 1992.

Snyder TE, Krantz KE: Abdominal-retroperitoneal sacral colpo-pexy for the correction of vaginal prolapse, *Obstet Gynecol* 77:944, 1991.

Sutton GP, Addison WA, Livengood CH, et al: Life-threatening hemorrhage complicating sacral colpopexy, *Am J Obstet Gynecol* 140:836, 1981.

Tancer ML, Fleischer M, Berkowitz BJ: Simultaneous colpo-recto-sacropexy, *Obstet Gynecol* 70:951, 1987.

TeLinde RW: Prolapse of the uterus and allied conditions, *Am J Obstet Gynecol* 94:444, 1966.

Timmons MC, Addison WA, Addison SB, et al: Abdominal sacral colpopexy in 163 women with posthysterectomy vaginal vault prolapse and enterocele, *J Reprod Med* 37:323, 1992.

Timmons MC, Kohler MF, Addison WA: Thumbtack use for control of presacral bleeding, with description of an instrument for thumbtack application, *Obstet Gynecol* 78:313, 1991.

Ulmsten U, Ekman G, Giertz G, et al: Different biochemical composition of connective tissue in continent and stress incontinent women, *Acta Obstet Gynecol Scand* 66:455, 1987.

Zeitlin MP, Lebherz TB: Pessaries in the geriatric patient, *J Am Geriatr Soc* 40:635, 1992.

PART FOUR

Specific Conditions

CHAPTER 19

Detrusor Instability and Hyperreflexia

Mickey M. Karram

Prevalence and Incidence
Etiology
  Idiopathic detrusor instability
  Neurologic disease
  Bladder outlet obstruction
  Psychosomatic
  Urine in the proximal urethra
  Inflammation
  Instability following pelvic surgery
  Orgasm
  Detrusor hyperactivity with impaired contractility
Clinical Features
Physical Examination
Investigation
  Urinalysis and culture
  Voided volume chart
  Urodynamic tests
Management
  Nonsurgical management
  Surgical treatment
Mixed Incontinence

The unstable bladder is one that contracts involuntarily or that can be made to contract involuntarily. Urinary incontinence secondary to this condition occurs in many patients without any other recognizable abnormalities. Bladder instability represents the sec-ond most common cause of incontinence in women after genuine stress incontinence.

Bladder instability was described initially by Hodg-kinson et al in 1963 when they observed this condition in approximately 8% of their patients with urinary incontinence. Over the years, many terms have been used to describe involuntary detrusor contractions: *unstable bladder, detrusor instability, motor urge incontinence, spastic bladder, hyperreflexic bladder, detrusor dyssynergia, hypertonic bladder, automatic bladder, systolic bladder* and *uninhibited bladder.* Standardization of definitions and diagnostic criteria has allowed for more specific categorization and terminology. Currently two terms are accepted by the International Continence Society (ICS) for use in describing an overactive detrusor. The first, *unstable bladder* or *detrusor instability*, is a condition in which the bladder is objectively shown to contract, either spontaneously or with provocation, during the filling phase of a cystometrogram in a neurologically intact female while the patient is attempting to inhibit micturition. Unstable detrusor contractions may be asymptomatic or they may cause abnormal symptoms, most commonly urgency, frequency, and urge incontinence. The second term, *detrusor hyperreflexia*, is defined as detrusor overactivity due to disturbances of the nervous control mechanisms. This term should be used only when the bladder dysfunction can be explained by objective evidence of a relevant neurologic disorder. This chapter reviews the characteristics, clinical presentation, diagnosis, and management of detrusor instability and hyperreflexia in women.

PREVALENCE AND INCIDENCE

Recent epidemiologic data suggest that the prevalence of urinary incontinence is higher in the general population than has been previously appreciated. However, the true prevalence, incidence, and spontaneous regression rates of detrusor instability are still unknown because the condition cannot be diagnosed clinically. Many patients have involuntary detrusor contractions noted on cystometry, but are completely asymptomatic. Turner-Warwick reported that the lowest prevalence of instability is found in people between the ages of 10 and 30 with an overall prevalence in the general population of approximately 10%. He noted that, after the age of 30, the prevalence increases with age, partly due to cerebrovascular deterioration in older patients.

Currently, the best data available are by Diokno et al who performed cystometrograms on 169 randomly selected, community-dwelling women and found 7.9% to have detrusor instability. This represented 4.9% of continent women and 12.2% of incontinent women.

The prevalence is much higher in elderly hospitalized or nursing home patients. Ouslander et al found detrusor instability or hyperreflexia in 46% of 135 elderly incontinent women. A review by Abrams of urodynamic findings in 2124 women found detrusor instability in 38% of women over 65 years of age and in only 27% of those under 65 years.

The prevalence of detrusor instability in women who present for evaluation of incontinence ranges from 10% to 55%. Webster et al noted detrusor instability to be a contributing factor in incontinence in 73 of 133 (55%) women referred for evaluation. Forty-five percent of patients with prior failed surgery for stress incontinence were noted to have detrusor instability. Walters and Shields found detrusor overactivity in 31% of incontinent women referred for urodynamic testing. Twenty-two percent had isolated detrusor instability, 14% had mixed detrusor instability and stress incontinence, and 2% had detrusor hyperreflexia.

ETIOLOGY

The two factors known to produce involuntary contraction of the detrusor muscle are outflow obstruction and neurologic dysfunction. A great deal of speculation has focused on the cause of detrusor instability in nonobstructed, neurologically intact patients. A variety of diverse factors have been implicated (see accompanying box) and are discussed in the following sections.

Idiopathic Detrusor Instability

With our current diagnostic capabilities, greater than 90% of women with this condition appear to have no other recognizable pathology. Kinder and Mundy studied detrusor muscle strips in vitro from patients with detrusor instability and from normal, continent subjects. The unstable muscle strips showed an increased response to direct electrical stimulation and an increase in sensitivity to stimulation with acetylcholine. In vivo, this response would correspond to a higher sensitivity of efferent neurologic activity or to a lower level of acetylcholine release necessary to initiate a detrusor contraction. It is not clear, however, whether this supersensitivity of the detrusor smooth muscle cell membrane is due to a relative cholinergic denervation or to reduced inhibitory or modulatory neurologic activity, possibly mediated by vasoactive intestinal polypeptide (VIP). VIP is a 28-amino acid neuropeptide with powerful relaxant effects on smooth muscle. It is abundant in normal human bladders and

---

Conditions Possibly Associated With the Development of Detrusor Instability and Detrusor Hyperreflexia

Idiopathic
Neurologic disease
Bladder outlet obstruction
    Pelvic organ prolapse
    Posturethropexy
Psychosomatic disease
Urine in proximal urethra
Inflammation
Previous pelvic surgery
Orgasm
Detrusor hyperreflexia with impaired contractility

markedly decreased in the bladders of patients with detrusor instability. It has been hypothesized that deficiency of this substance or a similar neuroregulatory peptide is the key to development of unstable bladder activity.

Neurologic Disease

Detrusor hyperreflexia is associated with neurologic lesions of the suprasacral cord and higher centers. These lesions block the sacral reflex arc from the cerebral cortex and other higher centers that are crucial to both voluntary and involuntary inhibition of the bladder. In this group of patients, involuntary detrusor contractions usually are associated with appropriate relaxation of the urethral sphincter, as there is preservation of long tracts from the pontine region. Neurologic conditions resulting in detrusor hyperreflexia include multiple sclerosis, dementia, cerebrovascular disorders, and Parkinson's disease.

Multiple Sclerosis

Multiple sclerosis (MS) is a disease of unknown etiology characterized by varying neurologic signs and symptoms; it usually affects patients between 20 and 40 years of age. Demyelinating plaques in the white matter of the cerebral cortex, cerebellum, brain stem, spinal cord, and optic nerve may produce varied neurologic dysfunction and symptoms. MS is characterized by evidence of multiple lesions and usually a progressive course of bladder dysfunction. Plaques in the frontal lobe or in the lateral columns usually produce lower urinary tract dysfunction.

The incidence of bladder dysfunction as an initial symptom is 5%; however up to 90% of patients with MS show evidence of bladder dysfunction during the course of their disease. Approximately 60% of patients with lower urinary tract dysfunction show detrusor hyperreflexia on cystometry. Up to half of these patients demonstrate detrusor sphincter dyssynergia, and the others demonstrate adequate and appropriate sphincter relaxation. Approximately 30% of patients will be noted to have an underactive or areflexic detrusor. Table 19-1 summarizes the urodynamic findings in patients with MS.

Cerebrovascular Disease

Cerebrovascular disease affects 300,000 people per year in the United States. The disease is associated

TABLE 19-1 Summary of urodynamic findings in patients with MS

Authors	Patients (No.)	Hyperreflexia detrusor (%)	Underactive or areflexic detrusor (%)	Detrusor-sphincter dyssynergia (%)
Andersen and Bradley	51	63	33	30
Ketelaer et al	100	49		86
Bradley	301	62	34	72
Schoenberg et al	39	74		50
Blaivas et al	41	56	40	27
Piazza and Diokno	27	85	13	50
Beck et al	46	87		
Philp et al	52	99	0	88
Goldstein et al	84	76		50
Van Poppel et al	160	66	24	33
Awad et al	39	67		51
Peterson and Pederson	88	82	16	41
Hassouna et al	70	70	18	75
Gonor et al	64	78	20	12

From Fowler CJ, Betts CD, Fowler CG: Bladder dysfunction in neurologic disease. In Asbury AK, McKhann GM, McDonald WI, (eds): *Diseases of the nervous system clinical neurobiology*, vol 1, Philadelphia, 1992, WB Saunders.

with varying degrees of chronic disability, including bladder dysfunction. Atherosclerosis, arteritis, intracranial hemorrhage, and arterial malformations may be etiologic factors. Infarction of discrete areas of the frontal lobe, internal capsule, brain stem, or cerebellum can result in bladder dysfunction. During the initial phase of a cerebrovascular accident, urinary retention secondary to detrusor areflexia is common. During recovery, detrusor hyperreflexia with an appropriate sphincteric response usually occurs. Very rarely detrusor-sphincter dyssynergia results.

Parkinson's Disease

Parkinson's disease occurs in 100 to 150 per 100,000 persons. Onset usually occurs after the age of 50, and the course of the disease is progressive. The incidence of bladder dysfunction ranges from 40% to 70%. Parkinson's disease is associated with loss of pigmented neurons in the substantia nigra and locus ceruleus. In addition, there is loss of the neurotransmitter dopamine in the caudate nucleus, putamen, and globus pallidus. The etiology of these changes is unknown. Bladder dysfunction occurs in 40% to 70%, although it is rarely an initial manifestation. Cystometry, when abnormal, shows detrusor hyperreflexia. Obstructive symptoms occasionally can result from therapy with antiparkinsonian agents.

Dementia

Dementia is a diffuse deterioration in intellectual function manifested primarily by memory deficits and secondarily by changes in conduct. The etiologies of dementia include aging, severe head injury, encephalitis, presenile dementias (including Alzheimer's disease, Pick's disease, Jakob-Creutzfeldt disease), hydrocephalus, and syphilis. The mechanism of bladder dysfunction can be direct involvement of the cerebrocortical areas concerned with bladder control. It is sometimes also related to inattention to personal hygiene. Cystometric findings show detrusor hyperreflexia or areflexia, depending on the etiology and severity of the dementia.

Neoplasia

Brain tumors in the superior medial frontal lobe can result in bladder dysfunction. Cystometry generally shows some degree of detrusor hyperreflexia, as well as irritative voiding symptoms. Spinal cord tumors above the level of the conus medullaris and cervical spondylosis also can produce detrusor hyperreflexia.

Bladder Outlet Obstruction

Bladder outlet obstruction is found infrequently in women. When abnormal voiding patterns occur, they are usually due to poor detrusor function rather than to physical obstruction. However, obstructive voiding may contribute to detrusor instability that sometimes occurs with severe uterovaginal prolapse and after urethropexy procedures.

Although not directly relevant to the gynecologist, this condition often occurs in men with bladder outflow obstruction. Relief of the obstruction, whether due to bladder neck dysfunction, prostatic enlargement, or distal urethral stricture, usually leads to relief of the instability.

Psychosomatic

Frewen contends that once structural, organic, and infective causes have been excluded, 80% of idiopathic detrusor instability is psychosomatic. His report emphasizes the taking of a searching history, which often leads to a readily definable psychosomatic etiology. Although patients with detrusor instability probably have a higher incidence of psychologic abnormalities, whether these abnormalities are the cause or the result of detrusor instability is unclear.

Urine in the Proximal Urethra

After the study by Barrington in 1931, it was suggested that urgency results from the presence of urine in the proximal urethra. This theory has been the subject of considerable controversy as some studies have reported objective data to support it, while others have found urine in the proximal urethra to be a nonspecific finding. Sutherst and Brown studied 50 women by measuring urethral and detrusor pressures during and after injection of fluid into the urethra at various bladder capacities. None of the cases demonstrated any change in detrusor activity, even in patients who were objectively shown to have bladder instability on previous cystometry. Beck et al (1976), on the other hand, reported a series of surgical cures in patients who had been shown to have detrusor instability and evidence of bladder neck funneling on radiographic studies. They postulated that the funneling of urine into the proximal urethra caused detrusor instability and that the majority of symptoms resolved by correction of this funneling with anterior colporrhaphy. Clearly, more data are needed to resolve this issue.

Inflammation

Inflammation of the bladder mucosa, with or without associated bacteriuria, has been suggested as a cause of bladder instability. Bhatia and Bergman performed urodynamic studies on women with acute urinary tract infections before treatment. Half of those with urodynamic evidence of detrusor instability had stable cystometrograms after the infection was treated.

Contrary to this, Bates et al reported on more than 2000 patients examined by video-cystography on whom culture and sensitivity studies of mid-stream urine specimens were performed. They found that of 35 patients infected at the time of the study, only three had non-neuropathic detrusor instability.

Instability After Pelvic Surgery

The correlation between detrusor instability and pelvic surgery is confusing and at times unexplainable. Studies on patients operated on for stress incontinence who had stable cystometrograms preoperatively note that 7% to 27% will develop detrusor instability postoperatively. Postoperative detrusor instability is more common in patients with previous bladder neck surgery and in those with coexistent detrusor instability and sphincteric incompetence preoperatively.

Radical pelvic surgery, hysterectomy, and pelvic prolapse surgery can at times result in an unstable bladder. Partial denervation of the bladder during the operative process with subsequent development of detrusor dysfunction is currently the most accepted theory.

Orgasm

Orgasm may be an etiologic factor in detrusor instability. The exact pathogenesis is unknown, but patients sometimes experience urgency or urge incontinence associated with a gush of urine during climax. Treatment is the same as with idiopathic detrusor insta-

bility; sexual counseling and education frequently are helpful.

Detrusor Hyperactivity With Impaired Contractility

Resnick and Yalla noted that there exists a subgroup of women with detrusor instability resulting in incontinence, but these patients cannot effectively empty their bladders when attempting to void. Detailed urodynamic testing revealed that impaired contractility caused impaired emptying and may represent the last stage of detrusor instability, in which there is a deterioration of detrusor function.

CLINICAL FEATURES

The fundamental feature of an unstable bladder is that it contracts involuntarily. This contraction causes the sensation of impending voiding or urgency. If urgency regularly occurs before the bladder is full, frequency results. If frequency occurs at night, nocturia occurs. If the patient is unable to resist the involuntary contraction, urge incontinence results. Thus the typical clinical presentation involves urgency, frequency, nocturia, and urge incontinence, with urgency being the cardinal symptom.

Frequency is related to fluid intake and should always be verified with a voided volume diary. Nocturia is a symptom only if the desire to void wakes the patient from sleep. Patients who awake for other reasons and decide to urinate are not categorized as having nocturia.

These symptoms are not exclusive to bladder instability. According to Bates et al, motor urgency is the occurrence of these symptoms in the presence of uninhibited detrusor contraction. Sensory urgency is the occurrence of these symptoms secondary to a hypersensitive, yet stable, bladder. Sensory urgency occurs in bladder irritative states, such as infection, urethral syndrome, interstitial cystitis, and carcinoma in situ.

Less common symptoms of detrusor instability include bedwetting, which occurs in about one third of patients, and voiding difficulty. Patients may feel urgency and then rush to relieve themselves, only to find that they have difficulty voiding. This difficulty may occur because the detrusor contraction that gave the patient urgency has subsided, and the patient now has difficulty initiating another contraction to adequately void.

Pain is not a common symptom of women with detrusor instability. Pain with a full bladder in conjunction with urgency and frequency is suggestive of a hypersensitive bladder condition, such as interstitial cystitis.

When obtaining the urologic history, it is important to inquire into the patient's personal, family, social, sexual, and environmental history. As previously mentioned, Frewen emphasized that the stimulus for bladder activity is not a local one, but is central in origin and influenced by psychologic, social, and environmental factors. Great care must be exercised in obtaining a psychiatric history. The suggestion of a psychiatric basis for the problem may be extremely harmful to the doctor-patient relationship, making subsequent trust and compliance difficult.

Numerous studies have evaluated the accuracy of diagnosing detrusor instability based on symptoms alone. Farrar et al noted that patients who complained only of stress incontinence with no other symptoms usually were found to have stable bladders. If they complained of urgency, frequency, and/or nocturia in addition to the stress incontinence, the incidence of detrusor instability increased. If urgency and urge incontinence accompanied stress incontinence, the bladder was unstable 80% of the time. Patients who complained of frequency, nocturia, urgency, and urge incontinence without any stress incontinence were all noted to have an unstable bladder. Eighty percent of patients who complained of incontinence upon getting out of a chair or of constant wetness regardless of any provoking factor were noted to have detrusor instability.

Walters and Shields studied clinical symptoms in 106 consecutive, incontinent women. The urologic symptom frequencies showed marked overlap among answers to individual questions and urologic diagnoses. Of the ten questions studied, only two—sensory urgency and enuresis—were associated with overactive detrusor function. Sensory urgency was frequently found in both groups, including 71% of women with genuine stress incontinence; however, only 9% of women in the detrusor instability group had no sensory urgency, making genuine stress incontinence more likely in incontinent women with no symptom of urgency. A recent history of enuresis was strongly associated with overactive detrusor function and uncommon (8%) in the genuine stress incontinence group. When enuresis is present, empiric medical or behavioral therapy for unstable bladder may be appropriate.

PHYSICAL EXAMINATION

General physical and neurologic examinations should be performed, as in all incontinent patients. Anal sphincter tone and perineal sensation, as well as anal cutaneous and bulbocavernosus reflex tests, are the most important aspects of the neurologic examination. It is unusual, however, for a neurologic examination to reveal unsuspected neuropathy.

Characteristically, idiopathic detrusor instability produces no physical signs that are pathognomonic for the disease. Careful bimanual and speculum examinations should be performed on all patients. In addition, an examination should be conducted to identify the presence or absence of the sign of urinary incontinence. The examination is best accomplished if the patient has a full bladder. If incontinence occurs simultaneous with a rise in intraabdominal pressure, as with coughing, it is most likely due to sphincteric weakness (genuine stress incontinence). On the other hand, if it occurs shortly after the cough and is of a more prolonged nature, it is most likely due to an uninhibited bladder contraction precipitated by the cough. If incontinence cannot be demonstrated in the supine position, the patient should be asked to stand and again undergo various provocative maneuvers.

INVESTIGATIONS
Urinalysis and Culture

Because the symptoms of urinary infection and other irritative bladder conditions commonly mimic detrusor instability, urinalysis should be performed before further investigation is initiated. As previously mentioned, bacteriuria may cause bladder instability and will sometimes resolve after the infection has been treated. Urine cytology should be performed to rule out neoplasia in patients with chronic bladder irritative symptoms, particularly elderly patients and those with microscopic hematuria.

Voided Volume Chart

A chart of the timing and volume of intake and output is indispensable for corroborating the patient's history and symptomatology. Typically, a patient with an unstable bladder will void different volumes of urine at different intervals, whereas patients with sensory urgency tend to void consistently small volumes at fairly regular intervals. We usually ask patients to keep a 48-hour chart, usually over a weekend so as to avoid the possible interference of the pressures of work. Follow-up charts are also useful to provide evidence to both patient and physician of a response to treatment. This procedure is particularly important when bladder retraining is used for treatment.

Urodynamic Tests
Cystometry

Cystometry is the mainstay of investigation for bladder storage function and is the only method of objectively diagnosing detrusor instability or hyperreflexia. The first ICS report on standardization of terminology of the lower urinary tract in 1976 stated that, to make the diagnosis of unstable bladder, contractions must be noted to exceed 15 cm H_2O on filling cystometry. Since then, many studies have noted that contractions less than 15 cm H_2O also can produce symptoms. The ICS has subsequently changed the definition to state that any rise in true detrusor pressure that is not thought due to bladder compliance can be termed an overactive detrusor. If detrusor overactivity occurs in the absence of a neurologic lesion, it is termed an unstable bladder. These findings may be symptomatic or asymptomatic.

Coolsaet et al investigated 334 women with either isolated detrusor instability or coexistent detrusor instability and genuine stress incontinence and noted that 87 of the 334 (26%) women had contractions of less than 15 cm H_2O during cystometry. In this group, 7% were asymptomatic, 10% had subthreshold detrusor instability leading to urinary incontinence, and 85% had symptoms of urgency and frequency. This

study clearly showed that contractions of a magnitude less than 15 cm H_2O are clinically significant.

The rise in pressure that occurs on cystometry may be phasic (i.e., a pressure rise followed by a pressure fall) or constant. Many investigators believe that the latter situation should be termed a low compliance bladder because it is sometimes secondary to conditions resulting in changes in the passive elastic properties of the bladder wall, such as interstitial or radiation cystitis. Fig. 19-1 reviews the various cystometric patterns that can be seen in patients with detrusor instability.

During the cystometric evaluation of patients with suspected detrusor instability, one must use provoking stimuli if detrusor instability is not elicited during filling. Sometimes the provocation necessary to reproduce a detrusor contraction cannot be performed in a laboratory setting. This problem has been demonstrated in numerous ambulatory monitoring studies in which symptomatic patients were noted in the urodynamic laboratory to have normal bladder filling, but, when monitored on a continuous basis, uninhibited contractions were elicited.

Testing should always be performed with the patient in a sitting or erect position, as supine filling cystometry alone will fail to uncover a significant proportion of unstable bladders. Other provoking factors are coughing, straining, heel-bouncing, jogging in place, listening to running water, and placing the patient's hands under running water. Fig. 19-2 is a urodynamic tracing from a patient with cough-provoked detrusor instability.

The terminal bladder contraction completes the cystometrogram. In a patient without neurologic or urologic disease, this contraction requires voluntary facilitation by the patient. If the patient can suppress the terminal contraction, the controlling central nervous system reflexes are intact.

Urethral Pressure Studies

These studies add little to the diagnosis of detrusor instability or to the differentiation of patients with stress incontinence from those with urgency incontinence. If simultaneous urethrocystometry is performed during filling, the diagnosis of urethral instability or uninhibited urethral relaxation can be made.

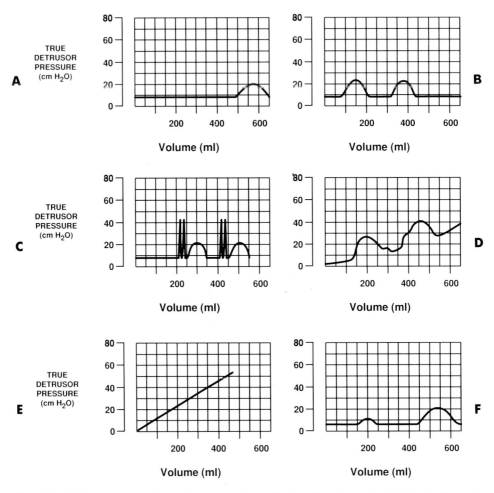

Fig. 19-1 Various cystometric patterns noted in patients with detrusor instability. **A,** Normal filling cystometry with voluntary terminal contraction. **B,** Phasic involuntary detrusor contractions that return to baseline. **C,** Cough-provoked detrusor instability. **D,** Phasic contractions with steady rise in detrusor pressure. **E,** Steady rise in detrusor pressure (low compliance bladder). **F,** Subthreshold detrusor instability with voluntary terminal contraction.

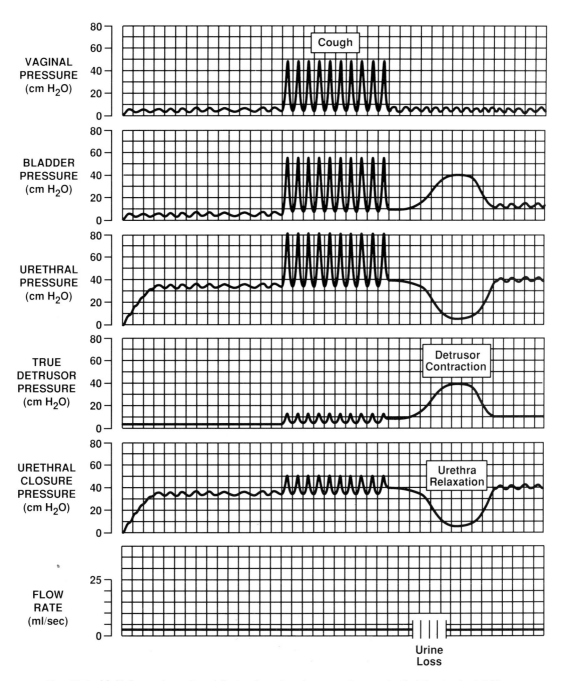

Fig. 19-2 Multichannel urodynamic tracing showing cough-provoked detrusor instability. Note visual loss of urine occurs a few seconds after the last cough in conjunction with an involuntary bladder contraction and complete urethral relaxation.

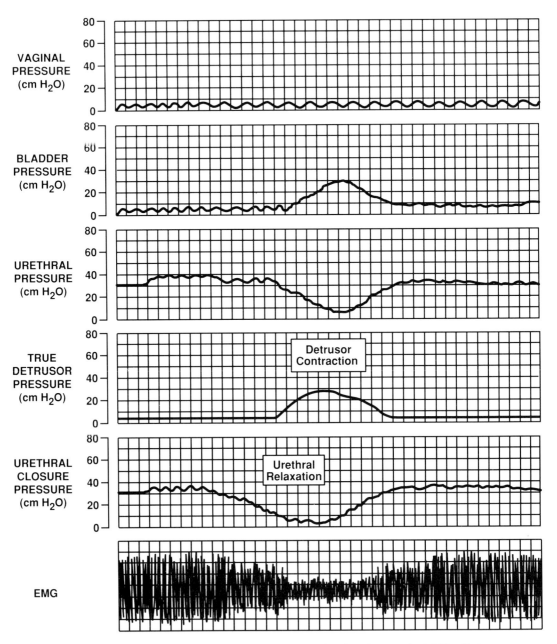

Fig. 19-3 Multichannel subtracted urethrocystometry showing detrusor instability. Note urethral relaxation and quieting of EMG activity.

Detrusor contractions are almost always preceded by a drop in urethral pressure (Fig. 19-3). A study by Bergman et al studied urethral pressure tracings in 72 women with detrusor instability to learn whether urethral pressure changes may be the cause, rather than the effect, of bladder contractions. They noted that patients had one of two patterns with regard to urethral pressure change. The first pattern demonstrated uninhibited bladder contraction that preceded any change in urethral pressure; the second pattern noted a urethral pressure drop of greater than or equal to 20 cm H_2O 2 to 5 seconds before the detrusor contraction. Patients who had urethral relaxation before the detrusor contractions responded better to alpha-sympathomimetic drugs, whereas those patients without urethral pressure changes responded more favorably to anticholinergic drugs.

Electromyography

Electromyography (EMG) gives information only on activity of the external striated urethral sphincter muscles. Its potential value in patients with detrusor instability is to document voluntary control of this sphincter, as well as demonstrate that the external sphincter and detrusor muscle function in a coordinated fashion (Fig. 19-4). Mayo found that 48% of patients with idiopathic detrusor instability exhibited reflex relaxation of the sphincter at the time of a detrusor contraction. This observation is important because these patients are probably unable to voluntarily contract the external sphincter at the moment of the detrusor contraction, thus inhibiting urine loss. Spontaneous sphincter relaxation can also be detected during EMG studies, leading to the diagnosis of uninhibited urethral relaxation. However, I believe the sole use of external sphincter EMG studies is for the diagnosis of detrusor-external sphincter dyssynergia, which is a rare condition and occurs only in patients with neurologic disease. EMG adds little to the evaluation and management of neurologically intact female patients.

Bethanechol Supersensitivity Test

Ordinarily, one should attempt to perform all urodynamic studies in the absence of pharmacologic interference. Medications often must be discontinued 24

to 48 hours before any urodynamic tests are performed. Pretest administration of some pharmacologic agents, however, may improve the interpretability of cystometric studies. Bethanechol chloride, which has acetylcholine-like activity and acts on the postganglionic parasympathetic effector cells to enhance contractility of the bladder, has been used for this purpose. Although it has minimal effect on a normal bladder, an unstable bladder, whether idiopathic or neurogenic in origin, demonstrates detrusor contractions after the administration of this compound. It has been used to identify patients who are suspected of having detrusor instability which cannot be elicited on provocative cystometry. To perform the test, 2.5 mg of bethanechol chloride is administered subcutaneously, and the cystometrogram is repeated approximately 30 minutes later.

Endoscopy

The indications for cystoscopy in patients suspected of having detrusor instability are microscopic hematuria and abnormal urine cytology. Cystoscopy should also be performed when the diagnosis is in doubt and other conditions, such as interstitial cystitis, need to be ruled out.

MANAGEMENT

Incomplete understanding of the cause(s) of detrusor instability has lead to several diverse treatment plans. Comparison of various methods is difficult because of differences in patient population, methods of diagnosis, cystometric techniques, and follow-up protocols. Broadly, the management of detrusor instability is separated into surgical and nonsurgical modalities (see accompanying box).

Nonsurgical
Bladder Retraining Drills

This method of therapy institutes a program of scheduled voiding with progressive increases in the interval between each void. Therapy is based on the assumption that conscious efforts to suppress sensory stimuli will reestablish cortical control over an uninhibited bladder, thus reestablishing a normal voiding pattern. This mode of therapy has been studied most thor-

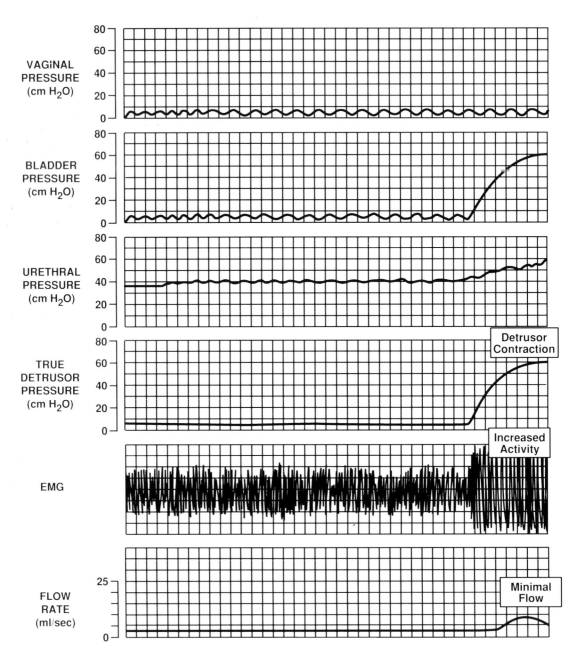

Fig. 19-4 Multichannel urodynamic tracing showing detrusor-external sphincter dyssynergia. As patient tries to void, an increase in EMG activity is associated with a strong bladder contraction, rise in urethral pressure, and minimum urine flow.

Treatment Methods For Detrusor Instability and Detrusor Hyperreflexia

Nonsurgical Methods

Bladder retraining
Biofeedback
Psychotherapy
Functional electrical stimulation
Drug therapy

Surgical Methods

Bladder distention
Phenol injections
Selective sacral blockade
Sacral neurectomy
Transvaginal resection of inferior hypogastric pelvic nerve plexus
Bladder transection
Augmentation cystoplasty
Urinary diversion

oughly by Frewen and by Fantl et al. In several studies, Frewen reported success rates of approximately 80%. His protocol, however, included primarily in-hospital behavioral management and concurrent pharmacologic therapy. Fantl et al reported on 92 patients with objective evidence of detrusor instability treated by bladder drill, with or without anticholinergic therapy. Cure rates were the same in both groups: 83% in patients treated with bladder drill and drugs versus 79% in patients treated with bladder drill alone. These high cure rates with bladder retraining drills have been substantiated by other authors.

The technique used for bladder retraining involves giving the patient insight into the nature of her dysfunction. Drawings demonstrating cerebral cortical inhibitory effect over bladder reflexes can be shown to the patient to assist in explaining the lower urinary tract dysfunction. The patient's own cystometric tracing also can be shown to her to illustrate the dysfunction.The patient then is taught scheduled voidings at timed intervals, which can vary from 15 minutes to 1 hour, according to the patient's own frequency and/or incontinence intervals. We usually start patients at voiding intervals of 30 to 60 minutes. They

are given preprinted cards, which they maintain daily. Voiding events (daily and nightly), involuntary leaking episodes, and occurrences that precipitate incontinence should be checked. The patients are instructed to make an earnest effort to follow the schedule. They should try to suppress urgency and void only at the scheduled times. At these times, the patient is asked to attempt to void regardless of the presence or absence of urinary urgency. Schedules are not followed during sleeping hours. Follow-up visits are scheduled every 1 to 2 weeks, at which time the cards are reviewed with the patient. Micturition intervals are increased periodically by 15 to 60 minutes, according to the response. A 6- to 12-week treatment program is anticipated in most cases.

Enthusiastic patient contact, reassurance, good long-term support and follow-up are important. The degree of patient compliance is predictive of success. Because the success rate is so good and this mode of therapy involves relatively low cost, bladder retraining drills should be the first line of therapy in patients with detrusor instability.

Biofeedback

Biofeedback is a form of patient reeducation in which a closed feedback loop is created so that one or more of her normally unconscious physiologic processes are made accessible to her by auditory, visual, or tactile signals. An attempt is made to modify the physiologic process by manipulating the signal presented to the patient. This method has been used with some success in the treatment of autonomic dysfunctions, hypertension, and cardiac dysrhythmias. Cystometry is explained to the patient, the test is begun, and an audible signal is used to let the patient know that her bladder pressure is rising. The tone of the signal varies according to the amount of bladder pressure rise. The patient also visualizes the urodynamic tracing throughout the test. The bladder is repeatedly filled while the patient attempts to inhibit detrusor contractions. Individual treatment sessions are approximately 1 hour and are repeated weekly for up to 8 weeks.

Cardozo et al have reported 81% subjective and objective improvement with biofeedback. They noted that biofeedback was not as successful in patients with severe detrusor instability, particularly in women with large detrusor contraction occurring at small volumes. Burgio et al reduced incontinence episodes by 85% in patients with biofeedback and by 94% in patients with both sensory and motor urge incontinence. Patients need to be highly motivated to improve with this form of therapy.

Psychotherapy

The possible psychosomatic origin of this condition has been discussed. Hafner et al studied psychotherapy as a method of treatment in 26 patients with urgency, frequency, and urge incontinence. Patients were treated with six 1-hour sessions of group psychotherapy. Approximately one third of the patients benefitted considerably, one third refused treatment or ceased treatment prematurely, and one third improved slightly or not at all. MacCaulay et al randomized 50 patients with detrusor instability or sensory urgency to receive bladder retraining drills, propantheline bromide, or psychotherapy. Patients who received psychotherapy showed significant improvement, and no patient had more than minor incontinence at follow-up; however, urinary frequency was unaffected.

Functional Electrical Stimulation

Functional electrical stimulation (FES) works by stimulating the afferent limb of the pudendal reflex arc, resulting in an increase in pelvic floor and urethral striated muscle contractility. In addition, stimulation of the afferent portion of the pudendal nerve can result in the reflex inhibition of detrusor contractility. Clinical studies have supported this finding for patients with hyperreflexic bladders, as well as those with idiopathic detrusor instability. Some patients with detrusor instability respond to FES after having been refractory to behavioral and pharmacologic therapies. The main difficulty with FES is patient acceptance of intravaginal or transrectal stimulation. Patients must wear these devices for several hours each day, and many patients reject this for psychologic or aesthetic reasons. The dismal results of Leach and Bavendam in using the Incontan transrectal stimulating device— a 94% dropout rate in a study of 36 patients—clearly points out these limitations.

More recently, investigators have studied the ef-

ficacy of intermittent maximal electrical stimulation in treating incontinence. With this form of therapy, a short period of stimulation (for example, 30 minutes) is given to the patient at maximum tolerable intensity and the treatment continued over several weeks. Eriksen et al reported a trial involving acute short-term maximal pelvic floor electrical stimulation of 48 patients with idiopathic detrusor instability. Each received 20 minutes of simultaneous vaginal and anal electrical stimulation for an average of seven treatments. Initial clinical and urodynamic cures were observed in 50% of patients, and significant improvement occurred in an additional 33%. At 1-year follow-up, persistent positive therapeutic effects were found in 77% of patients. In another study, Plevnik et al treated 30 patients with detrusor instability with maximal electrical stimulation at home for 20 minutes per day for 30 days. A cure was noted in 29%; an additional 22% reported improvement. Bent et al noted a significant subjective improvement in 69% of patients with detrusor instability, using a regimen of 15 minutes of maximal stimulation twice daily for 6 weeks.

The role of FES as therapy for detrusor instability is still evolving. Although currently not a first-line therapy, it may benefit certain groups of patients who have failed multiple treatment regimens.

Drug Therapy

Although behavior modification improves or cures most patients with detrusor instability, pharmacologic therapy remains the most popular mode of treatment. A number of pharmacologic agents are effective. Because the etiology of detrusor instability is unknown, however, the response to treatment is often unpredictable and side effects are common with effective doses.

In general, drugs improve detrusor instability by inhibiting the contractile activity of the bladder. These agents can be broadly classified into anticholinergic drugs, calcium channel blockers, tricyclic antidepressants, musculotropic drugs, and a variety of other less commonly used drugs (Table 19-2).

Anticholinergic agents. A variety of anticholinergic drugs are effective in the management of detrusor instability, although certain agents have more specific activity on the detrusor muscle than on other

---

TABLE 19-2   Pharmacologic therapy for detrusor instability

Mechanism of action	Name of drug	Minimum and maximum dosage	Potential side effects	Contraindications
Anticholinergic	Propantheline bromide	15 mg BID to 30 mg QID	Anticholinergic effects (dry mouth, blurred vision, drowsiness, tachycardia, constipation)	Glaucoma, intestinal obstruction, cardiac dysrhythmia, myasthenia gravis
Smooth muscle relaxant, anticholinergic, local anesthetic	Oxybutynin chloride	2.5 mg BID to 5 mg QID	Anticholinergic effects	as above
	Flavoxate hydrochloride	100 mg BID to 200 mg QID	Anticholinergic effects	as above
Smooth muscle relaxant (antispasmodic)	Dicyclomine hydrochloride	10 mg BID to 40 mg QID	Anticholinergic effects	as above
Calcium channel blocker	Nifedipine	10 mg BID to 120 mg QD	Edema, hypotension, flushing, dizziness, nausea, abdominal pain, rash, weakness, palpitation	Congestive heart failure, coronary artery disease, hypotension, narrow angle glaucoma
Calcium channel blocker, anticholinergic	Terodiline hydrochloride	12.5 mg BID to 25 mg BID	Edema, hypotension, flushing, dizziness, nausea, abdominal pain, rash, weakness, palpitation	Congestive heart failure, coronary artery disease, hypotension, narrow angle glaucoma
Tricyclic antidepressant, anticholinergic, alpha-adrenergic agonist, antihistaminic	Imipramine hydrochloride	25 mg QD to 75 mg BID	Anticholinergic effects, orthostatic hypotension, hepatic dysfunction, mania, cardiovascular effects (especially in the elderly)	Glaucoma, intestinal obstruction, cardiac dysrhythmia, myasthenia gravis, monoamine oxidase inhibitors prohibited

cholinergically innervated organs. One of the earliest anticholinergic agents used for detrusor instability was methantheline bromide. Use of this drug for peptic ulcer disease led to acute urinary retention in some patients. This reaction prompted urologists to use it for refractory cases of urgency and frequency, with good preliminary results. Propanthaline bromide, a related but more potent compound, was later found to be as efficacious as methantheline bromide in controlling this condition, but with fewer side effects.

For many years, propantheline bromide was the treatment of choice for detrusor instability and the drug to which most other new compounds were compared. Numerous trials have shown this drug to inhibit involuntary detrusor contractions and to increase bladder capacity. The dose is 15 to 30 mg orally three to four times a day. Side effects are those of parasympathetic blockade: dry mouth due to suppression of the salivary or pharyngeal secretions, constipation due to decreased gastrointestinal motility, tachycardia due to vagal blockade, and transient blurring of vision from blockade of the sphincters of the iris and ciliary muscles of the eye. Dry mouth is the most common side effect; others are likely to occur with higher drug doses. In general, the maximum dose is usually determined by patient tolerance to side effects rather than by other forms of toxicity. These drugs should be used with caution in patients with narrow-angle glaucoma and in patients with significant cardiac dysrhythmias.

Emepronium bromide is an anticholinergic agent whose potentially dangerous side effects have prevented it from becoming a popular medication. However, Massey and Abrams studied a new formulation, emepronium carageenate, in a dose titration trial. They noted that symptoms improved with increasing total daily doses without serious side effects. This improvement was confirmed by urodynamic data. Therefore, this drug may hold some promise for treatment of detrusor instability.

Musculotropic agents. Smooth muscle relaxant drugs used for detrusor instability include oxybutynin chloride (Ditropan, Marion Laboratories, Inc., Kansas City, Mo), dicyclomine hydrochloride (Bentyl, Lakeside Pharmaceuticals, Cincinnati, Ohio) and flavoxate hydrochloride (Urispas, SmithKline Beecham Consumer Products, Pittsburgh, Pa).

Oxybutynin chloride is probably the most effective drug currently available for the treatment of detrusor instability. It is a tertiary amine compound that possesses strong musculotropic, antispasmodic, and local anesthetic effects in addition to having moderate anticholinergic and antihistaminic properties. This drug is marketed specifically for urologic indications and is prescribed in a dose of 2.5 to 10 mg one to four times daily. It is also available in a liquid suspension, which is suitable for use in children and elderly persons. Diokno and Lapides have demonstrated the effectiveness of this drug in reducing the amplitude and frequency of detrusor contractions and in increasing cystometric bladder capacity in patients with detrusor hyperreflexia. In a placebo-controlled trial, 30 unselected patients with detrusor instability underwent treatment. Symptomatic improvement was achieved

in 69% of those receiving oxybutynin chloride and in only 8% receiving placebo. Urodynamic improvement occurred in one half of the patients on oxybutynin chloride. Seventeen (57%) of the patients suffered side effects; in five, side effects were so severe that the drug was discontinued.

Numerous clinical trials have confirmed that symptoms of urgency, frequency, and urge incontinence are significantly improved or eradicated in a large proportion of patients using oxybutynin chloride. It is effective for both neuropathic and idiopathic detrusor instability. Some patients, however, will be unable to tolerate its anticholinergic side effects.

Dicyclomine hydrochloride is an alternative to oxybutynin chloride when side effects of the latter are intolerable. Dicyclomine is usually used to treat gastrointestinal disorders. It has few side effects, but is considerably less effective than oxybutynin chloride in the management of detrusor instability.

Flavoxate hydrochloride inhibits phosphatide esterase activity and increases intracellular cyclic adenosine diphosphate, a mediator of smooth muscle relaxation. Published data on this drug does not support its effectiveness in the treatment of detrusor instability, even though it is still commonly used in clinical practice.

Imipramine hydrochloride. The tricyclic antidepressant, imipramine hydrochloride (Tofranil, Geigy Pharmaceuticals, Ardsley, NY), improves bladder storage significantly. This medication appears to improve bladder hypertonicity or compliance rather than uninhibited contractions. It has been prescribed for treatment of enuresis in children for many years. The drug is given in a dose of 25 mg, one to three times a day for adults and 5 to 10 mg, four times a day for children. Single nightly doses can be given in patients for the treatment of nocturnal enuresis. As compared to placebo, the drug causes a statistically significant improvement in frequency of bedwetting. It has a complex pharmacologic action, with anticholinergic, antihistaminic, and local anesthetic properties. It also increases bladder outlet resistance, due to a peripheral blockade of noradrenaline uptake. Due to this dual action, the drug also may be effective for patients with combined stress incontinence and detrusor instability. The side effects are anticholinergic, as well as tremor and fatigue. One must also be aware of the cardio-vascular side effects that can occur in elderly patients, the most common of which is orthostatic hypotension.

Calcium channel blockers. Terodiline hydrochloride is a calcium channel blocker that has been used extensively for detrusor instability in Europe, but is not yet available in the United States. Numerous clinical trials have demonstrated that the drug increases bladder capacity and volume and decrease symptoms of urgency and frequency in patients with detrusor instability, as compared to placebo. Tapp et al reported on 70 patients who had completed a double-blind, placebo-controlled, multicentered, dose-titrated study of terodiline for idiopathic detrusor instability. Drug treatment led to significant decreases in voiding frequency, incontinence episodes, and urgency with a significant increase in voided volume. Although urodynamic parameters tended to improve when compared with those of placebo, these improvements were not statistically significant. Terodiline also has been shown to be effective in patients with sensory urgency when used in conjunction with bladder retraining drill. The dose is 25 to 50 mg per day in divided doses.

In addition to its calcium antagonistic activity, terodiline appears to have an antimuscarinic effect that tends to predominate in low concentrations, whereas the calcium antagonist effect is added at higher concentrations. Side effects include dry mouth, visual blurring, dizziness, and specific calcium antagonistic effects such as headache, ankle swelling, tremor, and jitteriness. In general, however, it is well tolerated and seems to have fewer anticholinergic side effects than oxybutynin chloride. Terodiline is a promising new drug, which it is hoped will be available soon in the United States.

Other agents. Other drugs that have been shown to possibly inhibit bladder contractility include beta-adrenergic agonists, such as clenbuterol and terbutaline. These drugs have been shown in animal studies to increase bladder capacity; however, their role in the management of detrusor instability in humans is uncertain. In addition, alpha-adrenergic antagonists and prostaglandin synthetase inhibitors reduce bladder capacity in animals; however, no significant benefit has been reported in humans.

Synthetic vasopressin, DDAVP (l-desamino-8-D-arginine vasopressin), decreases urine production. It is given in doses of 20 to 40 μg intranasally as a spray or snuff at bedtime. This dose has been shown to decrease urine production by up to 50%. Ramsden et al showed that DDAVP was superior to placebo in reducing the number of bedwetting episodes in 21 severely enuretic patients. Hilton and Stanton found the drug produced fewer nightime voids, as compared to placebo, in 25 women with nocturia. This drug is helpful in patients with troublesome nocturnal urinary symptoms, but is contraindicated in patients with hypertension, ischemic heart disease, or congestive heart failure.

Certain considerations should always be kept in mind regarding drug therapy for detrusor instability: (1) each drug should be given for at least 6 weeks before deeming it a failure, as the onset of benefit may, at times, be delayed; (2) drug doses must be titrated, based on subjective response and the presence or absence of side effects; (3) if one drug is not beneficial, it is worth trying other drugs with different modes of action or combining drugs; (4) placebo effects are high and may be present in as many as 50% of patients; and (5) detrusor instability is a relapsing and remitting condition, and treatment may need to be adjusted accordingly.

Surgical Treatment

If conservative management (i.e., bladder retraining, pharmacologic management and electrical stimulation) fails to control detrusor instability, surgery may be indicated. Procedures include bladder distention, subtrigonal injection of phenol, selective sacral blockades, selective sacral neurectomy, transvaginal denervation of the bladder, bladder transection, augmentation cystoplasty, and urinary diversion.

Bladder distention involves stretching the bladder under epidural anesthesia for about 2 hours, in four half-hour periods with a short break between each. Distention should produce a hydrostatic pressure equal to the systolic blood pressure. Although initial studies were promising, recent reports have been less enthusiastic, with success rates of only about 10%. The only complication reported is bladder rupture, which occurs in 52% of cases.

Transvaginal infiltration of the pelvic plexus with

phenol was described by Ewing et al as a less traumatic alternative to bladder transection. Initial studies reported success rates in the 60% range for refractory detrusor instability and detrusor hyperreflexia. A more recent study by Wall and Stanton reported on a series of 28 patients with refractory urge incontinence who underwent a total of 40 transvesical phenol injections. Only eight patients (29%) achieved a significant response, and all relapsed during the 22-month follow-up period.

Another similar denervation procedure is selective blockade of the sacral pelvic nerves, which involves the injection of a local anesthetic into the foramina of sacral segment S3. Permanent neurolysis can be obtained by the injection of 6% aqueous phenol. The few studies on this procedure have reported variable results. Awad et al developed a similar technique using a cryoprobe instead of phenol injections. They reported good or excellent results in 16 of 17 patients with idiopathic detrusor instability. Mean duration of follow-up was 4.8 months. The technique was safe; temporary sensory disturbances were the only side effects.

Selective sacral neurectomy is a neurosurgical procedure that involves identification of the sacral roots through a limited sacral laminectomy. Electrical stimulation is used to determine which of the roots should be sectioned, as judged by the effect of stimulation on intravesical pressure. Usually the S3 root is divided bilaterally. Studies on this procedure have reported good results on small numbers of patients.

The Ingelman-Sundberg procedure is a transvaginal partial denervation of the bladder originally described in 1959. In this procedure the inferior hypogastric pelvic nerve plexus is resected after a preliminary local anesthetic block has indicated the likelihood of a successful outcome. Successful outcomes have been reported in 50% to 80% of patients.

Bladder transection was initially described by Turner-Warwick and Ashken in 1967. This operation involved complete transection of the bladder above the trigone and ureteric orifices and division of all inferior lateral communications. The largest series was reported by Mundy who noted a 74% subjective cure rate at 1-year follow-up.

Augmentation cystoplasty also has been used for resistant cases of detrusor instability. The bladder is bisected almost completely and a patch of gut, usually ileum, equal in length to the circumference of the bisected bladder (almost 25 cm), is sewn in place. The operation often cures the symptoms of detrusor instability but results in inefficient voiding. Patients may have to learn to strain to void or resort to clean intermittent self-catheterization. Mundy and Stephenson reported on a series of 40 patients treated by "clam" ileocystoplasty. Thirty-six (90%) were cured of their symptoms, and 30 were able to void spontaneously and efficiently.

For those women with severe detrusor instability or hyperreflexia in whom all other methods of treatment have failed, urinary diversion via an ileal conduit may be considered as a last resort. This mode of therapy is particularly useful in young disabled patients with severe neurologic dysfunction.

MIXED INCONTINENCE

Detrusor instability can coexist with genuine stress incontinence in up to 30% of patients. Karram and Bhatia treated 52 women with coexistent genuine stress incontinence and detrusor instability. Of these, 27 underwent colposuspension and 25 were given oxybutynin hydrochloride together with imipramine and/or estrogen. Of those who were surgically treated, 59% were cured and 22% improved; of those who were given medical treatment, 32% were cured and 28% improved. This study suggests that medical management reduces the need for surgical intervention. If patients fail medical management and bladder neck surgery is recommended, the patient should understand that the postoperative course of detrusor instability is somewhat unpredictable.

SUMMARY

Detrusor instability is a common condition characterized by multiple symptoms, some of which are embarrassing and may cause an increasingly restricted lifestyle. A lack of understanding of the pathophysiology of this condition is reflected in the numerous methods of currently available treatments. It is important to elicit the patient's main complaints and aim treatment accordingly. Although complete, indefinite cure is rare, the majority of patients can achieve significant reduction of their symptoms. As the pathophysiology of detrusor instability becomes better understood, it is hoped that there will be significant advances in management.

BIBLIOGRAPHY

Prevalence and Incidence

Abrams P: Detrusor instability and bladder outlet obstruction, *Neurourol Urodyn* 4:317, 1985.

Arnold EP, Webster JR, Loose H, et al: Urodynamics of female incontinence: factors influence the results of surgery, *Am J Obstet Gynecol* 117:805, 1973.

Diokno AC, Brown MB, Brock BM, et al: Clinical and cystometric characteristics of continent and incontinent noninstitutionalized elderly, *J Urol* 140:567, 1988.

Hodgkinson CP, Ayers MA, Drukker BH: Dyssynergic detrusor dysfunction in the apparently normal female, *Am J Obstet Gynecol* 87:717, 1963.

Ouslander J, Staskin D, Raz S, et al: Clinical versus urodynamic diagnosis in an incontinent geriatric female population, *J Urol* 137:68, 1987.

Sand PK, Hill RC, Ostergard DR: Incontinence history as a predictor of detrusor instability, *Obstet Gynecol* 71:257, 1988.

Sand PK, Hill RC, Ostergard DO: Supine urethroscopic and standing cystometrogram as screening methods for the detection of detrusor instability, *Obstet Gynecol* 70:57, 1987.

Turner-Warwick RT: Observations on the function and dysfunction of the sphincter and detrusor mechanism, *Urol Clin North Am* 6:13, 1979.

Walters MD, Shields LE: The diagnostic value of history, physical examination, and the Q-Tip cotton swab test in women with urinary incontinence, *Am J Obstet Gynecol* 159:145, 1988.

Webster GD, Sihelnik SA, Stone AR: Female urinary incontinence: the incidence, identification and characteristics of detrusor instability, *Neurourol Urodyn* 3:235, 1984.

Etiology

Anderson JT, Bradley WE: Bladder and urethral innervation in multiple sclerosis, *Br J Urol* 48:193, 1976.

Awad SA, Gajewski JB, Sogbein SK, et al: Relationship between neurological and urological status in patients with multiple sclerosis, *J Urol* 132:499, 1984.

Barrington FJ: The component reflexes of micturition in the cat, *Brain,* 54:177, 1931.

Beck RP, Armsch D, King C: Results in treating 210 patients with detrusor overactivity incontinence of urine, *Am J Obstet Gyncol* 125:593, 1976.

Beck RP, Warren KG, Whitman P: Urodynamic studies in female patients with multiple sclerosis, *Am J Obstet Gynecol* 139:273, 1981.

Bhatia NN, Bergman A: Cystometry: unstable bladder and urinary tract infection, *Br J Urol* 58:134, 1986.

Blaivas JG, Bhimani G, Labib KB: Vesicourethral dysfunction in multiple sclerosis, *J Urol* 122:342, 1979.

Bradley WE: Urinary bladder dysfunction in multiple sclerosis, *Neurology* (Minneapolis) 28 (9 Pt 2):52, 1978.

Cardozo LD, Stanton SL, Williams JE: Detrusor instability following surgery for genuine stress incontinence, *Br J Urol* 51:204, 1979.

Cucchi A: Detrusor instability and bladder outflow obstruction. Evidence for a correlation between the severity of obstruction and the presence of instability, *Br J Urol* 61:420, 1988.

Frewen WK: An objective assessment of the unstable bladder of psychosomatic origin, *Br J Urol* 50:246, 1978.

Goldstein I, Siroky MB, Sax DS, et al: Neurourologic abnormalities in multiple sclerosis, *J Urol* 128:541, 1982.

Gonor SE, Carroll DJ, Metcalfe JB: Vesical dysfunction in multiple sclerosis, *Urology* 25:429, 1985.

Gu J, Restorick JM, Blank MA, et al: Vasoactive intestinal polypeptide in the normal and unstable bladder, *Br J Urol* 55:645, 1983.

Hassouna M, Lebel M, Elhilali M: Neurologic correlation in multiple sclerosis, *Neurourol Urodyn* 3:73, 1984.

Hilton P: Urinary incontinence during sexual intercourse: a common, but rarely volunteered, symptom, *Br J Obstet Gynaecol* 95:377, 1988.

Ketelaer P, Leruitte A, Vereecken RL: Striated urethral and anal sphincter electromyography during cystometry in multiple sclerosis, *Electromyogr Clin Neurophysiol* 17:427, 1977.

Khan Z, Bhola A, Starer P: Urinary incontinence during orgasm, *Urology* 21:279, 1988.

Kinder RB, Mundy AR: Inhibition of spontaneous contractile activity in isolated human detrusor muscle strips by vasoactive intestinal polypeptide, *Br J Urol* 57:20, 1985.

Kinder RB, Mundy AR: Pathophysiology of idiopathic detrusor instability and detrusor hyper-reflexia: in vitro study of human detrusor muscle, *Br J Urol* 60:509, 1987.

Kinder RB, Restorick JM, Mundy AR: Vasoactive intestinal polypeptide in the hyper-reflexic neuropathic bladder, *Br J Urol* 57:289, 1985.

Petersen T, Pederson E: Neurourodynamic evaluation of voiding dysfunction in multiple sclerosis, *Acta Neurol Scand* 69:402, 1984.

Philp T, Read DJ, Higson RH: The urodynamic characteristics of multiple sclerosis, *Br J Urol* 53:672, 1981.

Piazza DH, Diokno AC: Review of neurogenic bladder in multiple sclerosis, *Urology* 14:33, 1979.

Ramsden PD, Smith JC, Pierce JM, et al: The unstable bladder — fact or artefact? *Br J Urol* 49:633, 1977.

Rees DLP, Whickham JEA, Whitfield HN: Bladder instability in women with recurrent cystitis, *Br J Urol* 50:524, 1978.

Resnick NM, Yalla SV: Detrusor hyperactivity with impaired contractile function, *JAMA* 257:3076, 1987.

Resnick NM, Yalla SV, Laurino E: The psychophysiology of urinary incontinence among institutionalized elderly persons, *N Engl J Med* 320:1, 1989.

Schoenberg HW, Gutrich J, Banno J: Urodynamic patterns in multiple sclerosis, *J Urol* 122:648, 1979.

Sutherst JR, Brown M: The effect on the bladder pressure of sudden entry of fluid into the posterior urethra, *Br J Urol* 50:406, 1978.

Van Poppel H, Vereecken RL, Leruitte A: Neuro-muscular dysfunction of the lower urinary tract in multiple sclerosis, *Paraplegia* 21:374, 1983.

Diagnosis

Awad SA, McGinnis RH: Factors that influence the incidence of detrusor instability in women, *J Urol* 130:114, 1983.

Bates CP, Whiteside CG, Turner-Warwick RT: Synchronous cine/pressure/flow cystourethrography with special reference to stress and urge incontinence, *Br J Urol* 42:714, 1970.

Bent AE, Richardson DA, Ostegard DR: Diagnosis of lower urinary tract disorders in postmenopausal patients, *Am J Obstet Gynecol* 145:218, 1983.

Bergman A, Koonings PP, Ballard CA: Detrusor instability. Is the bladder the cause or the effect? *J Reprod Med* 34:834, 1989.

Bhatia NN, Bradley WE, Haldeman S: Urodynamics: continuous monitoring, *J Urol* 128:963, 1982.

Bradley WE, Timm GE: Cystometry VI. Interpretation, *Urology* 2:231, 1976.

Cantor TJ, Bates CP: A comparative study of symptoms and objective urodynamic findings in 214 incontinent women, *Br J Obstet Gynaecol* 87:889, 1980.

Cardozo LD, Stanton SL: Genuine stress incontinence and detrusor instability: a review of 200 cases, *Br J Obstet Gynaecol* 87:184, 1980.

Coolsaet BLRA: Bladder compliance and detrusor activity during the collection phase, *Neurourol Urodyn* 4:263, 1985.

Coolsaet BLRA, Blok C, van Venrouij GEFM, et al: Subthreshold detrusor instability, *Neurourol Urodyn* 4:309, 1985.

Diokno AC, Wells TJ, Brock BM, et al: Urinary incontinence in elderly women: urodynamic evaluation, *J Am Geriatr Soc* 35:940, 1987.

Eastwood HDH, Warrell R: Urinary incontinence in the elderly female: prediction in diagnosis and outcome of management, *Age Aging* 13:230, 1984.

Farrar DJ, Whiteside CG, Osborne JL, et al: A urodynamic analysis of micturition symptoms in the female, *Surg Gynecol Obstet* 141:875, 1975.

Griffiths CJ, Assi MS, Styles RA, et al: Ambulatory monitoring of bladder and detrusor pressure during natural filling, *J Urol* 142:780, 1989.

Haylen BT, Sutherst JR, Frazer MI: Is the investigation of most stress incontinence really necessary? *Br J Urol* 61:147, 1989.

Hilton P, Stanton SL: Algorithmic method for assessing urinary incontinence in elderly women, *Br Med J* 282:940, 1981.

Jeffcoate TNA, Francis WJA: Urgency incontinence in the female, *Am J Obstet Gynecol* 94:604, 1966.

Korda A, Krieger M, Hunter P, et al: The value of clinical symptoms

in the diagnosis of urinary incontinence in the female, *Aust NZ J Obstet Gynaecol* 27:149, 1987.

Kulseng-Hanssen S, Klevmark B: Ambulatory urethro-cysto-rectometry: a new technique, *Neurourol Urodyn* 7:119, 1988.

Lockhart JL, Sherrel F, Weinstein D, et al: Urodynamics in women with stress and urge incontinence, *Urology* 20:333, 1982.

Low JA, Mauger GM, Drajovic J: Diagnosis of the unstable detrusor: comparison of an incremental and continuous infusion technique, *Obstet Gynecol* 65:99, 1985.

Mayo ME: Detrusor hyperreflexia: the effect of posture and pelvic floor activity, *J Urol* 119:635, 1978.

Ouslander J, Leach G, Abelson S, et al: Simple versus multichannel cystometry in the evaluation of bladder function in an incontinent geriatric population, *J Urol* 140:1482, 1988.

Sutherst JR, Brown MC: Comparison of single and multichannel cystometry in diagnosing bladder instability, *Br Med J* 288:1720, 1984.

Turner-Warwick RT: Some clinical aspects of detrusor dysfunction, *J Urol* 113:539, 1975.

Webster GE, Older RA: The value of subtracted bladder pressure measurements in routine urodynamic studies, *Urology* 16:656, 1980.

Treatment-Behavioral

Burgio KL, Whitehead WE, Engel BT: Urinary incontinence in the elderly: bladder-sphincter biofeedback and toileting skills training, *Ann Intern Med* 103:507, 1985.

Cardozo LD, Abrams PD, Stanton SL, et al: Idiopathic bladder instability treated by biofeedback, *Br J Urol* 50:512, 1978.

Cardozo LD, Stanton SL: Biofeedback: a 5-year review, *Br J Urol* 56:220, 1984.

Cardozo LD, Stanton SL, Hafner J, et al: Biofeedback in the treatment of detrusor instability, *Br J Urol* 50:250, 1978.

Fantl JA, Hurt WG, Dunn LJ: Detrusor instability syndrome: the use of bladder retraining drills with and without anticholinergics, *Am J Obstet Gynecol* 140:885, 1981.

Ferrie BG, Smith JS, Logan D, et al: Experience with bladder training in 65 patients, *Br J Urol* 56:482, 1984.

Freeman RM, Baxby K: Hypnotherapy for incontinence caused by the unstable detrusor, *Br Med J* 284:1831, 1982.

Frewen WK: A reassessment of bladder training in detrusor dysfunction in the female, *Br J Urol* 54:372, 1982.

Frewen WK: Role of bladder training in the treatment of the unstable bladder in the female, *Urol Clin North Am* 6:273, 1979.

Hadley EC: Bladder training and related therapies for urinary incontinence in older people, *JAMA* 256:372, 1986.

Hafner RJ, Stanton SL, Guy J: A psychiatric study of women with urgency and urgency incontinence, *Br J Urol* 49:211, 1977.

Jarvis GJ: A controlled trial of bladder drill and drug therapy in the management of detrusor instability, *Br J Urol* 53:565, 1981.

MacCaulay AJ, Stern RS, Holmes DM, et al: Micturition and the mind: psychological factors in the aetiology and treatment of urinary symptoms in women, *Br Med J* 294:540, 1987.

Millard RJ, Oldenburg BF: The symptomatic, urodynamic, and

psychodynamic results of bladder re-education programs, *J Urol* 130:715, 1983.

Pengelly AW, Booth CM: A prospective trial of bladder training as treatment of detrusor instability, *Br J Urol* 52:463, 1980.

Treatment-Functional Electrical Stimulation

Bent AE, Sand PK, Ostergard DR: Transvaginal electrical stimulation in the treatment of genuine stress incontinence and detrusor instability, *Neurourol Urodyn* 8:363, 1989.

Eriksen BC, Bergmann S, Eik-Nes SH: Maximal electrostimulation of the pelvic floor in female idiopathic detrusor instability and urge incontinence, *Neurourol Urodyn* 8:219, 1989.

Fall M: Does electrostimulation cure urinary incontinence? *J Urol* 131:664, 1984.

Fall M, Ahlstrom K, Carlsson C, et al: Contelle: pelvic floor stimulation for female stress-urge incontinence: a multicenter study, *Urology* 27:282, 1986.

Fossberg E: Urge incontinence treated with maximal electrical stimulation, *Neurourol Urodyn* 7:270, 1988.

Leach GE, Bavendam TG: Prospective evaluation of the Incontan transrectal stimulator in women with urinary incontinence, *Neurourol Urodyn* 8:231, 1989.

McGuire EJ, Shi-Chun Z, Horwinski R, et al: Treatment of motor and sensory detrusor instability by electrical stimulation, *J Urol* 129:78. 1983.

Merrill D: The treatment of detrusor incontinence by electrical stimulation, *J Urol* 122:515, 1979.

Plevnik S, Janez J: Maximal electrical stimulation for urinary incontinence. Report of 98 cases, *Urology* 14:638, 1979.

Plevnik S, Janez J, Vrtenik P, et al: Short-term electrical stimulation: home treatment for urinary incontinence, *World J Urol* 4:24, 1986.

Treatment-Drug Therapy

Andersen JR, Lose G, Norgaard M, et al: Terodiline, emepronium bromide, or placebo for treatment of female detrusor overactivity? A randomized, double-blind, cross-over study, *Br J Urol* 61:310, 1988.

Barker G, Clenning PP: Treatment of the unstable bladder with propantheline and imipramine, *Aust NZ J Obstet Gynaecol* 27:152, 1987.

Blaivas JG, Labib KB, Michalik SJ, et al: Cystometric response to propantheline in detrusor hyperreflexia: therapeutic implications, *J Urol* 124:259, 1980.

Briggs RS, Castleden CM, Asher MJ: The effect of flavoxate on uninhibited detrusor contractions and urinary incontinence in the elderly, *J Urol* 123:665, 1980.

Brooks ME, Braf ZF: Oxybutynin chloride (Ditropan) — clinical uses and limitations, *Paraplegia* 18:64, 1980.

Cardozo LD, Stanton SL: An objective comparison of the effects of parenterally administered drugs in patients suffering from detrusor instability, *J Urol* 122:58, 1979.

Cardozo LD, Stanton SL, Robinson H, et al: Evaluation of flur-

biprofen in detrusor instability, *Br Med J* 280:281, 1980.

Cardozo LD, Stanton SL: A comparison between bromocriptine and indomethacin in the treatment of detrusor instability, *J Urol* 123:399, 1980.

Castleden CM, Duffen CM, Gulati RS: Double-blind study of imipramine and placebo for incontinence due to bladder instability, *Age Aging* 15:299, 1986.

Diokno AC, Lapides J: Oxybutynin: a new drug with analgesic and anticholinergic properties, *J Urol* 108:307, 1977.

Farrar DJ, Osborne JL: The use of bromocriptine in the treatment of the unstable bladder, *Br J Urol* 48:235, 1976.

Finkbeiner AE, Bissada NK, Welch LT: Uropharmacology: part VI. Parasympathetic depressants, *Urology* 10:503, 1977.

Fischer-Rasmussen W, Korhonon M, Bossberg E, et al: Evaluation of long-term safety and clinical benefit of terodiline in women with urgency/urge incontinence: a multicentre study, *Scand J Urol Nephrol Suppl* 87:35, 1984.

Gajweski JB, Awad SA: Oxybutynin versus propantheline in patients with multiple sclerosis and detrusor hyperreflexia, *J Urol* 135:966, 1986.

Gruneberger A: Treatment of motor urge incontinence with clenbuterol and flavoxate hydrochloride, *Br J Obstet Gynaecol* 91:275, 1984.

Holmes DM, Montz FJ, Stanton SL: Oxybutynin versus propantheline in the management of detrusor instability. A patient-regulated variable dose trial, *Br J Obstet Gynaecol* 96:607, 1989.

Kohler FP, Morales P: Cystometric evaluation of flavoxate hydrochloride in normal and neurogenic bladders, *J Urol* 100:729, 1968.

Levin RM, Staskin DR, Wein AJ: The muscarinic cholinergic binding kinetics of the human urinary bladder, *Neurourol Urodyn* 1:221, 1982.

Macfarlane JR, Tolley D: The effect of terodiline on patients with detrusor instability, *Scand J Urol Nephrol Suppl* 87:51, 1984.

Massey JA, Abrams P: Dose titration in clinical trials. An example using emepronium carrageenate in detrusor instability, *Br J Urol* 58:125, 1986.

Molsey CV, Stephenson TP, Brendler CB: The urodynamic and subjective results of treatment of detrusor instability with oxybutynin chloride, *Br J Urol* 52:472, 1980.

Stanton SL: A comparison of emepronium bromide and flavoxate hydrochloride in the treatment of urinary incontinence, *J Urol* 110:529, 1973.

Tapp A, Fall M, Norgaard J, et al: Terodiline: a dose-titrated, multicenter study of the treatment of idiopathic detrusor instability in women, *J Urol* 142:1027, 1989.

Thompson IM, Lauvetz R: Oxybutynin in bladder spasm, neurogenic bladder, and enuresis, *Urology* 8:452, 1976.

Ulmsten U, Ekman G, Andersson KE: The effect of terodiline treatment in women with motor urge incontinence. Results from a double-blind study and long-term treatment, *Am J Obstet Gynecol* 153:619, 1985.

Wein AJ: Drug therapy for detrusor instability: where are we? *Neurourol Urodyn* 4:337, 1985.

Treatment-Surgery

Awad SA, Flood HD, Acker KL, et al: Selective sacral cryoneurolysis in the treatment of patients with detrusor instability/hyperreflexia and hypersensitive bladder, *Neurourol Urodyn* 6:307, 1987.

Blackford HN, Murray K, Stephenson TP, et al: Results of transvesical infiltration of the pelvic plexuses with phenol in 116 patients, *Br J Urol* 56:647, 1984.

Clarke SJ, Forster DM, Thomas DG: Selective sacral neurectomy in the management of urinary incontinence due to detrusor instability, *Br J Urol* 51:510, 1979.

Delaere KPJ, Debruyne FMJ, Michiels HGE, et al: Prolonged bladder distention in the management of the unstable bladder, *J Urol* 124, 334, 1980.

Ewing R, Bultitude MI, Shuttleworth KED: Subtrigonal phenol injection for urge incontinence secondary to detrusor instability in females, *Br J Urol* 54:689, 1982.

Ingelman-Sundberg A: Urge incontinence in women, *Acta Obstet Gynecol Scand* 54:153, 1975.

Ingelman-Sundberg A: Partial bladder denervation for detrusor dyssynergia, *Clin Obstet Gynecol* 21:797, 1978.

Lucas MG, Thomas DG, Clarke S, et al: Long-term follow-up of selective sacral neurectomy, *Br J Urol* 61:218, 1988.

McGuire EJ, Savastano JA: Urodynamic findings and clinical status following vesical denervation procedures for control of incontinence, *J Urol* 132:87, 1981.

Mundy AR: The surgical treatment of urge incontinence of urine, *J Urol* 128:481, 1982.

Mundy AR: Long-term results of bladder transection for urge incontinence, *Br J Urol* 55:642, 1983.

Mundy AR: The surgical treatment of detrusor instability, *Neurourol Urodyn* 4:352, 1985.

Mundy AR, Stephenson TP: "Clam" ileocystoplasty for the treatment of refractory urge incontinence, *Br J Urol* 57:641, 1985.

Opsomer RJ, Klarskov P, Holm-Bentzen M, et al: Long-term results of superselective sacral nerve resection for motor urge incontinence, *Scand J Urol Nephrol* 18:101, 1984.

Rosenbaum TP, Shah PJR, Worth PHL: Trans-trigonal phenol — the end of an era? *Neurourol Urodyn* 7:294, 1988.

Torrens MJ: The role of denervation in the treatment of detrusor instability, *Neurourol Urodyn* 4:353, 1985.

Turner-Warwick RT, Ashken MH: The functional results of partial, subtotal and total cystoplasty with special reference to ureterocaecocystoplasty, selective sphincterotomy, and cystocystoplasty, *Br J Urol* 39:3, 1967.

Wall LL, Stanton SL: Transvesical phenol injection of pelvic nerve plexuses in females with refractory urge incontinence, *Br J Urol* 63:465, 1989.

Mixed Incontinence

Karram MM, Bhatia NN: Management of coexistent stress and urge urinary incontinence, *Obstet Gynecol* 73:4, 1989.

Lockhart JL, Vorstman B, Politano VA: Anti-incontinence surgery in females with detrusor instability, *Neurourol Urodyn* 3:201, 1984.

McGuire EJ, Lytton B, Kohorn E, et al: The value of urodynamic testing in stress urinary incontinence, *J Urol* 124:256, 1980.

McGuire EJ, Savastano JA: Stress incontinence and detrusor instability/urge incontinence, *Neurourol Urodyn* 4:313, 1985.

McGuire EJ: Bladder instability and stress incontinence, *Neurourol Urodyn* 7:563, 1988.

CHAPTER **20**

Frequency, Urgency, and Painful Bladder Syndromes

Mickey M. Karram

Urethral Syndrome
    Etiology
    Diagnosis
    Treatment
Sensory Urgency
    Etiology
    Diagnosis
    Management
Interstitial Cystitis
    Etiology
    Diagnosis
    Treatment
    Surgical methods

Frequency, urgency, and other irritative bladder symptoms, in the absence of obvious pathology or infection, are frequently encountered in gynecologic and urologic practices. A wide spectrum of disease may be present in such a patient. These diseases may vary from very mild symptoms which require only reassurance and behavior modification, to extremely distressing symptoms, which require radical surgical therapy. When obvious pathology has been ruled out, these symptoms have historically been categorized under one of three categories: urethral syndrome, sensory urgency, and early stages of interstitial cystitis. These conditions are poorly understood and poorly

defined; their etiology remains obscure and therapy is empiric and erratic. Whether these conditions are various forms of the same disease or truly separate entities is currently unknown. With these caveats in mind, the following is a review of the literature on these conditions.

URETHRAL SYNDROME

There is no universally accepted definition for the urethral syndrome, and it is probably best to regard it as a diagnosis of exclusion. The term *urethral syndrome* has been used to describe a symptom complex that can include dysuria, frequency, urgency, suprapubic discomfort, and voiding difficulties in the absence of any objective findings of urethral or bladder abnormalities. It has been estimated that these lower urinary tract symptoms account for approximately 5 million office visits per year in the United States.

Etiology

The etiology of this condition is controversial. Popular hypotheses have included infection, urethral obstruction, urethral spasm, and hypoestrogenism, as well as psychogenic, neurologic, traumatic, and allergic causes.

Because infection is thought by many to be the most important etiologic agent of the urethral syndrome, it has been studied the most thoroughly. Most proponents of an infectious etiology base their arguments on the following:

1. The traditional criterion used in interpreting a urinary culture has been the presence of growth greater than or equal to 10^5 bacteria/ml. It is now well appreciated that 20% to 40% of women with lower urinary tract infection-like symptoms can have as little as 10^2 bacteria/ml.

2. Routine urine cultures do not reveal the presence of fastidious organisms and other noncoliform bacteria. These organisms require special collection, culturing, and incubation techniques for detection and identification.

3. Some investigators have speculated that the posterior urethra may be a site of infection because the short female urethra is surrounded by dense arborizing paraurethral glands. However, microbiologic substantiation of bacteria in the urethra is difficult.

Stamm et al (1980) have presented the best evidence to support the role of infection in urethral syndrome. These authors noted the presence of *Chlamydia trachomatis* in 11 of 59 women with acute urethral syndrome. These 11 women constituted more than one third of patients with urethral syndrome and sterile urine. Furthermore, 10 of the patients had pyuria (≥ 8 leukocytes/mm^3). Thus almost two thirds of patients with sterile pyuria had chlamydial infection, which suggests that chlamydia organisms may be an important cause of urethral syndrome in some populations.

Several other organisms have also been proposed as potential pathogens, including lactobacilli, *Staphylococcus saprophyticus*, corynebacteria, as well as other fastidious organisms such as *Ureaplasma urealyticum* and *Mycoplasma hominis*. However, data to substantiate correlation between clinical symptoms and the presence of these organisms are lacking. When Gillespie et al compared 41 patients diagnosed as having urethral syndrome to 42 control patients, no difference in the incidence of infection caused by *C. trachomatis*, lactobacilli, or other fastidious organisms was found. The number of leukocytes in urine was also similar in both groups.

In addition, it has been stated empirically that the urethral syndrome is secondary to an infectious etiol-

ogy due to the endoscopic subjective findings of urethritis and pseudomembranous trigonitis. These observations, however, have never been substantiated in any controlled trials. Furthermore, because these findings are not present in all individuals having urethral syndrome or in all patients with true bacterial cystitis, their significance is obscure. Finally, follow-up endoscopy to document their disappearance in patients who do improve has not been reported. When not artifactual, these endoscopic findings are of interest; however, they hardly support the concept of an inflammatory infectious etiology.

Spasms of the external urethral sphincter has also been postulated as a potential cause of the urethral syndrome. Three groups of investigators have reported results of this finding. Each group suggested that multiple factors may be responsible for these observations, including a functional etiology in many patients. Gratifying responses to therapy with diazepam, electrical stimulation, behavior modification, and biofeedback do little to support a true neurogenic etiology as opposed to a psychogenic etiology. Urodynamic studies in these patients present a picture that can be produced voluntarily in the neurologically intact individual and thus provide meager evidence to support an underlying neurogenic etiology.

Other evidence supports a psychogenic etiology for urethral syndrome. This theory is supported by higher scores of hysteria and hypochondriasis on Minnesota Multiphasic Personality Inventory (MMPI) in patients with urethral syndrome when compared with scores of age-matched control subjects (Carson et al). It has not yet been established, however, whether these findings are contributory or merely a consequence of an organic disease.

Early investigators supported the idea of obstruction secondary to stenosis of the urethra as a cause of urethral syndrome. However, the criteria for diagnosing urethral stenosis are inconsistent, histologic studies claiming to document periurethral fibrosis are not reproducible, and finally mechanical calibration of this ordinarily collapsible tube may be more a measure of distensibility than true resistance to flow.

Hypoestrogenism can be an etiologic factor in postmenopausal women with lower urinary tract dysfunction. The urethra is embryologically derived from the urogenital sinus, and its lower two thirds are covered by stratified squamous epithelium. Studies have shown that estrogen supplementation in postmenopausal women can decrease the symptoms of urgency as well as those of dysuria and frequency. Studies have also shown that senile urethritis is a definite diagnostic entity. Exfoliative cytologic studies in patients before and after estrogen therapy show a maturation change from transitional to intermediate squamous epithelium.

Diagnosis

Because the diagnosis of urethral syndrome is one of exclusion, a fairly extensive work-up is at times necessary. A thorough history is important. As previously mentioned, common complaints are frequency, urgency, dysuria, and suprapubic pressure. Other less frequent symptoms include bladder or vaginal pain, urinary incontinence, postvoid fullness, and dyspareunia. The patient should be questioned about the onset and duration of symptoms as well as about any provoking factors such as sexual intercourse. It is also helpful to obtain a urolog in which the patient keeps a record of fluid intake as well as frequency and amount of both daytime and nighttime voidings.

A general physical and neurologic examination should be performed with emphasis on examination of the back and confirmation of normal sensory and motor function. A local neurologic examination to obtain an anal reflex should document that the S-2, 3, 4 sacral spinal cord segments are intact. Examination to assess any anatomic abnormalities including the presence of significant pelvic relaxation, urethral hymenal fusion, and urethral caruncle should be performed in addition to bimanual examination to rule out pelvic masses. A catheterized urine specimen should always be obtained to rule out lower urinary tract infection. Urethral and cervical cultures for chlamydia should be obtained if the patient is sexually active or has sterile pyuria. Other wet smears and cultures of the vaginal area also should be performed as indicated.

Cystourethroscopy

The purpose of an endoscopic evaluation is to rule out diseases of similar symptomatology, since the obser-vation of urethral and trigonal erythema is not diagnostic of this condition. Because interstitial cystitis is likely to be the source of lower irritative symptoms in the presence of sterile cytologically unremarkable urine, it is probably best to perform an endoscopic examination under full anesthesia. This will also allow the performance of urethral and bladder biopsies if indicated. Other conditions that need to be ruled out include urethral and bladder diverticula and premalignant and malignant lesions of the bladder.

Urodynamic Studies

A cystometric evaluation is helpful in patients who have significant frequency and urgency. If the patient can comfortably be filled to normal bladder capacity and has normal bladder compliance, the conditions of detrusor instability, interstitial cystitis, and sensory urgency can be excluded. Uroflowmetry is a simple noninvasive test that can be performed to objectively confirm symptoms of voiding dysfunction. Should this instrumentation be unavailable, the average flow rate can be determined by dividing the amount voided by the time taken to void. Normal flow ratio should be greater than 15 mm/second. The total volume should be voided within 20 seconds, and the volume voided should be no less than 150 ml to preserve the accuracy of this test.

Psychiatric Testing

We do not routinely obtain a psychiatric evaluation unless we infer that symptoms are related to emotionally charged events. If MMPI studies are obtained, they should be backed up with sophisticated interpretation and a psychiatric interview.

Treatment

Many different forms of therapy have been advocated for the urethral syndrome. Because the etiology is obscure, no single therapy has been universally effective. We believe these patients are best divided into two groups. The first group consists of those patients whose symptoms are thought due to an infectious etiology. These are patients who, on urine culture, may have infection with less than 10^5 bacteria/ml or patients who have sterile pyuria. Patients who are noted to have urinary tract infection with a low bacteria count should be appropriately treated with antibiotics, based on sensitivity reports. If the patient is young and sexually active and has sterile pyuria or is suspected of having a chlamydia infection, a 10-day course of tetracycline should be given. Stamm et al (1981) published a double-blind, randomized trial comparing the efficacy of doxycycline versus placebo in the treatment of acute urethral syndrome. Sixty-two women completed the study, and overall, doxycycline was significantly more effective than placebo in subjectively improving the symptoms of dysuria and frequency. If symptoms are not improved and pyuria is not relieved, the second-line drug is erythromycin. Maskell et al have found this antibiotic to be active against most of the anaerobes that can be responsible for this disease as well as chlamydia and ureaplasma. If symptoms are still not relieved or if pyuria persists, a more detailed work-up for sterile pyuria must be undertaken, which eliminates causes such as microbacterial infections, stones, or tumors.

Some data support the continuous long-term use of low-dose antimicrobial prophylaxis in patients with these symptoms and a documented history of recurrent urinary tract infections. Kraft and Stamey in 1977 showed that some patients with a recurrent bacteriuria occasionally will experience irritable voiding symptoms when their urine is uninfected and then develop documented bacteriuria within several months.

If no infectious etiology is documented or suspected, patients must be individualized. We believe that all postmenopausal patients, whether or not they have objective evidence of estrogen deficiency, should be given a trial of local estrogen therapy. We prefer to start the patient on a form of estrogen vaginal cream (2 g/day) for approximately 8 weeks, followed by continuous oral estrogen.

If no improvement is noted after antimicrobial therapy, estrogen therapy, or both, the clinician is faced with a therapeutic dilemma. Our next line of therapy is to perform successive urethral dilations in conjunction with anterior vaginal wall massage (Fig. 20-1). The rationale for this mode of therapy is that the dilators are rigid instruments with which obstructed, inflamed, or infected urethral glands may be massaged through the anterior vaginal wall. In a recent study by Bergman et al in which 60 patients with a diagnosis

of urethral syndrome were randomly assigned to receive either placebo (20 patients), a 10-day course of tetracycline (20 patients), or three successive urethral dilations (20 patients), a 75% subjective improvement was noted in the urethral-dilation group. This cure rate was significantly higher than that in both placebo and tetracycline-treated groups. An objective improvement in uroflowmetry occurred only in the group treated with serial urethral dilation. Recently, Rutherford et al published data showing that cystoscopy alone was as effective as cystoscopy plus urethral dilation in the treatment of women with recurrent frequency and dysuria.

Numerous other modes of therapy have also been advocated. These treatments include nonsurgical modes of therapy in the form of biofeedback, psychotherapy, antiinflammatory agents, and bladder instillations including dimethylsulfoxide (DMSO) and silver nitrate. Reports of results with anticholinergics, alpha-adrenergic blockers, and skeletal muscle relaxants suggest that these drugs control the underlying urodynamic abnormalities previously described. Kaplan et al and Schmidt and Tanagho used skeletal muscle relaxants or electrostimulation combined with biofeedback techniques (women were shown uroflow and electromyographic [EMG] studies) and noted dramatic improvement in almost all patients.

More invasive therapy has included various forms of surgery to eliminate urethral stenosis, fulgurations, scarification, resection, and cryosurgical procedures. Reported results with each modality vary. The major problems with the studies are the use of nonrigid criteria to determine diagnosis and a too brief or unreported therapeutic response and duration of follow-up. Nonetheless, a large retrospective study performed by Carson et al and a prospective series by Mabry et al demonstrated 30% to 60% of patients undergoing surgical treatment experience improvement.

The most impressive findings of all these studies was that the best results (85% in Carson et al and 100% in Zufall [1978]) occurred in patients managed by observation only. Although these women probably had milder symptoms than those undergoing specific therapy, high rates of spontaneous remission must be considered in evaluating results of any treatment.

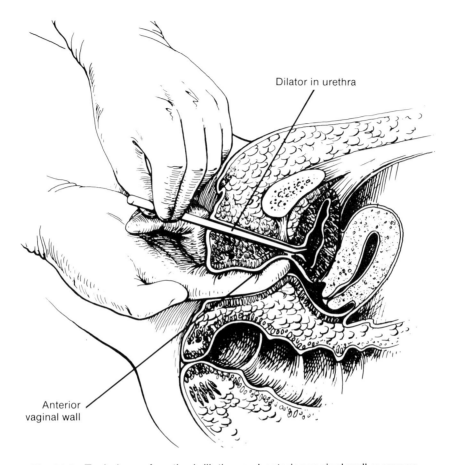

Dilator in urethra

Anterior
vaginal wall

Fig. 20-1 Technique of urethral dilation and anterior vaginal wall massage.

In conclusion, treatment for this condition should always be oriented initially toward a conservative approach, as it is usually as effective as surgery, far less expensive, and less subject to risk.

SENSORY URGENCY

The International Continence Society defines urgency as a strong desire to void accompanied by a fear of leakage or a fear of pain. This fear may be associated with two types of dysfunction. Urgency with cystometric evidence of an overactive detrusor muscle is termed *motor urgency,* whereas urgency that occurs at abnormally low volumes during filling cystometry without objective evidence of detrusor overactivity is

thought to be due to a hypersensitive detrusor and is thus termed *sensory urgency.* The problem with this definition is that there are no agreed upon, standardized cystometric parameters to differentiate normal sensation from hypersensation. Jarvis et al defined their group of patients with frequency and painful urgency using urodynamic criteria as abnormal if a first sensation of filling occurred at less than 75 ml of saline and maximum cystometric capacity was less than 400 ml in the presence of a stable detrusor. It has been empirically stated that a normal first sensation of filling should occur at 50 to 150 ml with a first urge to void at between 200 and 300 ml and maximum capacity between 400 and 700 ml. Because these values are based on a subjective response from a patient during an unphysiologic testing session, however, it is difficult to define absolute cystometric parameters.

For the same reasons the incidence of sensory urgency is unclear. One study noted a 6% incidence in 558 patients with incontinence and other symptoms who underwent cystometry.

Etiology

Little is known about the etiology of this condition. The aspect of sensory urgency that has been studied most is psychologic origin. Hafner et al noted that psychotherapy resulted in considerable improvement in one third of 26 patients. They also noted that during all the interviews, no patient left the room because of urgency. In a study of a mixed group of patients, MacCaulay et al found that patients with sensory urgency were more anxious than those with genuine stress incontinence. Although those with detrusor instability were equally anxious, the sensory urgency patients scored higher on hysteria scales.

Frewen has proposed that frequency and urgency possibly initiate detrusor instability rather than being symptoms due to the condition. Jarvis, on the other hand, has noted that sensory urgency does not always progress to detrusor instability, nor is detrusor instability invariably proceeded by sensory urgency. It has also been proposed that this is an early form of interstitial cystitis, even though current histologic investigations performed for this condition are negative.

Diagnosis

After performing a detailed history and general physical and neurologic examinations to rule out any systemic or neurologic illnesses to explain the patient's lower urinary tract dysfunction, the patient should record a 3-day to 1-week urinary diary. This diary is useful to corroborate the patient's symptoms by giving an objective measure of the diurnal and nocturnal frequency. The patient is requested to record her fluid intake and measure her urinary output. She is also instructed to note any episodes of incontinence or urgency. After this diary is reviewed, simple factors such as excessive fluid intake can be easily managed.

The patient should then undergo a cystometric eval-

uation to confirm the diagnosis. Sensory urgency should be considered a cystometric diagnosis even though the parameters of normality have not been fully agreed upon. Our criteria are more stringent than Jarvis' criteria. We have used a maximum cystometric capacity of less than 300 ml in the absence of any rise in true detrusor activity to define the condition of sensory urgency. Once the condition has been diagnosed on cystometry, cystoscopy under general anesthesia with biopsies of any suspicious area should be performed to rule out interstitial cystitis premalignant or malignant lesions, and any other intravesical pathology that could be producing the patient's symptoms.

Although used in Europe, urethral electric conductance (UEC), originally described by Plevnik et al, has obtained little popularity in the United States. The test relies on urothelium and urine having different electric impedance. The test is performed by using a specially designed conductivity catheter that can be used to detect opening of the bladder neck. The conductivity catheter is a 7 French silastic catheter with two gold-plated brass electrodes 1 mm apart and 1 mm mounted near the tip. A nonstimulatory current of 20 mV is applied across the electrodes and the conductivity recorded in microamps (μA) on a UEC catheter. The conductivity measurements are made with the patient lying supine with 250 ml normal saline in the bladder and the UEC catheter placed to record at the bladder neck mechanism. Using this technique the maximum deflection at rest (MDR) can be measured. When this test was performed in asymptomatic patients and compared to those with sensory urgency, the MDR had a much lower range in asymptomatic patients than in those with sensory urgency. A level of 36 μA distinguished the symptomatic from the asymptomatic group, with a highly significant difference between the value of MDR.

Management

The variety of types of therapy that have been proposed for the management of this condition indicates the lack of knowledge regarding the etiology. In addition, because no standard objective method of diagnosis exists, one must view therapies cautiously.

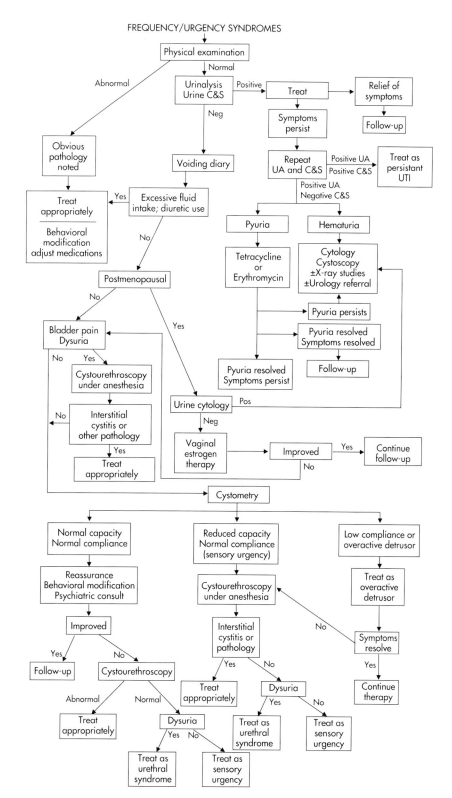

Fig. 20-2 Algorithm for diagnosis and management of frequency/urgency syndromes.

Management areas studied include certain drug therapies, as well as bladder drill, psychotherapy, biofeedback, and electrical stimulation.

Drug studies have included studies using anticholinergic drugs as well as bromocriptine and sedatives. Propantheline was studied in a mixed group of patients with detrusor instability and sensory urgency who were randomly allocated to one of three groups. Those given propantheline 15 mg three times a day for 3 months showed a modest improvement in frequency of micturition. In a group of 20 patients with sensory urgency, Klarskov et al compared terodiline and bladder drill to placebo and bladder drill in a double blind cross-over comparison. Treatment was given for a 3-week period with a 1-week washout before the cross-over. A significant decrease in urinary frequency and number of episodes of incontinence occurred in the terodiline-treated group. On urodynamic testing, bladder capacity and first sensation of filling both increased. After terodiline was withdrawn, 30% of the patients had a relapse of symptoms.

Since bromocriptine has been reported to produce symptomatic relief in bladder instability, O'Boyle and Parsons performed a double-blind randomized cross-over trial of bromocriptine against placebo in 14 patients with primary vesical sensory urgency. No therapeutic advantage was noted with bromocriptine over placebo.

Frewen (1972) reported that treatment by sedation and anticholinergic drugs was efficacious in both cases of urgency of micturition and urgency incontinence. He reported on 100 patients treated with emepronium and diazepam. At the end of 1 year, 80 patients were continent but half of these had some residual urgency. Elder and Stephenson used the same regimen and reported a 50% success over a 3-year period. In a mixed group of 65 women with detrusor instability and sensory urgency, Ferrie et al used the Frewen technique combining sedation with anticholinergic therapy as well as bladder retraining. In those with sensory urgency, favorable results were reported, prompting the authors to suggest that this regimen should be the primary treatment for sensory urgency.

A recommended algorithm for the diagnosis and management of frequency/urgency syndromes is shown in Fig. 20-2.

INTERSTITIAL CYSTITIS

Interstitial cystitis is one of the most disabling nonmalignant conditions encountered in medicine. It is an enigmatic condition of unknown etiology and confused management, which was initially described by Skene in 1887.

Secondary to poor diagnostic criteria, it is difficult to estimate the true incidence of this condition. The prevalence of diagnosed interstitial cystitis in the United States is currently estimated at 20,000 to 90,000 cases, with as many as five times that number undiagnosed. Interstitial cystitis occurs much more frequently in women than men, with a predominance of about 10:1. Although this condition can be seen in women of all ages, including young girls, the majority of patients are between 40 and 60 years of age.

Etiology

Although interstitial cystitis has been recognized for many years, the etiology remains obscure. A number of potential causes have been postulated, but none have been conclusively proven. Infection, lymphatic obstruction, psychosomatic dysfunction, neurogenic disorders, and allergic and autoimmune etiologies have all been investigated. Currently, the most accepted theory is autoimmune. This theory is supported by the presence of deposits of various immunoglobulins in the mucosa and submucosa of interstitial cystitis bladders and the presence of antibladder antibodies in the serum of patients with interstitial cystitis. There are two types of autoimmune disease: organ-specific, such as thyroiditis, and nonorgan-specific, such as systemic lupus erythematosus. Interstitial cystitis falls between these two types by being organ-specific with no organ-specific antibodies.

Several features of interstitial cystitis are common to other autoimmune diseases: (1) 90% of patients are female; (2) there is an increased incidence of systemic lupus, rheumatoid arthritis, polyarteritis nodosa, scleroderma, and autoimmune thyroiditis in patients with interstitial cystitis; (3) allergies to drugs occur in these patients in 20% to 70% of cases; (4) a positive antinuclear antibody is detected in 50% to 85% of patients; (5) histologic changes in the bladder include infiltration of lymphocytes, plasma cells, mast cells, and eosinophils in varying degrees, which are all consistent with connective tissue disease; and (6) most therapies to treat autoimmune disease have at some time been used to treat interstitial cystitis with varying degrees of success. Recent data by Anderson et al, however, have shed doubt on an autoimmune process being responsible for this condition, as they found antibladder antibodies in 75% of patients with interstitial cystitis and in 40% of controls. The difference was not statistically significant. Furthermore, they made the point that if an autoimmune response directed against bladder tissue were responsible for the disease, the relief of all symptoms after urinary diversion without cystectomy would not be expected nor would the recurrence of interstitial cystitis-like lesion in the intestinal segments of patients who had undergone augmentation cystoplasty. They believe that the immunologic changes represent a response to tissue damage due to some other mechanism.

The detection of antibodies both in the serum and in bladder biopsies from patients with interstitial cystitis probably means we are measuring a degree of injury to the bladder. A similar development of autoantibodies to epithelium occurs after burns to the skin. Whatever the cause, interstitial cystitis produces a chronic inflammatory state with a mixed cellular infiltrate of macrophages and plasma cells. Thus it is speculated that this process is responsible for the subsequent damage to the bladder and activation of the immune system in a manner analogous to inflammatory changes elsewhere in the body. If the autoimmune system does play a role in interstitial cystitis, it may be either a primary role that causes the condition or a secondary response to a local inflammation.

Another theory proposed by Parsons et al is that these patients have a dysfunctional epithelium that does not remain impermeable. This defect potentially permits urinary constituents to diffuse into subepithelial tissues. They have created this defective epithelium by using protamine sulfate to impair bladder surface impermeability in normal subjects. The impaired epithelium leaked urea and caused marked urgency and frequency. No one knows why epithelial leaks occur. An autoimmune phenomenon, inflammatory mediators, or an undefined viral problem have all been proposed.

Diagnosis

Diagnosis is based on a typical symptom complex, characteristic cystoscopic findings, and histologic evaluation of biopsy specimens.

The typical presentation has been described as an irritable bladder in an irritable patient. Symptoms, which are commonly severe and disabling, include diurnal and nocturnal frequency, as well as urgency, dysuria, hematuria, and suprapubic or perineal pain partially relieved by voiding. A recent study has also noted that these patients suffer from psychic helplessness, inadequacy in coping with problems, and sexual problems. The severity of symptoms can be quite varied and does not necessarily correlate with cystoscopic findings. The onset of the disease is often acute, mimicking urinary tract infection, and many of these patients will have received several courses of antibiotics before being diagnosed.

Physical examination is generally normal, although some investigators have described anterior vaginal wall tenderness on pelvic examination. Urinalysis may demonstrate microhematuria without pyuria or may be completely normal. Urine cytologic studies are invariably normal.

Cystometric studies usually reveal decreased bladder capacity secondary to severe pain. Early in the disease, bladder compliance is normal but as bladder wall fibrosis sets in, small intravesical volumes may produce abnormally high intravesical pressure.

Radiologic contrast studies play very little if any part in the diagnosis of interstitial cystitis. However, they are useful in excluding other lower urinary tract pathology.

Cystoscopy is the most important diagnostic measure. Because the functional bladder capacity is frequently limited by severe discomfort, cystoscopy under local anesthesia may not demonstrate any gross abnormalities and should thus be performed under general anesthesia to demonstrate the typical mucosal abnormalities. The bladder should initially be distended at 70 cm H_2O pressure and then emptied and distended a second time. The early findings of interstitial cystitis include submucosal hemorrhages and linear cracking of the mucosa. Glomerulation and fine trabeculation of the bladder wall may be seen with linear mucosal scarring in more advanced disease. The classic Hunner's ulcer is rarely seen and is by no means essential to make the diagnosis. The box below reviews early and late cystoscopic findings in patients with interstitial cystitis.

Although the diagnosis of interstitial cystitis is made on the basis of symptomatology and cystoscopic finding, bladder biopsies should be performed to exclude other conditions such as carcinoma in situ, tuberculosis, schistosomiasis (bilharziasis), radiation cystitis, and chronic infectious cystitis. To date no evidence suggests that interstitial cystitis is a prema lignant condition.

The histologic appearances of interstitial cystitis are nonspecific. The most consistent features are submucosal edema and vasodilation. There are varying degrees of fibrosis in the mucosa with infiltration by round cells as well as plasma cells and eosinophils. It has been proposed that the mast cell count is increased and in severe cases, large areas of epithelium are lost. Some think that a histologic estimation of the mast cells present in the detrusor muscle is of value in establishing the diagnosis.

A recent workshop sponsored by the National Institute of Arthritis, Diabetes, Digestive and Kidney Diseases published its concensus criteria for the diagnosis of interstitial cystitis (see accompanying box).

Treatment

Because the etiology of this condition is uncertain, treatment is empiric, difficult, and unsatisfactory; and a myriad of various treatments have been reported (see accompanying box). Oral drugs have been used very extensively. Proponents of the autoimmune etiology have used steroids and azathioprine, reporting successful results in approximately 50% of patients. Other drugs have been used with varying degrees of success, including anticholinergics, antispasmodics, nonsteroidal antiinflammatories, tranquilizers, and narcotics. More recently oral sodium pentosanpoly-

---

Most Common Cystoscopic Findings in Interstitial Cystitis

Early

1. Petechial submucosal hemorrhage (glomerulations)
2. Splotchy hemorrhages
3. Bloody drainage of fluid

Late

1. Decreased bladder capacity
2. Fissures, linear scars
3. Hunner's ulcers

Consensus Criteria for Diagnosis of Interstitial Cystitis

Automatic exclusions:
  <18 years old
  Benign or malignant bladder tumors
  Radiation cystitis
  Tuberculous cystitis
  Bacterial cystitis
  Vaginitis
  Cyclophosphamide cystitis
  Symptomatic urethral diverticulum
  Uterine, cervical, vaginal, or urethral cancer
  Active herpes
  Bladder or lower ureteral calculi
  Waking frequency < 5 times in 12 hours
  Nocturia < 2 times
  Symptoms relieved by antibiotics, urinary antiseptics, urinary analgesics (for example, phenazopyridine hydrochloride)
  Duration < 12 months
  Involuntary bladder contractions (urodynamics)
  Capacity > 400 ml, absence of sensory urgency
Automatic inclusions:
  Hunner's ulcer
Positive factors:
  Pain on bladder filling relieved by emptying
  Pain (suprapubic, pelvic, urethral, vaginal, or perineal)
  Glomerulations on endoscopy
  Decreased compliance on cystometrogram

Bladder distention is defined arbitrarily as 80 cm H_2O pressure for 1 minute. Two positive factors are necessary for inclusion in the study population. Substratification at the conclusion of the study by bladder capacity with the patient under anesthesia was less than and greater than 350 ml.

sulfate has been described as an effective therapy for interstitial cystitis. This compound is a synthetic analog of a sulfonated glycosaminoglycan, which is the natural compound found on the inner surface of the bladder mucosa. In interstitial cystitis this protective mucin layer is lost, and the oral or intravesical administration of Elmiron has been shown to replace the protective surface mucin. A recent study by Parsons and Mulholland noted that when Elmiron was compared to placebo in a double-blind fashion there was significant improvement in subjective parameters (pain, urgency, frequency, and nocturia) as well as objective improvement in average voided volumes in the Elmiron-treated group.

Most patients with interstitial cystitis have at some stage during treatment had hydrostatic bladder distention. The probable mechanism is that prolonged distention produces detrusor ischemia, which results in degeneration of nerves within the bladder wall. The

---

Treatment Modalities for Interstitial Cystitis

I. NONSURGICAL
  A. Systemic Therapy
    • Immunosuppressives (corticosteroids, azathioprine)
    • Antihistamines
    • Antiinflammatories
    • Sodium pentosanpolysulfate
  B. Local Therapy
    • Bladder distention
    • Instillation therapy (DMSO, oxychlorosene sulfate, silver nitrate)
    • Functional electrical stimulation
II. SURGICAL
  A. Endoscopic Procedures
    • Transurethral resection and fulguration
    • Nd:YAG laser
  B. Open Surgical Treatment
    • Denervation procedures (presacral neurotomy, selective sacral neurectomy, cystolysis, etc.)
    • Bladder augmentation procedures
    • Urinary diversion

---

clinical response is often dramatic but not long-lived, probably as a result of axonal regeneration. Intravesical drugs have also been used. Oxychlorosene (Clorpactin) was first used by Wishard et al in 1957 who noted a subjective success rate of 70%. Another study, which had a 6-year follow-up, noted that the treatment continues to be effective, although further courses are usually needed. Clorpactin has also been associated with cystoscopic evidence of healing of the bladder lesions. Instillation of Clorpactin requires general anesthesia. One liter of 0.4% oxychlorocine is freshly prepared in the operating theater just before use. The patient is catheterized and the solution is instilled by infusion under a hydrostatic pressure of 10 cm H_2O until the bladder is full. The bladder is then emptied and installations are repeated until 1 liter of solution has been used. Usually, the second and third instillation are performed at 4-week intervals to allow urothelium to regenerate.

Dimethyl sulfoxide (DMSO) has also been shown to be useful in the treatment of interstitial cystitis. This method eliminates the need for general anesthesia. The patient is catheterized and 50 ml of 50% solution of DMSO is instilled into the bladder. This solution is retained for 15 to 30 minutes, after which the bladder is emptied by voiding. Treatment is given at 2 weekly intervals until symptomatic relief is obtained at which time the intervals between treatment are increased appropriately. This therapy to date has been thought to be simple, effective, and inexpensive, with symptomatic improvement in up to 70% of patients. A recent study, however, has looked at the in vitro effects of DMSO on bladder function. These experiments performed in rabbits noted a negative effect on multiple parameters including compliance, capacity, and contractile and functional responses to field stimulation. This study would seem to indicate that the symptomatic improvement provided by DMSO cannot be attributed to a beneficial effect on bladder function. It is more likely that the improvement noted with DMSO is related to its local anesthetic properties. This study also raises the issue of possible deleterious effects on the bladder, which may become clinically evident only after a prolonged time period.

Another noninvasive mode of therapy is electrical

stimulation. This therapy can be achieved by placing electrodes on the lower abdomen or transvaginally. Although a favorable response has been reported, it involves long-standing treatment, in some cases, up to 1.5 years.

Surgical Methods

Surgical methods of treatment should be reserved only to those resistant cases that have failed conservative therapy. These methods can be classified broadly into endoscopic or open surgeries. Endoscopically, ulcers may be fulgurated or resected. Although this technique is not recommended as the sole treatment, it may be helpful in some cases. More recently, some investigators have advocated the use of the Nd:YAG laser to treat affected areas. Shanberg et al reported on five patients who were followed for 3 to 15 months after laser therapy and who had no recurrent symptoms. Local injection of hydrocortisone, saline, and heparin in and around the ulcer has been reported to be helpful. The duration of remission with hydrocortisone is not known, but it can be repeated as many times as required.

Open surgery should be reserved as a last resort in patients who have not responded to other forms of therapy. The various methods include partial cystectomy, intestinal cystoplasty, cystolysis, and cystoplasty and urinary diversion with or without cystectomy. Webster and Maggio reported on 19 patients with interstitial cystitis symptoms intractable to conservative management who underwent supratrigonal cystectomy and substitution enterocystoplasty. Twelve were cured of the pain and frequency, four improved, and three failed to improve and underwent urinary diversion. Preoperative features did not predict outcome, although poor results occurred more often in those who, under anesthesia, had large bladder capacities and those who had postoperative voiding difficulty requiring self-catheterization.

Partial cystectomy alone is of limited value. It involves resection of the diseased part of the bladder, but there is no guarantee that the disease will not recur in the bladder remnant. It also results in a small bladder with its associated symptoms. The end stage of interstitial cystitis is often a contracted bladder, but this can be overcome by augmentation cystoplasty. If

the bladder is not contracted, some investigators have suggested cystolysis as the treatment of choice. In this procedure the bladder is freed from its surrounding tissues down to the trigone posteriorly by dividing the superior and ascending branches of inferior vesical nerves. This technique presumably divides most of the sensory pathways to the upper part of the bladder. Neurosurgical techniques to denervate the bladder have enjoyed some popularity. These include presacral neurectomy, postsacral rhizotomy, and anterior lateral cordotomy.

SUMMARY

Urethral syndrome, sensory urgency, and interstitial cystitis are poorly understood conditions. Whether they are truly separate entities or varying degrees and presentations of the same disease is unknown. Symptoms of frequency, urgency, and bladder pain in the absence of obvious infection represent therapeutic challenges for the practicing gynecologist and urologist. Until more is known about the pathogenesis of these conditions, treatment will remain empiric. These patients have distressing symptoms and thus require much time, information, and reassurance. Future research may lead to more objective diagnostic modalities and more effective treatment regimens.

REFERENCES

Urethral Syndrome

Bergman A, Karram MM, Bhatia NN: Urethral syndrome. A comparison of different treatment modalities, *J Reprod Med* 34:157, 1989.

Bodner DR: The urethral syndrome, *Urol Clinics North Am* 15:699, 1988.

Boreham P: Cryosurgery for the urethral syndrome, *J R Soc Med* 77:111, 1984.

Bump RC, Copeland WE: Urethral isolation of the genital mycoplasmas and *Chlamydia trachomatis* in women with chronic urologic complaints, *Am J Obstet Gynecol* 152:38, 1985.

Carson CC, Osborne D, Segura JW: Psychologic characteristics of patients with female urethral syndrome, *J Clin Psychol* 35:312, 1979.

Carson CC, Segura JW, Osborne DM: Evaluation and treatment of the female urethral syndrome, *J Urol* 124:609, 1980.

Cox CF: The urethra and its relationship to urinary tract infection: the flora of the normal female urethra, *South Med J* 59:621, 1966.

Farrar DJ, Whitside CG, Osborne JD, et al: A urodynamic analysis of micturition symptoms in the female, *Surg Gynecol Obstet* 141:875, 1975.

Folsom AI, Alexander JC: Referred pain from the female urethra, *J Urol* 31:731, 1934.

Gallagher DJ, Mongomerie JZ, North JD: Acute infections of the urinary tract and the urethral syndrome in general practice, *Br Med J* 1:622, 1965.

Gillespie WA, Henderson EP, Linton KB, et al: Microbiology of the urethral (frequency and dysuria) syndrome. A controlled study with 5-year review, *Br J Urol* 64:270, 1989.

Kaplan WE, Firlit CF, Schoenberg HW: The female urethral syndrome: external sphincter spasm as etiology, *J Urol* 124:48, 1980.

Kraft JK, Stamey TA: The natural history of symptomatic recurrent bacteriuria in women, *Medicine* 56:55, 1977.

Mabry EW, Carson CC, Older RA: Evaluation of women with chronic voiding discomfort, *Urology* 18:244, 1981.

Maskell R, Pead L, Allen J: The puzzle of "urethral syndrome": a possible answer, *Lancet* 1:1058, 1979.

Parkes AC, Boreham P: Cryosurgery for the urethral syndrome: preliminary communication, *J R Soc Med* 73:428, 1980.

Raz S, Smith RB: External sphincter spasticity syndrome in female patients, *J Urol* 115:443, 1976.

Reiser C: A new method of treatment of inflammatory lesions of the female urethra, *JAMA* 204:378, 1968.

Richardson FH: External urethroplasty in women: technique and clinical evaluation, *J Urol* 101:719, 1969.

Rutherford AJ, Hinshaw K, Essenhigh DM, et al: Urethral dilatation compared with cystoscopy alone in the treatment of women with recurrent frequency and dysuria, *Br J Urol* 61:500, 1988.

Schmidt RA: The urethral syndrome, *Urol Clin North Am* 12:349, 1985.

Schmidt RA, Tanagho EA: Urethral syndrome or urinary tract infection? *Urology* 18:454, 1981.

Shirley SW, Stewart BH, Mirelman S: Dimethyl sulfoxide in treatment of inflammatory genitourinary disorders, *Urology* 11:215, 1978.

Smith PJ: The management of the urethral syndrome, *Br J Hosp Med* 22:578, 1979.

Splatt AJ, Weedon D: The urethral syndrome: experience with the Richardson urethroplasty, *Br J Urol* 49:173, 1977.

Splatt AJ, Weedon D: The urethral syndrome: morphological studies, *Br J Urol* 53:263, 1981.

Stamm WE, Running K, McKevitt M, et al: Treatment of the acute urethral syndrome, *N Engl J Med* 304:956, 1981.

Stamm WE, Wagner KF, Amsel R, et al: Causes of the acute urethral syndrome in women, *N Engl J Med* 303:409, 1980.

Tait J, Peddie BA, Bailey RR, et al: Urethral syndrome (abacterial cystitis)—search for a pathogen, *Br J Urol* 57:522, 1985.

Wilkens EGL, Payne SR, Pead PJ, et al: Interstitial cystitis and the urethral syndrome: a possible answer, *Br J Urol* 64:39, 1989.

Youngblood VH, Tomlin EM, Davis JB: Senile urethritis in women, *J Urol* 78:150, 1957.

Zufall R: Ineffectiveness of treatment of urethral syndrome in women, *Urology* 12:337, 1978.

Zufall R: Treatment of urethral syndrome in women, *JAMA* 184:138, 1963.

Sensory Urgency

Elder DD, Stephenson TP: An assessment of the Frewen regimen in the treatment of detrusor dysfunction in females, *Br J Urol* 52:467, 1984.

Ferrie BG, Smith JS, Logan D, et al: Experience with bladder training in 65 patients, *Br J Urol* 56:482, 1984.

Fischer-Rasmussen W, Multicentre Study Group: evaluation of long-term safety and clinical benefit of terodiline in women with urgency/urge incontinence. A multicentre study, *Scand J Urol Nephrol Suppl* 87:35, 1984.

Frewen WK: A reassessment of bladder training in detrusor dysfunction in the female, *Br J Urol* 54:372, 1982.

Frewen WK: The management of urgency and frequency of micturition, *Br J Urol* 52:367, 1980.

Frewen WK: Urgency incontinence, *J Obstet Gynaecol Br Commonw* 79:77, 1972.

Frewen WK: Urgency incontinence, *Br J Sex Med* 3:21, 1976.

Hafner RJ, Stanton SL, Guy J: A psychiatric study of women with urgency and urgency incontinence, *Br J Urol* 49:211, 1977.

Jarvis GJ: The management of urinary incontinence due to primary vesical sensory urgency by bladder drill, *Br J Urol* 54:374, 1982.

Klarskov P, Gerstenberg TC, Hald T: Bladder training and terodiline in females with idiopathic urge incontinence and stable detrusor function, *Scand J Urol Nephrol* 20:41, 1986.

MacCaulay AJ, Stern RS, Holmes DM, et al: Micturition and the mind: psychological factors in the aetiology and treatment of urinary symptoms in women, *Br Med J* 294:540, 1987.

McGuire EJ, Shi-Chung Z, Horwinski ER, et al: Treatment of motor and sensory detrusor instability by electrical stimulation, *J Urol* 129:78, 1983.

O'Boyle PJ, Parsons KF: Primary vesical sensory urgency. A clinical trial of bromocriptine, *Br J Urol* 51:200, 1979.

Peattie AB, Plevnik S, Stanton SL: The use of bladder neck electric conductance (BNEC) in the investigation and management of sensory urge incontinence in the female, *J R Soc Med* 81:442, 1988.

Plevnik S, Brown M, Sutherst JR, et al: Tracking of fluid in the urethra by simultaneous electric impedance measurement at three sites, *Urol Int* 38:29, 1983.

Interstitial Cystitis

Anderson JB, Parivar F, Lee G, et al: The enigma of interstitial cystitis—an autoimmune disease? *Br J Urol* 63:58, 1989.

Fall M, Johansson SL, Aldenborg F: Chronic interstitial cystitis: a heterogenous syndrome, *J Urol* 137:35, 1987.

Fall M, Johansson SL, Vahlne A: A clinicopathological and virological study of interstitial cystitis, *J Urol* 133:771, 1985.

Freedman AI, Wein AJ, Whitmore K, et al: In vitro effects of intravesical dimethylsulfoxide, *Neurourol Urodyn* 8:277, 1989.

Freiha FS, Stamey TA: Cystolysis: a procedure for the selective denervation of the bladder, *J Urol* 123:360, 1980.

Gillespie WA, Henderson EP, Linton KB, et al: Microbiology of the urethral (frequency and dysuria) syndrome. A controlled study with 5-year review, *Br J Urol* 64:270, 1989.

Hanno PM, Buehler J, Wein AJ: Use of amitriptyline in the treatment of interstitial cystitis, *J Urol* 141:849, 1989.

Holm-Bentzen M, Lose G: Pathology and pathogenesis of interstitial cystitis, *Urology* 29:8, 1987.

Hunner GL: Elusive ulcer of the bladder: further notes on a rare type of bladder ulcer with a report of 25 cases, *Am J Obstet Gynecol* 78:374, 1918.

Keltikangas-Jarvinen L, Auvinen L, Lehtonen T: Psychological factors related to interstitial cystitis, *Eur Urol* 15:69, 1988.

Lynes WL, Flynn SD, Shortliffe LD, et al: Mast cell involvement in interstitial cystitis, *J Urol* 138:746, 1987.

MacDermott JP, Charpied GC, Tesluk H, et al: Can histological assessment predict the outcome in interstitial cystitis? *Br J Urol* 67:44, 1991.

McGuire ES, Lytton B, Carnog SL: Interstitial cystitis following colocystoplasty, *Urology* 2:28, 1973.

Messing EM: The diagnosis of interstitial cystitis, *Urology* 29:4, 1987.

Messing EM, Stamey TA: Interstitial cystitis: early diagnosis, pathology and treatment, *Urology* 12:381, 1978.

Oravisto KJ: Epidemiology of interstitial cystitis, *Ann Chir Gynaecol* 64:75, 1975.

Oravisto KJ: Interstitial cystitis as an autoimmune disease: a review, *Eur Urol* 6:10, 1980.

Oravisto KJ, Alfthan OS: Treatment of interstitial cystitis with immunosuppression and chloroquine derivatives, *Eur Urol* 2:82, 1976.

Oravisto KJ, Alfthan OS, Jokinen EJ: Interstitial cystitis: clinical and immunological findings, *Scand J Urol Nephrol* 4:37, 1970.

Parsons CL, Koprowski PF: Interstitial cystitis: successful management by increasing urinary voiding intervals, *Urology* 37:207, 1991.

Parsons CL, Schmidt JD, Pollen JJ: Successful treatment of interstitial cystitis with sodium pentosanpolysulfate, *J Urol* 130:51, 1983.

Parsons CL, Mulholland SG: Successful therapy of interstitial cystitis with pentosan polysulfate, *J Urol* 138:513, 1987.

Perez-Marrero R, Emerson LE, Feltis JT: A controlled study of dimethyl sulfoxide in interstitial cystitis, *J Urol* 140:36, 1988.

Sant GR, Ucci AA, Alroy J: Bladder surface glycosaminoglycans (GAGs) in interstitial cystitis (abstract), *J Urol* 135:175a, 1986.

Shanberg AM, Baghdassarian R, Tansey LA: Treatment of interstitial cystitis with neodymium: YAG laser, *J Urol* 134:885, 1985.

Shanberg AM, Malloy T: Treatment of interstitial cystitis with neodymium:YAG laser, *Urology* 29:31, 1987.

Summary of the National Institute of Arthritis, Diabetes, Digestive and Kidney Diseases Workshop on Interstitial Cystitis, National Institutes of Health, Bethesda, Maryland, August 28-29, 1987, *J Urol* 140:203, 1988.

Webster GD, Galloway N: Surgical treatment of interstitial cystitis: indications, techniques, and results, *Urology* 29:34, 1987.

Webster GD, Maggio MI: The management of chronic interstitial cystitis by substitution cystoplasty, *J Urol* 141:287, 1989.

Wishard WN, Nourse MH, Mertz JHO: Use of Clorpactin WCS-90 for relief of symptoms due to interstitial cystitis, *J Urol* 77:420, 1957.

Witherow RN, Gillespie L, McMullen L, et al: Painful bladder syndrome—a clinical and immunopathological study, *Br J Urol* 64:158, 1989.

Worth PHL: The treatment of interstitial cystitis by cystolysis with observations on cystoplasty: a review after seven years, *Br J Urol* 52:232, 1980.

CHAPTER 21

Voiding Dysfunction and Retention

Linda M. Partoll

Normal Voiding
Voiding Dysfunction
    Prevalence
    Clinical presentation and diagnosis
    Classification
    Etiologies
Urinary Retention
    Acute urinary retention
    Chronic urinary retention
Treatment of Voiding Dysfunction and Retention
    Pharmacologic
    Surgical
    Intermittent self-catheterization

The lower urinary tract functions as both a storage and eliminatory unit. Storage and voiding are both possible because pressure gradients reflexedly change as needed. Voiding dysfunction occurs when the balance of pressure shifts more toward the storage function than the voiding function. In the end stage, voiding dysfunction can progress to urinary retention. This chapter discusses normal and abnormal voiding, urinary retention, and treatment modalities.

NORMAL VOIDING

Bladder control is learned during childhood and usually is taken for granted thereafter. The control and actual mechanics of normal voiding, however, involve an intricate neurophysiologic network, and an abnormality at any level can lead to voiding dysfunction. Required components of this control network include normal function of the central and peripheral nervous systems; a normal bladder wall and detrusor muscle; and normal anatomy and function of the bladder neck, urethra, and pelvic floor.

A brief review of the neurophysiology of micturition will help clarify how voiding occurs. A more detailed overview is found in Chapter 2.

Voiding is controlled by the summation of input from four different areas: cerebral cortex, brain stem, sacral spinal cord, and peripheral innervation. Of these areas, the brain stem, primarily the pons, is the most important as detrusor and sphincter activity are coordinated here in the pontine micturition center.

The cerebral cortex provides both conscious and unconscious control of the micturition reflex. Cortical control allows humans to dampen the micturition reflex until it is socially acceptable. The cortical input that controls voiding is quite complex, as evidenced by the variety of symptoms noted in patients suffering from cortical lesions. Depending on the location of the lesions, patients may suffer from urgency and urge incontinence or from urethral spasticity and retention. Patients may or may not have social concerns about their incontinence.

The pontine reticular formation accepts input from the peripheral nerves, the sacral spinal cord, and var-

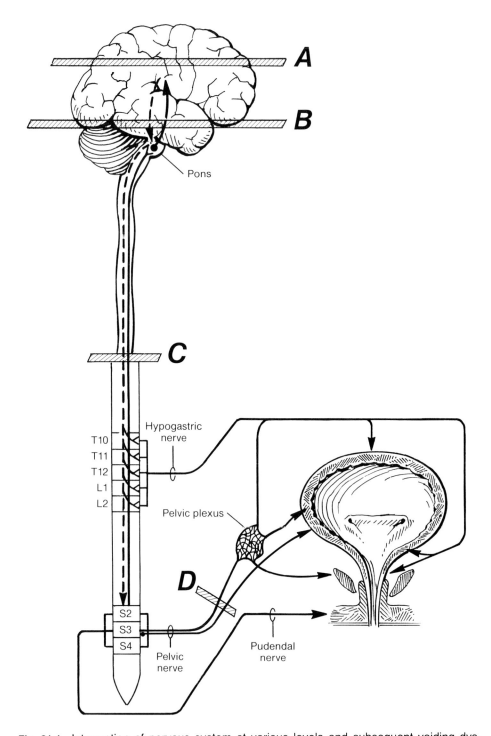

Fig. 21-1 Interruption of nervous system at various levels and subsequent voiding dysfunction. *A,* Lesions in higher cortical centers have various effects, including inability to voluntarily postpone voiding, urge incontinence, enuresis, urethral spasm, and loss of social concern about incontinence. *B,* Suprapontine lesions result in involuntary detrusor contractions with coordinated urethral relaxation. *C,* High spinal cord (upper motor neuron) lesions lead to detrusor hyperreflexia without coordinated urethral relaxation (detrusor-sphincter dyssenergia). *D,* Lower motor neuron lesions cause detrusor areflexia.

ious cortical centers and then coordinates detrusor and sphincter activity so that normal voiding can occur. Suprapontine lesions often result in involuntary voiding via a detrusor contraction with coordinated urethral relaxation.

Sacral spinal cord segments S2, S3, and S4 contain detrusor motor neurons that control micturition. Lesions between the sacral spinal cord and the brain stem tend to produce simultaneous uncoordinated contraction of the detrusor and external urethral sphincter, described as detrusor-sphincter dyssynergia.

Peripheral innervation is carried out via both sympathetic and parasympathetic fibers. Sacral parasympathetic fibers are the primary motor supply to the detrusor. Parasympathetic neurons have their cell bodies in the sacral spinal cord; the preganglionic fibers travel via the pelvic nerves to synapse in ganglia in and near the bladder wall. The cell bodies of sympathetic preganglionic neurons are located in the thoracolumbar spinal cord; they synapse in the inferior mesenteric and hypogastric ganglia. Their postganglionic fibers either synapse with parasympathetic fibers in or near the bladder wall, allowing for interaction between sympathetic and parasympathetic systems, or they terminate directly in the detrusor and urethral musculature. A simplified schematic diagram of bladder innervation and the effects of lesions at various levels is found in Fig. 21-1.

Normal voiding is accomplished by relaxation of the urethra, followed by a sustained contraction of the detrusor so that the bladder completely empties. This process begins when bladder distention causes stimulation of bladder wall pressure sensors. After cortical inhibition of the reflex is released, the micturition reflex is activated. The reflex is carried out in two steps: (1) relaxation of the periurethral striated musculature and pelvic floor muscles, resulting in a decrease in intraurethral pressure and funneling and descent of the bladder neck; and (2) a coordinated contraction of the detrusor, increasing intravesical pressure to surpass urethral pressure. Urine flow results, reaching a peak flow rate of 25 to 30 ml/sec. Brain stem modulation of the arc instructs the bladder how long to contract so that the bladder empties completely. When voiding is complete, the detrusor muscle is reflexively inhibited, and intravesical

and intraurethal pressures return to prevoiding levels. Normal voiding, therefore, is characterized by a sharp start, a smooth sustained flow, and a sharp conclusion. The urodynamic features of normal voiding are seen in Fig. 21-2.

VOIDING DYSFUNCTION

Voiding dysfunction and urinary retention represent points in a spectrum of incomplete voiding. Patients who have incomplete emptying progress from being asymptomatic to having symptomatic voiding difficulty to acute or chronic urinary retention. The mortality of this condition is low, as patients rarely progress to upper tract dilation and renal failure, but the morbidity is significant.

Prevalence

The actual prevalence of voiding dysfunction in women is difficult to estimate because only those referred to specialty clinics are fully evaluated. Stanton et al reported on 600 women referred to a clinic for various urologic symptoms. Voiding difficulty was confirmed in 25.5% of patients over 65 years old, in 13.6% of patients less than 65 years old, and in 16.5% of patients overall. Osborne reported that 21% of patients presenting to a clinic with urinary problems complained of symptoms suggestive of voiding dysfunction, but the diagnosis was confirmed in only one third of patients. Of the 159 women seen with symptoms consistent with voiding dysfunction, 44.5% had detrusor hyperreflexia, 44.5% had detrusor areflexia, and 11% had normal studies.

Clinical Presentation and Diagnosis

Patients with voiding dysfunction present with a variety of symptoms, including a weak stream, incomplete emptying, straining to void, and urinary frequency. Urinary retention can also lead to overflow incontinence. Unfortunately, these symptoms are relatively nonspecific; there is little correlation between symptoms and urodynamic findings.

A thorough evaluation is required in most patients with dysfunctional voiding symptoms. The history includes inquiring about prior voiding dysfunction postoperatively or postpartum, neurologic complaints or

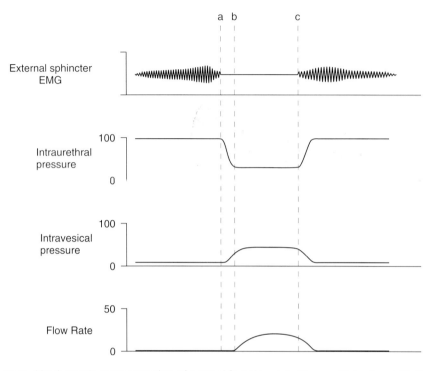

Fig. 21-2 Urodynamic representation of normal female micturition. *a,* Voluntary initiation of voiding with relaxation of external urethral sphincter and pelvic floor muscles and associated decrease in urethral pressure. *b,* Intraurethral pressure equals intravesical pressure and urine flow is initiated. *c,* Voluntary termination of voiding. (From Walters MD: *Obstet Gynecol Clin North Am)* 16:773, 1989.)

conditions, drug use, previous pelvic surgery, and general health problems such as diabetes and hypothyroidism. The physical examination must include pelvic, neurologic, and mental status examinations.

Diagnostic studies can be simple or complex, depending on the amount of disability and the need for making an exact (versus general) diagnosis. Basic screening studies include measurement of residual urine volume after voiding and uroflowmetry. Sophisticated diagnostic studies include simultaneous measurement of intraabdominal, intravesical, and intraurethral pressures, often combined with sphincter electromyography; alternatively video-cystourethrography can be performed (see Chapter 7).

In women with dysfunctional voiding, the urine flow rate is low (less than 15 ml/sec), and postvoid residual urine volume is often high. The following diagnostic criteria have been suggested by Massey and Abrams to diagnose voiding dysfunction: a maximum flow rate (Qmax) of less than 15 ml/sec with a residual urine volume greater than 100 ml on two occasions; or any two of the following: flow rate less than 12 ml/sec, detrusor pressure at peak flow (PFP) > 50 cm H_2O, urethral resistance (PFP/Qmax^2) greater than 0.2, and "significant" residual urine in the presence of elevated PFP or urethral resistance.

Classification

The International Continence Society (ICS) established a classification of lower urinary tract dysfunction. This classification divides abnormalities into those of the storage and voiding phases. In the voiding phase, detrusor and urethral function are examined separately, as shown in the accompanying box. An underactive detrusor denotes a detrusor contraction that is of inadequate strength or duration (or both) to

---

International Continence Society Classification of Voiding Phase Dysfunction

---

Detrusor Function During Voiding

1. Normal
2. Underactive
3. Acontractile

Urethral Function During Voiding

1. Normal
2. Obstructive
   a. Overactive
   b. Mechanical

Causes of Voiding Dysfunction and Retention

Neurologic (see box p. 304)

Lesions of the brain
Lesions of the spinal cord
Autonomic lesions
Local pain reflex

Pharmacologic (see Table 21-1)

Inflammatory

Acute urethritis
Acute cystitis
Acute vulvovaginitis
Primary herpes simplex virus infection

Obstructive

Extramural
    Impacted pelvic or vaginal mass
    Uterovaginal prolapse
Intramural
Intralumenal
Detrusor-sphincter dyssynergia

Endocrine

Hypothyroidism
Diabetes mellitus

Overdistention, Iatrogenic

Postoperative
Postpartum

Psychogenic

Nonneurogenic neurogenic bladder
Psychiatric disorder
    Hysteria
    Depression
    Schizophrenia

---

empty the bladder efficiently. Detrusor areflexia is defined as acontractility due to an abnormality of nervous control and denotes the complete absence of a centrally coordinated contraction.

Etiologies (see Box)
Neurologic

Urinary retention secondary to detrusor or urethral dysfunction is often caused by a neurologic lesion. As discussed earlier, neurologic lesions can cause voiding dysfunction in several ways. Although one cannot predict with complete accuracy the symptoms that a particular lesion will cause, certain patterns of dysfunction have been observed after certain insults. In review, cortical lesions result in urinary retention or in the inability to inhibit the micturition reflex. Lesions above the brain stem tend to result in detrusor hyperreflexia. Infrapontine lesions tend to result in detrusor-sphincter dyssynergia. A list of neurologic disorders that cause voiding difficulty and retention is shown in the box on p. 304.

Voiding dysfunction is common after cerebrovascular accidents. Urodynamic evaluation of 33 patients after cerebrovascular accidents revealed involuntary bladder contractions in 26 and poor bladder contractions in 7. Correlation of bladder dysfunction with anatomic location of the brain injury was inconclusive.

Patients experiencing prolonged postoperative voiding dysfunction after radical pelvic surgery can also be classified as having neurologic lesions, as their primary lesion is peripheral denervation of the bladder

and urethra secondary to surgical dissection. This lesion is frequently seen in women undergoing abdominoperineal resection of the rectum or radical hysterectomy. Over 50% of patients after radical hysterectomy report persistent urinary complaints, including voiding dysfunction, incontinence, and decreased sensation. Due to the anatomic location of the pelvic parasympathetic nerves and sympathetic plexi,

Neurologic Disorders Causing Voiding Dysfunction and Retention

Lesions of the Brain

Cerebrovascular disease
Parkinsonism
Multiple sclerosis
Concussion
Brain tumor
Shy-Drager syndrome

Lesions of the Spinal Cord

Spinovascular disease
Conus medullaris or cauda equina tumors
Prolapsed intervertebral disk
Spinal stenosis
Spinal arachnoiditis
Tabes dorsalis
Multiple sclerosis
Spinal cord injury
Dysraphic lesions

Lesions of Autonomic and Peripheral Innervation

Autonomic neuropathy
Sacral agenesis
Spinal cord injury
Diabetes mellitus
Tabes dorsalis
Pernicious anemia
Herpes zoster
Radical pelvic surgery

TABLE 21-1   Drugs that can cause voiding dysfunction and retention

Drug	Decreases bladder contractility	Increases outlet resistance
Atropine-like agents	+	
Ganglionic blockers	+	
Musculotropic relaxants (antispasmodics)	+	
Calcium antagonists	+	
Antihistamines	+	
Theophylline	+	
Phenothiazines	+	
Tricyclic antidepressants	+	+
Alpha-adrenergic agonists		+
L-dopa		+
Amphetamines		+

neurologic damage and subsequent voiding dysfunction occur more commonly after rectal surgery than uterine surgery.

The effect of simple abdominal hysterectomy on bladder function and urinary symptoms is unclear; conclusions of the few objective studies are contradictory.

Pharmacologic

Numerous classes of drugs can have detrimental effects on voiding. Any drug that inhibits bladder contractility or increases outlet resistance can result in incomplete emptying (Table 21-1). Clinically obvious voiding difficulty is not seen in most patients using these drugs; symptoms usually appear in patients who already have borderline voiding dysfunction. Any drug that interferes with the action of acetylcholine at vesical cholinergic receptors can result in voiding dysfunction. These drugs include anticholinergic agents, tricyclic antidepressants, and ganglionic blockers (e.g., mecamylamine). Alpha-adrenergic stimulants (e.g., epinephrine) increase urethral tone and can impair voiding by increasing outflow resistance.

Epidural anesthesia causes temporary retention primarily by inhibiting afferent neuronal transmission from the bladder, thereby decreasing the sensation of bladder fullness and the urge to void.

Inflammatory

Acute inflammation or infection of the bladder, urethra, vulva, or vagina can cause dysfunction via localized pain and edema. This reaction is seen in the immediate postoperative period as well as with various inflammatory processes. Primary herpes simplex virus infection can cause radiculitis with subsequent detrusor underactivity.

Obstruction

Urethral or vesical neck obstruction is the most common cause of voiding dysfunction in men; however, it is rare in women. Massey and Abrams reported that evaluation of 5948 women referred to a urodynamic unit revealed obstruction in only 163 patients (2.7%), although the classic symptoms of hesitancy, poor stream, and incomplete emptying were present in 40%. Causes of obstruction can be extramural (23.9%), intramural (73.6%), or intraluminal (2.5%). Extramural causes include pelvic or vaginal masses such as myomata, retroverted gravid uterus, and hematocolpos. Genital prolapse must be severe to cause enough urethral distortion so that obstruction occurs. Intramural causes include urethral stenosis, acute urethral edema, and chronic fibrosis secondary to surgery or radiation. Condylomata and urethral cancer are causes of intraluminal obstruction.

Voiding difficulty is frequently noted after bladder neck surgery, especially in patients who preoperatively void with no detrusor contraction in association with low flow rates. This is probably due to a certain amount of obstruction at the bladder neck.

Obstruction can also be due to urethral sphincter activity; in fact, the most common cause of urethral obstruction in women is failure of the distal urethra to relax during voiding. An actual sphincteric contraction may also occur, causing obstruction. In the worst situation, a detrusor contraction occurs simultaneously with sphincteric contraction; this condition is called detrusor-sphincter dyssynergia.

Detrusor-sphincter dyssynergia occurs only in patients with neurologic lesions, particularly high spinal cord lesions. Functional obstruction occurs despite high detrusor pressures. The degree of dysfunction depends on the contractile strength of the detrusor— as long as the detrusor can overcome urethral resistance, some amount of voiding can occur. An obstructed flow pattern usually is observed on uroflowmetry. Urethrovesical backwash, ureterovesical reflux, and high residual urine volumes all lead to recurrent infection. Treatment is aimed at inhibiting the detrusor hyperreflexia with drug and behavioral therapy. One can also attempt to effect relaxation of the external striated sphincter with alpha-sympathetic antagonists, such as prazosin and phenoxybenzamine, or to relax the pelvic floor musculature with centrally acting muscle relaxants, such as baclofen, dantrolene, or diazepam.

Endocrine

Endocrine causes of detrusor dysfunction include hypothyroidism and diabetes mellitus, both of which can cause a peripheral neuropathy in poorly controlled patients.

Overdistention

Overdistention, especially iatrogenic overdistention, is an often preventable cause of voiding dysfunction. Even one episode of overdistention can lead to a large hypotonic bladder. Overdistention can occur because of poorly managed acute or chronic retention. Patients at risk for overdistention, whether because of a longstanding disease process or a temporary situation such as surgery, must be carefully monitored for adequate urine output.

Psychogenic

Although psychogenic causes of voiding dysfunction are well known, it should be considered a diagnosis of exclusion. Criteria for the diagnosis are no detectable neurologic or other significant organic disease, positive correlation of psychiatric symptoms and the onset of voiding dysfunction, and clinical response to psychotherapy and pharmacologic treatment. Psychiatric disorders sometimes seen with voiding dysfunction include hysteria, depression, and schizophrenia.

Nonneurogenic neurogenic bladder is a voiding dysfunction with a behavioral etiology and is not attributable to a neurologic lesion. The precise psychiatric disorder is unclear and the clinical presentation varied, but the urodynamic findings are fairly precise. External urethral sphincter electromyogram (EMG) studies of patients with a true neurogenic bladder and detrusor-sphincter dyssynergia show an increase in EMG activity before and during the upslope of a detrusor contraction, and EMG activity quiets on the downslope. In contrast, EMG studies in patients with nonneurogenic neurogenic bladder show quieting of the external sphincter EMG before and during the upslope of a detrusor contraction and augmented EMG activity during the downslope of the detrusor contraction. EMG tracings in normal voiding show a quieting of activity before and during a detrusor contraction.

URINARY RETENTION

Inability to fully empty the bladder secondary to any of the mechanisms previously discussed can lead to urinary retention. Retention occurs either acutely or chronically. In either case, a thorough investigation into the cause of retention is required, as urinary retention may be a harbinger for a serious underlying problem.

Urinary retention can present in different ways; the symptoms usually reflect the degree to which retention occurs. Symptoms include a feeling of not being able to fully empty when voiding, lower abdominal pain or pressure, a complete inability to void, and incontinence secondary to urinary overflow.

Acute and chronic urinary retention are discussed separately, but it is important to note that there is considerable overlap in the causes of both.

Acute Urinary Retention

Traditional teaching about acute urinary retention in women suggests that it is a rare phenomenon with the commonest cause being psychogenic disturbances. This theory has been refuted in several recent studies; acute retention is now more commonly recognized as the initial symptom for an underlying disease process.

The causes of acute retention can be categorized as follows: postoperative or postpartum, neurologic, obstructive, psychogenic, and idiopathic. An obstruction can be gynecologic or urologic in nature. Doran and Roberts reviewed 103 women with acute urinary retention; the etiology of retention was determined to be postoperative or postpartum in 58 (56%), obstruction in 24 (23%), inflammation/infection in 7 (7%), neurologic in 7 (7%), psychogenic in 3 (3%), and "other" in 4 (4%).

It is well-known that women often cannot void postoperatively. There are many reasons for this phenomenon, for example, not being aware of bladder distention secondary to anesthesia or analgesia, local inflammation and tissue edema, pain or fear of pain with voiding, and bladder and/or urethral denervation. Urinary retention is also frequently seen postpartum and may be due to periurethral edema, obstetric lacerations, or bladder desensitivity because of epidural anesthesia. With extensive pelvic operations

such as radical (Wertheim) hysterectomy, postoperative urinary dysfunction can be especially severe and prolonged. Prevention of postoperative and postpartum urinary retention is very important. The bladder may be permanently damaged by even one incident of severe overdistention.

The frequency of neurologic causes of acute retention emphasizes the importance of a thorough neurologic examination. The most common neurologic cause is multiple sclerosis. Other causes include transverse myelitis, sacral agenesis, traumatic paraplegia, senile dementia, and peripheral neuropathy secondary to diabetes mellitus, vitamin deficiency, or hypothyroidism.

Obstruction of the urethra is much less common in women than men, but it can cause acute urinary retention. Obstruction may be due to a pelvic or vaginal mass imparting extrinsic pressure on the urethra or bladder neck, or it may be due to localized edema of these same structures. Urethal stenosis in women is rare.

Acute retention has been described with primary infection of genital herpes (Elsberg syndrome). It is believed that infection causes a sacral myeloradiculitis, resulting in a motor and sensory neuropathy. In most cases, bladder function is restored in 4 to 10 days. Occasionally, urinary retention may last as long as 5 to 7 weeks; in these cases a suprapubic catheter is recommended.

Psychogenic retention is most common in women with a prior history of psychiatric illness, although it can be the initial symptom. It is seen in women suffering from disorders such as hysteria, depression, and schizophrenia.

Chronic Urinary Retention

It was once thought that chronic urinary retention in women was usually due to vesical neck obstruction, and bladder neck resection was a common treatment. It has since been shown urodyanamically that detrusor failure is the most common cause of chronic retention. Detrusor failure is often due to neurologic derangement, with multiple sclerosis again being most common. In a reported series of 37 women with chronic retention, the cause of detrusor failure was determined to be idiopathic in 24 patients and neurologic in only 13 patients. The idiopathic causes included psychiatric disorders and surgery.

TREATMENT OF VOIDING DYSFUNCTION AND RETENTION

Treatment of voiding dysfunction depends on the cause of the dysfunction. Patients with obstructive voiding due to causes such as a pelvic mass should be treated with surgical removal of the impinging mass. Other causes of dysfunction, such as infection, condylomata, and urethral cancer, should be treated accordingly.

Prompt treatment of acute retention is important not only for relief of symptoms, but also to prevent further deterioration of bladder function. A chronically overdistended bladder can lead to upper urinary tract dilation and subsequent deterioration of renal function. The primary treatment goal is to establish bladder drainage. Drainage may be accomplished initially via a transurethral or suprapubic catheter. The catheter should be left in place until the patient can void spontaneously. In some patients with acute urinary retention, a one-time catheterization is all that is required. In others, especially postoperative patients, prolonged drainage is required. In these cases, simple observation should be used, as function usually returns spontaneously.

Pharmacologic

Detrusor underactivity or areflexia is difficult to treat effectively. Pharmacologic therapy has produced mixed results. Cholinergic agents such as bethanechol chloride have been the backbone of treatment for more than 30 years. Recent controlled studies, however, have demonstrated that both subcutaneous and oral bethanechol has no effect on flow rate or residual volume. Similarly, oral bethanechol has no beneficial effects in paralyzed patients with neuropathic bladders. Khanna suggested that poor therapeutic results with bethanechol chloride are due to its nicotinic effect on urethral smooth muscle. We believe that there is no indication for use of bethanechol in patients with voiding dysfunction.

Alpha-adrenergic blockers such as phenoxybenzamine have been used to decrease urethral resistance. Khanna reported a significant improvement in 26 of 31 patients treated with both bethanechol and phenoxybenzamine. In contrast, Murray states that women, unlike men, have no evidence of adrenergic innervation of the bladder neck, and that alpha-adrenergic blockers are not helpful in clinical practice.

Anticholinesterase inhibitor agents, such as distigmine bromide, act as parasympathomimetic agents so that the amount of acetylcholine available is increased by inactivation of acetylcholinesterase. Distigmine bromide has been reported to prevent postoperative urinary retention; however, it has not been successful in treating patients with neuropathic bladders.

Prostaglandin F_2 (PGF_2) and prostaglandin E_2 (PGE_2) cause contraction of isolated strips of detrusor muscle in animals. The clinical effectiveness of PGF_2 and PGE_2 in humans is controversial. Bultitude et al and Desmond et al reported improved voiding in women with detrusor failure after a single intravesical instillation of PGE_2. Intravesical instillation of PGF_2 postoperatively was also shown to reduce urinary retention, urinary tract infection, and required hospital days with no side effects. In contrast, Andersson et al were unable to show that PGE_2 had any beneficial effects in women with voiding disorders. Likewise, Delaere et al could not demonstrate a significant benefit with either PGE_2 or PGF_2.

Postmenopausal women may develop rigid, atrophic, or stenotic urethras due to inadequate levels of endogenous estrogens. The presence of intraurethral estrogen receptors and cytologic changes in urethral epithelia after estrogen therapy support the use of estrogen for relief of urinary symptoms in postmenopausal women. A significant decrease in voiding difficulty symptoms was found by Hilton and Stanton using intravaginal estrogen cream and by Versi and Cardozo with estradiol implants.

Surgical

Cystoscopy and urethral dilation are the primary surgical treatments for women with voiding dysfunction. Extreme dilation is not required and may cause urinary incontinence. Massey and Abrams showed that dilation to 36 French with estrogen replacement as needed resolved voiding dysfunction in 76% of women with intramural causes of dysfunction. In patients with neuropathic sphincteric obstruction, Otis urethrotomy/sphincterotomy was beneficial in less than 50% of the patients treated with this modality. With the advent of intermittent clean self-catheterization, there are few indications for more radical procedures, as they may lead to incontinence.

Intermittent Self-Catheterization

Clean, intermittent self-catheterization (ISC), introduced by Lapides et al in 1972, has become the mainstay of treatment for patients with severe dysfunction. Patients are taught to catheterize themselves using a clean (not sterile) catheter. Sterile urine is maintained in 45% to 90% of patients using sterile technique, and in 39% to 65% using a clean technique. Urinalysis of 38 patients using ISC showed that 67% had 10+ WBC/hpf (white blood cells per high power field); on urine culture, 14% were sterile, 43% had nonsignificant growth, and 43% had significant bacterial growth. Suppressive antibiotics are not used, and infection is treated as it occurs. It is imperative that ISC be introduced to the patient in a positive and supportive manner; the benefits of avoiding surgery, the elimination of an external device, and preservation of renal function should be stressed. This technique is discussed in detail in Chapter 29.

A permanent transurethral catheter is the last resort in nonsurgical treatment, as it carries the often inevitable risks of bladder and urethral irritation, bladder calculi formation, and urinary tract infection that can lead to fatal sepsis in debilitated individuals.

CONCLUSION

Our understanding of voiding dysfunction in women is far from complete. It is important to elucidate voiding patterns before surgery, when retention occurs, and when dysfunctional symptoms are present, remembering that voiding dysfunction may be a harbinger of another disease process. Treatment depends on the etiology of dysfunction. In patients in whom voiding dysfunction is attributed to obstruction, relief of the obstruction and/or urethral dilation will usually

improve the patients' symptoms. However, when the voiding dysfunction or retention is secondary to an underactive or areflexic detrusor, and treatment of the primary disease does not improve voiding function, then management usually consists of ISC. Clean, intermittent self-catheterization should be considered for all women with chronic voiding dysfunction and retention.

REFERENCES

Andersson KE, Hendriksson L, Ulmsten U: Effects of prostaglandin E$_2$ applied locally on intravesical and intraurethral pressures in women, *Eur Urol* 4:366, 1978.

Barrett DM: The effect of oral bethanechol chloride on voiding in female patients with excessive residual urine: a randomized double-blind study, *J Urol* 126:640, 1981.

Bhatia NN, Bergman A: Urodynamic predictability of voiding following incontinence surgery, *Obstet Gynecol* 63:85, 1984.

Bultitude MI, Hills NH, Shuttleworth KED: Clinical and experimental studies on the action of prostaglandins and their synthesis inhibitors on detrusor muscle in vitro and in vivo, *Br J Urol* 48:631, 1976.

Cameron MD: Distigmine bromide (Ubretid) in the prevention of postoperative retention of urine, *J Obstet Gynaecol Br Commonw* 73:847, 1966.

Dean AM, Worth PHL: Female chronic urinary retention, *Br J Urol* 57:24, 1985.

Delaere KP, Thomas CM, Moonen WA, et al: The value of intravesical prostaglandin E$_2$ and F$_2$ in women with abnormalities of bladder emptying, *Br J Urol* 53:306, 1981.

Desmond AD, Bultitude MI, Hills NH, et al: Clinical experience with intravesical prostaglandin E$_2$, *Br J Urol* 53:357, 1980.

Doran J, Roberts M: Acute urinary retention in the female, *Br J Urol* 47:793, 1976.

Garber SJ, Christmas TJ, Rickards D: Voiding dysfunction due to neurosyphillis, *Br J Urol* 66:19, 1990.

Greenstein A, Matzkin H, Kaver I, et al: Acute urinary retention in herpes genitalis infection, *Urology* 31:453, 1988.

Hemrika DJ, Schutte MF, Bleker OP: Elsberg syndrome: a neurologic basis for acute urinary retention in patients with genital herpes, *Obstet Gynecol* 68:37S, 1986.

Hilton P, Stanton SL: The use of intravaginal oestrogen cream in genuine stress incontinence, *Br J Obstet Gynaecol* 90:940, 1983.

Iosif CS, Batra S, Ek A, et al: Estrogen receptors in the human female lower urinary tract, *Am J Obstet Gynecol* 141:817, 1981.

Jaschevatzky OE, Anderman S, Shalit A, et al: Prostaglandin F$_2$ for prevention of urinary retention after vaginal hysterectomy, *Obstet Gynecol* 66:244, 1985.

Khanna OP: Disorders of micturition: neuropharmacologic basis and results of drug therapy, *Urology* 8:316, 1976.

Khanna OP: Non-surgical therapeutic modalities. In Krane RJ,

Siroky MB, editors: *Clinical neurourology,* Boston, 1979, Little, Brown.

Khan Z, Starer P, Yang WC, et al: Analysis of voiding disorders in patients with cerebrovascular accidents, *Urology* 25:265, 1990.

Krane RJ, Siroky MB, editors: Clinical neurourology, ed 2, Boston, 1991, Little, Brown.

Lapides J, Diokno AC, Silber SJ, et al: Clean intermittent self-catheterization in the treatment of urinary tract disease, *Br J Urol* 56:379, 1984.

Mainprize TC, Drutz HP: The Marshall-Marchetti-Krantz procedure: a critical review, *Obstet Gynecol Surv* 43:724, 1988.

Massey JA, Abrams PH: Obstructed voiding in the female, *Br J Urol* 61:36, 1988.

Mundy AR: An anatomical explanation for bladder dysfunction following rectal and uterine surgery, *Br J Urol* 54:501, 1982.

Murray K: Medical and surgical management of female voiding difficulty. In Drife JO, Hilton P, Stanton SL, editors: *Micturition,* London, 1990, Springer-Verlag.

Osborne JL: Urodynamics and the gynecologist, Aleck Bourne Lecture, 1981.

Paviakis A, Wheeler JS, Krane RJ, et al: Functional voiding disorders in females, *Neurourol Urodyn* 5:145, 1986.

Philip NH, Thomas DG: The effect of distigmine bromide on voiding in male paraplegic patients with reflex micturition, *Br J Urol* 52:492, 1980.

Philip NH, Thomas DG, Clarke SJ: Drug effects on the voiding cystometrogram: a comparison of oral bethanechol and carbachol, *Br J Urol* 52:484, 1980.

Preminger GM, Steinhardt JM, Fried FA, et al: Acute urinary retention in female patients: diagnosis and treatment, *J Urol* 130:112, 1982.

Roberts M, Smith P: Nonmalignant obstruction of the female urethra, *Br J Urol* 40:694, 1968.

Rudy DC, Woodside JR: Non-neurogenic neurogenic bladder: the relationship between intravesical pressure and the external sphincter electromyogram, *Neurourol Urodynam* 10:169, 1991.

Silva PD, Berberich W: Retroverted impacted gravid uterus with acute urinary retention: report of two cases and a review of the literature, *Obstet Gynecol* 68:121, 1986.

Smith P: Age changes in the female urethra, *Br J Urol* 44:667, 1972.

Smith PH, Turnbull MB, Currie DW, et al: The urological complications of Wertheims's hysterectomy, *Br J Urol* 41:685, 1969.

Stanton SL, Ozsoy C, Hilton P: Voiding difficulties in the female: prevalence, clinical and urodynamic review, *Obstet Gynecol* 61:144, 1983.

Stanton SL: Voiding difficulties and retention. In Stanton SL, editor: *Clinical gynecologic urology,* St Louis, 1984, Mosby–Year Book.

Tanagho EA, Miller ER: Initiation of voiding, *Br J Urol* 42:175, 1970.

Tammela T, Kontturi M, Kaar K, et al: Intravesical prostaglandin F_2 for promoting bladder emptying after surgery for female stress incontinence, *Br J Urol* 60:43, 1987.

Versi E, Cardozo LD: Oestrogens and lower urinary tract function. In Studd JWW, Whitehead MI, editors: *The menopause,* Oxford, 1988, Blackwell Scientific Publications.

Wein AJ, Barrett DM: Voiding function and dysfunction, Chicago, 1988, Year Book Medical Publishers.

Wein AJ, Mallory TR, Shofer F, et al: The effects of bethanechol chloride on urodynamic parameters in normal women and in women with significant residual urine volumes, *J Urol* 124:397, 1980.

CHAPTER 22

Lower Urinary Tract Infection

Mickey M. Karram

Prevalence
Definitions
Pathogenesis
   Host defense mechanisms
   Host susceptibility factors
Clinical Presentation
Microbiology of Urinary Tract Infection
Diagnosis of Bacteriuria
   Urine microscopy
   Office urine kit
   Urine culture
   Cystourethroscopy
   Radiologic studies
   Urodynamic studies
Differential Diagnosis
Management of Lower Urinary Tract Infection
   Asymptomatic bacteriuria—is treatment necessary?
   First infection or infrequent reinfections
   Recurrent infections
Sexual Intercourse and Diaphragm Use
Catheter-Associated Infection
Lower Urinary Tract Instrumentation
Pyelonephritis

Despite newer diagnostic and treatment modalities, urinary tract infections in women continue to represent a significant health care problem. They are among the most common infections treated by primary care physicians and account for approximately 5.2 million office visits per year. The health care cost of diagnosis,

antimicrobial treatment, and subsequent management of women with urinary tract infections has been estimated to exceed $1 billion annually.

The proper management of these patients, although often simple, has recently been challenged by: (1) the introduction of new antimicrobial agents, (2) the advent of single-dose therapy, (3) the recognition of additional lower urinary tract pathogens such as *Staphylococcus saprophyticus* and *Chlamydia trachomatis*, (4) the realization that many women with acute cystitis may have fewer than 10^5 colony forming units (cfu)/ ml in urine cultures, and (5) the understanding that certain women with infection-like symptoms will have sterile urine and will ultimately be diagnosed with either urethral syndrome or interstitial cystitis.

PREVALENCE

Approximately 5 million cases of acute cystitis occur annually in the United States. Urinary tract infections are more prevalent among women than among men (ratio of $8:1$), probably secondary to an anatomically short urethra, which is in proximity to a large bacterial reservoir within the introital tract and along the vaginal vestibule.

The incidence of urinary tract infections increases with age. At 1 year, there is a 1% to 2% incidence of bacteriuria in females; upper urinary tract pathology directly correlates with these infections. As many as 50% of these patients will show abnormalities on intravenous pyelograms, i.e., scarring and either ipsilateral reflux or some obstructive disease. After 1 year of age, the infection rate decreases to approximately 1% and continues to decrease until puberty. The incidence of urologic pathology associated with these infections also progressively decreases. With the introduction of sexual activity and pregnancy, the incidence rises and continues to increase with age. Between the ages of 15 and 24, the prevalence of bacteriuria is about 2% to 3% and increases to about 10% at the age of 60, 20% after the age of 65, and 25% to 50% after the age of 80 (Fig. 22-1).

Approximately 2% of all patients admitted to a hospital acquire a urinary tract infection during their stay, which accounts for 500,000 nosocomial urinary tract infections per year. One percent of these infections become life-threatening. Instrumentation or catheterization of the urinary tract is a precipitating factor in at least 80% of these infections.

DEFINITIONS

Before discussing urinary tract infections, an understanding of generally accepted definitions is essential, as the commonly used terminology can, at times, be confusing.

Cystitis indicates inflammation of the bladder, and can be used as a histologic, bacteriologic, cystoscopic,

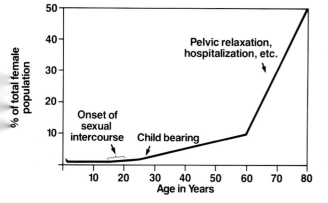

Fig. 22-1 Prevalence of bacteriuria in females as a function of age. *(From Karram MM: Lower urinary tract infection. In Ostergard DR, Bent AE (eds): Urogynecology and urodynamics, Baltimore, 1991, Williams & Wilkins.)*

or clinical term. Most commonly, it produces symptoms of urinary frequency and dysuria. Bacterial cystitis needs to be differentiated from nonbacterial cystitis (i.e., radiation-induced, interstitial, etc).

Urethritis refers to inflammation of the urethra and usually requires an adjective for modification (i.e., chlamydia, nonspecific, etc). In the female, symptoms of urethritis are indistinguishable from those of cystitis.

Trigonitis is inflammation or localized hyperemia of the trigone. This term is commonly used to describe the normal cobblestoned or granular appearance of the trigone and floor of the vesical neck. Failure to recognize that this epithelium is part of the normal embryologic development, plus lack of experience in cystoscopic examinations of normal women without bladder symptoms, is probably responsible for the frequent use of the terms *trigonitis* and *granular urethral trigonitis*.

The term *pyelonephritis* should be limited to the clinical description of patients with chills, fever, and flank pain, which is reasonably specific for an acute bacterial infection of the kidney. Other than this application, the term has limited use because a variety of renal diseases, including infarction and obstruction, produce identical histologic pictures in the renal cortex.

Bacteriuria implies the presence of bacteria in the urine. The term can include both renal and bladder bacteria. Symptomatic bacteriuria can have as few as 10^2 (cfu)/ml, whereas asymptomatic bacteriuria requires the growth of $\geq 10^5$ cfu/ml.

Prophylactic antimicrobial therapy refers to the prevention of reinfection of the urinary tract by the administration of drugs. It assumes bacteria have been completely eliminated before prophylaxis is initiated.

Suppressive antimicrobial therapy refers to the suppression of an existing infection that the physician is unable to eradicate. This suppression may result in sterile urine or it may reduce (suppress) the bacteria without achieving sterile urine.

Chronic is a poor term, as it defies clear definition and should thus be avoided whenever possible.

Complicated is commonly used in clinical antibiotic trials in an effort to distinguish simple from recurrent infections.Complicated is a poor term unless the unusual circumstances of the urinary tract are presented in detail for each entry.

Reinfection is infection occurring after cessation of therapy with a different strain of microorganism or a different serologic type. The source of recurrent bladder infection usually comes from outside the urinary tract.

Relapse implies consecutive urinary infection caused by the same bacterial strain, as opposed to bacterial reinfection. It is a useful term when used to describe consecutive infections, regardless of the time lapse between each of the infections. Unfortunately, some investigators use the term with a 2-week or less limitation between recurrences, implying that the kidney is the site of bacterial relapse, when, in reality, reinfections from the urethra or vagina can also readily recur within 2 weeks.

Persistence of bacteria implies the continued presence of the same infecting microorganisms isolated at the start of treatment. This may be caused by several factors, including resistance of the organism to antimicrobial therapy, inadequate concentrations of the drug in the serum or urine, inadequate dosage of the drug, poor patient compliance, or, most important, an underlying structural or functional abnormality harboring bacteria.

Superinfection is the appearance of organisms during treatment that are different from the originally isolated organisms.

PATHOGENESIS

The normal female urinary tract is remarkably resistant to infection. Although certain risk factors for developing urinary tract infections have been identified (see accompanying box), it remains unclear why some women are more prone than others to infection.

The pathogenesis of urinary tract infections in the female has been postulated to involve three primary mechanisms: hematogenous, lymphatic, or ascending extension of organisms directly from the rectum (Fig. 22-2). Hematogenous dissemination is the principal route by which staphylococcus organisms seed the kidney. This seeding leads to pyelonephritis and may

---

Known Risk Factors for Urinary Tract Infection

   I. Advanced Age
  II. Inefficient Bladder Emptying
      A. Pelvic relaxation
          1. Large cystocele with high residuals
          2. Uterovaginal prolapse resulting in obstructive voiding
      B. Neurogenic bladder, i.e., diabetes mellitus, multiple sclerosis, spinal cord injury, etc
      C. Drugs with anticholinergic effects
 III. Decreased Functional Ability
      A. Dementia
      B. Cardiovascular accidents
      C. Fecal incontinence
      D. Neurologic deficits
  IV. Nosocomial Infections
      A. Indwelling catheters
      B. Hospitalized patients
   V. Physiologic Changes
      A. Decreased vaginal glycogen and increased vaginal pH in women
  IV. Sexual Intercourse
      A. Diaphragm use

---

possibly be an important route for *Escherichia coli* in patients who do not have vesicoureteral reflux.

Retrograde (ascending) infection is the most widely accepted mechanism and appears to be important in the management of infections. Susceptibility probably depends on the inoculum size, the virulence properties of the invading microorganism, and the status of the host defense mechanisms. These host mechanisms are found in the urine and vagina and throughout the female urinary tract.

Ascending infection is characterized by a stepwise process whereby urinary pathogens initially colonize the periurethral tissue. If bacteria become established in the urethra, symptomatic or asymptomatic infection of the bladder occurs. If these organisms are able to overcome the host defense mechanisms in the bladder efficiently, they may ascend into the ureters and reach the kidneys, where another phase of host defense awaits bacteria gaining access to the renal parenchyma.

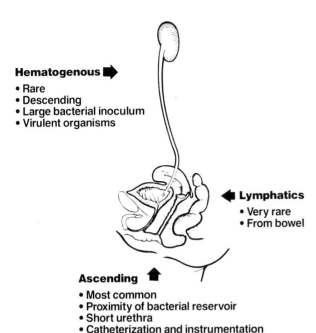

Hematogenous ▶
- Rare
- Descending
- Large bacterial inoculum
- Virulent organisms

◀ **Lymphatics**
- Very rare
- From bowel

Ascending ▲
- Most common
- Proximity of bacterial reservoir
- Short urethra
- Catheterization and instrumentation

Fig. 22-2 Pathways of bacterial entry into the urinary tract. *(From Karram MM: Lower urinary tract infection. In Ostergard DR, Bent AE (eds):* Urogynecology and urodynamics, *Baltimore, 1991, Williams & Wilkins.)*

Host Defense Mechanisms
Urine

Urine has important defense mechanisms against infection. Bacterial inhibitory factors include high or low osmolality, high urea concentration, high organic acid concentration, and low pH. A dilute urine with high osmolality, especially when associated with low pH, will inhibit bacterial growth by inhibiting phagocytosis and decreasing the reactivity of complement. In general, anaerobic bacteria and other fastidious organisms that make up a majority of the urethral flora will not multiply in urine; however, urine usually supports growth of nonfastidious bacteria.

Vaginal, Periurethral, and Perineal Colonization

The antibacterial defense mechanisms of the vaginal walls and periurethral area are important in preventing the progression of microorganisms from the rectum to the bladder. Normally, this area is colonized by gram-positive bacteria, lactobacillus, and diphtheroids (organisms that grow very poorly in urine and do not cause urinary tract infections). A number of studies have shown that females with recurrent cystitis will first colonize their vaginal introitus and periurethral area with Enterobacteria before the onset of the symptoms of cystitis and then will be at risk for infection until this colonization reverses to normal. Acidity of vaginal secretions may contribute to vaginal resistance to coliform bacteria. In premenopausal women, the vaginal pH is usually near 4.0. This acidic pH prohibits the growth of organisms such as *E. coli*, but promotes growth of the normally present organisms, such as lactobacillus, which interferes with the growth of uropathogens. High vaginal pH seems to be associated with the growth of enterobacteria.

Normal Periodic Voiding

Periodic voiding is one of the most important bladder defense mechanisms. In one study by Cox and Hinman the introduction of 10 million bacteria into normal male bladders failed to establish infection, as the organism rapidly cleared by voiding, diluting with fresh urine, and voiding again. Voiding displaces infected urine with sterile urine and flushes out bacteria attached to desquamated uroepithelial cells.

Prevention of Bacterial Adherence

The ability of organisms to bind to epithelial cells has been shown to correlate with their ability to infect the urinary tract. The ascending loop of Henle secretes Tamm-Horsfall protein, which is a uromucoid, rich in mannose. This protein may inhibit bacterial adherence and trap bacteria in the urine, allowing them to be flushed from the urinary tract. In addition, the presence of immunoglobulins in the urine and glycosaminoglycan in the bladder lining may be important factors in blocking bacterial adherence. The reduction of glycosaminoglycan probably plays a role in recurrent cystitis.

Host Susceptibility Factors
Bacterial Adherence

Microbial adherence to mucosal cells is considered to be a prerequisite to colonization and infection. As previously mentioned, in the majority of women, when these organisms enter the urethra and bladder, they do not adhere and are easily washed away. In persons susceptible to urinary tract infections, the organisms will quickly lock into the defective epithelial cells. The fecal flora is almost invariably the source of the infecting organisms, with the major pathogens being *E. coli*, although *Staphylococcus epidermidis*, enterococci, *Klebsiella*, and *Proteus* can sometimes be identified (Fig. 22-3).

The interaction of the mucosal and bacterial cells probably depends on both mucosal receptors and some type of attachment mechanism used by the bacteria. *E. coli* has been studied more than other bacteria and has been shown to possess surface organelles (adhesions) that mediate attachment to specific host receptors. These structures, called pili, can be present in large numbers on the microbial cell. Two types have been identified that appear to be important in urinary infections. Type I pili seek mannose as a receptor and are isolated from individuals with cystitis. These structures are present on most Enterobacteria and appear to be necessary for mucosal colonization. They tend to bind with a low affinity and their presence is not correlated highly with pathogenicity. Type II pili are mannose-negative or "p pili" and adhere to the P blood group. *E. coli* strains possessing p fimbriae are more virulent and are more likely to cause pyelonephritis than are strains without them.

Schaeffer et al (1981) studied the adherence of *E. coli* to vaginal epithelial cells in women who had experienced at least three urinary tract infections in the past year and in a control group. They found greater adherence in the study patients than in the controls; the increased adherence persisted despite temporary remission in the controls. The vaginal cells of those receiving a sustained course of antimicrobials showed less adherence than did the vaginal cells of patients who were not on antibiotics. If the antibiotics were discontinued, adherence returned and reinfection usually occurred. In another study, Schaeffer et al (1979) noted that adherence tends to be higher during the early, estrogen-dependent phase of the menstrual cycle.

High-risk women with recurrent urinary tract infections may be genetically prone to recurrent infec-

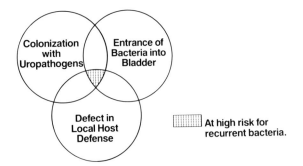

Fig. 22-3 Factors determining host risk and susceptibility to bacterial cystitis in normal females with anatomically normal urinary tracts. *(From Karram MM: Lower urinary tract infection. In Ostergard DR, Bent AE (eds):* Urogynecology and urodynamics, *Baltimore, 1991, Williams & Wilkins.)*

tion because they have a higher prevalence of the HLA-A3 subtype than do women who have never had urinary tract infections. Recent work also suggests that women of blood group B or AB, who are nonsecretors of blood group substances, have a significantly higher risk of developing infections compared with women of other blood groups.

Thus these genetic differences at the cellular level seem to influence bacterial adherence and make certain women more prone to urinary tract infections. These differences also influence the anatomic level of the infections.

Sexual Intercourse

In women, sexual intercourse appears to be a major determinant for bacterial entry into the bladder. Prospective studies have shown that many urinary tract infections develop the day after sexual intercourse. Both the frequency and recency of sexual intercourse increase the risk of cystitis. Women who have engaged in sexual intercourse within the previous 48 hours have a 60-fold increased risk of infection over women who have not. This increase appears to occur through inoculation of periurethral bacteria into the bladder during active intercourse. Women who have not colonized their vaginal and periurethral areas with coliform bacteria will introduce normal vaginal flora (i.e. *Lactobacillus*, diphtheroids or *S. epidermidis*) that do not produce infection and are rapidly cleared with voiding. In the colonized women, however the pathogenic organisms, such as *E. coli*, will infect the bladder.

Another commonly overlooked factor is the use of diaphragms. Studies have confirmed that diaphragm users are at increased risk of urinary tract infection, even after statistically controlling for sexual activity and history of previous urinary tract infection. The mechanism is unknown; however, it may be related to urethral obstruction caused by the diaphragm. Diaphragm users also have reduced vaginal colonization with lactobacillus, but coliforms are isolated three times more often in diaphragm users than in women using other contraceptive methods.

Systemic Factors

Diabetics are prone to develop neurogenic bladder dysfunction and severe vascular disease, both of which can predispose to urinary tract infections. Other genetic problems commonly associated with urinary tract infections are gouty nephropathy, sickle cell trait, and cystic renal disease.

The explanations for the pathogenesis of urinary tract infections apply only to those women who have normal urinary tracts. Bacteria in the presence of obstruction, stones, or a neurogenic bladder do not need special invasive properties other than the ability to grow in urine.

CLINICAL PRESENTATION

Signs and symptoms of urinary tract infection in women are diverse. It is helpful to distinguish lower urinary tract infection (cystitis) from upper tract infection (pyelonephritis) to aid in the selection of proper antimicrobial therapy and to plan appropriate follow-up.

Cystitis and associated urethral irritation are usually manifested by lower urinary tract irritative symptoms such as dysuria, frequency of small amounts of urine, urgency, nocturia, suprapubic discomfort, low backache, and flank pain. Occasionally, mild incontinence and hematuria may occur at the end of voiding. The urine rarely will be grossly bloody. Systemic symptoms, such as fever and chills, are usually absent.

Upper urinary tract infections involving the renal pelvis, calyces, and parenchyma will commonly present with fever, chills, malaise, and occasionally (especially in elderly patients) nausea and vomiting. Costovertebral angle tenderness and flank pain are usually present. There will be colicky pain if acute pyelonephritis is complicated by either a renal calculus or a sloughed renal papilla secondary to diabetic or analgesic nephropathy.

MICROBIOLOGY OF URINARY TRACT INFECTIONS

Urinary tract infection in the nonpregnant female is usually due to enteric strains of gram-negative aerobic organisms. *E. coli* accounts for approximately 80% of the community-acquired infections, with other organisms being responsible for a disproportionate number of infections compared with their frequency in stool flora. *Klebsiella* species cause about 5% of infections, whereas *Enterobacter* and *Proteus* species each cause approximately 2% of infections outside the hospital. *Serratia marcescens* and *Pseudomonas aeruginosa* are almost always nosocomial and are due to omission of infection control practices, usually after urethral catheterization or manipulation. Although anaerobes are present in abundance in the feces of normal individuals, they are rarely the cause of urinary tract infection. The oxygen tension in urine probably prevents their growth and persistence within the urinary tract. *S. saprophyticus* is the second most common pathogen isolated from young women with acute cystitis and accounts for approximately 10% of these cases. *S. epidermidis* is a frequent cause of nosocomial urinary tract infection in catheterized patients and is frequently resistant to antibacterial agents. Other gram-positive organisms, including the group B and group D streptococcus, cause 1% to 2% of urinary tract infections.

DIAGNOSIS OF BACTERIURIA

Before performing any tests to document the presence or absence of pathogenic bacteria in the urine, the method of urinary collection must be considered. Considerable care must be taken in the collection of urine from ambulatory women. Kass has published results demonstrating that one whole voided urine specimen with a colony count of greater than 10^5 cfu/ml has only an 80% chance of representing true infection. Three specimens increased the odds to 95%. Even when intelligent, educated patients are given clear, detailed instructions for collection of urine, errors can occur. Certain patients, due to physical disability or obesity, are simply unable to obtain a clean voided specimen without assistance. When necessary, to avoid these limitations, specimens can be obtained via urethral catheterization; or the patient can void in the lithotomy position on an examining table after the perineum is cleaned with soap and water, while the nurse collects a midstream specimen; or bladder urine can be aspirated suprapubically. Although urethral catheterization is the most time-honored method, it is not without risks. Reports have noted that catheter-induced infection rates range from 1% in young healthy women to as high as 20% in hospitalized women.

Urine Microscopy

Microscopic analysis of urine is an easy and valuable method of evaluating women with symptoms of urinary tract infection. A thorough microscopic examination of an uncentrifuged sample of urine can detect the presence of significant bacteria, leukocytes, and red blood cells. If infection with greater than 10^4 cfu/ml is present, the finding of one or more bacteria on a gram-stained urine specimen correlates highly with the presence of urinary tract infection, having a sensitivity of 80% and a specificity of 90% with a positive predictive value of approximately 85%. Thus, a Gram stain of the urine is useful in detecting abundant bacteriuria, but is of little help in infection with colony counts of less than 10^4 cfu/ml.

Fresh, unspun urine can also be quantitatively assessed with a hemacytometer for the number of white blood cells. The hemocytometer is positioned on the microscope stage. The number of leukocytes are counted in each of 9 large squares, divided by 9 and multiplied by 10 to yield the number of white blood cells per milliliter. Pyuria is defined as greater than 10 leukocytes per milliliter. Pyuria is present in nearly all women with acute urinary tract infection. Studies note the presence of pyuria to be 80% to 95% sensitive

(even when bacteria counts are less than 10^4) and 50% to 75% specific for the presence of urinary tract infection. It is also of value to ascertain whether red blood cells are present. Microscopic hematuria is found in about 50% women with acute urinary tract infection and is rarely present in patients who have dysuria due to other causes.

Office Urine Kits

If expertise for office microscopy is not available or feasible, it is reasonable to substitute a rapid diagnostic test for bacteriuria, pyuria, and hematuria, although, in general, these tests are less accurate than microscopy. The most common rapid detection test is the nitrite test, which depends on the conversion of urinary nitrate to nitrite by bacterial action. Numerous test kits are available (N-multisticks, N-multisticks C, and N-multisticks-SG, Ames Division, Miles Laboratory; Chemstrip 9 and Chemstrip LN from Boehringer Maenhein Diagnostics; and Kyotest 8 Fe from Kyoto Diagnostics). The test is often integrated with an esterase test that suggests the presence of pyuria by a color change caused by esterase found in leukocytes. The sensitivity of these tests is directly related to the bacterial counts. Wu et al showed a sensitivity of only 22% in infections with 10^4 to 10^5 cfu/ml versus 60% for greater than 10^5 cfu/ml. The test should be performed on concentrated first-morning-voided specimens. It has been suggested that false-negative results are more common if the test is used as a sampling technique at other times during the day. False-negative results can also occur in infections due to enterococci, as they do not convert nitrate to nitrite, and in the presence of certain dyes such as bilirubin, methylene blue, or phenazopyridine, as they may interfere with the interpretation of the test. Some authorities believe that these are good screening tests for asymptomatic bacteriuria, whereas others believe that the high false-negative rate limits their value.

Other rapid detection tests, such as filter methods, i.e., Back-T-Screen (Marion Laboratories, Inc, Kansas City, Mo), concentrate a specific quantity of urinary sediment on a filter of controlled pore size. One milliliter of urine is mixed with 3 ml of a diluent containing glacial acetic acid and other ingredients that dissolve crystals and increase adherence of bacteria and leukocytes. The diluted mixture is then passed through the filter and rinsed with a diluent. A safranin dye that stains the bacteria and leukocytes is then used, and a decolorizer is added to remove excess dye. Resulting colors are compared with a reference to quantitate the presence of bacteria and leukocytes. The sensitivity of these tests for urine infected with 10^4 to 10^5 cfu/ml is from 34% to 65%. As the number of organisms increases to greater than 10^5, the sensitivity also increases to 79% to 85%. The specificity of this test at lower bacterial counts is approximately 75%. The main advantage of these tests is a more reliable detection of smaller numbers of bacteria at the expense of lower specificity. This test is a good screening method because it detects both bacteria and pyuria.

Urine Culture

In the patient who has clinical signs of acute lower urinary tract infection and is noted to have pyuria, bacteriuria, or hematuria on one of the previously mentioned office tests, it is reasonable to initiate antibiotic therapy without obtaining a urine culture. However, if one of the screening techniques is deemed inappropriate or inconclusive, the patient has recurrent infection that has not been subjectively relieved with previous antibiotics, or if signs and symptoms are consistent with upper urinary tract infection, then a bacterial culture and sensitivity should be performed.

Traditionally a growth of 10^5 cfu/ml must be present to consider the culture positive. This criterion is based on studies demonstrating that the finding of greater than 10^5 cfu/ml on two consecutive urine cultures distinguishes women with asymptomatic bacteriuria or pyelonephritis from those with contaminated specimens.

The use of this cutoff, however, has two limitations. First, 20% to 40% of women with symptomatic urinary infections will present with fewer than 10^5 cfu/ml. This presentation is probably secondary to a slow doubling time of bacteria in urine combined with frequent bladder emptying from persistent irritation. A study by Stamm et al proposed that the best diagnostic criteria for culture detection in young symptomatic women is 100 cfu/ml or more, not 100,000 cfu/ml. The second limitation of the 10^5 cutoff is

overdiagnosis. In the original studies by Kass, a single culture of 10^5 cfu/ml or more had a 20% chance of representing contamination. Because patients who are susceptible to infection will often carry large numbers of pathogenic bacteria on the perineum, contamination of an otherwise sterile urine can at times occur. For this reason, care in the collection of the urine specimen must again be emphasized.

Although methods of obtaining cultures in the office are available, most clinicians use commercial laboratories. One should be familiar with the individual laboratory policy of reporting culture results. Some laboratories report any culture of fewer than 10^5 cfu/ml as negative and often report only the predominant organism in mixed cultures. Because many clinical laboratories now use rapid culture techniques that rely on photometric detection of the products of bacterial metabolism, many of the results fail to detect lower levels of bacteriuria that may be clinically significant. Sensitivity testing is also usually obtained via commercial laboratory, even though office tests have been described (i.e., broth dilution method, plate dilution method, disc diffusion method). The disadvantages of sensitivity testing are the long time involved (typically 24 to 48 hours), the absence of processing control by the referring physician, and the relatively high cost (approximately $18 to $20 per test).

Cystourethroscopy

Indications for endoscopic evaluation in women with urinary tract infection are controversial. In their study of 74 cystoscopies performed in women with two or more previous infections, Fowler and Pulaski noted that the only abnormality that altered treatment was the presence of a urethral diverticulum in three cases.

Engel et al reviewed 153 women who had undergone cystoscopy for urinary tract infection. Although abnormalities were noted in 62% of the cases, 84% of these abnormalities were inflammatory and presumably secondary to prior infection. Only one abnormality, a colovesical fistula, had an effect on treatment. Cystoscopy under local anesthesia has basically no risk and occasionally reveals findings useful in subsequent patient management. Thus cystoscopic examination should be considered in patients with recurrent or persistent lower urinary tract infection.

Radiologic Studies

Although it has long been believed that urinary tract infection constitutes one of the important indications for urography, the use of routine intravenous pyelogram (IVP) in women with otherwise uncomplicated infection has recently been challenged. The minimal (1% to 2%) yield of the IVP makes it an inefficient and expensive method to identify underlying disease. The cost of detecting a single significant and treatable urologic disorder has been estimated at $9000. Nevertheless, we believe the IVP is a valuable diagnostic test when there is (1) a history of previous upper urinary tract infection; (2) a history of childhood urinary tract infections; (3) a history of recurrent infections caused by the same organism, particularly if the organism is urea splitting, such as *Proteus mirabilis*, as these organisms are frequently associated with infected stones; (4) infection associated with painless hematuria; (5) a history of stones or obstruction, or (6) bacterial evidence of rapid recurrence suggesting bacterial persistence or an enterovesical fistula.

A voiding cystourethrogram or a double balloon catheter study should be performed if a urethral diverticulum is thought to be contributing to recurrent infections. Signs and symptoms of urethral diverticulum include leakage of urine, postvoid dribbling, and the finding of pus or pain on palpation and massage of the urethra.

Urodynamic Studies

Urodynamic studies, involving a range of procedures from simple cystometry and flow studies to complicated video-urodynamic studies, are sometimes useful to demonstrate abnormal bladder contraction and emptying. A vicious cycle of repeated lower urinary tract infections can lead to an obstructed voiding pattern, with high residual urine volumes that resulting from spasm of the external striated urethral sphincter secondary to infection or to the pain of acute cystitis. These tests can be helpful in patients with recurrent urinary tract infection who have neurologic disease or a history of pelvic or spinal surgery.

DIFFERENTIAL DIAGNOSIS

When the history or laboratory findings are not consistent with urinary tract infection, other causes of lower urinary tract symptoms must be considered. Vaginitis is a major cause of lower urinary tract symptoms, with *Trichomonas* and *Candida* the most commonly implicated organisms. Dysuria is also a common presenting symptom in sexually transmitted diseases, particularly *C. trachomatis* and, less commonly, herpes simplex virus or *Neisseria gonorrhoeae*. Some patients can distinguish internal from external dysuria. Discomfort that is centered inside the body is more commonly associated with urinary tract infection or chlamydial urethritis, whereas pain that starts when the urine flows across the perineum is more commonly associated with vaginitis or herpetic infection. Frequency, urgency, and voiding small amounts of urine are common in urinary tract infection and in sexually transmitted diseases, but are rare in vaginitis. Virtually all women with acute symptomatic urinary tract infection have pyuria and about half have microscopic hematuria. Pyuria can also exist in patients with urethritis secondary to sexually transmitted diseases, but is not present in vaginitis. Hematuria is not a feature of either sexually transmitted diseases or vaginitis; thus its presence strongly suggests cystitis. Postmenopausal women may have dysuria secondary to estrogen deficiency causing desiccation of the urethra and vaginal mucosa. The term *urethral syndrome* has been used to describe a group of women who are not estrogen-deficient and who complain of persistent lower urinary tract symptoms in spite of negative urine, vaginal, and urethral cultures. A full discussion of this condition is presented in Chapter 20. A suggested approach to the evaluation and management of women with dysuria is shown in Fig. 22-4.

MANAGEMENT OF LOWER URINARY TRACT INFECTION

General measures such as rest and hydration should always be emphasized in women with urinary tract infection. Hydration will dilute bacterial counts and perhaps destroy cell-wall-deficient bacterial strains.

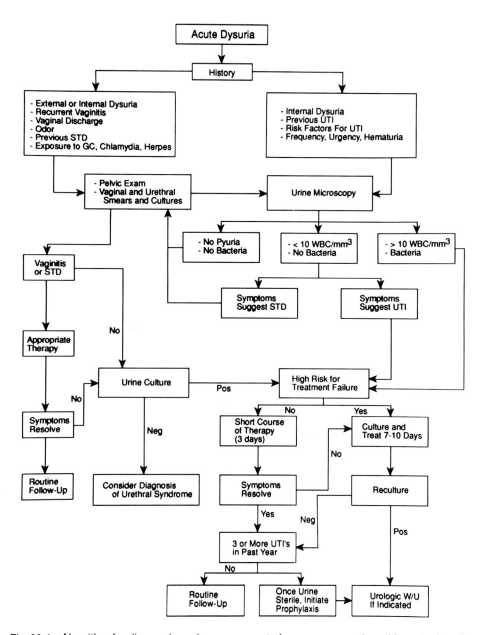

Fig. 22-4   Algorithm for diagnosis and management of women presenting with acute dysuria.

Acidification of the urine is helpful only in recurrent infections and in patients taking methenamine compounds, as the antibacterial activity of these agents is maximal at a pH of 5.5 or less. Urinary analgesic agents such as phenazopyridine hydrochloride (Pyridium) help relieve pain and burning on urination. If prescribed, they should be used for only 2 to 3 days along with a specific antibacterial agent.

General factors that influence the selection of antimicrobial agents for the treatment of urinary tract infections include the efficacy and the cost of the agent, the anticipated incidence and severity of adverse effects, and the dosing interval. Because the fecal flora is the reservoir for most organisms causing the infection, ideally a drug should be prescribed that has little or no effect on these microbes. These bacteria should not be altered because 20% of women with simple cystitis will have a recurrence shortly after stopping medication. A drug can alter bacteria in the bowel by either passing through the gastrointestinal tract without being absorbed or by having a high serum level. It is also important that a drug maintain a low serum level so as not to cause disruption of flora in other parts of the body, such as the vagina. If a drug appropriately matched to bacterial sensitivity causes a yeast vaginitis, the subsequent therapy for the vaginitis will increase patient morbidity and raise the cost of therapy. In addition, vaginitis precipitated by the antibiotic could lead to a vaginitis-cystitis cycle that may be difficult to treat.

The preceeding therapeutic goals should be kept in mind when treating these infections, as there are many misconceptions about commonly prescribed antibiotics. For example, ampicillin and tetracycline are both frequently prescribed for simple cystitis, but they have an incidence of yeast vaginitis that approaches 25% and 75%, respectively. Both drugs are excreted unchanged in the fecal stream and have stool levels three times that of urine. Nitrofurantoin, on the other hand, has excellent activity against *E. coli* and has no significant serum level. It has a 19-minute serum half life and is metabolized in every tissue in the body, resulting in no significant changes in fecal or vaginal flora. For this reason, no increase in bacterial resistance to nitrofurantoin has occurred after 30 years of use in the United States. Generic nitrofurantoin has a high incidence of gastrointestinal upset, whereas the trade form of the drug, Macrodantin, is well tolerated by the gastrointestinal tract. In theory, nitrofurantoin is an excellent antibiotic for simple cystitis.

The most common sulfonamide preparation used for urinary tract infections is the combination of trimethoprim with sulfamethaoxazole (TMP-SMX, Bactrim, Septra). These drugs have become popular in the management of urinary tract infections due to their broad range of activity against uropathogens, low incidence of adverse effects, twice daily dosage, and infrequent occurrence of bacterial resistance. Nevertheless, these agents have been shown to have a moderate effect on bowel and vaginal flora.

A group of synthetic quinolone derivatives related chemically to nalidixic acid recently have been introduced as antibacterial agents for urinary tract infections. Derivatives include norfloxacin, ciprofloxacin, enoxacin, pefloxacin, and amifloxacin. These agents are more active than nalidixic acid against gram-negative urinary tract pathogens. In addition, they have an expanded antibacterial spectrum that includes *P. aeruginosa* and gram-positive bacteria (e.g., staphylococci, enterococci). All of these agents are administered orally, with parental formulations available for some (e.g., ciprofloxacin). Although the drugs are associated with few adverse effects they are not used routinely due to their cost. Because they have little advantage for uncomplicated infections over more standard agents such as nitrofurantoin or TMP-SMX, they should be reserved for use in patients with resistant infections or as an alternative to parental antibiotics in complicated infections. Tables 22-1 and 22-2 list the dose, toxicity, and spectrum of antimicrobial activity for some of the commonly prescribed oral antibiotics.

Asymptomatic Bacteriuria: Is Treatment Necessary?

By definition, asymptomatic bacteriuria is the recovery of $\geq$ to 10^5 cfu/ml of a single bacterial species in at least two consecutive clean-catch urine specimens in the absence of clinical symptoms. Little is known about the natural history of untreated bacteriuria in women; most are treated once the diagnosis is made. Two studies have compared antibiotic treatment to placebo in women with asymptomatic bacteriuria. Both noted that 60% to 80% of patients will spontaneously clear their infection, whether they are treated or receive placebo. Although the long-term effects of asymptomatic bacteriuria are not completely known, there seems to be no association with renal scarring, hypertension, or progressive renal azotemia.

TABLE 22-1 Dosage and toxicity of antibiotics commonly used in the treatment of urinary tract infections

Drug	Oral dose and frequency	Minor toxicity	Major toxicity
*TMP-SMX	1 tab BID	Allergic	Serious skin reactions, blood dyscrasia
Nitrofurantoin	50-100 mg q 6-8 hr	GI upset	Peripheral neuropathy, pneumonitis
Ampicillin	250-500 mg q 6 hr	Allergic, candidal overgrowth	Allergic reactions, pseudomembranous colitis
Tetracycline	250-500 mg q 6 hr	GI upset, skin rash, candidal overgrowth	Hepatic dysfunction, nephrotoxicity
Cephalexin	250-500 mg	Allergic	Hepatic dysfunction
Norfloxacin	400 mg q 12 hr	Nausea, vomiting, diarrhea, abdominal pain, skin rash	Convulsions, psychoses, joint damage

*Trimethoprim-sulfamethoxazole.

TABLE 22-2 Spectrum of antimicrobial activity against common lower urinary tract pathogens

Organisms	TMP-SMX	Nitrofurantoin	Ampicillin	Tetracycline	Cephalexin	Carbenicillin	Gentamicin	Norfloxacin
E. coli	+ +	+ +	+ +	±	+ +	+ +	+ +	+ +
Pseudomonas	−	−	−	−	−	+ +	+ +	+ +
Klebsiella	+ +	±	−	±	+ +	−	+ +	+ +
Proteus	+ +	−	+ +	−	+ +	+ +	+ +	+ +
Enterobacter	+ +	−	−	−	−	+ +	+ +	+ +
Enterococcus	−	±	+ +	+ +	±	−	−	+ +
Staphylcoccus	−	±	+ +	+	+ +	+ +	+	+ +
Serratia marcescens	+	−	−	−	−	−	+ +	+ +

+ + Excellent.
+ Good.
± Occasionally effective.
− Resistant.

One definite indication for the screening and treatment of asymptomatic bacteriuria is pregnancy. Numerous double-blind trials have shown that antibiotic treatment will significantly reduce the risk of both pyelonephritis and low-birthweight babies.

To date, there is no definite advantage to treating asymptomatic bacteriuria in the nonpregnant women. However, recent studies have shown a significant association between asymptomatic urinary tract infection and overall mortality in elderly persons. Whether this association is a false-positive result or whether bacteriuria is serving as a marker for a chronic disease that was the actual cause of death needs to be determined by further studies.

First Infections or Infrequent Reinfections

Many treatment regimens have been reported for initial therapy of simple cystitis, ranging from one dose to two or more weeks of medication. Cystitis is a superficial infection of the bladder mucosa that rarely invades the lamina propria. Studies have shown that 30% of patients with simple cystitis can be cured by a simple bladder irrigation with a 10% neomycin solution. The longer treatment regimens were instituted, however, in an attempt to prevent relapse rates, which occur in about 20% of patients treated for cystitis. Almost all of these relapses are attributable to colonization of the vaginal walls and urethra with gram-negative bacteria that continued to grow on the perineum or reappeared when the drug was stopped. Relapse does not indicate that the prescribed drug has failed to eradicate the bacteriuria.

Numerous studies in the literature evaluate single-dose therapy in the management of acute, uncomplicated cystitis. A recent randomized trial of single-dose versus 10 days of TMP-SMX noted a significantly higher treatment failure rate after single-dose therapy 13 days after the initiation of therapy; however, when these patients were reevaluated at 6 weeks, the recurrence rates in the two groups were essentially the same. Penicillins and cephalosporins are less effective than TMP-SMX in a single dose, compared to a 7- to 10-day regimen. Single-dose TMP-SMX also is more effective than single-dose penicillin or cephalosporin in women with subclinical renal involvement, as noted by the presence of antibody-coated bacteria in the urine.

Besides the obvious advantages of patient compliance and cost, single-dose therapy has significantly fewer adverse effects compared to conventionally used 7- to 10-day regimens. Six percent to 8% of patients treated with single-dose TMP-SMX noted moderate to severe gastrointestinal side effects; symptomatic yeast vaginitis occurred in 2% to 4% percent of patients, and allergic reactions occurred 1% to 2% percent of patients. These side effects were two to four times more common after 7 to 10 days of TMP-SMX.

Due to the high initial recurrence rate, we have adopted a 3-day course of therapy to achieve most of the advantages of the single-dose therapy and avoid the higher adverse effects of the 7- to 10-day therapy. Nitrofurantoin and TMP-SMX have been our first-line drugs in patients with simple cystitis; amoxicillin or cephalosporins are used in patients with allergies to the first-line drugs, in resistant cases, or in patients

manifesting significant side effects. Single-dose therapy or a short course of therapy should be considered only in patients who are at low risk for treatment failures. Seven to 10 days of therapy are indicated for patients who have (1) systemic diseases such as diabetes mellitus, (2) history of acute pyelonephritis, (3) history of a treatment failure in the last 6 months, (4) history of childhood urinary tract infections, or (5) known structural abnormalities of the urinary tract.

Whether some form of objective assessment of the patient's urine is necessary after therapy is controversial. Traditional teaching has been to perform one, or sometime even several, posttherapy urine cultures to confirm the successful eradication of bacteria. However, it is rare for a patient to become asymptomatic after therapy, but continue to colonize bacteria in the urine. It has been estimated that the routine use of cultures to detect infrequent cases of asymptomatic bacteriuria after therapy for simple cystitis can cost up to $2000 per case. Few of these cases, when left undetected, will result in acute pyelonephritis. For this reason, patients with acute simple cystitis who have complete resolution of their symptoms do not require posttreatment urinary assessment. In those patients whose urinary symptoms persist beyond the 3 days of therapy, however, a urine culture and sensitivity should be obtained. Persistence of symptoms suggests the possibility that either the initial diagnosis of urinary tract infection was incorrect, or that the patient's infection is secondary to a resistant organism that was present from the onset of therapy or has developed during initial therapy. In cases of resistance, a 7- to 10-day course of a sensitive antibiotic should then be prescribed.

Recurrent Infections

Approximately 75% of all women who experience a urinary tract infection will subsequently experience less than one infection per year; however, 25% of women will develop almost three infections per year. These women comprise 50% of all women presenting with acute urinary tract infections.

Once the urine has been sterilized by appropriate antimicrobial therapy, the pattern of culture-documented reinfection or recurrence is helpful in the subsequent management of these patients (Fig. 22-5). It

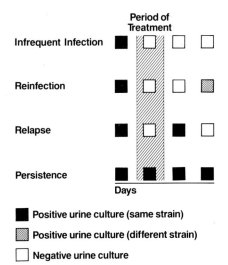

Fig. 22-5 Natural history of urinary tract infection. *(From Karram MM: Lower urinary tract infection. In Ostergard DR, Bent AE (eds):* Urogynecology and urodynamics, *Baltimore, 1991, Williams & Wilkins.)*

can also be used to classify patients with different infectious etiologies; to identify those who require further urologic evaluation; and to plan a specific, predictable, appropriate mode of therapy. The most common type of recurrence is a reinfection by different bacteria from the initially infecting strain. Even though the infections may be caused by the same species (e.g., *E. coli*), the organisms can usually be differentiated on the basis of colonial morphology and antimicrobial sensitivities. These infections are almost invariably due to a recurrent ascending infection from the vaginal introital area. That is not to say that the same organism cannot be the cause of reinfection, as the same strain can exist in the introital area for many months and cause multiple reinfections. Sexual intercourse and occult urinary tract abnormalities may also facilitate reinfection and must always be considered in these patients.

As previously mentioned, a less common form of recurrence which has been termed *relapse*, is characterized by reappearance of the original infecting strain in the urine, usually, but not necessarily, within 2 weeks after finishing therapy. Traditional teaching has been that relapsing infections are due to inade-

quately treated upper urinary tract infections. Recent studies, however, have noted that reinfection from the vaginal introital area can occur within a 2-week period. Relapsing infection from an upper urinary tract source or an infected stone should be suspected if the same organism is repeatedly isolated 7 to 10 days after treatment with an antimicrobial agent to which the organism is sensitive. In many of these patients, one cannot obtain sterile urine; thus these infections are termed bacterial persistence (see accompanying box). Endoscopic and radiographic evaluations must be selectively performed in cases of relapse or persistence of infection.

Because the fecal flora is the ultimate source of the majority of recurrent urinary tract pathogens, oral antimicrobial agents used to treat these patients should not alter rectal flora. Sulfonamides, penicillins, tetracyclines, and cephalosporins in full dosages can cause fecal flora to become rapidly resistant, not only to the original drug, but also to other antimicrobial agents by means of transfer of extra-chromosomal plasmids. Other drugs, such as the quinolones or nitrofurantoin, cause very little resistance, as they have minimal effects on fecal flora. The goal of management of reinfected urine is to achieve sterile urine; therefore, antimicrobial agents should be administered in doses sufficient to exceed by a wide margin the minimal concentration required to inhibit growth. If the dose is inadequate, resistant organisms develop in about 10% of the cases, which complicates the treatment of these already resistant patients.

Most patients with recurrent urinary tract infections

Correctable Urinary Tract Abnormalities Causing Persistent Bacteriuria

1. Urethral diverticulum
2. Infected stone
3. Significant anterior vaginal wall relaxation
4. Papillary necrosis
5. Foreign body
6. Duplicated or ectopic ureter
7. Atrophic pyelonephritis (unlateral)
8. Medullary sponge kidney

are treated with low-dose, continuous prophylaxis. This regimen is highly cost-effective and is recommended as the initial form of therapy in women who have frequent reinfections. Its success depends on using an antimicrobial agent that has minimal or no adverse effect on the fecal flora and that can be administered in a small dosage. Once the urine has been completely sterilized by a full-dose course of therapy, nightly therapy can be initiated with one of many different drugs (Table 22-3). Nitrofurantoin, 100 mg, or cephalexin, 250 mg, are both effective. These drugs do not cause resistance in the fecal flora, however, vaginal colonization with sensitive bacteria continues. Their efficacy depends on nightly bactericidal activity in the urine against sensitive reinfecting organisms. The efficacy of cephalexin depends on use of a minimal dose. If it is given four times a day in full doses, it gives rise to resistant strains; a dose of 250 mg nightly is effective. TMP-SMX in a dose of 50 mg is active, not only because of bactericidal activity against urinary bacteria, but also because TMP diffuses in the vaginal fluid at a concentration bactericidal to most urinary pathogens. Low-dose TMP-SMX or TMP alone causes resistance in about 10% of rectal cultures. Cinoxacin in a dose of 250 to 500 mg/day also has been shown to be effective in prophylactic therapy. This synthetic antimicrobial agent is chemically similar to nalidixic acid and shares its activity against common gram-negative uropathogens. Its advantages include a high urinary concentration that does not cause plasmid-mediated multiple drug resistance in the fecal flora.

The majority of patients will continue to maintain

sterile urine while on prophylactic therapy, although break-through infections may occur infrequently and should be treated with full-dose antimicrobial therapy. We empirically continue the prophylactic therapy for approximately 6 months and then follow the patient off therapy with frequent cultures. Approximately 30% of women will be free of infection for at least the subsequent 6 months. Unfortunately, remission does not necessarily reflect a complete cure. If reinfection occurs, it must be managed by reinstitution of low-dose nightly prophylaxis.

Self-start intermittent therapy is an alternative to continuous prophylactic therapy in patients with recurrent urinary tract infections. With this form of treatment, the patient is given a dipslide and instructed to perform a urine culture when she has symptoms of a recurrent urinary tract infection. She then empirically begins a 3-day course of full-dose antimicrobial therapy; usually one of the previously mentioned antibiotics is used. Full-dose nitrofurantoin, cinoxacin, or norfloxacin is an excellent choice. Norfloxacin seems to be an ideal drug for self-start therapy. It has a broader spectrum of activity in comparison to any other oral agent and is comparable to or better than most available parental antimicrobial agents. In addition, it is active against many resistant bacteria and has a low rate of spontaneous mutation to resistant organisms. In a multicentered comparative study of over 350 patients with urinary tract infections, the percentage of strains susceptible to norfloxacin was 99%, as compared to 90% for TMP-SMX. In addition, the percentage of bacteriologic cures was significantly greater with the norfloxacin (compared to TMP-SMX) and side effects were minimal.

With self-start therapy the patient is instructed to bring the urine culture to the physician's office the day of or the day after she believes the infection begins. A repeat culture is then performed, also via dipslide method, approximately 7 days after the completion of therapy. The cost of this therapy is thus limited to two inexpensive dip-slide cultures and a short course of antimicrobial therapy. If the patient's symptoms do not respond to the initial antimicrobial drug, a repeat culture and sensitivity are performed and therapy is adjusted accordingly. If the initial culture was negative, other causes of lower urinary tract symptoms

TABLE 22-3   Oral antimicrobial agents useful for prophylactic prevention of recurrent urinary tract infections

Agent	Dosage
Nitrofurantoin	100 mg
Cephalexin	250 mg
*TMP-SMX	50 mg
Cinoxacin	250-500 mg

*Trimethoprim-sulfamethoxazole.

must be pursued. This technique is particularly attractive for women with less frequent infections who are willing to play an active role in their diagnosis and management.

Finally, a small percentage of patients with recurrent urinary tract infections are at high risk for serious morbidity and renal scarring from bacteriuria because of pregnancy, diabetes mellitus, congenital abnormalities, and obstructive uropathy. The primary care physician should carefully watch for such patients, as prompt therapy, appropriate referral, and careful follow-up are mandatory.

SEXUAL INTERCOURSE AND DIAPHRAGM USE

If a patient's history suggests that reinfections are preceded by intercourse, she may take a single antimicrobial tablet before or after intercourse. Vosti first demonstrated that nitrofurantoin given after coitus prevented urinary tract infection. More recently, Pfau et al showed that TMP-SMX, nalidixic acid, nitrofurantoin, and sulfonamides were all effective in preventing recurrent urinary tract infections when given to young sexually active women whose infections occurred postcoitally. Compared with continuous low-dose prophylaxis, this approach may reduce medication costs and side effects and lessen the emergence of resistant bacterial strains.

If possible, a woman who has recurrent urinary tract infections and uses a diaphragm should consider another method of contraception. If a change is not feasible, it should be determined whether symptoms of urinary obstruction occurs with the diaphragm in place. If such symptoms occur, it should be ascertained whether the diaphragm is too large. Women in this category should also be advised to void as promptly as possible after intercourse.

CATHETER-ASSOCIATED INFECTION

Catheter-associated urinary tract infection is the most common nosocomial infection and the most frequent source of bacteremia in hospitalized patients. A recent study by Platt et al demonstrated a threefold increase in mortality in these patients. The relationship between bacteriuria and mortality is uncertain. Risk factors of catheter-associated infection are advanced age, female sex, and an increasing degree of underlying illness.

The pathogenesis of catheter-associated urinary infection has not been studied as well as that of urinary tract infection of noncatheterized patients. Points of bacterial entry, however, have been identified and include introduction of bacteria residing in the urethra into the bladder at the time of catheterization, subsequent entry of bacteria colonizing the urethra meatus along the mucus sheath external to the catheter, and ascent of bacteria within the catheter lumen itself. The relative proportion of infections occurring through these different routes of entry have not been determined. Prospective studies have demonstrated that organisms causing infection in catheterized patients can be identified in the urethral or rectal flora 2 to 4 days before the onset of bacteriuria in 70% of women. Until more is known about the pathogenesis of nosocomial bacteriuria, the bulk of preventive efforts should continue to focus on aseptic care of the urinary catheter (see accompanying box).

There has been no demonstrable efficacy of local antimicrobial ointments applied to the meatal junction, despite the apparent association of meatal colonization with subsequent infection. The use of antimicrobial irrigants has also been ineffective in reducing the prevalence of bacteriuria. Although systemic antimicrobial agents reduce the occurrence of bacteriuria for the first few days of catheterization, their use is not widely recommended because the benefit accrued—reduction of asymptomatic bacteriuria—may not be worth the cost and attendant risk of development of resistant microorganisms.

Prevention of Bladder Infection in Elderly Long-Term Catheterized Patients

1. Monitor urine level in bag every 4 hours. Exchange catheter if cessation of flow for 4 hours.
2. Fluid intake of 1.5 L/day.
3. Avoid catheter manipulations.
4. Exchange catheter if infection is suspected.
5. Exchange catheter every 8 to 12 weeks.

All patients with chronic indwelling catheters develop bacteriuria. As long as the catheter system is a closed functioning system and the patient has no local or systemic symptoms or signs, however, there is no advantage to treatment with systemic antibiotics. On the other hand, 10% of elderly patients with indwelling catheters develop bacteremia and gram-negative septicemia, a serious disease with a 20% to 50% mortality rate. These patients must be promptly identified, as they require hospitalization and vigorous systemic antibiotic therapy. A traumatic event consisting of obstruction, manipulation, or removal of an inflated indwelling bladder catheter often precedes the onset of urosepsis. In addition to antibiotic therapy, it is essential to establish free flow of urine for the catheterized patient with acute urosepsis. The complications of concomitant bacteremia (shock, adult respiratory distress syndrome, disseminated intravascular coagulation, and gastric hemorrhage) must be readily recognized and appropriately managed. Certain measures can be taken to prevent these life-threatening complications in patients with chronic indwelling catheters (see box p. 325). Catheters should be checked every 4 hours by experienced personnel to assure proper drainage and to prevent formation of any encrustations within the tubing of the catheter, and indwelling catheters should be changed every 8 to 12 weeks depending on whether they are silicon- or Teflon-coated. Again, it must be emphasized that the most important preventive measure is complete asepsis in the insertion of the catheter and in the care of patients with chronic indwelling catheters.

LOWER URINARY TRACT INSTRUMENTATION

Whether patients undergoing lower urinary tract instrumentation for diagnostic or therapeutic purposes need prophylactic antibiotics is an unresolved issue. A recent prospective, double-blind, placebo-controlled study noted that during urodynamic evaluation, endoscopic evaluation of the lower urinary tract, or urethral dilation, patients receiving placebo had a significantly higher infection rate than did those receiving either one dose of cephadroxal or three does of nitrofurantoin. Thus we routinely administer prophylactic antibiotics to patients after lower urinary tract instrumentation.

PYELONEPHRITIS

A comprehensive discussion of pyelonephritis is beyond the scope of this chapter. It is sufficient to say, however, that certain patients who appear to have typical signs and symptoms of acute cystitis will harbor subclinical upper urinary tract infection. These patients require aggressive therapy—usually a minimum of 10 days of antimicrobial therapy. At times they will require hospitalization and intravenous antibiotic therapy. As in cystitis, 70% of cases of pyelonephritis are secondary to *E. coli* infection. Patients with acute pyelonephritis usually have high-titer bacteriuria and, unless obstruction is present, microscopic examination of the urine should demonstrate bacteria and leukocytes. If symptoms are relatively mild and the patient is highly reliable, treatment of mild pyelonephritis with oral agents on an outpatient basis is an acceptable approach. The drug of choice is TMP-SMX because it has high tissue levels, and a wide spectrum of activity against coliform organisms and bacterial resistance is relatively uncommon. However, patients who exhibit toxicity, who are unable to take oral medications, who have any complicating factors, or who are not entirely reliable should be hospitalized and treated initially with parenteral antibiotics.

BIBLIOGRAPHY
Prevalence

Mulholland SG: Controversies in management of urinary tract infection, *Urology* (Suppl) 27:3, 1986.

National Center for Health Statistics: ambulatory medical care rendered in physicians' offices. United States 1975, *Adv Data* 12:1, 1977.

Rolleston GL, Shannon FT, Utley WLF: Relationship of infantile vesico-ureteric reflux to renal damage, *Br Med J* 1:460, 1970.

Turck M, Stamm W: Nosocomial infection of the urinary tract, *Am J Med* 70:651, 1981.

Winberg J, Anderson HJ, Bergstrom T, et al: Epidemiology of symptomatic urinary tract infection in childhood, *Acta Paediatr Scand* (Suppl) 252:3, 1974.

Pathogenesis

Cox CE, Hinman F: Experiments with induced bacteriuria, vesical emptying and bacterial growth on the mechanism of bladder defense to infection, *J Urol* 86:739, 1961.

Cox LE, Lacy SS, Hinman F: The urethra and its relationship to urinary tract infection. II. The urethral flora of the female with recurrent urinary tract infection, *J Urol* 99:632, 1968.

Eden CS, Eriksson B, Hanson LA: Adhesion of *Escherichia coli* to human uroepithelial cells in vitro, *Infect Immun* 18:767, 1977.

Fihn SD, Johnson L, Pinkstaff C, Stamm WE: Diaphragm use and urinary tract infection. Analysis of urodynamic and microbiologic factors, *J Urol* 136:853, 1986.

Fihn SD, Latham RH, Roberts P, et al: Association between diaphragm use and urinary tract infection, *JAMA* 253:240, 1985.

Foxman B, Frerichs RR: Epidemiology of urinary tract infection: I. Diaphragm use and sexual intercourse, *Am J Public Health* 75:1308, 1985.

Iwahi T, Abe Y, Nakao M, et al: Rule of type I fimbriae in the pathogenesis of ascending urinary tract infection induced by *Escherichia coli* in mice, *Infect Immun* 39:307, 1983.

Kaye D: Antibacterial activity of human urine, *J Clin Invest* 47:2374, 1968.

Kinane DF, Blackwell CC, Brettle, et al: ABO blood group, secretor state and susceptibility to recurrent urinary tract infection in women, *Br Med J* 285:7, 1982.

McCabe WR, Jackson GR: Treatment of pyelonephritis: bacterial, drug & host factors in success or failure among 252 patients, *N Engl J Med* 272:1037, 1965.

Nicolle LE, Harding GKM, Preiksaitis J, Ronald AR: The association of urinary tract infection with sexual intercourse, *J Infect Dis* 146:579, 1982.

Orskov I, Ferencz A, Orskov F: Tamm-Horsfall protein or uromucoid is the normal urinary slime that traps type I fimbriated *Escherichia coli.* Letter to the editor, *Lancet* 1:887, 1980.

Parsons CL: Prevention of urinary tract infection by the exogenous glycosaminoglycar sodium pertosan polysulfate, *J Urol* 127:167, 1982.

Parsons CL, Greenspan C, Moore SW, et al: Role of surface mucin in primary antibacterial defense of bladder, *Urology* 9:48, 1977.

Parsons DL, Schmidt JD: Control of recurrent lower urinary tract infections in the postmenopausal women, *J Urol* 128:1224, 1982.

Reid G, Sobol JD: Bacterial adherence in the pathogenesis of urinary tract infection: a Review, *Rev Infect Dis* 9:470, 1987.

Schaeffer AJ: Recurrent urinary tract infections in women: pathogenesis and management, *Postgrad Med* 81:51, 1987.

Schaeffer AJ, Amundsen SK, Schmidt LN: Adherence of *Escherichia coli* to human urinary tract epithelial cells, *Infect Immunol* 24:753, 1979.

Schaeffer AJ, Jones JM, Dunn JK: Association of in vitro *Escherichia coli* adherence to vaginal and buccal epithelial cells with susceptibility of women to recurrent urinary-tract infections, *N Engl J Med* 304:1062, 1981.

Schaeffer AJ, Radvany RM, Chmiel JS: Human leukocyte antigens in women with recurrent urinary tract infections, *J Infect Dis* 148:604, 1983.

Stamey TA, Sexton CC: The role of vaginal colonization with entero- bacteriaceae in recurrent urinary infections, *J Urol* 113:214, 1975.

Stamey TA, Timothy MM: Studies of introital colonizations in women with recurrent urinary infections. I. The role of vaginal pH, *J Urol* 114:261, 1975.

Strom BL, Collins, West SL, et al: Sexual activity, contraceptive use, and other risk factors for symptomatic and asymptomatic bacteriuria, *Ann Intern Med* 107:816, 1987.

Vaisanen V, Elo J, Tallgreen LG, et al: Mannose-resistant haemagglutination and P antigen recognition are characteristic of *Escherichia coli* causing primary pyelonephritis, *Lancet* 2:1366, 1981.

Microbiology

Bailey RR: Significance of coagulase-negative staphylococcus in urine, *J Infect Dis* 127:179, 1973.

Hovelius B: Urinary tract infections caused by *Staphylococcus saprophyticus* recurrences and complications, *J Urol* 122:645, 1979.

Kass EH: Bacteriuria and diagnosis of infections of the urinary tract, *Arch Intern Med* 100:709, 1967.

Lewis JF, Brake SR, Anderson DJ, Vredeveld GD: Urinary tract infection due to coagulase-negative staphylococcus, *Am J Clin Pathol* 77:736, 1982.

Marrie T, Kwan C, Noble M, et al: *Staphylococcus saprophyticus* as a cause of urinary tract infections, *J Clin Microbiol* 6:427, 1982.

Maskell R: Importance of coagulase-negative staphylococci as pathogens in the urinary tract, *Lancet* 1:1155, 1974.

Nicolle LE, Hoban SA, Harding GKM: Characterization of coagulase-negative staphylococci from urinary isolates, *J Clin Microbiol* 17:267, 1983.

Schaeffer AJ: Recurrent urinary tract infections in women. Pathogenesis and Management, *Postgrad Med* 81:51, 1987.

Scllin M, Cooke DI, Gillespie WA, et al: Micrococcal urinary-tract infections in young women, *Lancet* 2:570, 1975.

Turck M, Goffe B, Petersdorf RG: The urethral catheter and urinary tract infection, *J Urol* 88:834, 1962.

Wallmark G, Arremark I, Telander B: *Staphylococcus saprophyticus:* a frequent cause of acute urinary tract infection among female outpatients, *J Infect Dis* 138:791, 1978.

Diagnosis

Bixler-Forell E, Bertram MA, Bruckner DA: Clinical evaluation of three rapid methods for the detection of significant bacteriuria, *J Clin Microbiol* 22:62, 1985.

DeLange, HE, Jones B: Unnecessary intravenous urography in young women with recurrent urinary tract infections, *Clin Radiol* 34:551, 1983.

Engel G, Schaeffer AJ, Grayhack JT, et al: The role of excretory urography and cystoscopy in the evaluation and management of women with recurrent urinary tract infection, *J Urol* 123:190, 1980.

Fair WR, McClennan BL, Jost RG: Are excretory urograms necessary in evaluating women with urinary tract infections? *J Urol* 121:313, 1979.

Fowler JE Jr, Pulaski T: Excretory urography, cystography, and cystoscopy in the evaluation of women with urinary tract infection, *N Engl J Med* 304:462, 1981.

Free AH, Free HM: Urinalysis: its proper role in the physician's office, *Clin Lab Med* 6:253, 1986.

Johnson JR, Stamm WE: Diagnosis and treatment of acute urinary tract infection, *Infect Dis Clin North Am* 1:773, 1987.

Kraft JK, Stamey TA: The natural history of symptomatic recurrent bacteriuria in women, *Medicine* 56:55, 1977.

Kunin CM: Detection, prevention and management of urinary tract infection, ed 4, Philadelphia, 1987, Lea & Febiger.

Mabeck CE: Studies in urinary tract infections. I. The diagnosis of bacteriuria in women, *Acta Med Scand* 186:35, 1969.

Mogensen P, Hansen LK: Do intravenous urography and cystoscopy provide important information in otherwise healthy women with recurrent urinary tract infection? *Br J Urol* 55:261, 1983.

Needham CA: Rapid detection methods in microbiology: are they right for your office? *Med Clin North Am* 71:591, 1987.

Newhouse, JH, Rhea JT, Murphy RX, et al: Yield of screening urography in young women with urinary tract infection, *Urol Radiol* 4:187, 1982.

Reid G: The office microbiology laboratory, *Urol Clin North Am* 13:569, 1986.

Schaeffer AJ: The office laboratory, *Urol Clin North Am* 7:29, 1980.

Stamm WE: Measurement of pyuria and its relation to bacteriuria, *Am J Med* 75:53, 1983.

Stamm WE, Counts GW, Running KR, et al: Diagnosis of coliform infection in acutely dysuric women, *N Engl J Med* 307:463, 1982.

Wu TC, Williams EC, Koo SY, et al: Evaluation of three bacteriuria screening methods in a clinical research hospital, *J Clin Microbiol* 21:796, 1985.

Youngblood VH, Tomlin EM, Williams JO, Kimmelstiel P: Exfoliative cytology of the senile female urethra, *J Urol* 79:110, 1958.

Management

Bailey RR, Abbott GD: Treatment of urinary tract infection with a single dose of amoxicillin, *Nephron* 18:316, 1977.

Britt MR, Garibaldi RA, Miller WA, et al: Antimicrobial prophylaxis for catheter-associated bacteriuria, *Antimicrob Agent Chemother* 11:240, 1977.

Brumfitt W, Faiers MC, Franklin INS: The treatment of urinary infection by means of a single dose of cephaloxidine, *Postgrad Med J* 46:65, 1970.

Buckwold FJ, Ludwid P, Godfrey KM, et al: Therapy for acute cystitis in adult women: randomized comparison of single-dose sulfasoxazole vs trimethoprim-sulfamethoxazol, *JAMA* 247:1839, 1982.

Burke JP, Garibaldi RA, Britt MR, et al: Prevention of catheter-associated urinary tract infections, *Am J Med* 70:655, 1981.

Burke JP, Jacobson JA, Garbaldi RA, et al: Evaluation of daily meatal care with poly-antibiotic ointment in prevention of urinary catheter-associated bacteriuria, *J Urol* 129:331, 1983.

Childs SJ, Goldstein EJ: Ciprofloxacin as treatment for genitourinary tract infection, *J Urol* 141:1, 1989.

Evans DA, Kass EH, Hennekens CH, et al: Bacteriuria and subsequent mortality in women, *Lancet* 1:156, 1982.

Fang LST, Tolkoff-Rubin NE, Rubin RH: Efficacy of single-dose and conventional amoxicillin therapy in urinary tract infection localized by the antibody-coated bacteria technic, *N Engl J Med* 298:413, 1978.

Fihn SD: Single-dose antimicrobial therapy for urinary tract infections: "Less is more"? or "Reductio ad absurdum"? *J Gen Intern Med* 1:62, 1986.

Fihn SD, Johnson C, Roberts PL, et al: Trimethoprim sulfamethoxazole for acute dysuria in women: a double-blind, randomized trial of single-dose versus 10-day treatment, *Ann Intern Med* 108:350, 1988.

Garibaldi RA, Burke JP, et al: Meatal colonization and catheter-associated bacteriuria, *N Engl J Med* 303:316, 1980.

Garibaldi RA, Burke JP, Dickman ML, Smith CB: Factors predisposing to bacteriuria during indwelling urethral catheterization, *N Engl J Med* 291:215, 1974.

Goldstein EJ, Alpert ML, Najem A: Norfloxacin in the treatment of complicated and uncomplicated urinary tract infections: a comparative multicenter trial, *Am J Med* 82:65, 1987.

Greenberg, RN, Sanders CV, Lewis AC, et al: Single-dose cefaclor therapy of urinary tract infection: evaluation of antibody-coated bacteria test and C-reactive protein assay as predictors of cure, *Am J Med* 71:841, 1981.

Hoener B, Patterson SE: Nitrofurantoin disposition, *Clin Parmacol Ther* 29:808, 1981.

Hooper DC, Wolfson JS: The fluoroquinolones: pharmacology, clinical uses and toxicities in humans, *Antimicrob Agents Chemother* 28:716, 1985.

Kalowski S, Rudford N, Kincaid-Smith P: Crystalline and macrocrystalline nitrofurantoin in the treatment of urinary tract infection, *N Engl J Med* 290:385, 1974.

Kraft JK, Stamey TA: The natural history of symptomatic recurrent bacteriuria in women, *Medicine* 56:55, 1977.

Lee C, Ronald AN: Norfloxacin: its potential in clinical practice, *Am J Med* 82:27, 1987.

Mabeck CE: Treatment of uncomplicated urinary tract infection in non-pregnant women, *Postgrad Med* 48:69, 1972.

Martinez FC, Kindrachuk RW, Thomas E, et al: Effect of prophylactic low dose cephalexin on fecal and vaginal bacteria, *J Urol* 133:994, 1985.

Mayer TR: UTI in the elderly: how to select treatment, *Geriatrics* 35:67, 1980.

Mayrer AR, Andriole VT: Urinary tract antiseptics, *Med Clin North Am* 66:199, 1982.

McCabe WR, Jackson GR: Treatment of pyelonephritis: bacterial, drug and host factors in success or failure among 252 patients, *N Engl J Med* 272:1037, 1965.

Neu HC: Quinolones: a new class of antimicrobial agents with wide potential uses, *Med Clin North Am* 72:623, 1988.

Parsons CL: Urinary tract infections in the female patient, *Urol Clin North Am* 12:355, 1985.

Pfau A, Sacks T, Englestein D: Recurrent urinary tract infections in premenopausal women. Prophylaxis based on an understanding of the pathogenesis, *J Urol* 129:1152, 1983.

Platt R: Adverse consequences of acute urinary tract infections in adults, *Am J Med 82* (suppl 6B):47, 1987.

Platt R, Polk BF, Murdock B, Rosner B: Mortality associated with nosocomial urinary tract infection, *N Engl J Med* 307:736, 1982.

Reed MD, Blumer JL: Urologic pharmacology in the office setting, *Urol Clin North Am* 15:737, 1988.

Rubin RH, Fang LST, Jones SR, et al: Single-dose amoxicillin therapy for urinary tract infection, *JAMA* 244:561, 1980.

Sabbaj J, Hoagland VL, Shih WJ: Multiclinic comparative study of norfloxacin and trimethoprim-sulfamethoxazole for treatment of urinary tract infections, *Antimicrob Agents Chemother* 27:297, 1985.

Schaeffer AJ: Recurrent urinary tract infections in women. Pathogenesis and management, *Postgrad Med* 81:51, 1987.

Schultz HJ, McCaffrey LA, Keys TF, Nobrega FT: Acute cystitis: a prospective study of laboratory tests and duration of therapy, *Mayo Clin Proc* 59:391, 1984.

Sisca TS, Heel RC, Romankiewicz JA: Cinoxacin: a review of its pharmacological properties and therapeutic efficacy in the treatment of urinary tract infections, *Drugs* 25:544, 1983.

Stamey TA, Condy M, Mihara G: Prophylactic efficacy of nitrofurantoin macrocrystals and trimenthoprim-sulfamethoxazole in urinary infections: biologic effects on the vaginal and rectal flora, *N Engl J Med* 296:780, 1977.

Stamm WE, Counts GW, McKevitt M, et al: Urinary prophylaxis with trimethoprim and trimethoprim-sulfamethoxazol: efficacy, influence on the natural history of recurrent bacteriuria, and cost control, *Rev Infect Dis* 4:450, 1982.

Stamm WE, McKevitt M, Counts GW, et al: Is antimicrobial prophylaxis of urinary tract infections cost effective? *Ann Intern Med* 94:251, 1981.

Tolkoff-Rubin NE, Weber D, Fang LST, et al: Single dose therapy with trimethoprim-sulfamethoxazole for urinary tract infection in women, *Rev Infect Dis* 4:443, 1982.

Vosti KL: Recurrent urinary tract infections: prevention by prophylactic antibiotics after sexual intercourse, *JAMA* 231:934, 1975.

Warren JW, Platt R, Thomas RJ, et al: Antibiotic irrigation and catheter-associated urinary tract infections, *N Engl J Med* 299:570, 1978.

Weinstein L, Madoff MA, Samet CM: The sulfonamides, *N Engl J Med* 263:793, 1960.

Wise R, Griggs D, Andrews JM: Pharmokinetics of the quinolones in volunteers: a proposed dosing schedule, *Rev Infect Dis* 10(suppl 1):S83, 1988.

Wolfson JS, Hooper DC: The fluoroquinolones: structures, mechanisms of action and resistance, and spectra of activity in vitro, *Antimicrob Agents Chemother* 28:581, 1985.

Wong ES, Hooton TM: Guidelines to prevention of catheter-associated urinary tract infection, *Infect Control* 2:125, 1980.

Wong ES, McKevitt M: Running K, et al: Management of recurrent urinary tract infections with patient-administered single-dose therapy, *Ann Intern Med* 102:302, 1985.

CHAPTER 23

Lower Urinary Tract Fistulas

Thomas E. Elkins
Christopher Fitzpatrick

Historical Perspectives
Epidemiology and Etiology
Classification
Presentation, Investigation and Preoperative
  Preparation
Surgical Repair
  Anesthesia and position
  Instruments and materials
  Vaginal repair
  Abdominal repair
  Urinary diversion
Complications
Prevention

HISTORICAL PERSPECTIVES

The earliest evidence of vesicovaginal fistula was recorded by Professor DE Derry in the mummified remains of Queen Henhenit, one of the wives of King Mentuhotep II of Egypt (11th Dynasty, circa 2050 BC). In his dissection of the mummy at the Cairo School of Medicine in 1923, Derry noted a large vesicovaginal fistula in the presence of a severely contracted pelvis; he concluded that the fistula was a consequence of obstructed labor. Hippocrates (460-377 BC) recognized the problem of urinary incontinence after confinement but offered no clue as to its cause. In his textbook, 'Al Kanoun,' the celebrated Persian physician Avicenna (980-1037) was the first

to recognize that urinary incontinence after difficult labor was due to communication between the bladder and vagina.

No further reference to vesicovaginal fistula appeared until 1597 when both Felix Platter of Basle and Luiz de Mercado of Valladolid separately reviewed the problem but offered no constructive therapeutic advice. Zacharin states that the term *fistula* was first used by de Mercado instead of the usual term *ruptura*.

In 1663, Hendrik Von Roonhuyse of Amsterdam published *Medico-Chiurgical Observations about the Infirmities of Women*. Commonly thought of as the first textbook on operative gynecology, this text was translated into English in 1676. The fourth chapter is entitled "Rupture of the Bladder; the Signs, Causes, Prognostics and Cure Thereof." Von Roonhuyse proposed a revolutionary surgical technique for the closure of vesicovaginal fistulas based on the following principles: lithotomy position, good exposure of the fistula with a vaginal speculum, marginal denudation of the fistula edge using a fine scissors or knife, and approximation of the denuded edges with "stitching needles of stiff swans' quills." There is no record that Von Roonhuyse operated on patients using this technique. In 1752 a medical text by the Swiss physician Johann Fatio was posthumously published, which recorded two successful fistula repairs performed by Fatio himself in 1675 and 1684 using Von Roonhuyse's technique.

Volter in 1687 suggested that sutures should be

interrupted, and he introduced the use of a retention urinary catheter. During this same period Pietro DiMarchettis claimed complete cures using cautery. In later years Monteggia, Dupuytren, and others also recommended cautery.

The nineteenth century was the dawn of a new era in the surgical treatment of vesicovaginal fistula. In 1834, Jobert de Lamballe successfully repaired a small number of fistulas using pedicled skin-flaps *(autoplastic vaginale par la methode indienne)*. A second technique *(autoplastie par glissment ou par locomotion)* later enabled him to close a greater number of fistulas. This technique involved dissecting the bladder from the cervix and vagina with the additional use of curved releasing incisions in the vagina to facilitate mobilization and low-tension closure.

In a letter to the Boston Medical and Surgical Journal in August, 1838, John Peter Mettauer of Virginia stated that he had successfully repaired a vesicovaginal fistula about the size of a half dollar piece using lead wire. This was the first successful repair in the United States.

On June 21, 1849, in a small eight-bed infirmary on Perry Street, Montgomery, Alabama, James Marion Sims operated on a young slave woman named Anarcha for the thirtieth time. Using the genupectoral position, a bent pewter spoon as a vaginal speculum, and reflected light from a mirror, Sims denuded the fistula edge, closing the defect in one layer with fine silver wire applied with leaden bars and perforated shot. On the eighth day, Sims reexamined the patient and noted that the wound was well healed. In 1852, he published his classic paper "On the treatment of vesicovaginal fistula" in the *American Journal of Medical Sciences*. He deprecated both cautery as advocated by Dupuytren for small fistulae and obturation of the vulva as practiced by Vidal De Cassis (whereby the bladder and vagina are converted into a common reservoir for urinary and menstrual discharge). Sims insisted on liberal use of opium for perioperative analgesia and stressed the importance of postoperative bladder drainage with a urethral catheter. He later designed a silver sigmoid-shaped, self-retaining catheter for this purpose. In 1853 Sims moved to New York and in 1855 he became chief surgeon in the newly built Woman's Hospital, where he was later joined by a brilliant young assistant, Thomas Addis Emmet. Sims and Emmet worked closely together, Emmet perfecting many of his mentor's techniques.

In his text *Vesico-vaginal Fistula from Parturition and Other Causes with Cases of Recto-vaginal Fistula,* published in 1868 and dedicated to Sims, Emmet reported on 270 consecutive patients treated in the Woman's Hospital: 200 were cured; 65 were improved, and 5 were considered incurable. Emmet eventually succeeded Sims at the Woman's Hospital. Probably his greatest contribution to obstetric care was his insistence that frequent catheterization of the bladder in labor, together with the judicious use of forceps for second-stage delay, would prevent the majority of labor-related vesicovaginal fistulas.

In 1861, Maurice Collis of Dublin advocated the flap-splitting technique whereby the anterior vaginal wall is widely dissected from the bladder with separate closure of the two defects. This method was later popularized by Mackenrodt in Berlin.

In the 1880s and 1890s, Trendelenburg and Von Dittel reported failed attempts at fistula repair using extraperitoneal and intraperitoneal suprapubic approaches respectively. Schuchardt also devised a parasacral incision, which permitted better access to high fistulas, particularly when associated with vaginal stenosis.

The discovery of antibiotics and the development of general and regional anesthesia contributed significantly to the surgical treatment of vesicovaginal fistulas in this century. Other notable milestones included urethral reconstruction using lateral vaginal flaps and labium minus grafts (Noble, 1901), suprapubic intraperitoneal repair of posthysterectomy, high vesicovaginal and rectovaginal fistulas (Kelly, 1902), partial colpocleisis for posthysterectomy vesicovaginal fistulas (Latzko, 1914, 1942), urethral reinforcement using pelvic floor muscles (Martius, 1928), pedicled gracilis muscle flaps (Garlock, 1928), bulbocavernosus flaps (Martius, 1942), pubococcygeus, bulbocavernosus, rectus abdominis and gracilis muscle flaps (Ingleman-Sundberg, 1960), publication of *The Vesico-Vaginal Fistula* (Moir, 1961), the use of pedicled omental flaps in the repair of extensive veiscovaginal fistulas (Kircuta and Goldstein, 1972), urethral reconstruction (Symmonds, 1978; Tanagho et al, 1972, 1981), the foundation of the Second Fistula Hospital in Addis Ababa, Ethiopia in 1975, and the report of 1789 fistulae over an 11-year period from Nigeria (Ward, 1980).

EPIDEMIOLOGY AND ETIOLOGY

The vast majority of vesicovaginal fistulae that occur in the developing world are due to obstetric causes; elsewhere abdominal surgery, particularly simple total abdominal hysterectomy, is the major cause. Of 377 cases reported by Lawson from Ibadan, Nigeria, 369 (97.9%) were obstetric (343 of these being a consequence of obstructed labor); of 166 cases also reported by Lawson from the United Kingdom, 116 (69.9%) were related to surgery and 21 (12.6%) to obstetrics.

Urinary tract injuries can occur with pelvic surgery performed by even the most experienced surgeons. Although some series have shown ureteral injury to occur in 0.5% to 2.5% of patients undergoing hysterectomy, others have shown an injury rate to both bladder and ureter of 0.05% of 35,000 pelvic operations. In the developed world, the incidence is low. However, worldwide the problem is vast in developing countries.

In an 1989 report by Nnabugwu-Otensanya from Zaria, Nigeria, 41% of fistula patients were under 15 years of age; all were primiparae whose labors had resulted in stillborn infants. All had been ostracized by their husbands, families, and communities. Many had waited 5 years or more for primary surgical repair.

Our knowledge of the prevalence of vesicovaginal fistulas in the developing world is based on women treated in hospitals. The prevalence is likely to be considerably underestimated, as few women are aware that the condition is treatable. In addition, the social isolation that many suffer as a result of their incontinence renders it difficult for them to learn about appropriate care. Few district hospitals have the staff, equipment, or expertise to manage the problem. Poverty, long distances, and long waiting lists deter women from traveling to major centers.

Prolonged impaction of the presenting fetal part against a distended edematous bladder eventually leads to pressure necrosis and fistula formation. Absent or untrained birth attendants, reduced pelvic di-

mensions (due to early childbearing, chronic disease, malnutrition, and rickets), uncorrected inefficient uterine action, malpresentations, hydrocephalus, and introital stenosis secondary to tribal circumcision all contribute to obstructed labor. Fistulas also may be caused by the use of forceps, decapitation hooks, cranial perforators, cranioclasts, and surgical abortion. They are also associated with symphysiotomy, the practice of Gishiri cuts (i.e., an incision in the anterior vaginal wall, made for a variety of obstetric and gynecologic ills), and the use of traditional postpartum vaginal caustics. Vesicovaginal fistulas may follow cesarean section or cesarean hysterectomy, particularly in the presence of distorted anatomy (e.g., massive fibroids) and surgical inexperience. Obstetric fistulas are characterized by considerable necrosis, sloughing, tissue loss, and cicatrization. They are also associated with a wide range of other problems: stillbirth, ruptured uterus, rectovaginal fistula, third- and fourth-degree laceration, vaginal stenosis, bladder calculi, symphyseal chondritis/osteitis, pelvic infection, foot-drop, anemia, hypoalbuminemia, amenorrhea, divorce, ostracization, depression, and suicide.

In a more contemporary setting, Lee et al, reviewed 303 women with genitourinary fistulas who were treated in the Mayo Clinic. In 225 patients (74%) the fistula resulted from gynecologic surgery for a benign condition, most commonly fibroids, dysfunctional uterine bleeding, prolapse, incontinence, carcinoma in situ, endometriosis, and ovarian cysts. Malignant conditions were responsible in 42 patients (14%). Ureterovaginal fistulas were associated in particular with radical hysterectomy. Fistulas as a consequence of simple hysterectomy is most often due to overvigorous blunt dissection of the bladder from the uterus and cervix resulting in an unrecognized tear. Necrosis due to clamp or suture injury may also be responsible. The posthysterectomy fistula is usually located above the interureteric ridge, medial to both ureteral orifices. Unlike obstetric fistulas, massive tissue loss is uncommon.

Vesicovaginal fistulas may also be caused by pelvic radiotherapy. Slowly progressive endarteritis from radiation exposure may cause tissue necrosis that interferes with initial and subsequent repair attempts. They may present several years after treatment and represent major management problems because of marked tissue fibrosis, contracture fixity, and devascularization. It is essential to histologically rule out cancer recurrence in these lesions.

Miscellaneous causes of vesicovaginal fistulas include gynecologic malignancy, lymphogranuloma venereum, tuberculosis, syphilis, bladder calculus, retained vaginal foreign body, and trauma. Although schistosomiasis only rarely causes fistula formation, infection may make fistula closure more difficult and healing less certain.

CLASSIFICATION

Obstetric vesicovaginal fistulas may be classified in a number of ways. An anatomic classification proposed by many is as follows:

1. *Juxta-urethral:* involving the bladder neck and proximal urethra with damage to the sphincteric mechanism, occasionally with total urethral loss and fixity to bone
2. *Mid-vaginal:* without involvement of the bladder neck or trigone
3. *Juxtacervical:* opening into the anterior vaginal fornix or cervical canal with possible distal ureteral involvement
4. *Massive:* a combination of the first three fistulas with dense scarring and fixity to bone and often with ureteral involvement at the fistula margins and prolapse of the bladder through the large defect.
5. *Compound:* involving rectovaginal, or ureterovaginal, as well as vesicovaginal fistulas
6. *Vesicocervical or vesicouterine:* usually following cesarean sections.

Another classification of obstetric fistulas proposed by Mahfouz involves consideration of the site of obstruction during labor. Therefore, juxtacervical fistulas result from obstruction at the pelvic inlet, mid-vaginal fistulas result from obstruction at the level of the ischial spines, and suburethral/urethral fistulas result from pelvic outlet obstruction.

A newer classification being proposed for obstetric fistulas in developing countries is aimed at fistula repair training programs. This classification separates fistulas on a functional basis according to those that

---

Functional Classification of Difficult or High-risk Fistulas

1. >4-5 cm in diameter
2. Involvement of
   Urethra
   Ureter(s)
   Rectum
3. Juxtacervical fistulas with incomplete visualization of the superior edge
4. Previous failed repair(s)

From Elkins TE et al: *Int J Urogynecol*, 1993, in press.

---

are most difficult to repair and have the most significant complications and those that are relatively simple to repair (see box). This approach allows general repair efforts to expand among nonfistula specialists and for appropriate referrals to be made to specialty centers.

Gynecologic vesicovaginal fistulas are generally separated into those resulting from radiation therapy and those that are postsurgical, along with individual anatomic descriptions.

PRESENTATION, INVESTIGATION, AND PREOPERATIVE PREPARATION

Blood-stained urine on the completion of pelvic surgery may indicate an intraoperative vesicovaginal fistula. Thereafter, patients may present with continuous leakage of urine per vaginam after an interval of days, weeks (surgical and obstetrical fistulae), or even months or years (radiotherapy-related fistulas). If the fistula is very small, leakage may be intermittent or related to a full bladder or particular body position.

Collection of fluid from the vagina in suspected cases and measurement of its urea concentration may confirm it as urine. A thorough speculum examination of the vagina, urethrocystoscopy, and intravenous urogram are recommended in most cases where they are available.

Instillation of methylene blue into the bladder will stain vaginal swabs in the presence of a vesicovaginal fistula. Unstained wet swabs may indicate a ureterovaginal fistula, which may be confirmed by intravenous indigo carmine, intravenous urography, or cystoscopic retrograde urography. Use of methylene blue intravenously must be chosen with caution because of the risk of methemoglobinemia, a rare but serious complication. Occasionally, a fistula is so small that leakage of dye occurs only with a full bladder and Valsalva maneuver.

At cystoscopy the size, site, and number of fistulae and the state of the local tissues are carefully noted. Key points include proximity to the bladder neck urethral sphincter, and ureteral orifices together with the presence of tissue edema, slough, infection, induration, scarring, and fixity to bone. Water cystoscopy may not be possible in cases with large fistulae. Placing the patient in the genupectoral position will allow the bladder to fill with air, thus permitting dry cystoscopy. Bladder calculi and nonabsorbable sutures should be removed. Urine should be examined microscopically, cultured, and treated if infected. In areas of endemic schistosomiasis, cystoscopic biopsies may need to be performed. Associated local problems such as rectovaginal fistulas, anal sphincter disruption, vaginal stenosis, and ammoniacal dermatitis must be documented and treated.

If a vesicovaginal fistula is diagnosed within 7 days of occurrence, is less than 1 cm in diameter, and is unrelated to malignancy or irradiation, bladder drainage alone for up to 4 weeks may cure between 12% and 80% of such lesions, but the outcome is unpredictable. Cystoscopic cauterization of small lesions may also be successful. Standard management of vesicovaginal fistula dictates an interval from injury to repair of 3 to 6 months in surgical and obstetic fistulae and up to 1 year in radiation-induced fistulas to allow for resolution of necrosis and inflammation. If there is an associated rectovaginal fistula, a transverse colostomy performed 2 to 3 months before fistula repair may be helpful.

Krantz has championed the early closure of small fistulas as soon as they are identified postoperatively. Fearl and Keizur used serial cystoscopy in 20 patients to determine suitability for fistula repair; surgery was performed on average 2 to 4 months earlier than if they had used empiric intervals, with no decrease in success rates. Corticosteroids and nonsteroidal antiinflammatory drugs have been used by some to facilitate early surgery but their efficacy has not been proved. Herbert and Vaughn recommended that the appropriate time for repair should be individualized based on endoscopic evidence of healing. When the fistula site and adjacent tissues are pliable, noninflamed, epithelialized, and free of granulation tissue and necrosis, little is gained by waiting longer.

Patients awaiting surgical repair need considerable psychologic support. Leakage from small fistulas may be controlled by frequent voiding and the use of tampons, perineal pads, or silica-impregnated incontinence pants. A vaginal diaphragm with a watertight attachment to a urinary catheter can collect urine from larger fistulas into a leg bag. Long-term indwelling catheters should be avoided.

Ammoniacal dermatitis is treated with sitz baths and zinc oxide barrier ointment. Oral or vaginal estrogen will improve urogenital tissue integrity in oophorectomized or postmenopausal women before attempts at surgical repair. In malnourished patients, a high-protein diet, vitamin and trace element supplements, and the correction of anemia are essential before surgical repair.

All patients with vesicovaginal fistula need a thorough physical examination. Examination under anesthesia may be necessary to identify tissue edges and to plan surgical approaches in the case of large or obscure vesicovaginal fistulas.

SURGICAL REPAIR

The majority of vesicovaginal fistulas can be closed transvaginally. This method is primarily described in this chapter. In the series of 303 cases reported by Lee et al, 80% were repaired transvaginally irrespective of fistula size, number, or history of previous repairs. Surgery should not be performed during menstruation, given the increased tissue vascularity at this time.

Anesthesia and Position

Methods of suitable anesthesia include epidural, low spinal, and general. Small fistulas may be repaired under local anesthesia with or without sedation. For proximal urethral or bladder neck fistulas, Lawson's position may be used. The patient is placed prone on the operating table with her knees apart and her ankles raised and supported in stirrups, with the table in reversed Trendelenburg position. Alternatively, a "jackknife" position may be used in which the patient is placed prone with the hips abducted and well flexed, the table being "jackknifed" at this point. For higher fistulas, an exaggerated lithotomy position with standard Trendelenburg position provides optimal access; we prefer this position for all vaginal approaches. Labial retraction sutures and, if necessary, an episiotomy or Schuchardt's incision may improve exposure.

Instruments and Materials

Adequate light, appropriate instruments, and materials are mandatory. Instruments most useful include Chassar Moir, Church, or Kelly fistula scissors, fine Allis forceps, Sims skin hooks, Sims or Breisky retractors, fine-tipped suction tips, and long-handled scalpels with No. 11 and 15 blades. Although no single suture material has proven superiority, the use of 2-0 and 3-0 polyglycolic acid on CT-2 needles is favored by many for closure of all layers. The use of fine monofilament nylon for vaginal closure (with delayed removal at 3 to 4 weeks) also remains popular. In the developing world the choice of instruments and materials in many centers remains strongly influenced by local supplies and financial constraints.

Vaginal Repair

The use of stay sutures close to the fistula margin or the insertion and inflation of a pediatric-sized Foley catheter through the fistula tract into the bladder helps to evert the fistula edge and improves descent and stability for dissection. Very small fistulas may require gentle dilation using lacrimal duct probes and small dilators to allow insertion of the catheter (Fig. 23-1). Infiltration of tissues with normal saline or 1/200,000 adrenaline solution may also help with dissection and reduce oozing. Concern has been raised about an increase in infection rates after adrenaline use in vaginal surgery, so many surgeons use only saline.

If the fistula encroaches on the ureteral orifices, the orifices should be identified and catheterized at the outset. If identification proves difficult, intravenous indigo carmine with or without furosemide may be helpful.

The classic method of fistula repair involves split

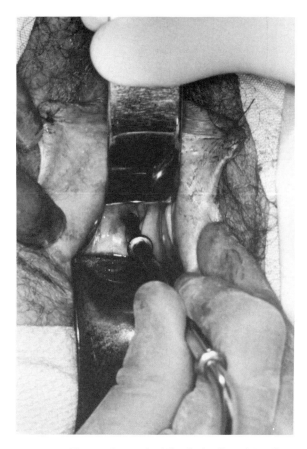

Fig. 23-1 The vesicovaginal fistula is dilated to allow insertion of a pediatric Foley catheter through the fistula and into the bladder. Use of a catheter helps to evert the fistula edge, thus improving descent and stability for dissection.

flap dissection, mobilization of tissue planes, absolute hemostasis, and low-tension closure (Fig. 23-2). A circumscribing vaginal (usually vertical) incision is made along the long axis of the fistula. The subvaginal plane is dissected in all directions, taking care to avoid excessive dissection, which may result in avascular necrosis. If the fistula tract is small, it can be excised; if large and fibrotic, the edges can be freshened. Overexcision of fistula edges may result in too large a defect and in intracystic hemorrhage from bladder edges postoperatively. This can cause catheter blockage, bladder distention, and failure of the repair. If mobilization proves difficult, radical or circumferential vaginal incisions, made at a distance from the

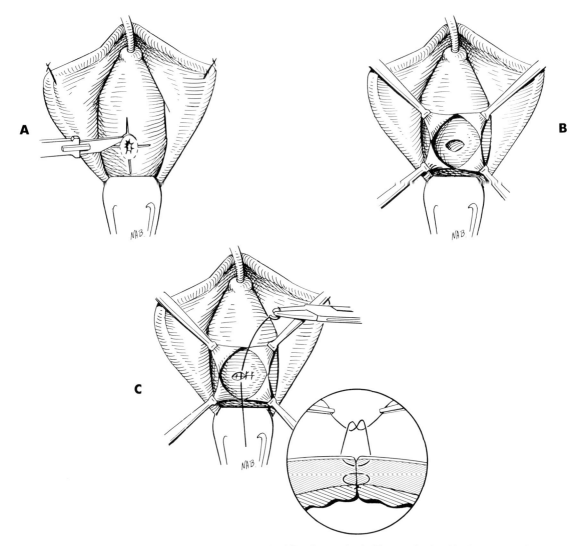

Fig. 23-2 Vaginal approach to vesicovaginal fistula repair: **A**, The vaginal epithelium around the fistula is sharply excised. **B**, The vaginal wall is mobilized off the bladder in preparation for layered closure. **C**, The bladder wall is closed transversely in 2 layers, using interrupted sutures.

fistula, may facilitate both mobilization and low-tension closure. Once hemostasis is achieved, these incisions are left open.

Bladder closure in the trigonal area should be in a transverse direction; vertical closure may draw the ureteral orifices toward the midline and obstruct them. Before closure of large defects, Zacharin recommends bilateral attachment of healthy bladder wall to the ischiopubic periosteum to stabilize the bladder and thereby protect the repair postoperatively. The bladder is closed using submucosal interrupted Lembert sutures, placed 3 mm apart and at a similar distance from the fistula edge. They should be tied so as to coapt the tissue without strangulation. Purse-string closure may compromise blood supply at tissue edges and is not recommended. A second layer of interrupted

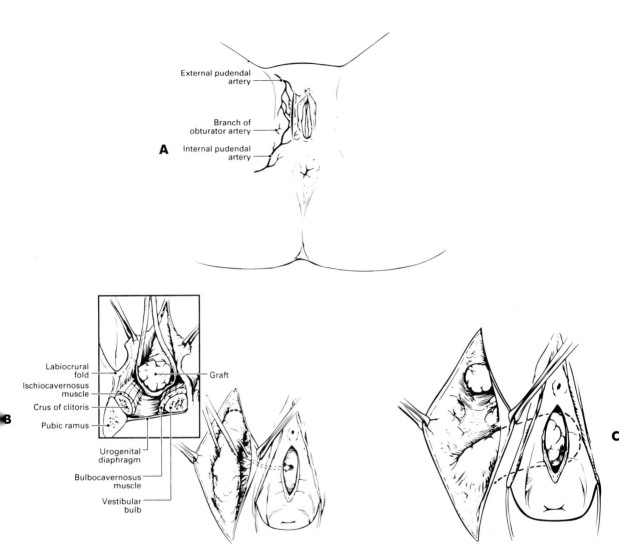

Fig. 23-3 Technique of modified Martius graft for vesicovaginal fistula repair. **A,** Blood supply of the Martius graft region; **B,** anatomic structures adjacent to the Martius graft; **C,** tunneling of the Martius graft into position over the closed fistula. *(From Elkins TE, DeLancey JOL, McGuire EJ: Obstet Gynecol 75:727, 1990.)*

sutures closes the bladder muscularis and reduces tension on the first layer. The vagina may be closed in one or two layers using interrupted sutures, the outside layer being mattressed.

If the fistula is recurrent, large, due to radiotherapy, or involving the bladder neck and urethra, a Martius, rectus muscle, or gracilis muscle graft may be tunneled subcutaneously and anchored between the bladder and vaginal walls. The function of these grafts is to introduce a new blood supply, separate the bladder and vaginal suture lines, provide support, and obliterate dead space. A modified Martius graft technique is shown in Fig. 23-3.

The integrity of the repair may be tested by the instillation of methylene blue or indigo carmine into the bladder, but care must be taken to avoid distention.

A vaginal pack may be inserted for 24 hours postoperatively, particularly if vaginal relaxing incisions are used. The bladder is drained for 10 to 14 days, depending on the fistula size. If some leakage persists at 14 days, further drainage for 7 more days may occasionally result in closure. Placing the patient in the prone position for 24 to 48 hours after surgery may prevent pressure from the catheter on the repair suture line before bladder mucosal integrity is restored. Fixation of the transurethral catheter externally is important, especially in suburethral fistulas. Extreme efforts to hydrate the patient are important postoperatively to autoirrigate the bladder, which avoids clot formation, catheter obstruction, bladder distention, and repair disruption. While catheterized, the patient is maintained on prophylactic antibiotics. Coitus is postponed for at least 6 weeks.

The Latzko technique of partial colpocleisis may be used for repair of posthysterectomy vesicovaginal fistulas with cure rates of between 93% and 100% at the first attempt. A simple procedure, it has the advantage of short operating time, minimal blood loss, and low postoperative morbidity. Vaginal shortening is not a problem unless the vagina is already shortened. The technique is significantly different from the classic method of fistula repair described earlier. The vaginal mucosa in the Latzko operation is mobilized around the fistula margin in the shape of an ellipse, at least 2.5 cm in all directions, with closure of the subvaginal tissue and vaginal mucosa using 2-0 or 3-0 interrupted sutures. The posterior vaginal wall thus becomes part of the posterior bladder wall; eventually it reepithelializes with transitional epithelium. Coitus is deferred for at least 3 months.

Juxtacervical fistulas, which may follow cesarean section, may be repaired vaginally if the cervix can be drawn down to provide access. Alternatively, an abdominal approach is warranted. Although rarely necessary, repair may be facilitated by concomitant hysterectomy.

Fistulas involving the bladder neck and proximal urethra may follow anterior colporrhaphy or surgery for suburethral diverticula. Most commonly, however, they are a consequence of prolonged labor and thus complicated by considerable tissue loss and fixity to bone. Because of sphincter destruction, postoperative continence remains a considerable challenge. Noble

originally described urethral reconstruction using bilateral vaginal flaps tubularized around a catheter, the resultant defect being covered by labial skin grafts. Moir used suburethral buttress sutures to improve continence. Symmonds achieved continence in 14 out of 20 patients with significant urethral destruction by constructing a small-caliber urethra around a size 10 to 12 French Foley catheter using contractile tissues that had retracted into the urethral roof, and using Martius grafting and retropubic suspension at a later date if necessary. Morgan et al, reported success in eight of nine patients using a combined abdominovaginal approach with urethral reconstruction from residual urethral tissue, Martius grafting, a Marlex suburethral sling, and labial skin flaps. Tubularized anterior bladder flaps also have been used with some success to achieve continence. Tanagho et al have convincingly shown that the concentrically arranged muscle fibers in the bladder directly adjacent to the internal urethral meatus can be used to create a neosphincter.

Abdominal Repair

The indications for abdominal repair of vesicovaginal fistulas include high inaccessible fistulas, multiple fistulas, involvement of the uterus and/or bowel, and the necessity for ureteral reimplantation. A midline incision facilitates omental grafting when required. The peritoneal cavity should be opened both to exclude adherent bowel and omentum and to allow omental grafting. O'Conor recommends bivalving the bladder. The ureteral orifices and fistula(s) are identified; the fistula is mobilized and closed using peritoneal or, more preferably, omental grafts interposed between the bladder and vaginal suture lines. The omental graft can be mobilized and lengthened by division and ligation of the omental attachments to the hepatic flexure and right half of the transverse colon, preserving enough branches of the gastroepiploic vessels to provide an adequate blood supply.

Rarely, a combined abdominovaginal repair is necessary. This procedure is most common with high juxtacervical fistulas that have a nonvisualized distal edge by the vaginal approach. The omentum may be sufficiently mobilized to allow paraurethral grafting within the vaginal operative field.

Ureteral fistulas may be treated by direct reimplantation or by using a Boari-Ockerblad flap, with suture line tension reduced by a bladder-psoas hitch (see Chapter 25). Occasionally, with gross ureteral destruction, ureteroureterostomy may be required.

Urinary Diversion

The most common indication for urinary diversion is total incontinence after successful anatomic repair of bladder neck/proximal urethral fistulae. Ureterosigmoidostomy was performed by Ward in 26 of 1789 cases. Occasionally, a fistula remains unrepaired after multiple attempts and urinary diversion is chosen. Most of these cases involve circumferential defects that include most or all of the urethra. Anal sphincter incontinence and rectovaginal fistula are absolute contraindications to ureterosigmoidostomy. Ileal conduit formation is not a feasible option in most developing countries. Cancerous fistulas should not be repaired; percutaneous nephrostomies may provide beneficial symptomatic relief when life expectancy is short.

COMPLICATIONS

Postoperative complications of vesicovaginal fistula repair surgery include vaginal stenosis, amenorrhea, small-bladder syndrome, hemorrhage, infection, suture-line breakdown, osteitis pubis, thromboembolism, fistula recurrence, stress urinary incontinence, and urge incontinence. Fistulas greater than 4 cm in diameter often present significant difficulty. Vesicovaginal fistulas occurring after radiotherapy may be further complicated by urethral dysfunction, detrusor areflexia and fibrosis, vesicoureteric reflux, and upper tract deterioration. Dyspareunia due to tenderness over the site of Martius grafts also has been reported. Metabolic disturbance and recurrent pyelonephritis may develop after ureterosigmoidostomy. After successful anatomic repair, elective cesarean section is strongly recommended for subsequent deliveries.

PREVENTION

Every year one-half million women die in the developing world from complications of pregnancy. For every mother that dies, between 10 and 15 are permanently damaged, many as a result of vesicovaginal fistula (World Health Organization, 1987). Epidemi-

ologic research is urgently required to identify those communities with a high prevalence of fistula and the characteristics of those women who are at high risk for bladder/urethral injury during labor. Preventative strategies include improvement of nutritional status (to lessen the prevalence of pelvic contraction), postponing pregnancy until pelvic maturity, maternity waiting homes, bladder drainage in labor, partographs and emergency transport systems for women in prolonged labor to centers staffed by skilled personnel, improved prenatal care, and universal education for women. Nonspecialists also should be trained to repair simple fistulas, with referral of complex cases to specialized fistula hospitals. Careful dose calculation, administration, source insertion and shielding, together with appropriate bladder drainage, reduce the risk of radiation-induced lower urinary tract fistulas. This complication may, nonetheless, arise many years later after a symptom-free interval. In the developed world, the majority of vesicovaginal fistulas could be prevented by careful dissection of the bladder from the uterus and cervix at the time of hysterectomy, careful placement of sutures and clamps during vaginal cuff closure, and the intraoperative recognition and repair of bladder trauma.

BIBLIOGRAPHY
Historical Perspectives

Collis MH: Further remarks upon a new and successful mode of treatment for vesicovaginal fistula, *Dublin Q J Med Sci* 31:302, 1861.

Derry DE: Note on five pelves of women in the eleventh dynasty in Egypt, *J Obstet Gynaecol Br Emp* 42:490, 1935.

DiMarchettis P: Observationum Medico-Chirurgicarum Rariorum Sylloge, *Patave,* 1675

Emmet TA: *Vesico-vaginal fistula from parturition and other causes with cases of recto-vaginal fistula,* New York, 1868, William Wood.

Falk HC: *Urological injuries in gynecology,* ed 2, Philadelphia, 1964, FA Davis.

Fatio J: Helvetisch-vernunstige Wehemutter. Basel, 1752

Garlock JH: The cure of an intractable vesicovaginal fistula by the use of a pedicled muscle graft, *Surg Gynecol Obstet* 47:255, 1928.

Ingelman-Sundberg A: Pathogenesis and operative treatment of urinary fistula in irradiated tissue. In Youssef AF (ed): *Gynecological urology,* Springfield, 1960, Charles C Thomas.

Jobert de Lamballe A-J: Traite des Fistules Vesico-Uterines, Paris, 1852, Balliere et Fils.

Kelly HA: The treatment of vesico-vaginal and recto-vaginal fistulae high up in the vagina, *Johns Hopkins Hosp Bull* 13:73, 1902.

Kircuta I, Goldstein AM: The repair of extensive vesico-vaginal fistulas with pedicled omentum: a review of 27 cases, *J Urol* 108:724, 1973.

Latzko W: Postoperative vesicovaginal fistulae: genesis and theory, *Am J Surg* 58:211, 1942.

Mackenrodt A: Die operative Heilung grosser Blasenscheidenfisteln, *Zentralbl Gynakol* 8:180, 1894.

Martius H: Die operative Wiederher-stellung der Volkommen fehlenden Harnrohre und des Schließmuskels derselben, *Zentralbl Gynakol* 8:480, 1928.

Martius H: Zur Auswahl der Harnnstel-und inkontinenz operation, *Zentralbl Gynakol* 32:1250, 1942.

Mettauer JP: Vesico-vaginal fistula, *Boston Med Surg J* 22:154, 1840.

Moir JC: *The vesico-vaginal fistula,* London, 1961, Balliere Tindall.

Noble CP: The new formation of the female urethra with report of a case, *Am J Obstet Gynecol* 43:170, 1901.

Schuchardt K: Eine Neue Methode der Gebarmutterexstirpation, *Zentralbl Chir* 20:1121, 1893.

Sims JM: On the treatment of vesico-vaginal fistula, *Am J Med Sci* 23:59, 1852.

Ward A: Vesicovaginal fistulas: a report of 1789 cases. Paper presented to the meeting of the Federation of International Gynaecology and Obstetrics World Congress, San Francisco, Calif, 1980.

Epidemiology and Etiology

Freda VC, Tacchi D: Ureteral injury discovered after pelvic surgery, *Am J Obstet Gynecol* 83(3):406, 1962.

Lawson J: Tropical obstetrics and gynecology III. Vesico-vaginal fistula—a tropical disease, *Trans R Soc Trop Med Hyg* 83:454, 1989.

Lee RA, Symmonds RE, Williams TJ: Current status of genitourinary fistula, *Obstet Gynecol* 72:313, 1988.

Nnabugwu-Otensanya BE: Social consequences of vesico-vaginal fistulae: Zaria experiences, Society of Obstetrics and Gynecology of Nigeria Conference, Calabar, September 5-8, 1989.

Solomons E, Levin EJ, Bauman JS, et al: A pyelographic study of ureteric injuries sustained during hysterectomy for benign conditions, *Surg Gynecol Obstet* 111(1):41, 1960.

Symmonds RE: Incontinence: vesicle and urethral fistulas, *Clin Obstet Gynecol* 27(2):499, 1984.

Classification

Elkins TE, Mahama E, O'Donnell KE, et al: Operative management of the high risk patient with obstetric vesicovaginal fistula, *Int J Urogynecol* 1992 (in press).

Hamlin RH, Nicholson EC: Reconstruction of urethra totally destroyed in labor, *Br Med J* 2:147, 1969.

Lawson JB: Birth-canal injuries, *Proc R Soc Med* 61:368, 1968.

Mahfouz NB: Urinary and faecal fistulae, *J Obstet Gynaecol Br Emp* 45:405, 1938.

Presentation, Investigation, and Preoperative Preparation

Collins CG, Pent D, Jones FB: Results of early repair of vesicovaginal fistula with preliminary cortisone treatment, *Am J Obstet Gynecol* 80:1005, 1960.

Falk HC, Orkin LA: Nonsurgical closure of vesicovaginal fistulas, *Obstet Gynecol* 9:538, 1957.

Falk HC: *Urological injuries in gynecology,* Philadelphia, 1984, FA Davis.

Carl CL, Kelzure LW: Optimum time interval from occurrence to repair of vesicovaginal fistula, *Am J Obstet Gynecol* 104:205, 1969.

Herbert DB, Vaughn ED: Vesicovaginal fistula: a therapeutic challenge, *Infect Surg* pp 130-9, 1985.

Krantz K: Personal correspondence and ACOG Video Festival, The American College of Obstetricians and Gynecologists Annual Meeting, Atlanta, May, 1988.

Latzko W: Postoperative vesicovaginal fistulae: genesis and theory, *Am J Surg* 58:211, 1942.

O'Conor VJ: Review of experience with vesico-vaginal fistula repair, *J Urol* 123:367, 1980.

Taylor JS, Henson AD, Rachow P, et al: Synchronous combined transvaginal-transvesical repair of vesicovaginal fistulas, *Aust NZ J Surg* 50:23, 1980.

Surgical Repair

Bissada NK, MacDonald D: Management of giant vesicovaginal and vesicourethrovaginal fistulas, *J Urol* 130:1073, 1983.

Elkins TE, DeLancey JOL, McGuire EJ: The use of modified Martius graft as an adjunctive technique in vesicovaginal and rectovaginal fistula repair, *Obstet Gynecol* 75:727, 1990.

Elkins TE, Ghosh TS, Tagoe GA, et al: Transvaginal urethral reconstruction from tubularized anterior bladder wall in the repair of obstetric fistulas, *Obstet Gynecol* 79(3):455, 1992.

Elkins TE, Drescher C, Martey JO, et al: Vesicovaginal fistula revisited, *Obstet Gynecol* 72:307, 1988.

Falk HC, Bunkin IA: The management of vesico-vaginal fistula following abdominal total hysterectomy, *Surg Gynecol Obstet* 93:404, 1951.

Hanash KA, Sieck U: Successful repair of a large vesicovaginal fistula with associated urethral loss using the anterior bladder flap technique, *J Urol* 130:775, 1983.

Herbert DB, Vaughn ED: Vesicovaginal fistula: a therapeutic challenge, *Infect Surg,* Feb:130, 1985.

Lawson JB: Vesical fistulae into the vaginal vault, *Br J Urol* 44:623, 1972.

Miller NF: The surgical treatment and postoperative care of vesicovaginal fistula, *Am J Obstet Gynecol* 44:873, 1942.

Morgan JE, Farrow GA, Sims RH: The sloughed urethra syndrome, *Am J Obstet Gynecol* 130:521, 1978.

Nichols DH, Randall CL: Vaginal surgery, ed 3, Baltimore, 1989, Williams & Wilkins.

O'Conor VJ: Repair of vesicovaginal fistula with associated urethral loss, *Surg Obstet Gynecol* 146:251, 1978.

Robertson JR: Vesicovaginal fistulas. In Slate WG (ed): *Disorders of the female urethra and urinary incontinence,* Baltimore, 1982, Williams & Wilkins.

Symmonds RE, Hill LM: Loss of the urethra: a report on 50 patients, *Am J Obstet Gynecol* 103(2):130, 1978.

Tanagho EA, Smith DR: Clinical evaluation of a surgical technique for correction of complete urinary incontinence, *J Urol* 107:402, 1972.

Tanagho EA: Bladder neck reconstruction for total urinary incontinence: 10 years of experience, *J Urol* 125:321, 1981.

Zacharin RF: *Obstetric fistula,* New York, 1988, Springer Verlag Wien.

Zoubek J, McGuire E, Nol F, DeLancey J: The late occurrence of urinary tract damage in patients successfully treated by radiotherapy for cervical carcinoma, *J Urol* 141:1347, 1988.

Prevention

American College of Obstetricians and Gynecologists: Genitourinary fistulas, *ACOG Technical Bulletin* No. 53, Jan 1985.

Thorton JG: Should vesicovaginal fistula be treated only by specialists? *Tropical Doctor* 16:78, 1986.

World Health Organization: Call to Action: Safe Motherhood Conference. Nairobi, February 10-13, 1987.

CHAPTER 24

Suburethral Diverticula

Laszlo Sogor

Historical Prespectives on Diseases of the Urethra
Pertinent Anatomy
Pathophysiologic Considerations
    Definition
    Etiologies
Incidence
Clinical Diagnosis
Diagnostic Techniques
    Radiography
    Endoscopy
    Sonography
    Urethral pressure profilometry
Surgical Treatment
    Historical review
    Suggested surgical techniques

The female urethra is a 4-cm long narrow membranous canal that extends from the bladder to the external orifice on the vulvar vestibule. Dysfunction of this tube leads to major disability, as has been recognized since ancient times. Obstruction of the urethra is life-threatening. Incontinence produces psychologic, emotional, and social consequences.

This chapter describes diseases of the urethra (especially those related to diverticula). It traces the history from antiquity to the present and offers insight into etiology. After reviewing the classic diagnostic methods, newer diagnostic modalities will be pre-

sented. Because cure of this condition is primarily surgical, several procedures are described.

HISTORICAL PERSPECTIVES ON DISEASES OF THE URETHRA

The first recorded evidence of interest and treatment specific to the urethra is found in the Ayuveda of Sucrutu, a Hindu treatise written around 500 BC. The Hindus at this time were treating strictures of the urethra by graduated dilators made of wood or metal, as well as treating other diseases of the urethra by injections. Hippocrates in 400 BC was the first to write about urethral abscesses. Cornelius Celcus at the beginning of the Christian century was the next to write definitively of urethral conditions.

Aside from the mention of urethral strictures and abscesses in the ancient literature, the first specific mention of urethral pathology in western literature occurred in Ambrose Pare's collected works (1575), wherein he wrote about the "skinny caruncles of womens privies." This condition also was observed by Morgagni during postmortem examination in a young girl. He described "from the orifice of the urethra a small reddish body was vominant and this one cut into longitudinally I perceived to be nothing else, but the internal code at that meatus." In 1750, Samuel Sharp noted "the excruciating torment and violent disorders caused by caruncles and I excised one with complete relief of symptoms."

The first description of an operation to treat diverticula in the English literature occurred in 1786 (Hey). In this report, a vaginal incision was made into the diverticulum cavity. The cavity was packed with lint resulting in a cure. A century later, Cullen reviewed the literature of the time and presented his first case (from Prof. H. Kelly's service at Johns Hopkins Hospital). Thirty-eight cases were summarized and possible etiologies of the various types of suburethral sacks were discussed. During the intervening years, many different terms were used to describe what we now include within the spectrum of suburethral diverticulum. These included urethrocele, urethral diverticulum, suburethral abscess, suburethral diverticulum, and urethrovaginal urinary pocket.

PERTINENT ANATOMY

The urethra is dorsal to the symphysis pubis and is embedded in the anterior wall of the vagina. The diameter when undilated averages 6 mm. It perforates through the perineal membrane, with its external orifice directly above the vaginal opening. The lining membrane has longitudinal folds and many small urethral glands that open into the urethra throughout its entire length. The largest of these are the periurethral glands of Skene. Skene's ducts open just within the urethral orifice, although the exact anatomic location is variable. The mucus coat is continuous externally with that of the vulva and internally with that of the bladder. It is primarily a stratified squamous epithelium, which becomes transitional near the bladder.

PATHOPHYSIOLOGIC CONSIDERATIONS

Definition

For practical considerations, a suburethral diverticulum is any fluid-filled mass along the anterolateral portions of the vagina, which can be shown to have direct communication with the urethra.

Etiologies
Congenital

Suburethral diverticula have been diagnosed in female patients from the age of 5 on through menopause. This fact, as well as case descriptions of male newborns with diverticula, make a compelling case for congenital etiology. Further support stems from histologic studies of dissected diverticular walls, wherein mucosa, submucosa, and a muscular coat can be found.

The specific congenital origin in general cannot be ascertained; however, several known structures may be etiologic, including remnants of Gartner's or wolffian duct cysts that rupture into the urethra. In addition, a faulty union of the longitudinal folds of the urethra may lead to suburethral diverticular cysts. Other theories have implicated cell rests that become cystic and ultimately perforate into the urethra.

Despite these theories, one must be careful to assign congenital etiology based simply on histology because a suburethral abscess that becomes sterile can become entirely reepithelialized from the urethra. If the patient is evaluated late in the course of events, a congenital etiology might be assigned, whereas in fact the condition was acquired.

Acquired

In this category birth trauma, infection, instrumentation, and urethral stones are of primary consideration. Many patients with diverticula give a previous history of prolonged, difficult labor. The presumption is that trauma occurs to the inferior wall of the urethra from the descending fetal head. The mechanism of damage is related possibly to necrosis and obstruction of Skene's duct. Some authors of older gynecologic texts, including TeLinde, mention infection as the primary etiology of suburethral diverticula. The most notable organism mentioned is gonococcus. The mechanism is identical to that seen with Bartholin's abscess, i.e., infection with subsequent suppuration of the periurethra and paraurethral glands. Because of the delicate nature of the urethral folds, any instrumentation has the potential for tearing through the epithelium and leading to false channels and pockets, which, over time, may become reepithelialized and filled with fluid, thus meeting criteria for suburethral diverticulum. Numerous reports in the literature report the presence of stones within suburethral diverticula. One thought is that the passage of stones through the urethra can, in some instances, lead to an erosion through the mucosal wall with incomplete reepithelialization of the erosion. A suburethral diverticulum

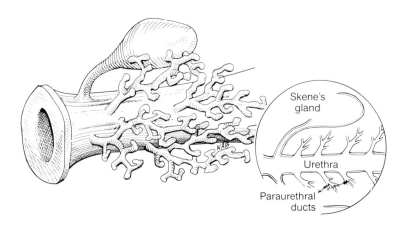

Fig. 24-1 Schematic diagram of the paraurethral glands and Skene's gland (after Huffman).

with a stone could form. Alternatively, the presence of a stone in a diverticulum may simply be a precipitate that forms after the diverticulum has formed from other etiologies.

Summary

Skene described two large ducts lying on each side of the urethra and related them to clinical problems. Although these structures were described as early as 1672 by deGraaf, our anatomic understanding of them and their potential role in diseases of the urethra became evident only after Huffman performed detailed studies of the development of periurethral glands in the human female. In his initial studies, Huffman performed wax model reconstructions of portions of the urethra and the uterovaginal anlage in fetuses from 50 to 224 mm, as well as six women. From these studies, the anlagen of periurethral glands were observed for the first time in a 50-mm fetus. These small buds arise from the ventral and lateral surfaces of the urethra above the müllerian tubercle. In adult urethras, the orifices of all the paraurethral and periurethral glands arise from the urethral mucosa itself. No glandular structures were observed arising from the urogenital sinus in the vaginal epithelium or in the vestibule. From the histologic appearances of these glands, one can conclude that they are homologues to that portion of the male prostate that develop cranial

to the mesonephric duct/urogenital sinus union.

Huffman continued his work using wax models of the duct systems surrounding the urethra (Fig. 24-1). From this work, we conclude that the distinction between paraurethral and periurethral glands is meaningless.

Everett pointed out the importance of gonococci in infections of the periurethral ducts and glands. Periurethral ducts and glands may play an important role in many cases of urethritis by acting as a nidus for many chronic infections of the female urethra and vagina. Organisms involved include gonococci, *Chlamydia trachomatis*, and *Trichomonas vaginalis*. The latter organism can use the urethral glands as a source for intractable vaginal infections. Other opportunistic organisms also can be involved. Whenever these glands become obstructed, small abscesses can form from which putrid material can be expressed through the urethra. These abscesses then "point" into the urethra and rupture into it, thereby forming a suburethral diverticulum. Therefore, an infectious etiology probably represents the majority of cases of suburethral diverticula.

Primary cysts of the periurethral duct system do occur. They are seen in histologic preparations, but are usually microscopic. If these cysts do enlarge, they generally produce small fluctuant tumors of the anterior vaginal wall, generally no larger than 2 or 3

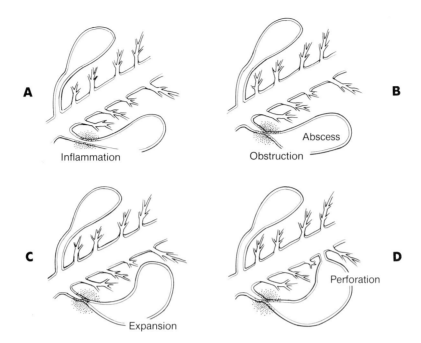

Fig. 24-2 Hypothetical mechanism of acquired suburethral diverticulum. **A,** An initial inflammatory response occurs in Skene's duct or one of the paraurethral ducts. **B,** An abscess forms within the gland or duct leading to obstruction of the gland neck. **C,** Expansion of the abscess. **D,** Perforation of the abscess into the urethra leading to diverticulum formation.

cm. They usually are asymptomatic and not appreciated on physical examination. Rarely, they may cause dyspareunia. Anterior and anterolateral wall cysts need to be differentiated from cysts of mesonephric or paramesonephric origin.

Netter, presumably using the work of Huffman and Krantz, presented color drawings of his conceptualization of periurethral and paraurethral gland structures. His discussion noted that the majority of glands tend to form an interdependent conducting system terminating in the large Skene's duct, which opens on either side of the midline just dorsal to the urethral meatus. He believed that these are remnant structures, which serve no specific purpose. Netter again noted the important view that their position predisposes them to infection, especially by gonococci. Their relatively poor drainage fosters the tendency of such infections to become chronic.

A model for cyst/abscess formation is demonstrated in Fig. 24-2.

INCIDENCE

Wharton and Kearns discussed 30 cases of suburethral diverticula in women at the Johns Hopkins Hospital between 1890 and 1949. The incidence for this condition was 1 in 2300 gynecologic admissions. The majority of these diverticula were reported within the most recent 10 years of the publication. Johnson reported no observations of a suburethral diverticulum in 140,000 admissions over a period of 10 years. After the lesion was called to the attention of the staff, nine proven cases were found over the subsequent year. MacKinnon et al reported 204 cases of suburethral diverticula between 1935 through 1955. Interestingly, they lamented that the standard urologic text failed to

TABLE 24-1   Frequency of symptoms in women with urethral diverticula

Symptom	Wharton and Kearns	Mackinnon et al	Hoffman and Adams	Davis and Robinson
Frequency	63%	66%	—	70%
Burning	63%	79%	35%	35%
Pain	40%	29%	30%	36%
Incontinence	30%	25%	42%	49%
Dyspareunia	13%	14%	12%	14%
Retention	6%	—	—	3%
Difficulty voiding	20%	32%	—	—
Hematuria	—	17%	11%	20%
Vaginal mass	—	12%	27%	—

list suburethral diverticulum as a condition that can be found in female patients. Furthermore, they noted that many teaching programs in both urology and gynecology overlooked this subject. No incidence figures were given in this publication. Davis and TeLinde reported an 8% rate. Bruning found three diverticula in 500 autopsy specimens for a 0.6% incidence. In response to this study, Anderson evaluated patients in Aarhus, Denmark using injection urethrography. He reported a 3% incidence of suburethral diverticula. Despite the approximate incidence of at least 3%, several modern gynecologic textbooks still fail to mention this entity.

CLINICAL DIAGNOSIS

Patients with suburethral diverticula can be asymptomatic or can have symptoms of chronic recurring cystitis with pain, burning, frequency, and dyspareunia. The main feature of these episodes is a refractoriness to medical treatment. In addition, a significant percentage of patients complain of difficulty voiding, postvoiding dribbling, urinary incontinence, or gross hematuria. Some patients notice a protruding tender vaginal mass. Rarely, obstruction of the urethra can ensue. Interestingly, the duration of symptoms is often quite long. Table 24-1 summarizes the clinical manifestations in several of the larger published series.

The most commonly described signs of suburethral diverticula are the presence of an anterior vaginal mass and the ability to express pus and/or urine from the

mass via the urethral orifice. Using these signs, Davis and TeLinde diagnosed diverticula correctly in 63% of their cases. Ancillary techniques were required for diagnosis because of failure to express fluid in the remainder of cases with an anterior vaginal mass.

DIAGNOSTIC TECHNIQUES
Radiography

The objective of all diagnostic methods is to demonstrate a urethral communication to a diverticular sac. Thomas in 1930 described a technique for female urethography using retrograde injection of iodized oil into the urethra. He used a simple syringe inserted into the urethral meatus. A variation on this technique was discussed by Taylor who used a Foley catheter with a distal silk ligature to tamponade the vesicourethral sphincter and prevent reflux. Other authors catheterized the diverticular orifice with ureteral catheters during urethroscopy and instilled radioopaque media. This procedure was difficult and often unsuccessful and led to failure of diagnosis in up to one third of cases.

Davis and Cian reported a new technique—positive-pressure urethrography—for the diagnosis of urethral diverticula, for which they constructed a special catheter. This system is similar to the one devised by Taylor to prevent bladder reflux; however, a sliding balloon was added to maintain the catheter in position as well as to tamponade the external meatus. In this fashion, the urethra became a closed tube, which could

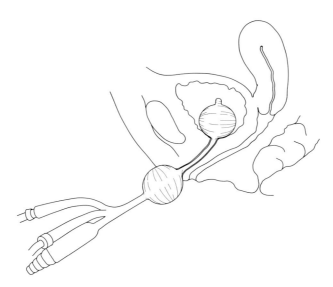

Fig. 24-3 Trattner double-balloon catheter. Proximal balloon inflates within bladder neck anchoring catheter and distal balloon occludes external meatus. Contrast fills urethra through slit seen between balloons. *(From Greenberg M, Stone D, Cochran ST, et al: Am J Radiol 136:259, 1981.)*

be injected with contrast medium under moderate pressure, permitting visualization of diverticula even with minute sinus tracts (Fig. 24-3). They reported four cases using this system and recommended that a urethrogram be obtained in any case of chronic urinary tract infection or suspected diverticulum. Surgical excision was facilitated by radiographic demonstration of the exact size and location of the lesion. They noted that occasionally several diverticula may be present concurrently, and that some diverticula may have more than one urethral orifice.

Voiding cystourethrograms performed under cinefluoroscopy have improved the diagnostic yield by 40%. No comparative studies between cinefluoroscopy and positive-pressure urethrography are available.

Endoscopy

Cystourethroscopy is the time-honored method of diagnosis for suburethral diverticula. Most urogynecologic articles recommend this diagnostic modality, *Campbell's Urology*, however, does not mention cystourethroscopy as a required diagnostic modality. Furthermore, Hoffman and Adams specifically note that endoscopic diagnosis has not been a routine part of their evaluation because many times the diverticular opening into the urethra is too small to be seen endoscopically. Cystourethroscopy alone is inadequate to establish the diagnosis because of the 30% to 40% false-negative rate. Therefore, a radiographic procedure should be added.

Sonography

With the advent of vaginal probe sonography, the evaluation of vaginal masses becomes feasible. We have used vaginal ultrasound to evaluate cases of proven suburethral diverticula. Although ultrasound can evaluate these cystic lesions quite satisfactorily, especially when they are distended, it cannot prove that they are true suburethral diverticula because of inadequate visualization of the connection into the urethra.

Urethral Pressure Profilometry

Suburethral diverticula can sometimes show a dip in urethral pressure on urethral pressure profile. This finding can be used to localize suburethral diverticular openings in relation to the area of maximal urethral closure pressure (MUCP). If the openings are distal to the MUCP, then diverticulectomy or marsupialization can be used for treatment with little risk of damage to the continence mechanism. If the openings are proximal to or at the MUCP, then diverticulectomy or partial ablation should be used with the attendant risk of urinary incontinence in cases complicated by noncure or fistula formation. Unfortunately, the biphasic pattern frequently is not observed in patients with proven diverticula.

Summary

We perform positive-pressure urethrography or voiding cystourethrography after physical examination raises suspicion for suburethral diverticulum. In this manner, adequate evaluation of the size and complexity of the diverticular sac(s) can be gleaned, as well as the location of all orifices. We do not believe that cystourethroscopy offers any additional diagnostic information before surgical resection.

SURGICAL TREATMENT

Historical Review

We do not know how the barbers of Europe approached acute suburethral diverticulum, but we suspect they practiced simple incision and drainage. As discussed previously, Hey opened into the sac per vaginum and then packed the diverticulum. It is fascinating that the two papers in *Urologic and Cutaneous Reviews* in 1937 and 1938 came to opposite conclusions as to the preferred method of surgical treatment. Young and McCrea concluded that simple vaginal incision of the pouch usually results in complete recovery in 2 to 4 weeks. Hunner recommended a diverticulectomy. He initiated the procedure by removing an oval piece of redundant vaginal mucosa overlying the diverticulum, followed by resection of the diverticulum.

Hunner later modified his operation to involve a simple midline incision with subsequent resection of the right vaginal margin. A de facto vaginal flap then was created from the left to the right to prevent the final row of sutures from overlapping the first two lines of closure. A purse-string suture was used to

close the fistulous opening into the urethral mucosa. Interrupted sutures brought the paraurethral fascial tissue together. The vagina was closed with silver wire. The bladder was catheterized and the vagina was packed with gauze.

Hoffman and Adams identified several important principles for successful suburethral diverticulum repair. These included complete removal of the sac and identification and closure of all openings into the urethra. They made a longitudinal incision over the diverticulum with dissection of the sac, subsequent entry into the sac, excision, and layer closure. In their series of 60 patients, 55 achieved excellent results. Stress incontinence developed in three patients, perhaps because the diverticula were located close to the bladder neck. Anterior colporrhaphy cured two of these patients.

O'Connor stressed several factors in repair of the diverticulum. Most notable was that the urethra is not readily separable from the anterior vaginal wall and thus there is no anatomic plane of cleavage.

Davis and Robinson reported on 120 cases of urethral diverticulum. The majority (98) were treated by transvaginal diverticulectomy encompassing removal of the sacs with layer closure of the urethra and vagina. They reported no cases of vesicovaginal fistula, one recurrent diverticulum, and four patients with urethrovaginal fistulas. Urethral strictures were not classified as a complication of the procedure, as many of their patients had preoperative strictures related to the diverticulum or repair.

Spence and Duckett presented their observations on suburethral diverticula, initially stressing complete excision of the diverticulum. They pointed out the importance of the division of the communication between the diverticulum and the urethra and the reconstruction of the urethra in layers overlying a urethral catheter. They also emphasized the value of using methylene blue dye to distend the diverticular cavity before the surgical procedure.

Spence and Duckett described an alternative surgical procedure that subsequently became known as the Spence procedure. Basically, this procedure is a marsupialization technique applicable only to distal diverticula. These authors reported resolution of the diverticula in all patients and no postoperative incontinence in seven of nine patients. This procedure currently is one of the most common repair operations for distal diverticula because of its relative ease and success.

An interesting approach was presented by Sholum et al, who made a semilunar incision beneath the urethral orifice, dissected underneath the vaginal mucosa to the diverticulum, and excised it. This technique avoided an extensive vaginal incision and its attendant difficulties. In this fashion, the vaginal epithelium remains intact over the area of excision of the diverticulum. These authors reported successful use of the method in 17 patients. They noted no difficulty in establishing an appropriate plane between the vagina and diverticulum. Although this procedure represents an interesting variation on excision of the sac, it is a rather difficult operation in practice, especially for proximal diverticula.

Proximal diverticula have a higher risk of bladder entry and its attendant propensity for vesicovaginal fistula formation and damage to the bladder neck, potentially resulting in stress incontinence. Because of these difficulties, Tancer et al reported a partial ablation technique for these difficult diverticula. In this procedure, the diverticular sac is dissected out vaginally, incised longitudinally, and entered. The main body of the diverticulum is excised, but no effort is made to enucleate the sac at its neck. The opening is closed side-to-side using No. 3-0 suture. A second layer of sutures is placed, which imbricates the urethral incision. The diverticular wall is then closed in a double-breasted fashion to bolster the previous closure and to obliterate the original cavity. Tancer et al performing this operation on 34 women over a 10-year period and reported no cases of urinary incontinence or fistula formation. This procedure has become a popular operation for proximal diverticula because of its high success rate and low frequency of urinary incontinence.

Suggested Surgical Techniques

Because multiple operations are available to correct suburethral diverticula, it is imperative to adjust the operation for the patient. Our primary operation is a diverticulectomy (Fig. 24-4). We use an inverted U-flap for the vaginal epithelium and a "vest-over-pants"

closure of the periurethral fascia to avoid overlapping sutures, and thereby diminish the incidence of urethrovaginal fistulas.

If the diverticulum is located in the proximal urethra near the bladder neck, we prefer to perform a partial ablation technique as described by Tancer et al to lower the risk of damage to the bladder neck and urethral sphincteric continence mechanism.

The Spence operation is indicated for diverticula in the distal urethra, distal to the area of maximal urethral closure pressure. This operation is very straightforward, but patients should be selected carefully to avoid the risk of postoperative incontinence.

The following are step-by-step descriptions of the three main operations for suburethral diverticula.

Diverticulectomy

1. After regional or general anesthesia, the patient is placed in lithotomy position. One to three doses of prophylactic antibiotics generally are used. Urethroscopy is performed before the surgery to localize the diverticular opening(s) into the urethra and to assure there are no other unsuspected findings.
2. A double-balloon catheter is placed into the urethra, and the balloons are set at the proximal and distal urethra and inflated. Sterile milk or methylene blue dye is injected into the catheter to inflate the urethra and diverticulum. This catheter is kept in place until the sac is entered so that it can be inflated periodically during dissection. It is also necessary to assure that the urethra or diverticular sac have not been entered inadvertently.
3. Hemostatic solution can be injected submucosally. An inverted U-shape incision is made over the diverticulum through the vaginal epithelium, which is then dissected off the urethra and periurethral tissue (Fig. 24-4, *A*).
4. A longitudinal incision is made carefully over the diverticular sac. The fascial tissue overlying and surrounding the diverticulum is completely dissected and mobilized (Fig. 24-4, *B* and *C*).
5. Dissection is continued around the sac until the neck is visualized. If the entire neck of the diverticulum is isolated, the diverticulum is ex-

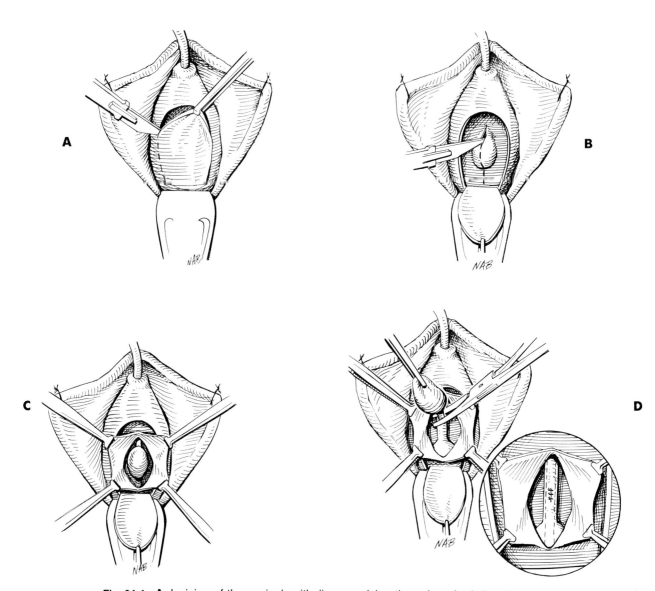

Fig. 24-4 **A**, Incision of the vaginal epithelium overlying the suburethral diverticulum, creating a ∪-shaped flap. **B**, Incision of the periurethral fascial tissue over the diverticular sac. **C**, Complete dissection and mobilization of the fascial tissue surrounding the suburethral diverticulum. **D**, A complete dissection of the suburethral diverticulum with its attendant neck. The sac is excised at its neck. *Insert*, Defect in the urethra after closure with fine, absorbable interrupted sutures.

Continued.

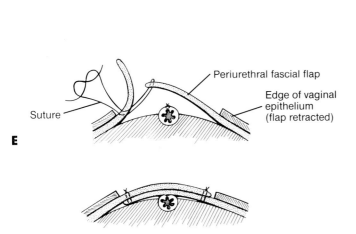

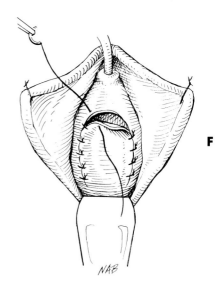

Fig. 24-4, cont'd. E, Demonstration of the "vest-over-pants" technique of closure of periurethral fascial tissue. **F,** Closure of the vaginal flap with interrupted No. 2-0, absorbable suture. We prefer to use interrupted suturing techniques to avoid tissue shortening.

cised from the urethra (Fig. 24-4, *D*). If the entire sac can not be mobilized, then the sac should be opened longitudinally and the inside of the diverticulum explored to note the condition of the tissue and the presence of other diverticular openings or sacculations. The sac then is excised at its neck. The urethral opening is closed longitudinally over a Foley catheter with interrupted, fine, delayed-absorbable suture (Fig. 24-4, *D,* and *inset*).

6. The periurethral fascia, which previously was developed into flaps bilaterally, is closed in a "vest-over-pants" fashion over the urethra (Fig. 24-4, *E*). This maneuver avoids suture lines that overlap the urethral repair.

7. The flap of vaginal epithelium is repositioned and the incision is closed with No. 2-0, absorbable, interrupted sutures (Fig. 24-4, *F*), used to avoid tissue shortening.

8. The vagina is generally packed for 1 day. Continuous urinary drainage may be carried out with a transurethral Foley catheter or suprapubic catheter for 2 to 5 days.

Partial Ablation Technique

1. The surgical steps for the partial ablation technique are the same as for diverticulectomy up to the point of identification and dissection of the intact diverticular sac.

2. The diverticulum is incised longitudinally; the sac is entered and explored. The opening into the urethra is identified.

3. The easily excisable portion of the sac, not including the neck of the diverticulum, is excised (Fig. 24-5). No effort is made to enucleate the sac at its neck or at the juncture with the urethra. The base and neck of the diverticulum is then closed side to side, using fine, interrupted, absorbable suture. A second layer of similar sutures is placed, which further imbricates the previous urethral defect.

4. The "vest-over-pants" periurethral fascial closure and closure of the vaginal epithelium are completed as for a diverticulectomy.

5. A bulbocavernosus muscle transplant, as described in Chapter 23, is optional for diverticulectomy or partial ablation.

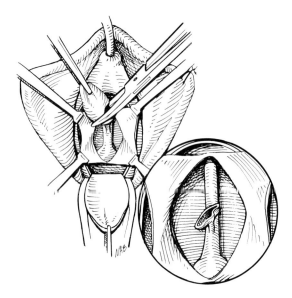

Fig. 24-5 Demonstration of the partial ablation technique for proximal diverticulum (as described by Tancer et al). In this technique, the diverticulum is excised and a portion of the base of the diverticulum and its neck are left intact and closed in an imbricating fashion with interrupted, fine absorbable suture.

Spence Procedure

1. The patient is positioned as for a diverticulectomy. A urethroscopy is performed to locate the diverticulum and its opening.
2. An Allis clamp is placed on the anterior vaginal wall opposite the diverticular orifice. One blade of the scissor is placed in the urethra and the other in the vagina. The scissor divides the floor of the diverticulum and the overlying vaginal epithelium, including the posterior urethra distal to the diverticulum.
3. Redundant flaps of diverticular sac and vaginal epithelium are trimmed.
4. A running, locking, delayed absorbable suture coapts the margins of the remaining lining of sac and adjacent vaginal epithelium. Both the bladder neck and the urethra proximal to the diverticular orifice are left untouched.

TABLE 24-2 Complications associated with repair of suburethral diverticula

Complication	Frequence of occurrence (%)
Recurrent urinary tract infection	5
Fistula	4
Recurrence	4
Stress incontinence	2
Stricture formation	1

Modified from Ginsburg DS, Genadry R: *Obstet Gynecol Surv* 39:1, 1984.

5. A vaginal pack and urethral catheter were used for 48 hours in the original article by Spence and Duckett; however, they are probably not necessary. This procedure usually can be performed on an outpatient basis.

Certainly, no surgical procedure is without difficulties and complications, and excision of suburethral diverticula by any method falls within this general dictum. Ginsberg and Genadry reviewed the literature to 1984. Their complication rates are summarized in Table 24-2.

SUMMARY

The suburethral diverticulum has a long history as a clinical problem for women. Diagnosis clearly depends on a heightened index of suspicion, as many of the symptomatologies can be attributed to other urogynecologic conditions. It is indeed unfortunate that to some extent our instruments inhibit the diagnosis itself. For example, the anterior blade of a bivalve speculum may hide a suburethral diverticulum. Generally, careful palpation of the urethra is not included in the instruction of bimanual examination. Palpation should be performed because the incidence of diverticula can be up to 3% in the general female population and can be readily diagnosed by a careful physical examination in up to two thirds of patients. Radiologic, endoscopic, and urodynamic techniques also can be used to diagnose and localize suburethral diverticula.

Variations on surgical procedures for this condition have been summarized. The major feature of the surgical procedures is careful dissection and excision of the sac with closure of the urethra and intervening spaces. With meticulous dissection and careful closure, success rates of better than 95% can be achieved with few complications.

BIBLIOGRAPHY

Anderson MJF: The incidence of diverticula in the female urethra, *J Urol* 98:96, 1967.

Asmussen M, Miller A: *Clinical gynecologic urology*, Boston, 1983, Blackwell Scientific Publications.

Benjamin J, Elliott L, Cooper JF, et al: Urethral diverticulum in adult female, clinical aspects, operative procedure and pathology, *Urology* 3:1, 1974.

Bhatia NN, McCarthy TA, Ostergard DR: Urethral pressure profiles of women with diverticula, *Obstet Gynecol* 58:375, 1981.

Bruning EJ: *Die Pathologie der Weiblichen Urethra und des Paraurethrium*, Berlin, 1959, Stuttgart.

Butler WJ: The diagnosis of urethra diverticula in women, *J Urol* 95:63, 1966.

Cullen TS: Abscess in the urethro-vaginal septum, *Bull Johns Hopkins Hosp* 5:45, 1894.

Davis BC, Robinson DG: Diverticula of the female urethra: assay of 120 cases, *J Urol* 204:850, 1970.

Davis HJ, Cian LG: Positive pressure urethrography: a new diagnostic method, *J Urol* 75:753, 1956.

Davis HJ, TeLinde RW: Urethral diverticula: an assay of 121 cases, *J Urol* 80:34, 1958.

Devine CJ: Surgery of the urethra. In Walsh PC, Gittes RF, Perlmutter AD, et al: *Campbell's urology*, ed 5, Philadelphia, PA, 1986, WB Saunders.

Drutz HP: Urethral diverticula, *Obstet Gynecol Clin North Am* 16:923, 1989.

Edwards EA, Beebe RA: Diverticula of the female urethra, *Obstet Gynecol* 5:729, 1955.

Everett HS: *Gynecologic and obstetrical urology*, Baltimore, 1944, Williams & Wilkins.

Folsom AI: Diseases of the urethra and penis. In *History of urology*, Baltimore, 1933, Williams & Wilkins.

Ginsburg DS, Genadry R: Suburethral diverticulum in the female, *Obstet Gynecol Surv* 39:1, 1984.

Greenberg M, Stone D, Cochran ST, et al: Female urethral diverticula: double-balloon catheter study, *Am J Radiol* 136:259, 1981.

Hey W: *Practical observations in surgery*, Philadelphia, 1805, Humphreys.

Hoffman MJ, Adams WE: Recognition and repair of urethral diverticula, *Am J Obstet Gynecol* 92:106, 1965.

Huffman JW: The development of the periurethral glands in the human female, *Am J Obstet Gynecol* 46:773, 1943.

Huffman JW: The detailed anatomy of the paraurethral ducts in the adult human female, *Am J Obstet Gynecol* 55:86, 1948.

Huffman JW: Clinical significance of the paraurethral ducts and glands, *Arch Surg* 62:615, 1951.

Hunner GL: Calculus formation in a urethral diverticulum in women. Report of three cases, *Urol Cutan Rev* 42:336, 1938.

Johnson CM: Diverticula and cysts of female urethra, *J Urol* 39:506, 1938.

Jones HW, Jones GS: *Novak's textbook of gynecology*, ed 10, Baltimore, 1981, Williams & Wilkins.

Keith LG, Ames BL: The female urethra. In Sciara JJ (ed): *Gynecology and obstetrics*, revised edition, Hagerstown, Md, 1987, Harper & Row.

Kistner RW: *Gynecology: principles and practice yearbook*, Chicago, 1983, Year Book Medical Publishers.

Krantz K: Anatomy of urethra and anterior vaginal wall, *Am J Obstet Gynecol* 62:374, 1951.

Kretschmer HL: Diverticula in the anterior urethra in male children, *Surg Gynecol Obstet* 62:634, 1936.

MacKinnon N, Pratt JH, Pool TL: Diverticulum of the female urethra, *Surg Clin North Am* 39:953, 1959.

Netter FH: The Ciba collection of medical illustrations, vol 2, *The reproductive system*, 1974.

O'Connor VJ: Surgery in the female urethra. In Glen JF, Boyce WH (eds): *Urologic surgery*, New York, 1969, Harper Norwell.

Reid DE, Ryan KG, Benirschke K: *Principles and management of human reproduction*, Philadelphia, 1972, WB Saunders.

Robertson J: Urethral diverticula. In Ostergard D, Bent A (eds): *Urogynecology and urodynamics*, ed 3, Baltimore, 1991, Williams & Wilkins.

Sholem SL, Wechsler M, Roberts M: Management of the urethral diverticulum in women: a modified operative technique, *J Urol* 112:485, 1974.

Skene AJ: The anatomy and pathology of two important glands of the female urethra, *Am J Obstet Gynecol* 13:265, 1880.

Slate WG: Lesions of the female urethra. In Pratt JH, Malek RS (eds): *Disorders of the female urethra and urinary incontinence*, Baltimore, 1978, Williams & Wilkins.

Spence HM, Duckett JW: Diverticulum of the female urethra: clinical aspects and presentation of a simple operative technique for cure, *J Urol* 104:432, 1970.

Tancer ML, Mooppan MU, Pierre-Louis C, et al: Suburethral diverticulum treatment by partial ablation, *Obstet Gynecol* 62:511, 1983.

Taylor WN: Urologists Correspondence Club Letters 16:37, 1950.

TeLinde RW: Surgical conditions of the vulva and the vagina. In *Operative gynecology*, ed 2, Philadelphia, 1953, JB Lippincott.

Thomas R: Examination of the female urethra, *Acta Radiol* 11:527, 1930.

Wharton LR, Kearns W: Diverticula of the female urethra, *J Urol* 63:1063, 1950.

Young BR, McCrea, LE: Urethrocele; urethral diverticulum; suburethral abscess in the female: roentgen appearance; treatment; review of the literature, report of a case, *Urol Cutan Rev* 41:91, 1937.

CHAPTER 25

Gynecologic Injury to the Ureters, Bladder, and Urethra: Recognition and Management

George W. Mitchell
Mark D. Walters

Prevention of Lower Urinary Tract Injury During Gynecologic Surgery
General principles
Adnexal surgery
Simple and radical abdominal hysterectomy
Vaginal hysterectomy
Cesarean section
Techniques to Recognize Lower Urinary Tract Injury During Gynecologic Surgery
Ureter
Bladder
Urethra
Postoperative Evaluation of Suspected Vaginal Fistulas
Techniques to Repair Intraoperative Lower Urinary Tract Injury
Distal ureter
Proximal two thirds of ureter
Bladder
Urethra

Injury to the urinary tract occurs during approximately 1% of gynecologic procedures. In a few instances this is deliberate, such as when the ureter must be freed from a trapped position or when the bladder must be opened to guide its dissection from the anterior uterine wall or to permit retrograde ureteral catheterization. In most cases, however, the injury is inadvertent. The avoidance of such injuries requires constant vigilance by the surgeon, although even great care is unlikely to achieve a perfect record over time. The likelihood of injury tends to be related to the difficulty of the operation, and sometimes it is advisable to seek help from those more experienced and with special expertise. Intraoperative recognition of the injury is of the utmost importance, as immediate repair is almost uniformly successful. This chapter discusses issues related to the prevention, recognition, and management of injuries to the lower urinary tract during obstetric and gynecologic surgery.

PREVENTION OF LOWER URINARY TRACT INJURY DURING GYNECOLOGIC SURGERY
General Principles

Many operations must be performed on an emergency basis or for serious disease for which treatment cannot be postponed. All that can be accomplished under those circumstances to prepare the patient for surgery is to regulate electrolytes and hematocrit and hope for the best. On the other hand, elective surgery should not be performed on individuals in poor condition, whether because of systemic disease, poor nutrition, or disordered mental state, unless the quality of life is so seriously affected that delay in treatment would cause prolongation of suffering.

Preoperatively, the coagulability of the patient's blood must be tested and, if found unsatisfactory, appropriate steps must be taken to alleviate the situation either before or at the time of surgery, particularly if the patient has a history of menorrhagia. Intraoperatively, the gynecologic surgeon should avoid clamping or ligating large volumes of tissue, which could incorporate ureter or bladder in the pedicle. It is desirable to clamp, suture, or cauterize only the smallest amount of tissue that encompasses a bleeding point or vascular pedicle. Repeated attempts to coagulate such large bleeding points can lead to extensive tissue damage in contiguous areas, which could include bladder or ureter.

The surgical setup is an important aspect of safe surgery and is often neglected. One cannot allow residents, nurses, or technicians to be responsible for having available and in good condition the equipment required for a specific operation. The necessary equipment should be assessed in advance and steps taken to see that it is on hand. Light sources are of particular importance and, if inadequate for a difficult dissection deep in the pelvis, should be supplemented by a flexible fiberoptic light or head lamp.

The incision must be of correct position and length for adequate exposure. The lower midline incision gives good pelvic exposure and can be extended around the umbilicus if access to the pelvic organs is unsatisfactory. Low transverse incisions are highly desirable for certain types of procedures, such as retropubic suspensions of the vesical neck, but they should not be used for cosmetic reasons if too little exposure could complicate the procedure and endanger the patient, particularly true when large uterine tumors or adnexal masses are encountered. This incision should give way to a muscle-cutting type of incision whenever greater exposure is needed.

Adnexal Surgery

Even the most experienced examiner cannot always tell whether a pelvic mass is of uterine or adnexal origin, or, if adnexal, whether it is benign or malignant. Despite the more frequent adjunctive use of computer tomography (CT) scans, ultrasound, Doppler flow, and tumor markers, uncertainty still may exist. In cases of cancer, advanced endometriosis, or the possible presence of some rare entity such as retroperitoneal tumor or fibrosis, intravenous pyelograms (IVP) should be performed. The usefulness of this procedure has been debated because studies have shown that routine IVP before surgery for pelvic tumors has been relatively nonproductive in terms of finding pathology or preventing injury. However, to detect ureteral obstruction as a result of pelvic disease and to assess the adequacy of renal function, it surpasses either CT scan or sonography. It is comforting to know in advance the function of both kidneys and the location of the obstruction of the ureter when present. A pelvic kidney may resemble a pelvic tumor by physical examination or CT scan, but it cannot escape detection by IVP. Should a mass of probable inflammatory nature be found on the left side only in an elderly person, the possibility of diverticulitis must be considered and either a barium enema or flexible sigmoidoscopy performed.

In the early days of radical hysterectomy and for many operations in which the compromise of ureters was feared, it was customary to insert retrograde ureteral stents to identify and possibly to protect the ureters during surgery. This custom has not been totally abandoned, but most surgeons today prefer the unencumbered ureter, believing that it will be more flexible, more easily retracted, and less susceptible to damage. Stents can always be introduced during surgery when the need arises. During a difficult dissection, however, being able to palpate the ureter is reassuring and, for the inexperienced surgeon, the use of stents may be necessary.

For major gynecologic surgery, a Foley catheter should be left in the bladder during the operation and kept on constant drainage. For any difficult operation or one involving the urinary tract directly, a catheter with separate channels that permits both filling and emptying should be used, with one channel connected to an overhead drainage bottle to permit rapid filling and the identification of bladder leaks. The size of the catheter should be compatible with the size of the urethra; 16 or 18 French usually is appropriate. The Foley bulb should be 10 ml, not 30 ml, as the latter, when filled, may be large enough to interfere with dissection of the bladder from the cervix or with manipulation around the vesical neck.

At the inferior level of a lower midline incision, the bladder may be pulled high by its peritoneal reflection as a result of incomplete emptying, ascites, tumor, or previous surgery, especially cesarean section. For this reason, the preperitoneal fat is carefully incised and retracted to expose the transparent peritoneum beneath. As the edge of the bladder is approached, the tissues become more vascular, which should serve as a warning that the vertical incision has progressed far enough caudally. To provide full exposure, it is sometimes necessary to cut the peritoneum obliquely toward the inguinal ligament and away from the bladder attachment. When a transverse incision is used, the peritoneum should be entered at a point as far cephalad as possible to avoid a direct cystotomy.

After entering the peritoneum, the first objective is to evaluate its contents, including fluid, blood, exudate, and the spread of disease over the surface. Appropriate specimens and cultures are sent to the laboratory. Next the upper abdomen is explored systematically, while the surgeon mentally catalogs the various organs according to a pattern that can be faithfully recorded at a later time. Careful palpation of the liver, gall bladder, pancreas, duodenum, stomach, and spleen comes first. With the index finger in the foramen of Winslow, the common duct and hepatic artery can be squeezed with the opposing thumb. The omentum and transverse colon are then pulled down and examined, and the hand is passed down the vena cava and aorta in a search for enlarged lymph nodes. Appropriate x-ray films should be available on the screen in the operating room.

Attention is then directed to the pelvic pathology that is the objective of the operation. If no adhesions are present, with the patient in Trendelenburg position the intestine is packed into the upper abdomen and retained by a retractor. A large tumor mass may have to be elevated into the incision and, if bowel adhesions are present, they must be carefully separated by sharp dissection with the aid of countertraction on adjacent

surfaces. It should now be possible to identify the type of pathology and decide on a course of action. Important variables such as whether the disease is benign or malignant and whether it is bilateral, the patient's age, the patient's future fertility potential and wishes, and the technical feasibility of the procedure should all be considered. The presence of an ovarian cyst or solid tumor on a long infundibulopelvic ligament invites rapid clamping and ligation of the pedicle. Care should be taken not to include a portion of the ureter in the ligature, as it is not infrequently drawn into the base of the infundibulopelvic ligament. Always first identify the ureter as it crosses the pelvic brim and passes close to the ovarian vessels in its course down the lateral pelvic wall. With one exception, the infundibulopelvic ligament should be ligated close to the ovarian pathology and as far from the pelvic wall as possible, regardless of whether the ovarian vein seems to be thrombosed. The only exception is that during a radical hysterectomy it is desirable to resect the infundibulopelvic ligament near the point of entrance of the ovarian vessels into the pelvis, being careful to free the ureter from its close attachment, to provide space for a proper node dissection.

Both benign and malignant ovarian and paraovarian tumors frequently are encased in adhesions and are bound either to the pelvic wall or to other organs within the pelvis. This dissection can be especially difficult when it is necessary to debulk the maximum possible amount of malignant tumor. Both the ureter and the bladder must be kept under constant surveillance during this dissection. This monitoring is best accomplished by identifying the ureter at or above the pelvic brim and following it down to where it blends with the pathology. In the majority of instances, the ureter is not invaded directly by adnexal disease and may be stripped away while still maintaining viability and patency. This stripping is accomplished with a combination of fine-pointed scissors and peanut dissectors while traction is made on the mass to be mobilized and resected.

Like the ureter, the bladder is seldom directly involved, but both its upper and lower surfaces may be encased by tumor. Under these circumstances, total tumor removal is impossible; but with less extensive disease, dissection under the bladder may be aided by

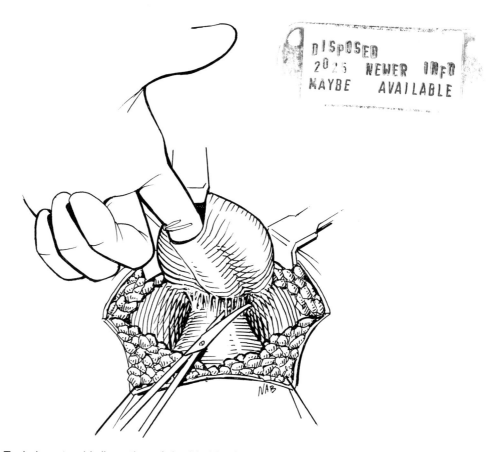

Fig. 25-1 Technique to aid dissection of the bladder from adjacent adherent structures. After a cystotomy incision, a finger in the bladder provides a proprioceptive guide to accurate dissection of the bladder from adjacent organs without further injury. Performing a cystotomy also gives the surgeon information about ureteral patency and position.

a high cystotomy incision. This is accomplished by instilling 300 ml of saline into the bladder and entering by a stab wound. A finger in the bladder provides a proprioceptive guide to accurate dissection without injury (Fig. 25-1). For disease that extends retroperitoneally or within the broad ligament, the approach is greatly simplified by cutting the round ligament first and mobilizing the mass from above downward.

In some instances the infundibulopelvic ligament is difficult to identify within the pelvis, and it becomes necessary to cut the peritoneum lateral to the colon, which is then mobilized medially to identify the ovarian vessels above the pelvic brim and separate them from the ureter. Once these vessels are clamped and ligated, the surgeon can count on a relatively bloodless field for further dissection. Remember never to cut or ligate any thick, cordlike structure without first determining that the ureter is separate from it.

Surgery for extensive endometriosis presents similar problems, but there are some differences. Because the ureter is often involved in the endometriotic process the retroperitoneal area must be investigated at the time of laparoscopy or laparotomy to make sure that it is not trapped. If a conservative operation is planned, this maneuver can be accomplished most easily by opening the peritoneum at its posterior reflection from the round ligament (with or without dividing the round ligament) and continuing the incision upward along the psoas muscle, being careful to avoid the infundibulopelvic ligament. While traction is maintained on the medial cut edge of the peritoneum, one finger is placed inside the retroperitoneal space with the thumb outside, or vice versa; the ureter, which is almost always adherent to this medial flap of peritoneum, can easily be palpated. As in the case of adnexal tumors, the ureter may be drawn from its usual path and distorted by disease, but it cannot escape detection either above or below the disease process and thus can be traced to its point of involvement. Endometriosis may invade the ureteral wall or even its lumen, but more often it surrounds and constricts the ureter by a fibrotic reaction and can lead to complete occlusion. Ovariectomy is unlikely to produce a beneficial effect on ureteral obstruction, although it will stop catamenial hematuria. Although possible, it is unlikely that postoperative treatment with gonadotropin-releasing hormone (GnRH) agonists will alleviate the fibrosis obstructing the ureter, and attempts to dissect the ureter from its endometriotic bed usually leave it damaged. For this reason, transection and reimplantation of the ureter into the bladder may be necessary.

Endometrial implants also are seen frequently on the peritoneal covering of the bladder but seldom invade the bladder lumen. At the time of laparotomy or laparoscopy, such implants may be handled by excision, fulguration, laser treatment, ovariectomy, or a combination of any two or three. As always, the management of direct bladder muscular involvement requires good judgment and careful technique.

Large adnexal tumors, uterine leiomyomas, or pregnancy tend to obstruct ureters by compression at the pelvic brim. In contrast, pelvic inflammatory disease that has progressed to the formation of tuboovarian abscesses can obstruct but seldom completely occludes the ureters along their lower third. Radiographs sometimes show lateral deviation of the ureters, which is, of course, impossible because they are against the pelvic wall; but they may be moved superiorly, inferiorly, or medially by their adherence to the inflammatory masses. The important issue is that their anatomic position is variable, leading to increased risk of trauma during dissection.

Most tuboovarian abscesses are treated medically, and few require surgery. When they do, removal of tubes, ovaries, and uterus is often the treatment of choice, although drainage is sometimes used in an attempt to conserve reproductive function. The urinary tract is at risk only when radical treatment is being applied, and either the ureters or the bladder may be traumatized, as the abscesses are usually located in the posterior pelvis behind the broad ligament and on top of the rectum, where blunt dissection is necessary. By manipulating the fingers of one hand beneath the mass near the base of the broad ligament, the abscesses are mobilized upward and peeled from their attachments to bladder and rectum. The ureters can usually be stripped off without difficulty as long as they can be identified and protected. This type of blunt dissection is easier to accomplish and safer when the disease is in an acute or subacute stage. Longstanding pelvic inflammatory disease is associated with dense adhesions, necessitating sharp dissection in areas where exposure is poor. Upward traction on the posterior bladder wall and filling of the bladder to identify the proper plane are good adjuncts to successful separation from pathology. The ureters must be identified along their entire courses both during and after organ dissection and removal.

Simple and Radical Abdominal Hysterectomy

Trauma to the lower urinary tract is approximately 10 times more common during abdominal hysterectomy than during adnexal surgery. The ureter is damaged generally as it passes beneath the uterine vessels or as it enters the bladder. Such injuries occur more frequently during radical hysterectomy because of pelvic lymph node dissection and because of the extensive mobilization of the ureters and bladder from the cervix and vaginal wall and the resulting devascularization. Preoperative IVP is essential before operations for uterine and cervical cancer, both for determining ureteral obstruction and position and the presence of congenital anomalies.

If a lymph node dissection is to be performed first, the peritoneum on either side is opened by cutting the round ligament and incising the lateral peritoneum over the psoas muscle to a level just beyond the peritoneal reflection of the cecum or the sigmoid colon.

The ureters on either side are palpated as they pass deep along the medial peritoneal flaps. These flaps of peritoneum, with the ureters attached, are dissected bluntly from the lateral pelvic walls over the great vessels down to the sacrum. The rectum and its mesentery, including the superior hemorrhoidal artery and vein, are mobilized bluntly from the surface of the sacrum and elevated so that a tape can be passed beneath them and the adjacent developed peritoneal flaps. The tape thus encompasses both ureters as well as the rectum. With the aid of the tape, these organs can be elevated and shifted from side to side away from the great vessels, permitting lymph node dissection without fear of injury to the ureters. When the bladder and rectum are to be mobilized from the cervix and vagina, the tape is removed, releasing the ureters. With this technique the ureters can be kept under direct vision at all times, reducing the likelihood of injury. As the radical operation progresses, the uterine vessels are ligated at their origin from the hypogastric artery and vein, the medial pedicle is retracted over the ureter, and the cardinal ligament is cut at its attachment to the pelvic wall. This separation of the ureter from its tunnel as it enters the bladder is accomplished by the careful placement of small right angle clamps along the roof of the tunnel perpendicular to the cervix, including only small amounts of this vascular tissue to avoid drawing the ureter into the subsequent ligature. Attempts to free the terminal ureter by sharp dissection without clamping are almost certain to cause heavy bleeding and require ligatures in an area where the chance of injury to ureter or bladder is great. With the proper technique, the ureter can be left attached to its peritoneal flap along most of its length and will retain most of its blood supply. With good visualization throughout the operative field, direct injury is unlikely.

Mobilization of the bladder from the cervix and anterior vaginal wall requires a combination of blunt and sharp dissection. A finger covered by one layer of gauze or a peanut dissector is helpful for the blunt dissection. The sharp dissection should be accomplished with fine scissors. If bleeding is well controlled, bladder muscle inadvertently left behind as the dissection proceeds downward can be spotted easily on the relatively pale vaginal wall. This finding tells the operator to shift the plane more toward the vaginal side. The presence of the Foley catheter balloon in the bladder also serves as a guide.

During simple hysterectomy for benign disease, trauma to the ureters is often due to attempts to control unexpected bleeding. This is most likely to occur in the region of the cardinal ligaments, when ligatures have failed to include the descending branch of the uterine artery or have slipped off their pedicles. If a single bleeding point is not clearly seen, the tendency is to clamp the bleeding area with a large clamp, which can easily include a portion of the ureteral wall. A more sensible approach is to grasp the offending pedicle or area between thumb and forefinger or with a noncrushing clamp, then release the hold enough to see the exact point from which the bleeding is originating. Once the area is identified, place the smallest clamp that will encompass the exact amount of tissue necessary. Such bleeding is never fulgurated, as surrounding tissue can be damaged and other ligatures burned loose.

The ureter runs only about 1.5 cm lateral to the cervix, and careless placement of clamps at the level of the uterine vessels and below can injure the ureter, especially if it is not in its usual position. Fig. 25-2 illustrates the technique of intraoperative palpation of the ureter in the cardinal ligament before clamping the uterine vessels. Complete downward mobilization of the bladder to the level of the anterior vaginal fornix and skeletonizing the uterine vessels by cutting the peritoneum of the posterior broad ligament allows the ureters to fall away. Clamps should be placed against the lateral wall of the cervix, and the incision should be with a knife close to the cervical side.

One successful technique for avoiding ureteral injury is an intracapsular enucleation of the cervix. A Y-shaped incision is made in the endopelvic fascia on the anterior wall of the cervix, allowing the placement of clamps inside the fascia. This ensures that the clamp is not in contact with the ureter.

At the end of the hysterectomy, some surgeons clamp completely across the vagina below the cervix before removing the uterus. When this approach is taken, it is essential that the bladder is mobilized for at least 5 mm below the level of the clamps to avoid incorporation of the bladder wall in the vaginal cuff

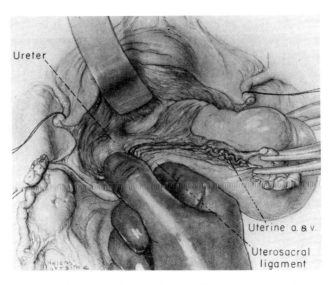

Fig. 25-2 Intraoperative demonstration of identification of the ureter before clamping the uterine vessels at the level of the uterosacral ligaments. (*From Burch JC, Lavely HT*: Transactions of the American surgical association, *Philadelphia, 1952, JB Lippincott.*)

ligatures. Similarly, when the vagina is first opened to remove the cervix and then closed with interrupted sutures, care must be exercised to avoid incorporating a portion of the bladder in one of the sutures. The same caution applies to those who leave the vagina open and cast a running, locking suture around the vaginal edge.

Peritonizing the pelvic floor after hysterectomy is probably unnecessary but is often undertaken because it leaves a neat appearance. There is risk involved in this procedure because it can include a ureter in the running stitch or pull the bladder muscle, rather than its peritoneal reflection, over the vaginal closure. Sutures placed near or in the urinary tract should always be absorbable and synthetic. If they impinge on the lumen, absorbable sutures are less likely than nonabsorbable sutures to give rise to stone formation.

Vaginal Hysterectomy

During vaginal hysterectomy, the chief problem is the separation of the bladder from the cervix and the anterior lower uterine segment. Although the base of the bladder is only loosely attached to the uterus and cervix, it is essential to find the right plane through which the bladder can be stripped away and mobilized up-ward. With heavy downward traction, the cervix is brought as low as possible in the vagina. The proper place to make the initial circumferential incision around the cervix can be determined by grasping the anterior vaginal wall and underlying bladder with an Allis clamp and drawing it upward away from the portio of the cervix. The point where the retracted vaginal mucosa does not rise from the cervix is the place to make the anterior incision.

In older patients, the cervix may be atrophic and the fornices obliterated, permitting the bladder to descend almost to the level of the cervical os. In such cases, the cervix is gently grasped close to the external os with Allis clamps and the incision made delicately not more than 1 cm from the os to avoid injuring the bladder. As the dissection between the bladder and cervix begins, heavy downward traction causes the thin fascia between the two organs to retract upward, permitting access to the vesicocervical space. The curved scissors' points are held downward against the uterus during the early part of this dissection. During the blunt dissection that follows, pressure is maintained against the uterine rather than the bladder side. Blunt dissection is best accomplished with a forefinger shielded by a single layer of gauze and should be kept strictly in the midline. Dissection should be stopped at intervals for inspection to be sure that no bladder muscle has been left on the uterine side. When no further resistance is encountered, the dissection should be at the level of the peritoneal attachment of the bladder to the uterus. After peritoneal entry, a retractor is inserted and kept in that position until the end of the operation. The upward pull on this retractor prevents injury to the bladder and holds the ureters out of harm's way.

Patients who have had one or more previous cesarean sections are at increased risk of cystotomy because the bladder tends to be more densely adherent to the uterus, and the peritoneal reflection of the bladder may have been drawn upward to cover the incision in the lower uterine segment. If vaginal hysterectomy is attempted after cesarean section, the bladder must be dissected with scissors, staying in the midline, and watching for the tell-tale evidence of bladder muscle left behind on the uterus.

If strict indications for the operation have been observed, a vaginal hysterectomy should require only three clamps on each side. With the bladder and ureters retracted upward, as previously noted, the first clamp should include both the uterosacral and cardinal ligaments and should pose no threat to the ureter. If the first clamp has been properly placed, the next level should be at the junction of the uterine vessels with the uterus. This clamp should be placed from below upward and then, by swinging the handle laterally, brought to a position lateral and at right angles to the uterus, securing both the main and ascending branches of the vessels. Placing the clamp parallel to the uterus or higher than necessary jeopardizes the ureter. Not including the ascending branch of the uterine artery can lead to bleeding, and attempts to clamp the bleeding vessel increases the risk of ureteral injury. Some vaginal surgeons have observed that it is possible to palpate the ureter during vaginal hysterectomy, but all may not have achieved this art. It is helpful to do one vaginal hysterectomy with stents in the ureters to understand their anatomic location.

The final clamp on the round and ovarian ligaments and on the isthmic portion of the fallopian tube together with the uteroovarian vessels is not in close enough proximity to the urinary tract to pose a prob-

lem. When unexpected bleeding occurs at any point in the operation, unhurried examination of the area and careful clamping of only the amount of tissue essential to provide hemostasis is essential. If bleeding is impossible to control and the anatomy is distorted by clot and damaged tissue, a tight pack followed by a laparotomy is preferabe to attempts at mass ligature from below.

During the anterior colporrhaphy that sometimes follows vaginal hysterectomy, damage to the urinary tract can come from three sources. The first is dissection in the wrong plane to free the bladder from the overlying vaginal wall, and the second is the tendency to carry the dissection too far laterally. In both instances heavy bleeding is likely to be the result, the first because of stripping the bladder adventitia from the muscle, and the second by penetrating beyond the inferior pubic ramus and urogenital diaphragm where there is a rich venous plexus. Abnormal bleeding leads to clamping, ligature, and cauterization, which may cause penetration, contusion, or anatomic distortion of the bladder base. Bleeding from the dissected vaginal flap at an early point in the operation clearly indicates that the bladder fascia and adventitia have been stripped away from the muscle and that the operator is in the wrong plane. Beginning again closer to the vaginal side corrects the error. The inferior border of the descending pubic ramus is an easily palpable landmark that shows that the dissection has proceeded far enough to permit an adequate plication, unless an additional suprapubic operation is planned to correct urinary stress incontinence.

The third and most serious potential cause of urinary tract injury during anterior colporrhaphy is the placement of plication sutures in and around the vesical neck. Sutures around the proximal and distal urethra may constrict and immobilize it, causing retention or difficulties with micturition. Partial obstruction can also occur if the sutures are placed too far laterally or in two layers at the level of the bladder neck. If placed too deep in the bladder wall, sutures can partially or completely obstruct the ureters. The crucial point to remember is that the Foley catheter bulb pulled downward to the vesical neck will clearly identify the point at which the initial suture should be placed. Lembert sutures should be placed in the bladder adventita, not in the vaginal submucosa, deep enough that the needle cannot be seen during its passage through about 1 cm of tissue. If undue tension is required to tie the sutures, they have been placed too far laterally.

After conventional vaginal hysterectomy and anterior colporrhaphy, urinary drainage may be by the transurethral or suprapubic route, the latter being the most popular. If suprapubic drainage is to be used, it is preferable to insert the catheter before the operation, whether the insertion is antegrade or retrograde to ensure that this important procedure is properly accomplished with the chief surgeon in attendance and that good drainage has been established. Filling the bladder or elevating it on an internal trocar for catheter insertion before surgery puts no strain on any suture line.

Posterior colporrhaphy after vaginal hysterectomy does not cause direct damage to the urinary tract but can cause postoperative urinary retention. Operations on the perineum and close to the levator muscles cause pain and spasm of the muscles, making it difficult for them to relax to initiate micturition. At times this inability to void may be long lasting, requiring both reassurance and local pain relief for cure.

Cesarean Section

In the days when retroperitoneal cesarean section was frequently necessary to avoid serious postpartum infection, injury to the bladder was common. Now that that operation is no longer necessary, injury to the bladder is uncommon but not unknown. The probable cause of some of these injuries may be haste to extract the baby, which is understandable. Dissection of the bladder to expose the lower uterine segment for uterine incision is sometimes associated with significant bleeding and rarely can result in cystotomy, especially if previous cesarean sections have been performed. If dissection is performed carefully, however, and no further than necessary, especially at the lateral margins, the bleeding should not require clamping and massive ligatures that are likely to damage the bladder or ureters. Extension of a transverse low segment incision into the uterine vessels necessitating rapid clamping or ligature can lead to damage of the ureters and, if this is suspected, their integrity should be tested

by techniques discussed later. Classic incisions and lower segment vertical incisions can extend directly into the bladder during a difficult delivery, and bladder competence must be assured before the operation is completed if this eventuality is even suspected.

Placenta percreta sometimes directly invades the bladder and can penetrate through to the mucosa; this unusual circumstance requires the assistance of an experienced urologist, as resection of a portion of the bladder may be necessary. The hysterectomy that follows this complication and other obstetric emergencies is likely to be associated with major hemorrhage and distortion of normal anatomy, increasing the risk of both ureteral and bladder damage. As long as these possibilities are addressed before the operation is concluded, the necessary steps can be taken to assure a final successful outcome.

The incision in the uterus must be closed with great care and with synthetic absorbable suture material. Disruption of this incision, associated with infection and/or minor bladder injury, can result in the formation of a vesicouterine fistula days or weeks later.

TECHNIQUES TO RECOGNIZE LOWER URINARY TRACT INJURY DURING GYNECOLOGIC SURGERY
Ureter

The next best thing to the prevention of urinary tract injury during surgery is its early diagnosis, preferably before the patient leaves the operating room. The technique of ureteral identification and palpation at various steps in gynecologic procedures has been discussed, but sometimes this technique is inadequate. Clear visualization of the ureter along most of its course is helpful; but disease, fat, bleeding, and congenital anomalies may interfere.

Inspection may reveal a ligature in or around the ureter that can easily be removed. When the injury is not so obvious and the approach is abdominal, the following steps can be taken in order of preference.

The bladder is filled with 300 ml of normal saline and opened retroperitoneally by a stab wound in its dome. The opening is enlarged by an incision vertically in the midline partially bisecting the bladder.

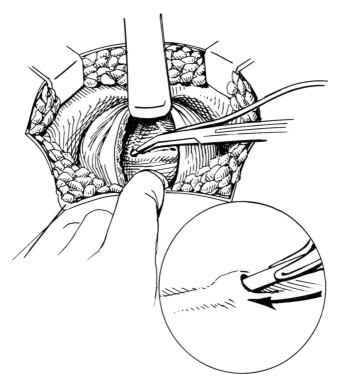

Fig. 25-3 Technique of passage of ureteral catheter after cystotomy has been performed.

With the ureteral orifices under direct observation as the sides of the bladder incision are retracted, an injection of indigo carmine dye is given intravenously. The appearance of dye from the ureter or ureters suspected of having been injured indicates patency. Should the dye fail to appear, a No. 5 whistle tip ureteral catheter or No. 8 pediatric feeding tube is inserted into the ureteral orifice and passed upward to identify the point of obstruction (Fig. 25-3). This maneuver can also be used to pass the stent through the obstruction and provide drainage during healing. It is possible that such an attempt may lead to perforation of the ureter and further difficulty; therefore, forceful attempts to push the catheter upward are contraindicated. Catheters with a memory tip that maintain position in the renal pelvis without being dislodged are more desirable as stents, but are sometimes difficult to pass through an obstruction.

Some surgeons are reluctant to open the bladder deliberately, and they prefer to reposition the patient for cystoscopy and bring in the necessary equipment. The cystoscopist can then observe the ureteral orifices as the dye is injected and can also attempt to pass catheters up the affected ureter. This method is satisfactory but requires more time and operating room disturbance; the choice depends on the individual surgeon.

A direct method for determining ureteral injury is to isolate the ureter at the pelvic brim between two Babcock clamps, make a small hole in the antimesenteric border with a No. 11 Bard-Parker blade, and insert a catheter antegrade to the point of obstruction or into the bladder. If the catheter is to be left in place, the ureteral opening is enlarged enough to permit the insertion of one end into the renal pelvis. In either case, the ureteral opening must be carefully closed with through-and-through fine interrupted sutures of absorbable synthetic material over the stent, and the area drained retroperitoneally at the conclusion of the operation.

Without opening the ureter at all, dye can be injected into it with a needle and syringe. Leakage in the pelvis denotes a ureteral laceration and failure of the dye to pass into the bladder suggests an obstruction.

When ureteral injury is suspected during vaginal surgery, the patient is in position to be evaluated directly by cystoscopy, and this is the method of choice. Dye injection followed by cystoscopic inspection or retrograde ureteral catheterization can be performed efficiently.

Bladder

During either abdominal or vaginal gynecologic surgery, injury to the bladder is most often detected by a gush of urine into the operative field. Sometimes the point of injury is occult, especially in a bloody field, and diagnostic procedures are necessary to ascertain the location and size of the hole. The bladder may also be damaged by sutures that penetrate through to the mucosa, but which, when tied, do not cause immediate leakage. This type of injury occurs during cesarean section, abdominal hysterectomy, and retropubic suspension operations for stress urinary incontinence. Lesser injury may involve the muscularis, but not the mucosa, and diagnosis can be made only by careful inspection.

Penetrating bladder injuries are best identified by transurethral injection of sterile dye or milk, which can be seen clearly against the surrounding tissues. Sterile milk may be obtained from pediatric sources and is somewhat preferable because it can be easily suctioned off without staining the tissues in the area. For all types of bladder injury, whether the result of vaginal or abdominal surgery, cystoscopy is invaluable. If the opening is extremely large, cystoscopy is limited by the inability of the bladder to contain a distending fluid; but in most circumstances it denotes accurate location of the opening, its size, and its relationship to the ureteral orifices. A suture in the bladder, which may not have been identified after

dye instillation, can be seen, cut, and possibly removed.

Urethra

Injury to the urethra during abdominal operations only occurs during retropubic surgery for stress urinary incontinence, especially with Marshall-Marchetti-Krantz (MMK) procedures. Vaginal injury to the urethra is usually due to sutures inappropriately placed along the urethra; this problem has been reported in about 0.3% of MMK procedures. Efforts to correct stress urinary incontinence by plication of the so-called pubourethral ligaments can, under unusual circumstances, either penetrate or irreparably constrict the urethra. Sling procedures and combined suprapubic and vaginal operations to elevate the vesical neck can interfere with urethral blood supply; in a few cases, slough of the distal urethra has resulted. If urethral damage of any kind is suspected, the best available technique is intraurethral inspection with a zero-degree panendoscope.

Intraoperative urethral damage results in immediate or long-term problems, which can lead to postoperative voiding dysfunction or to urethrovaginal fistula. Chronically, partial damage to the delicate neurovascular network along the urethra can result in compromised urethral function, which can lead to recurrent type III stress incontinence.

POSTOPERATIVE EVALUATION OF SUSPECTED VAGINAL FISTULAS

Postoperative vesicovaginal fistulas produce leakage of urine immediately postoperatively or several weeks after surgery. Any suspected vaginal fistula should be evaluated immediately to rule out ureteral involvement. The bedside or office evaluation of urine leakage through the vagina is shown in Fig. 25-4. This evaluation can give the surgeon a clear idea of the site of the fistula, or the results may be inconclusive. In either situation, endoscopy and IVP are usually necessary to determine the exact location of the fistula and to evaluate for ureteral patency. Posthysterectomy vesicovaginal fistulas almost always occur at the anterior aspect of the vaginal cuff. On cystoscopy, they appear

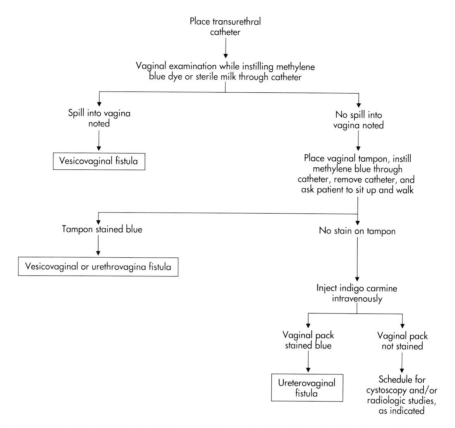

Fig. 25-4 Algorithm for the bedside or office evaluation of vaginal leakage of urine suggesting lower urinary tract fistula.

near the midline, above the interureteric ridge. Fistulas should be managed according to the recommendations outlined in Chapter 23.

TECHNIQUES OF REPAIR OF INTRAOPERATIVE LOWER URINARY TRACT INJURY
Distal Ureter

Ureteroneocystostomy

Damage to the ureter during gynecologic operations most often occurs within 4 cm of the entrance of the ureters into the bladder. If the damage cannot be rectified easily by removing an offending ligature and repositioning the ureter, the standard procedure to correct the damage is ureteroneocystostomy (Fig. 25-5). Perioperative prophylactic antibiotics should always

be given for these types of operations. The technique of ureteroneocystostomy is as follows:

1. The ureter is mobilized from its peritoneal attachment at the point of injury and severed proximally at a point where its blood supply and good condition can be guaranteed. The end of the severed ureter is cut obliquely to provide a larger opening.
2. The bladder is opened in the manner previously described and bisected vertically in the midline down close to the trigone.
3. The distal portion of the cut ureter is ligated close to its entrance into the bladder and, if possible, resected.
4. A small opening is made in the mucosa of the bladder on the side of the reimplantation as

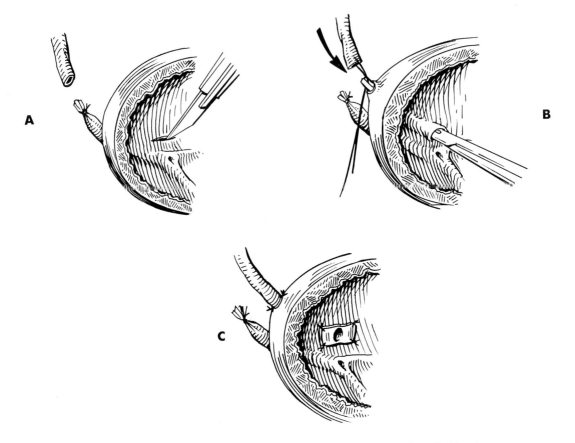

Fig. 25-5 Technique of ureteroneocystostomy with submucosal tunneling. **A,** After the ureter is divided and the distal stump ligated, an incision is made in bladder mucosa near the old ureteral orifice. **B,** The end of the ureter is tagged and pulled into the bladder lumen after a 2 cm submucosal tunnel is created with a curved clamp. **C,** The distal ureter is spatulated, everted, and sutured in four corners to the bladder mucosa. Several sutures are also placed to anchor the ureter to the bladder adventitia.

close as possible to the previous ureteral opening, and a small curved hemostat is passed through this opening and tunneled between the bladder mucosa and muscle about 1 cm toward the lateral pelvic wall. Another opening is made into the bladder from the outside over the opened tips of the hemostat.

5. A suture is attached to the proximal ureter, grasped by the hemostat, and pulled through the small cystotomy opening and through the tunnel between the mucosa and bladder muscularis into the bladder lumen.

6. The fish-mouthed ureteral opening with the long edge closer to the trigone is stitched to the bladder mucosa with interrupted sutures of fine absorbable synthetic material, passing through the full thickness of the ureteral wall.

7. To take the tension off the anastomosis, two or three sutures are placed outside of the bladder between the ureteral adventitia and bladder adventitia, taking care not to encroach on the ureteral lumen.

8. A ureteral stent with a memory tip is passed up the ureter into the renal pelvis to ensure

TABLE 25-1   Duration of ureteral catheter use

Injury*	Duration	Preremoval test
Minimum to extensive	At least 5-7 days	Cystogram/excretory urogram
Transection/resection	6-8 weeks	Cystogram/excretory urogram
Ureteroneocystostomy	At least 7 days	Cystogram

From Pettit PD: *Obstet Gynecol* 73:539, 1989.
*With minor injury (such as with sheath, needle, or crushing), no therapy other than drainage, hemostasis, antibiotics, and bladder drainage would be required.

patency during the healing process. Some surgeons prefer to have the stent in place during the anastomosis, but it can interfere with visualization. The other end of the ureteral catheter may be brought out through the urethra, where it can be attached to the Foley catheter. It can also be left lying in the bladder, or it can be brought out through the anterior abdominal wall where it is attached to a suprapubic catheter.

9. The bladder is closed with a running suture of No. 3-0, synthetic absorbable material, including the bladder mucosa and the inner muscular layer. A second layer of either a running or interrupted No. 3-0 suture is placed in the outer muscular layer and the serosa.

10. A suprapubic Foley or Malecot catheter is inserted through a separate stab incision in the bladder dome and surrounded by a purse-string suture before being brought out through the anterior abdominal wall. The combination of transurethral and suprapubic drainage for at least 24 hours reduces the chance that blood clots will obstruct the flow of urine from a single catheter and cause retention of urine.

11. The site of anastomosis is covered with the lateral pelvic peritoneum, concluding the operation.

The bladder is drained for 7 to 10 days and the ureteral catheter is left in place for 7 to 14 days after ureteroneocystostomy, as per surgeon's preference. If the distal end of the ureteral catheter was left in the bladder, cystoscopy would be necessary for removal. Postoperative pyelography and/or retrograde cystography showing no extravasation of dye should be ob-

tained before the ureteral catheter is removed. Recommendations for duration of ureteral catheter use for various ureteral operations as described by Pettit are shown in Table 25-1.

The technique of tunneling the ureter between the mucosa and the bladder muscle to the point of anastomosis is intended to prevent reflux during bladder emptying, but may not always be necessary. It is important that no tension is placed on the anastomotic site and when the proximal ureter is too short, a direct opening into the bladder and mucosa-to-mucosa anastomosis is advisable.

The ureter may also be "dunked" into the bladder without the need for a transvesical anastomosis. This technique is outmoded and is applicable only when speed is of the essence. Two sutures are placed in the split severed end of the proximal ureter, one at 12 and one at 6 o'clock, 2 mm from the end; and an opening is made in the filled bladder from the outside as close as possible to the proximal ureter. The four ends of the two ureteral sutures are attached to small free needles, and each needle is passed through the bladder opening and back out through the full thickness of the bladder wall close to the opening and about 5 mm apart. Traction on these sutures pulls the ureter into the bladder lumen, where it is fixed by tying each of the two sutures outside. The lower edge of the split ureter is positioned at 6 o'clock within the bladder and the upper edge at 12 o'clock. Sutures are taken between the ureteral adventitia as it enters the bladder and the bladder adventitia in order to close the opening completely and take the tension off the two stay sutures. As in the case of the transvesical anastomosis, a ureteral stent is inserted, with one end in the renal pelvis and the other in the bladder. The absence of a tunnel within the bladder and the lack of careful stitching in a mucosa-to-mucosa intravesical anastomosis may cause future reflux or obstruction at the point of entry.

Psoas Hitch

Proper management of ureteral injuries higher in the pelvis depends on the exact location and the type of injury. In general, serious damage to the ureter in most of its lower third is best treated by reimplantation into the bladder, as previously described. This procedure may be difficult, or even impossible, when the point to be bypassed is 4 to 5 cm away from the bladder, and the ureter cannot be sufficiently mobilized from above to draw it down for anastomosis without tension.

The psoas hitch (Fig. 25-6) is the best method for bringing these two organs together and is also the easiest to perform. The first step is a cystotomy large enough to admit one finger. With a forefinger in this opening the bladder is pushed toward the lateral pelvic wall as far as it can be easily stretched. Under ordinary circumstances this point can be to the bifurcation of the common iliac artery. While the bladder is being held in this position, at least two sutures of synthetic absorbable material are placed between the psoas muscle and the bladder wall, taking care not to damage the major vessels. The finger inside the bladder ensures that the lumen is not included in the stitch. With the bladder thus advanced and held in position, the ureter can be united with it by either of the two previously discussed techniques, the transvesical approach being preferable. Anatomic displacement of the bladder, even to this extent, does not result in loss of function. Implantation of the ureter into the bladder dome or whatever location is necessary generally is compatible with normal future ureteral and renal function.

Distal Neoureter Formation with Bladder Flap

A more intricate, technically difficult, and less effective method of relieving tension on the anastomosis is the formation of a neoureter from a flap of bladder (Fig. 25-7). This operation has a number of modifications (Boari, Ockerblad, Demel), but the general

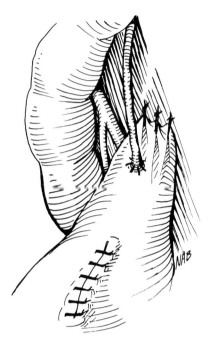

Fig. 25-6 Psoas hitch is used for distal ureteral injuries in which there is tension on the ureteroneocystostomy. This technique brings the bladder cephalad to relieve tension on the suture site.

principle consists of cutting a full-thickness strip across the dome of the bladder, about 1 cm wide and 5 or 6 cm long, leaving one end of the strip attached to its original position on the side where the ureteral injury occurred. A tube is formed by suturing together the edges of this strip, and the large opening in the dome of the bladder is closed in two layers. The end of the bladder tube is connected to the proximal ureter with interrupted through-and-through mucosa-to-mucosa sutures. The distal ureter can also be passed through a submucosal bladder wall tunnel to prevent urine reflux (Fig. 25-7, *B*). The site of anastomosis is extraperitonized, pulling it against the lateral pelvic wall.

This operation has a high complication rate due to the devascularization of the bladder flap and leakage at the anastomotic site. Because of the latter possibility, retroperitoneal suction drainage is maintained

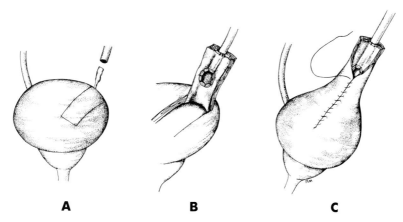

Fig. 25-7 Distal neoureter formation with bladder flap. **A,** Bladder flap to be created outlined on bladder. **B,** Flap created, ureter sewn in place via submucosal tunnel. **C,** Flap sewn into tube to close bladder defect. (*From Gillenwater JY, Grayhack JT, Howards SS, et al*: Adult and pediatric urology, *Chicago, 1987, Year Book Medical Publishers.*)

for at least the first 24 to 48 hours. A ureteral catheter stent is used as in the previous operations.

Proximal Two Thirds of Ureter
Ureteroureterostomy

Occasionally, a ureter is cut directly in its midportion, leaving clean proximal and distal ends. If the blood supply is good and any traumatized bits of tissue can be removed without shortening the ureter, an end-to-end anastomosis is feasible. Some surgeons advocate cutting each end of the ureter on a slant in order to enlarge the anastomotic lumen, but this technique is not necessary unless the ureteral lumen is very small. The anastomosis is performed over a catheter using through-and-through fine suture material with the stitches set 2 mm back from the ureteral edge; 4 or 5 such sutures are usually all that are necessary. The area is extraperitonized and drained.

Transureteroureterostomy

Relatively proximal ureteral injury can be treated by end-to-side anastomosis of the proximal end of the damaged ureter to the ureter on the other side. Urologists favor this method, and it seems to give good results, but it is not usually performed by gynecologic surgeons, possibly because of lack of experience and

because of the theoretical risk of threatening renal function on both sides.

The technique is not difficult. The proximal ureter on the damaged side is brought retroperitoneally beneath the mesentery of the rectum to a point where it can lie without tension adjacent to the undamaged ureter. It is easier to open the recipient ureter when it is stented, and the end-to-side anastomosis is completed with fine interrupted absorbable synthetic sutures. As in all other operations of this type, the vascularity of the transplanted ureter must be adequate, there can be no compression on the retroperitoneal tunnel through which it has passed, and there can be no tension on the anastomosis. Extraperitoneal drainage of the anastomotic site is required.

Cutaneous Ureterostomy

Extensive damage to major portions of the ureter, reaching to a high level cephalad and jeopardizing future renal function, may be treated in one of two ways—cutaneous ureterostomy and ileal transplant. It is likely that serious ureteral damage of this extent may have occurred during a protracted, difficult operation associated with considerable blood loss, and the patient's general condition requires speed to terminate the procedure. A skin ureterostomy may be necessary as a temporary life-saving measure when enough proximal ureter is left above the pelvic brim to be brought out through a stab wound in the flank, well away from the primary incision. The end of the proximal ureter is sutured to the skin and stented to prevent obstruction at the skin level. The extraperitoneal tunnel, through which the ureter is drawn, is made by incising both skin and fascia and passing a long Kelly clamp through the openings retroperitoneally down to the end of the proximal ureter. The clamp grasps a previously placed suture in the end of the ureter, and gentle traction is used to draw the ureter up through the tunnel to the point of junction with the skin. Cutaneous ureterostomies almost inevitably cause pyelonephritis long-term, and plans must be made for conversion to a less morbid type of procedure when the patient's condition permits.

Ileal Transplant Techniques

A second technique to replace large portions of damaged ureter is with a transplanted defunctionalized segment of ileum. This operation is extensive and should never be attempted by an inexperienced surgeon or when a lesser operation could be performed. A segment of ileum of appropriate length is removed from continuity, with its mesentery attached, and an end-to-end anastomosis of the severed proximal and distal ends of the intestine is performed, allowing the defunctionalized ileal segment to fall free on its mesentery. This part of the operation is most rapidly and efficiently done with the gastrointestinal anastomosis stapler. Being careful not to twist the mesentery, the surgeon mobilizes the defunctionalized segment toward the affected side and closes the proximal end of the segment with the stapler. An end-to-side ureterointestinal anastomosis is performed over a stent, using a full-thickness ureteral-wall-to-bowel-mucosa technique and interrupted absorbable sutures. The intestinal muscle is closed loosely around the implanted ureter.

An opening is made in the bladder dome large enough for a direct ileovesical anastomosis, which is then accomplished with fine interrupted absorbable sutures. The stent remains in place with one end in the renal pelvis and the other in the bladder or ex-

teriorized, as previously described. In a few cases, the intestine must be anastomosed to the renal pelvis. When this is necessary, both ends of the ileal segment are left open, the proximal one being anastomosed directly to the renal pelvis. When meticulously performed, this operation has produced good results, but it is not for the uninitiated.

Bladder

When inadvertent cystotomy occurs during abdominal surgery, the main problem is the proximity of the defect to the ureteral orifices. If the opening is high above the bladder base, as can be judged fairly accurately by the position of the Foley catheter, a simple repair can be achieved from the outside, using two layers of No. 3-0 absorbable sutures, each beginning at a point above the defect and continuing to a point just beyond. The first running suture includes the mucosa and about half of the muscularis of the bladder; the second layer is running or interrupted and includes the bladder muscularis and the adventitia.

Defects close to the bladder base require a second deliberate cystotomy from above to check accurately the position of the ureters with relation to the repair. The question of ureteral involvement in the defect must be settled immediately by catheterization of the suspected ureter or by dye injection and, if found incompetent, this ureter must be reimplanted through a separate opening, as noted earlier. Otherwise, the repair of the bladder is begun inside, where the ureteral orifices can be kept under direct vision while the first running suture is placed in the mucosa and muscularis. The second suture can be placed from the outside more conveniently, but this is a matter of the surgeon's preference.

After the bladder repair has been completed, it is tested with transurethral injection of sterile dye or milk. Postoperative drainage is best provided by both transurethral and suprapubic catheters for the first 24 hours because of the possibility of catheter blockage by blood clot.

Inadvertent cystotomy during vaginal hysterectomy poses a potentially more serious problem because the defect is likely to be close to the base of the bladder, and visualization of it is relatively limited.

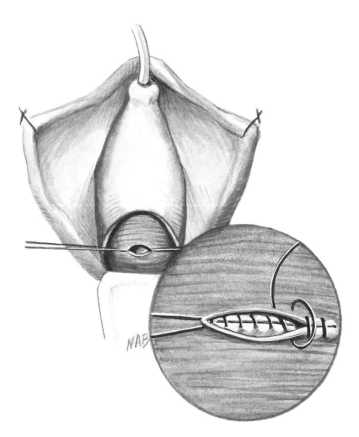

Fig. 25-8 Technique of vaginal repair of cystotomy. The defect is repaired in two layers: the first layer can be running or interrupted in the bladder mucosa and the inner muscularis; the second layer of sutures imbricates the first layer.

The cystoscope is always used to define the exact location of the defect and its relationship to the ureters. Because the opening will not permit bladder distention and because blood is present in the bladder as a result of the injury, the water must be kept running through the cystoscope until a clear view is obtained. The cystotomy is then closed in the manner noted earlier, using two layers of running sutures (Fig. 25-8). Adequacy of the repair is then tested with the transurethral injection of dye or milk. Such injuries usually occur at the beginning of the procedure, and there is no reason not to complete the operation afterward. Deferring bladder repair until the hysterectomy is finished is also acceptable.

Urethra

Intraoperative urethral injuries during conventional gynecologic surgery are practically unknown. Sutures incorrectly placed in the course of the retropubic urethropexy operations may involve the urethra, but this is seldom realized until the postoperative phase, unless cystoscopy is performed concurrently. If a stitch has been placed incorrectly, it is cut and removed. Perforation of the urethra during anterior colporrhaphy or needle urethropexy is a remote possibility and should give rise to no long-term difficulty, as it can be repaired easily by a simple purse-string or longitudinal closure of fine absorbable suture and a covering vaginal flap. A Martius graft as described in

Chapter 23 can also be used if blood supply to the injured area is inadequate.

SUMMARY

In summary, the cardinal principles of lower urinary tract repair are the following:

1. Early recognition
2. Adequate mobilization of the injured area to permit repair without tension
3. Evaluation of the competence of both ureters
4. Mucosa-to-mucosa anastomoses without tension
5. Stenting of ureteral anastomoses
6. Closure of bladder defects with running sutures
7. Testing all repairs with sterile dye or milk
8. Adequate drainage, either suprapubic, transurethral, or both
9. Postoperative pyelography and cystography, as indicated.

When these principles are followed, the urinary tract generally heals well.

REFERENCES

Boari A: Contributo spermentale alla plastica del-uretere, *A H Acad Sci Med Nat Ferrara* 68:149, 1884.

Corriere JN: Ureteral injuries. In Gillenwater JY, Grayhack JT, Howards SS, et al, editors: *Adult and pediatric urology,* Chicago, 1987, Year Book Medical Publishers.

Demel R: Ersatz des ureters durch eine Plastik aus der Harnblase (VorJäufige Mitteilung), Zentralbl Chir 41:2008, 1924.

Eisenkop SM, Richman R, Platt LD, et al: Urinary tract injury during cesarean section, *Obstet Gynecol* 60:591, 1982.

Hebert DB: How to avoid or minimize urologic injuries in surgery, *Contemp Obstet Gynecol* 22:213, 1983.

Hodgkinson CP, Eyler WR, Ayers MA: Dynamic topography of the lower ureter in vaginal hysterectomy, *Am J Obstet Gynecol* 89:111, 1964.

Hofmeister FJ: Pelvic anatomy of the ureter in relation to surgery performed through the vagina, *Clin Obstet Gynecol* 24:821, 1982.

Mann WJ, Arato M, Patsner B, et al: Ureteral injuries in an obstetrics and gynecology training program: etiology and management, *Obstet Gynecol* 72:82, 1988.

Mann WJ: Intentional and unintentional ureteral surgical treatment in gynecologic procedures, *Surgery* 172:453, 1991.

Mattingly RF, Thompson JD: *TeLinde's operative gynecology,* ed 6, Philadelphia, 1985, JB Lippincott.

Ockerblad NF: Reimplantation of the ureter into the bladder by a flap method, *J Urol* 47:845, 1947.

Penalver MA: Urinary tract injuries. In Hurt WG, editor: *Urogynecologic surgery,* Gaithersburg, 1992, Aspen Publishers.

Pettit PD: Double-J ureteral catheters in gynecologic surgery, *Obstet Gynecol* 73:536, 1989.

Piscatelli JT, Simel DL, Addison WA: Who should have intravenous pyelograms before hysterectomy for benign disease? *Obstet Gynecol* 69:541, 1987.

Redman JF: Anatomy of the genitourinary system. In Gillenwater JY, Grayhack JT, Howards SS, et al, editors: *Adult and pediatric urology,* Chicago, 1987, Year Book Medical Publishers.

Symmonds RE: Ureteral injuries associated with gynecologic surgery: prevention and management, *Clin Obstet Gynecol* 19:623, 1976.

Vaselli AJ, Bennett AH: Suture material in urologic and gynecologic surgery, *Infect Surg* 2:522, 1983.

Wheelock JB, Krebs HB, Hurt WG: Sparing and repairing the bladder during gyn surgery, *Contemp Obstet Gynecol* 23:155, 1984.

Wheelock JB, Krebs HB, Hurt WG: Ureteral laceration in gyn surgery—mostly preventable, *Contempt Obstet Gynecol* 24:155, 1984.

Witters S, Cornelissen M, Vereecken R: Iatrogenic ureteral injury: aggressive or conservative treatment, *Am J Obstet Gynecol* 155:582, 1986.

CHAPTER 26

The Effects of Gynecologic Cancer and Its Treatment on the Lower Urinary Tract

Paul P. Koonings

Urologic Complications of Genital Cancer
    General effects
    Cervical cancer
    Vulvar cancer
    Vaginal cancer
    Ovarian, fallopian tube, and endometrial cancer
Urologic Complications of Surgical Therapy
    Radical hysterectomy
    Radical vulvectomy
    Pelvic exenteration
    Vaginectomy
Urologic Complications of Radiation Therapy
Urologic Complications of Chemotherapy
    Cisplatin
    Cyclophosphamide
    Ifosfamide
Gynecologic Cancer: Hemorrhagic Cystitis and Its Treatment

Cancer strikes approximately one third of Americans during their lifetime. The latest statistics from the American Cancer Society predict over one-half million new cases of invasive cancer in women during 1993; genital cancers account for 25% of this total. Furthermore, it has been predicted that 1 in 10 female deaths will occur secondary to a gynecologic malignancy. As the population continues to age in developed countries, the gynecologist will see an increasing frequency of genital cancer. Hence, the gynecologist must have a working knowledge of both the evaluation and treatment of female cancer with its related urologic side effects.

The integral apposition of the urinary and genital tract places the former at risk for dysfunction when genital malignancy develops, especially lower genital cancer. Urogenital dysfunction can occur either secondary to the malignancy itself or from its treatment. Chemotherapy, irradiation, and surgery all have been implicated with both temporary and permanent urologic complications.

This chapter provides an overview of the effects of gynecologic cancer and its treatment on the urinary tract. The effects of genital cancer on the ureter, bladder, and urethra are discussed. Urogenital effects secondary to surgery, irradiation, chemotherapeutic agents, and hemorrhagic cystitis from a gynecologic cancer perspective are also described.

UROLOGIC COMPLICATIONS OF GENITAL CANCER

General Effects

The unique intimacy of the urinary and genital tracts accounts for the majority of urinary tract symptoms experienced when genital cancer occurs. Symptoms usually arise from one of two mechanisms. Invasion of the urinary tract from genital cancer accounts for a direct effect. A mass effect secondary to the genital cancer can produce an indirect effect on the urinary system. Rarely do paraneoplastic syndromes present with urinary dysfunction. Usually, the primary disease is responsible for the effects demonstrated by the urinary system, although metastatic disease may be responsible in some circumstances.

In general, involvement of the urinary system secondary to genital cancer portends a poorer prognosis, which is reflected in the majority of staging schemes presently used for genital cancer. Pathologic confirmation documenting invasion needs to be demonstrated for the large number of staging systems.

It is beyond the scope of this chapter to discuss the risk factors and histologic types involved with genital cancer. The reader is directed to a textbook of gynecologic cancer. Approximately 90% of the lower genital cancers are squamous in nature, with tobacco use and human papilloma virus representing major risk factors.

Cervical Cancer
Background and Staging

With the advent of the Papanicolaou smear, it was once hoped that routine screening would eliminate cervical cancer. Unfortunately, this scenario has not materialized, although the routine cervical cancer screening has apparently decreased the incidence of this disease. Nevertheless, it is important to realize that in 1993, the American Cancer Society predicts 13,500 new cases of invasive cervical cancer.

Evaluation of the urinary tract is the cornerstone of cervical cancer staging. Presently, cervical cancer staging is obtained from clinical examination alone. Under the auspices of the International Federation of Gynecology and Obstetrics (FIGO), the diagnostic tests listed in the accompanying box are permitted for staging. If possible, the pelvic examination should be

---

Diagnostic Tests Allowed by FIGO for Cervical Cancer Staging
Physical examination
Chest x-ray
Skeletal x-ray
Intravenous pyelogram
Barium enema
Biopsy
Cystoscopy
Proctoscopy

performed using anaesthesia. These tests take into account the usual routes by which cervical cancer spreads, including: (1) local invasion into the vagina, parametrium, bladder, rectum and (2) lymphatic spread, both local and distal.

Diagnostic tests, including computed tomography (CT), ultrasound (US), and laparoscopy may not be used for FIGO staging. These tests should be used when clinically indicated to individualize therapy for each patient.

The current FIGO strategy system is shown in the box on p. 375. The evaluation of the urinary tract is an essential step for accurate staging. Involvement of the urinary tract usually allows for a step-up in stage with a resultant decrease in 5-year survival as demonstrated in the 1988 FIGO report (Table 26-1).

Effects on the Urinary Tract

The central location of the cervix with reference to the lower urinary tract places the ureter, bladder, and urethra at risk of involvement when cervical cancer develops. Urinary dysfunction develops insidiously from either the primary disease or its lymphatic metastasis. The ureters are particularly vulnerable as their course through the pelvis brings them within millimeters of the cervix as they enter the parametria, a favored path of cervical cancer extension.

Involvement of the parametria due to the lateral spread of cervical cancer accounts for a large number of cases of ureteral obstruction. Obstruction is due to the mechanical effect of the adjacent tumor collapsing the tunnel. Direct ureteral invasion, as noted by van Nagell et al, is exceptional. Alternatively, ureteral

FIGO Staging for Carcinoma of the Cervix Uteri

Stage 0	Carcinoma in situ, intraepithelial carcinoma.
Stage I	Carcinoma is strictly confined to the cervix (extension to the corpus should be disregarded).
Stage II	Carcinoma extends beyond the cervix but has not extended to the pelvic wall. The carcinoma involves the vagina, but not as far as the lower third.
Stage III	Carcinoma has extended to the pelvic wall. On rectal examination, there is no cancer-free space between the tumor and the pelvic wall.
	Tumor involves the lower third of the vagina.
	All cases with a hydronephrosis or nonfunctioning kidney are included unless known to be due to other causes.
Stage IV	Carcinoma has extended beyond the true pelvis or has clinical involved the mucosa of the bladder or rectum. Bullous edema as such does not permit a case to be allotted to stage IV.

TABLE 26-1   FIGO staging of cervical cancer

Stage	N	5-year survival (%)
I	10,912	76
II	10,765	55
III	8255	31
IV	1386	7

obstruction occurs as the ureter enters the pelvis. Enlarged lymph nodes secondary to metastatic disease occlude the ureter at this juncture. Henriksen reported on 356 necropsies secondary to cervical cancer. These included both treated and untreated cases. Ureteral obstruction with resulting uremia was responsible for at least 50% of the cervical cancer deaths. Both processes of ureteral obstruction were described.

Ureteral obstruction may be unilateral or bilateral.

Unilateral obstruction may be completely asymptomatic. Other patients may present with flank pain, fever, and uremia secondary to urinary infection. Rapid deterioration of the affected kidney will occur unless resolution of the condition is imminent.

Unrecognized ureteral obstruction results in destruction of the involved kidney. Urine continues to be formed, causing increased intraluminal pressure adjacent to the renal pelvis. This development results in urinary dysfunction and the eventual loss of the kidney. Bricker and Crowley et al demonstrated that the rapidity and extent of kidney damage is due to several factors, such as the duration, level, and degree of obstruction; associated infection; and previous state of renal function.

Thus, the physician needs to rule out ureteral involvement when cervical cancer is suspected. Physical examination should include costovertebral palpation to detect renal tenderness or enlargement. Renal function tests should be obtained and checked for evidence of uremia. Electrolytes and an electrocardiogram will reveal if hyperkalemia and cardiac dysfunction are present. Patients with large cervical lesions (≥ 3 cm) should undergo timely evaluation of kidneys and ureters. Previously, the intravenous pyelogram (IVP) was the method of choice. Webb et al have shown that US is as sensitive in detecting ureteral obstruction as IVP. Because US is a less invasive diagnostic procedure and does not require dye administration, it should be the method of choice to diagnose ureteral obstruction. Furthermore, as Frolich et al pointed out in a study of 210 new cases of cervical cancer, US examination of the kidneys and ureters requires no patient preparation.

Once diagnosed, ureteral obstruction demands prudent and timely intervention. Each case should be managed individually, especially those with prior pelvic irradiation. Optimally, patients without renal failure should achieve relief of ureteral obstruction via the retrograde passage of double J-stents using cystoscopy. Once placed, their proper location should be confirmed with ultrasound. The urine should be routinely examined at regular intervals for bacteriologic infection and, if present, should be treated appropriately. Ureteral stents should be replaced according to the manufacturer's guidelines. Recommendations vary between 3 to 12 months depending on the composition of the stents.

Frequently, retrograde placement of ureteral stents is not possible. In these circumstances, placement of percutaneous nephrostomy tubes is a viable alternative. Ideally, US is the method of choice to guide placement. As Dudley et al reported, however, nephrostomy tubes are not a panacea and can be associated with serious complications resulting from both their placement and location. Placement has been associated with pneumothorax, severe hemorrhage, and even death. Long-term nephrostomy use is complicated by infection, blockage, and accidental removal. Fortunately, resolution of perinephric edema after nephrostomy tube use allows for placement of antegrade ureteral stents in a large number of cases. This approach is attempted 5 to 7 days after placement, thereby allowing discontinuation of the percutaneous nephrostomy tubes. The absence of a vesicovaginal fistula should be confirmed before ureteral stents are placed. Otherwise, urinary incontinence may result.

Patients with uremia secondary to ureteral obstruction present a more difficult challenge. Electrolyte abnormalities, especially hyperkalemia, should be reversed discriminately by the use of insulin, dextrose, and sodium bicarbonate to lower potassium levels, as well as the occasional use of calcium chloride to protect the heart from dysrhythmias. After these abnormalities have been recognized and appropriately treated, steps should then be taken to alleviate the obstruction as previously discussed.

Bladder invasion by cervical cancer indicates advanced disease. As noted in the staging system, mucosal involvement is mandatory for FIGO staging. During cystoscopy, bladder washings should be obtained for cytologic evaluation. Punch biopsies of suspicious areas need to be evaluated histologically. The number and location of the ureteral orifices should be noted and ureteral stents passed when appropriate. As previously mentioned, the presence of any fistulas should be considered.

Most patients with cervical cancer do not complain of bladder symptoms. When these symptoms are present, they arise from both mass effect and direct invasion of the bladder. Mass effect causes compression of the bladder resulting in nocturia and frequency.

Direct invasion occasionally produces vesicovaginal fistulas with hematuria.

Rarely, subvaginal extension of cervical cancer may involve the urethra. Subsequently, obstruction, fistula formation, and hematuria result. Urethroscopy with appropriate biopsies is usually diagnostic.

Vulvar Cancer
Background and Staging

Vulvar cancer represents approximately 5% of female genital cancers, although this proportion rises with age. The 1988 FIGO statistics represent 1815 cases of vulvar cancer with a peak age distribution at 70 years; 15% of these patients were premenopausal.

Unlike cervical cancer staging, vulvar cancer staging is surgical, as implemented in the 1989 revised FIGO classification. Previously, vulvar cancer staging had been based on clinical examination alone. The body of evidence confirmed that clinical examination, when compared to surgicopathologic staging, is a notoriously inaccurate means of assessing lymph node metastasis of the inguinal-femoral chains.

Involvement of the urinary tract is an integral component of the vulvar staging system (see box). Invasion of the urinary tract usually allows for an upstage. Mucosal involvement should be confirmed in these situations.

Effects on the Urinary Tract

Urinary symptoms rarely arise from vulvar cancer. Less than 10% of patients complain of dysuria. Urethral obstruction secondary to cancer is exceptional. Bladder invasion is usually due to greatly advanced disease, which may result in incontinence and hematuria. Other symptoms, including pain, discharge, and a mass, however, will usually bring the patient to the attention of a physician first.

Vaginal Cancer
Background and Staging

Vaginal cancer is the rarest of the female genital cancers in part because a primary malignancy that involves either the cervix or vulva and the vagina is not considered a vaginal cancer. Furthermore, when vaginal cancer develops, it is usually in the proximal and distal third of the vagina.

FIGO Staging for Carcinoma of the Vulva

Stage 0   Carcinoma in situ; intraepithelial carcinoma.

Stage I   Tumor confined to the vulva and/or perineum—2 cm or less in greatest dimension, no nodal metastasis.

Stage II   Tumor confined to the vulva and/or perineum—more than 2 cm in greatest dimension, no nodal metastasis.

Stage III   Tumor of any size with (1) adjacent spread to the lower urethra and/or the vagina, or the anus, and/or (2) unilateral regional lymph node metastasis.

Stage IVA   Tumor invades any of the following: upper urethra, bladder mucosa, rectal mucosa, pelvic bone, and/or bilateral regional node metastasis.

Stage IVB   Any distant metastasis including pelvic lymph nodes.

FIGO Staging for Carcinoma of the Vagina

Stage 0   Carcinoma in situ, intraepithelial carcinoma.

Stage I   Carcinoma is limited to the vaginal wall.

Stage II   Carcinoma has involved the subvaginal tissue but has not extended to the pelvic wall.

Stage III   Carcinoma has extended to the pelvic wall.

Stage IV   Carcinoma has extended beyond the true pelvis or has clinical involved the mucosa of the bladder or rectum; bullous edema as such does not permit a case to be allotted to stage IV.

Stage IVA   Spread of the growth to adjacent organs and/or direct extension beyond the true pelvis.

Stage IVB   Spread to distant organs.

International Federation of Gynecology and Obstetrics: Annual report on the results of treatment in gynecological cancer, vol 20, Stockholm, 1988, FIGO.

In the last three decades, diethylstilbestrol (DES) exposure has increased the incidence of vaginal adenocarcinoma. With the discontinuation of DES use, these rates will probably decline.

Vaginal cancer staging is clinical as shown in the accompanying box. Anterior lesions should be a signal to perform cystourethroscopy with cytologic washings and biopsy of any suspicious lesions. As in the cervical and vulvar staging, involvement of the urinary tract allows for upstaging.

Effects on the Urinary Tract

The central position of the vagina between the vulva and cervix allows for varied presentations when malignancy develops. Upper vault involvement may mimic cervical cancer-related urogenital problems (e.g., ureteral and bladder dysfunction). Evaluation of these problems has been discussed previously. Similarly, lower vaginal malignancy may duplicate the symptoms associated with vulvar cancer. Malignancy involving the mid-portion of the vagina may simulate either proximal or distal vaginal cancer depending on spread.

Ovarian, Fallopian Tube, and Endometrial Cancer

The ovary is one of the five leading cancer sites causing mortality in women. Despite the pelvic location and propensity for intraabdominal spread of ovarian cancer, dysfunction of the urinary tract is rare. Occasionally, mass effect of the tumor may compromise bladder capacity and cause ureteral dilation; however, bladder or ureteral mucosal invasion is uncommon. Unlike the majority of genital cancer staging systems, urinary tract involvement is not a consideration. Fallopian tube cancer, an even rarer entity, affects the urinary tract in a similar fashion. There is no official staging system for this cancer, and in general, ovarian cancer staging is applied.

Endometrial cancer is the most common female genital cancer in the United States. Early detection with a high index of suspicion has lead to a decline in the cancer death rate. Recently, FIGO has changed the staging system from clinical to surgical. Involvement of the bladder mucosa allows for upstaging as shown in the box. Symptomatic complaints arising from the urinary tract secondary to the malignancy are unusual unless a large mass is present or there is bladder invasion. If invasion is suspected, evaluation of the urinary tract with US may be indicated to rule out an obstructive problem.

UROLOGIC COMPLICATIONS OF SURGICAL THERAPY

Radical Hysterectomy

Since Professor Wertheim published his monograph "The extended abdominal operation for carcinoma uteri," originally in German, radical hysterectomy has emerged as the premier technique for treating early stage cervical and endometrial cancer when clinically indicated. With early stage disease, cure rates are excellent—well over 85% 5-year cure rates in selected populations. The procedure is fraught with hazards and pitfalls that may lead to major morbidity. Thus before selecting this option, the surgeon should be experienced with this technically demanding operation.

The incidence of urogenital fistulas, both ureterovaginal and vesicovaginal, after radical hysterectomy has decreased dramatically over the last century. In Wertheim's series of 500 patients, 32 (6.4%) developed a ureterovaginal fistula and 34 (6.8%) suffered from postoperative vesicovaginal fistulas. Infection leading to necrosis was the etiologic agent believed responsible for these complications.

In 1951, Meigs described 280 cases of radical hysterectomy. He reported a rate of ureterovaginal fistulas similar to Wertheim's a half-century earlier. The ureterovaginal fistulas rate was attributed to a compromised ureteral blood supply. Noteworthy is the low vesicovaginal fistula rate, only two instances in over 280 cases (<1%), a tremendous improvement over Wertheim's experience. No explanation was given for these disparate experiences.

Contemporary studies place the vesicovaginal and ureterovaginal fistula rates at approximately 1%. Larson et al described 223 patients who underwent radical hysterectomy with pelvic lymphadenectomy. Two patients (0.8%) developed a ureteral fistula, and one patient developed a ureteral stricture. Other recent

FIGO Staging for Carcinoma of the Corpus Uteri	
Stage IA	Tumor limited to endometrium.
Stage IB	Invasion to less than one-half the myometrium.
Stage IC	Invasion to more than one-half the myometrium.
Stage IIA	Endocervical glandular involvement only.
Stage IIB	Cervical stromal invasion.
Stage IIIA	Tumor invades serosa and/or adnexa, and/or positive peritoneal cytology.
Stage IIIB	Vaginal metastases.
Stage IIIC	Metastases to pelvic and/or paraaortic lymph nodes.
Stage IVA	Tumor invasion of bladder and/or bowel mucosa.
Stage IVB	Distant metastases including intraabdominal and/or inguinal lymph nodes.

studies have documented similar experiences.

Intraoperative recognition and respect for the ureter and bladder are paramount in avoiding a urogenital fistula. The course of the ureter should be visualized directly from its entrance into the pelvis to its termination into the bladder. Therefore, familiarity with pelvic anatomy and exposure of the retroperitoneal spaces is mandatory. Injury via avulsion, transection, ligation, crushing, and fulguration must be avoided. The ureter should not be handled directly. Resultant damage to the blood supply may account for subsequent fistula formation. Indirect ("no-touch") handling is attempted in all instances.

A variety of approaches has been used in an effort to avoid fistula formation. Green et al attached the ureter to the superior vesical artery. They believed that the artery would act as a stent for the ureter. Avoidance of hypogastric artery ligation has also been proposed as a method of decreasing fistula formation, although confirmatory data concerning efficacy are lacking. A comparison between these two techniques awaits study.

Intraoperative ureteral injuries that are identified

and properly treated immediately have excellent results. Distinguishing between reversible and nonreversible damage to the ureter may be difficult. If a question should arise, it is easier to correct the damage immediately than postoperatively.

Classic teaching divides ureteral repairs into those above and those below the pelvic brim. If a suprapelvic repair is required, direct ureteral anastomosis is attempted, which is facilitated by placement of a ureteral stent. Moreover, a closed suction drain in the abdominal area is recommended. Examples are ureteral-ureterostomy or transureteral-ureterostomy.

Ureteroneocystostomy is the usual ureteral repair performed in the pelvis. A nonrefluxing type should be attempted. Once again, a ureteral splint and closed suction drain for approximately 1 week is indicated. Longer drainage is recommended if the area has undergone previous irradiation.

If the bladder lumen is entered during surgery, early recognition with adequate repair is usually rewarded with an intact bladder. A two-layer closure using fine absorbable suture is indicated in most cases. If the laceration is near a ureteral orifice, cystoscopic evaluation is necessary. Judicious passage of ureteral stents should be considered to ensure patency in select cases. Bladder drainage is facilitated with either a transurethral or suprapubic catheter for approximately 1 week. A retroperitoneal drain is usually not required.

The majority of unrecognized ureterovaginal and vesicovaginal fistulas present 1 to 2 weeks postoperatively. Location and identification of the fistulas are essential in the subsequent management of the patient. Methylene blue, indigo carmine, or sterile milk are instilled initially into the bladder to determine if there is a vesicovaginal fistula. If no leak is identified, indigo carmine is given intravenously to determine whether a ureteral-vaginal fistula is present. IVP and cystoscopy also are used to locate the fistula.

Although the patient will desire immediate correction, most authorities recommend waiting 3 to 6 months before attempting a repair to allow for resolution of any inflammation and infection. A preemptive attempt at repair before inflammation resolves is a formula for surgical failure; subsequent repair will prove more difficult.

Several nonsurgical measures may be attempted during this waiting period. Occasionally, these measures alone will result in permanent resolution of the problem. The use of bladder drainage may keep dry a patient with a vesicovaginal fistula. A trial of suprapubic or Foley catheter occasionally produces permanent continence as smaller fistulas occasionally heal with simple urinary diversion. The use of "prophylactic" antibiotics during bladder drainage is controversial because resistant organisms emerge. Treatment of a specific bladder infection is recommended in most cases; however, no study has compared these two approaches in depth.

Retrograde placement of ureteral stents should be attempted in the presence of ureterovaginal fistulas. If cystoscopic guidance is unsuccessful, recent experience suggests that using a ureteroscope occasionally proves successful. This approach also can result in a resolution of this condition without major surgery.

Persistent fistulas require surgical repair. Nonvaginal approaches for vesicovaginal repair are seldom indicated. Meticulous technique is required; adequate mobilization of local tissue with a layered closure is successful in the majority of cases. Ureterovaginal fistulas require neoureterocystostomy in most instances.

Patients with vesicovaginal fistulas who were previously irradiated should be considered for graft placement to provide a fresh blood supply. Common techniques incorporate either the omentum or bulbocavernosus muscle. Recurrent or persistent malignancy needs to be ruled out in these cases.

Bladder dysfunction is the most common complaint after radical hysterectomy. Unfortunately, as normal micturition itself is not completely understood, the pathophysiology underlying postradical hysterectomy voiding disorder is even less well understood, although several theories attempt to explain the changes.

Neurologic dysfunction secondary to bladder denervation has been proposed as an etiology for postradical hysterectomy bladder dysfunction. Originally, Ramon-Lopez and Barclay suggested parasympathetic overdominance. Nerve regeneration was proposed to explain the resolution of this problem demonstrated over time in most patients. The use of parasympatholytic agents, however, could not correct the dysfunction, indicating involvement of another mechanism.

TABLE 26-2 Bladder changes after radical hysterectomy

Author	Total bladder capacity		Bladder compliance		Residual volume	
	<9 months	>9 months	<9 months	>9 months	<9 months	>9 months
Scotti et al	NS	NS	↓	↓	c	↑
Westby and Asmussen	NS	NS	c	c	↑	NS
Farquharson et al	↑	c	↓	c	↑	c
Vervest et al	↓	c	↓	c	↑	c
Forney*	↑	↑	c	c	↑	NS
Low et al	c	c	↓	↓	c	c
Carenza et al*	↑	c	c	c	c	c

*CO_2 cystoscopy.
NS, No change; *c*, not examined; ↓, decreased; ↑, increased.

Forney implicates sympathetic denervation in postoperative voiding dysfunction. He demonstrated that with partial resection of the cardinal ligament, less than half the patients developed a voiding disorder, whereas almost all patients with complete transection developed a voiding disorder. That sympathetic fibers transversed the cardinal ligament supported his belief. To strengthen this theory, Photopulos and Vander Zwaag reported on 102 patients with radical hysterectomy and 21 patients with modified radical hysterectomy. Although the patients with less extended radical surgery had less voiding disorders, no statistical difference could be demonstrated.

Edema, hematoma, and scar formation also have been postulated as contributing to bladder dysfunction. Seski and Diokno suggested that the surgical trauma alone adversely affects the detrusor muscle and paravesical tissue via these mechanisms. Resolution of postsurgical trauma accounted for the return to normal voiding.

In summary, the exact reason for the dysfunction is not known. A combination of the previous theories probably represent the cause. Further studies in this area will elucidate the origin of this difficult problem. Several urodynamic studies have examined bladder parameters after radical hysterectomy; most have been quite consistent (Table 26-2). Postoperatively, in both the short and long term, bladder compliance is decreased and is associated with bladder instability. Increased residual volume, at least in the short term, is also demonstrated. It is initially surprising that total bladder capacity is usually increased after radical hysterectomy when compliance is decreased. Most patients, however, have decreased bladder sensation with resultant overdistention, accounting for the increase in bladder capacity.

Because overdistention results in slower bladder recovery, bladder drainage is used routinely. Many different protocols have been suggested to treat this problem, each with advantages and disadvantages. Currently, we place a Foley catheter for a minimum of 2 weeks after radical hysterectomy. Afterwards, the patient undergoes weekly bladder challenges until the residual urine volume is less than 100 ml, at which time the Foley catheter is removed.

Urethral changes after radical hysterectomy have been documented by several urodynamic studies. Early findings include a decrease in functional length, which appears to resolve with time (Table 26-3); however, urethral pressure is adversely affected for a long time. Scotti et al commented on 12 patients, five of whom developed genuine stress urinary incontinence as documented by urodynamic evaluation. No relationship was demonstrated between the radicality of the procedure and the degree of urethrovesical dysfunction.

Prehysterectomy education of the patient regarding possible bladder dysfunction after surgery will help alleviate patient anxiety. The need for prolonged bladder catheterization after radical pelvic surgery generally should be explained preoperatively to the patient.

TABLE 26-3   Urethral changes after radical hysterectomy

Author	Functional urethral length		Maximal urethral pressure	
	<9 months	>9 months	<9 months	>9 months
Scotti et al	NS	NS	↓	↓
Westby and Asmussen	NS	NS	↓	↓
Farquharson et al	↓	↓	↓	c
Vervest et al	NS	c	NS	c
Forney*	c	c	↓	↓
Low et al	↓	↓	↓	↓
Carenza et al	↓	c	↓	c
Sasaki et al	NS	NS	↓	↓

*CO_2 cystoscopy.
NS, No change; *c*, not examined; ↓, decreased.

Radical Vulvectomy

Radical vulvectomy currently represents the gold standard in the treatment of vulvar cancer. Pioneers in developing and popularizing this procedure include Taussig and Way. Way treated over 600 cases of vulvar cancer covering three decades of practice.

Vulvar carcinoma has predilection for the periurethral area. Approximately 50% of vulvar cancers develop within 2 cm of the urethral orifice. Common sites include the labia majora and minora and clitoris. Because most authorities recommend a 2 cm margin of excision about the malignancy, the urethra is commonly in a vulnerable position, and physicians must be cognizant of lesions in this region. A careful, thorough examination of the vulvar area should be performed with every Pap smear and pelvic examination. The physician should not hesitate to perform vulvar biopsies. Early diagnosis, less radical surgery, and a better prognosis are the rewards of this approach.

Historically, under the tutelage of Taussig and Way, en bloc radical hysterectomy with groin node dissection has routinely been performed for this disease. These procedures have been referred to colloquially as trapezoid, butterfly, or Texas longhorn incisions. Partial urethral resection has been included as an occasional adjunct to this procedure, thus ensuring adequate tumor margins.

Misdirection of the urine stream is the most commonly encountered complaint. Reid et al described 41 patients who underwent vulvectomy, 27 (65%) of whom complained of significant urine spray. Similarly, of the 58 radical vulvectomies reported by Culame, 17% developed a spraying urine stream. Few reliable options are available to treat this distressing problem. Surgical correction often is unsuccessful. Different appliances resembling funnels have been placed in the urethra to direct flow, but results have not been encouraging.

Genuine stress urinary incontinence (GSUI) represents another major problem. The incidence varies between 4% to 51% as a sequela to vulvectomy. Cystocele, rectocele, and prolapse accompany GSUI in the majority of cases. Patients with preoperative GSUI are particularly at risk. Distal urethral resection increases both the incidence and severity of GSUI. Morley hypothesized that introital enlargement due to loss of pelvic support along with cicatrization were attributable causes. Unfortunately, few urodynamic studies have been performed in this area. The report by Reid et al appears to be the most exhaustive. They examined 21 patients who underwent major vulvar resection and performed both preoperative and postoperative urodynamic studies. In general the bladder urodynamics were unaffected by the surgery. On the other hand, urethral dynamics were adversely affected. A significant decrease in distal urethral pressure was demonstrated in those patients with resected urethral tissue. Overall, urethral length and pressure were decreased; however, statistical significance was not demonstrated.

During the last decade, attention has focused on individualized therapy for patients with vulvar cancer, including performing less radical vulvar surgery to obtain the same cure rate without the resultant morbidity. Burke et al using this technique noted no urinary dysfunction in their patients. Further experience will determine whether this technique may be expanded to other situations, thereby decreasing the likelihood of developing these urologic complications.

Pelvic Exenteration

Pelvic exenteration represents the last-resort effort to eradicate genital malignancy. The major indication is recurrent or persistent cervical cancer after therapeutic irradiation. Selected vulvar carcinomas comprise the majority of other indications.

There are three major types of pelvic exenteration: posterior, anterior, and total. A posterior exenteration is rarely indicated or performed. Experience has demonstrated that bladder and urethral performance is unsatisfactory in the majority of cases. Previously irradiated tissue, compromised blood supply, and denervation all contribute to this effect. The patient who undergoes this surgery is usually a bladder cripple, requiring diversion at a later date. Anterior and total pelvic exenteration both result in bladder extirpation; therefore, urinary diversion is an integral portion of this operation. Also associated with these procedures is removal of the urethra.

Two types of urinary diversion are commonly performed today: incontinent and continent. Incontinent urinary diversion is presently the most popular. Since Bricker revolutionized this procedure in 1950, the ileal conduit remains the standard. Transverse and sigmoid colon conduits are used in some centers. Proponents of the latter two conduits claim decreased complication rates when compared to the ileal conduits.

Jejunal conduits are to be avoided unless no other alternatives are available. They are associated with a high incidence of metabolic abnormalities, which include hyponatremia, hyperkalemia, and hyperchloremic acidosis. The length of jejunum is directly associated with the severity of the electrolyte imbalance.

Increasing familiarity with conduit formation has decreased the immediate postoperative complication rate to approximately 10%. These complications include fistulas, leaks, infection, and ureteral obstruc-

tion. Long-term complications include ureteral obstruction and chronic infection with resultant deterioration of renal function. Current recommendations include evaluation of renal function tests and urinalysis (including culture) at regular intervals. Renal ultrasound should be performed to detect obstruction once or twice a year and when clinically indicated.

Over the last decade, continent urinary diversions have become more popular. The Koch pouch is derived from 80 cm of ileum that has been detubularized and folded, forming a reservoir. Extensive research has demonstrated that a low-pressure reservoir is thereby created, thus obviating damage to the kidneys due to back pressure. Reservoir capacity is between 400 and 600 ml, allowing intermittent catheterization every 4 to 6 hours and obviating the need for a stomal bag. Recently, a modification of the procedure has been described that uses salvaged urethral tissue to connect to the reservoir, bypassing the need for an abdominal stoma. Numerous modifications and other alternative mechanisms also have been used, including the Mainz, Indiana, and Miami pouches. Experience with these alternative continent reservoirs is limited, as compared to the Koch pouch.

Current recommendations as to which procedure the patient should undergo vary. Urostomy formation should be tailored to suit each situation. Expertise and familiarity with each procedure should weigh in the final decision.

Vaginectomy

Vaginectomy is infrequently performed as the sole procedure. Rubin et al reported on 15 patients with vaginal carcinoma who underwent surgery for cure. Only one patient underwent radical vaginectomy alone. Treatment for vaginal malignancy located in the upper vagina is usually associated with a radical hysterectomy, whereas in the lower vagina, a vulvar excision is commonly included. Barclay reported on six patients who underwent vaginectomy (partial or total) alone and three additional patient who underwent adjuvant radiotherapy. The reason for therapy was vaginal cancer after hysterectomy for dysplasia. Preoperative and postoperative cystometric studies (unknown type) revealed no bladder dysfunction secondary to denervation. An effort was made during surgery to preserve 2 cm of vaginal epithelium or to place a split-thickness graft adjacent to the urethrovesical junction.

Experience has revealed that colpocleisis will place the patient at high risk for developing genuine stress incontinence. The resulting scarification apparently "straightens" the urethrovesical junction, resulting in a "leadpipe urethra." Reconstruction of the vagina, usually with split-thickness skin grafts, may help prevent this complication.

UROLOGIC COMPLICATIONS OF RADIATION THERAPY

Radiation therapy is an important tool in the treatment of genital cancer. The type of irradiation depends on a multitude of factors, including the location, stage, type, and extent of disease. Most clinical experience with radiation therapy is derived from the treatment of cervical cancer.

The proximate location of the bladder and ureters to the cervix makes these structures particularly vulnerable to the effects of radiation therapy. The advent of afterloading tandem and ovoids has reduced the incidence of radiotherapy complications. Afterloading allows time for precise application of the tandem and ovoids because sources are added after checking placement. Location of these structures is mandatory after the placement of radiotherapy guides, but before the sources are implemented. Radiation therapy, once completed, requires close follow-up to detect any active disease and complication. Vaginal dilators and local estrogen cream should be used when clinically indicated.

Radiation complications are divided into acute and chronic types. Acute radiation complications usually occur near the end of therapy. Field and fraction size are but two factors that affect the severity and number of acute urinary tract complications. Symptoms include frequency, dysuria, and, rarely, hematuria. Bacteriologic examination of the urine with appropriate treatment should be performed to rule out a urinary tract infection. Occasionally, bladder antispasmodics and analgesics are indicated. If symptoms are severe, a delay in therapy may be necessary.

Chronic radiation complications are more difficult to correct. The total amount of radiation given and

fraction size are positively associated with the level of chronic complications. Bladder constriction secondary to radiation fibrosis is particularly troublesome. Nocturia, frequency, and dysuria are common complaints of this entity.

One of the few urodynamic studies evaluating the effect of radiation on the bladder and urethra was conducted by Parkin et al. Symptoms including urgency and frequency were expressed by half the patients. Bladder capacity and volume required for first bladder sensation was decreased by 25% when compared to that of controls. Detrusor pressure was increased three times that of controls. Functional urethral length and urethral closing pressure were significantly decreased. Estrogen replacement or use was not discussed. The authors concluded that before assessing fibrosis, medical management for detrusor instability may be helpful. Furthermore, urinary tract infections should be evaluated and treated appropriately. Medical therapy is unrewarding in the majority of cases. Urinary diversion, a radical last resort, is curative.

Vesicovaginal fistulas develop in fewer than 5% of patients receiving radiation therapy for cervical cancer. Patients with large-volume disease extending along the anterior vaginal wall are particularly susceptible. Cushing et al demonstrated that 50% of these patients have active disease at the time of diagnosis. Hence, it is prudent to biopsy any suspicious areas to rule out persistent or recurrent cancer before surgery. Complete evaluation of the urinary system is also required.

Once malignancy is determined not to be present, repair may ensue. Meticulous preparation of the involved site includes the use of local vaginal creams and douches to clear necrotic debris and decrease inflammation. Successful repair usually includes providing a new blood supply to the affected area. Sources include the omentum and bulbocavernosus muscle. Concurrent urinary diversion should be considered for repair of recurrent fistulas. Hyperbaric oxygen therapy may assist in the repair of fistulas in this setting. Further work will determine whether this approach is truly beneficial.

Ureteral stricture due to radiation damage alone is rare. Only five cases were discovered by Slater and Fletcher among 1416 patients managed at the MD

Anderson Hospital. Parliament et al reported 10 cases of obstructive uropathy among 328 patients treated with curative intent. Only five patients had symptoms, including pain, malaise, and fatigue. The majority of strictures are located near the ureterovesical junction and surgical intervention is required in most cases. Ureterolysis alone is usually unsuccessful. Neoureterocystostomy or, rarely, urinary diversion is required in the majority of cases. Recurrent or persistent disease needs to be ruled out.

UROLOGIC COMPLICATIONS OF CHEMOTHERAPY

The armamentarium of chemotherapeutic agents continues to increase. Recognition of side effects affecting the urinary tract associated with each drug is important.

Cisplatin

Cisplatin is a widely used drug in gynecologic cancer. Extensive experience has shown that renal failure will develop unless therapy is closely monitored. Cisplatin causes renal insufficiency with electrolyte loss, which can become irreversible with continued use. Hydration with resultant increase in renal blood flow during therapy appears to blunt renal damage. Attention to electrolytes, especially magnesium and calcium, is required. Before embarking on each chemotherapy course, renal function tests should be obtained. If creatine clearance is less than 60 ml/min, alternate therapy should be considered. The concurrent use of nephrotoxic drugs (e.g., aminoglycosides) should be avoided.

Cyclophosphamide

Cyclophosphamide (CTX) is extensively used in the treatment of ovarian cancer. The major toxic side effect affecting the urinary tract is hemorrhagic cystitis. Acrolein, a metabolite of CTX, is believed responsible. Direct irritation of the urothelium results and is primarily localized to the bladder. Generous hydration with frequent bladder emptying decreases the incidence and severity of this complication. The use of N-acetylcysteine sulphonate (Mesna) is warranted in patients receiving high-dose CTX. This agent conjugates with acrolein, thereby preventing urothelial irritation. An ADH-type effect secondary to CTX is rarely seen. Close observation of electrolytes and fluid balance is recommended whenever this agent is administered.

Ifosfamide

Ifosfamide is an alkylating agent structurally similar to CTX. Metabolites formed secondary to its use are extremely toxic to the urothelium. Before the advent of Mesna, these side effects prevented the use of this agent. The mechanism of action is similar to that described for CTX. Additionally, high-dose ifosfamide has been associated with renal damage with resultant elevation of serum urea and creatinine. As with CTX, renal function should be closely monitored.

GYNECOLOGIC CANCER: HEMORRHAGIC CYSTITIS AND ITS TREATMENT

Hemorrhagic cystitis may arise from a constellation of agents or insults. Interestingly, the treatments of female genital cancer are more likely than the disease itself to cause hemorrhagic cystitis. Immediate causes of hemorrhagic cystitis include radical hysterectomy and extrafacial hysterectomy after radiation therapy. Difficult bladder dissection and rough handling of urogenital tissue compounds this problem. Scrupulous surgical technique with gentle manipulation is required to lessen the chance of this complication. Fortunately, when this scenario is responsible, this complication is mild and resolves in most cases spontaneously.

Another well-known cause of hemorrhagic cystitis is pelvic radiotherapy. Unlike surgical or chemotherapeutic-induced hematuria, hemorrhagic cystitis caused by irradiation has a delayed presentation. It can occur without warning 1 to 20 years after therapy. Unfortunately, there is no reliable method to determine which patients will develop this complication. A search for active malignancy with radiologic imaging techniques and cystoscopy is mandatory. Cystoscopy allows for the immediate fulguration of any observed active bleeding site. The mechanism explaining this hematuria is well described. It is believed to arise secondary to edema, followed by submucosal hemorrhage of the bladder muscle, which causes the epithelium to become friable, leading to spontaneous hemorrhage. The spectrum of hemorrhagic cystitis extends from subclinical to life-threatening.

Chemotherapeutic agents are frequently implicated as a cause of hemorrhagic cystitis in gynecologic oncology patients. The two prime causative agents are ifosfamide and cyclophosphamide. As previously discussed, the parent compound does not have a direct toxic effect on the urothelium; certain metabolic by-products (e.g., acrolein) are responsible for the development of hemorrhagic cystitis. Hemorrhage develops during or immediately after administration in most cases. The offending agent should be discontinued until an investigation is complete, including patient history, physical examination, and renal function tests. It is imperative to rule out an infective cause.

The treatment and evaluation of hemorrhagic cystitis begins with the removal of any bladder clots. This procedure is facilitated by the placement of a large-bore catheter with generous irrigation and evacuation. The use of cold water for bladder irrigation enhances efficacy. Occasionally, cystoscopic removal of clots is indicated, which also provides an opportunity for fulguration of observed bleeding points. A regimen that includes the removal of clots, irrigation, and treatment of any urinary tract infection is successful in the majority of cases.

Failure to stop bladder hemorrhage with these techniques requires the use of more intensive therapy. Alum has a variable success rate. A 1% solution instilled continuously usually requires less than 24 hours to correct the hemorrhagic cystitis. If unsuccessful, silver nitrate represents an alternative. A 1% solution is placed in the bladder for 10 to 20 minutes and then removed. Several instillations may be required.

Other chemical means include the use of phenol, ε-aminocaproic acid, and formalin. These treatments are associated with severe side effects, including death. Their use is indicated only in severe cases that do not respond to the previously discussed maneuvers. If a hyperbaric chamber is accessible, this treatment may be effective in persistent cases.

Selective vascular embolization is very effective. It is particularly indicated in the nonoperative patient. Side effects of this procedure include fever, pain, and

renal failure due to radiographic dye use. An experienced interventional radiologist is required for this procedure.

Urinary diversion is used once medical therapy has been exhausted without relief. Removing the bladder from the urinary circuit provides resolution of the condition in the majority of cases. The question of whether to create a continent or incontinent urostomy should be individually addressed in each case between the patient and her surgeon. Cystectomy is indicated for intractable cases.

SUMMARY

The field of gynecologic oncology has made rapid progress over the last century. Education, awareness, and better diagnostic tests have allowed for earlier diagnosis in several genital cancers. Improved surgical techniques, higher energy radiotherapy units, and increasing experience with chemotherapeutic agents have decreased urologic side effects, both during and after treatment. This trend should continue as more progress is made.

BIBLIOGRAPHY
Surgery

Ahlering TE, Kanellos A, Boyd SD, et al: A comparative study of perioperative complications with Koch pouch urinary diversion in highly irradiated versus nonirradiated patients, *J Urol* 139:1202, 1987.

Anthopoulos AP, Manetta A, Larson JE, et al: Pelvic exenteration: a morbidity and mortality analysis of a seven-year experience, *Gynecol Oncol* 35:219, 1989.

Barclay DL, Roman-Lopez JJ: Bladder dysfunction after Schauta hysterectomy, *Am J Obstet Gynecol* 123:519, 1975.

Bricker EM: Current status of urinary diversion, *Cancer* 45:2986, 1980.

Burke TW, Stringer A, Gershenson DM, et al: Radical wide excision and selective inguinal node dissection for squamous cell carcinoma of the vulva, *Gynecol Oncol* 38:328, 1990.

Carenza L, Nobili F, Giacobini S: Voiding disorders after radical hysterectomy, *Gynecol Oncol* 13:213, 1982.

Culame RJ: Pelvic relaxation as a complication of the radical vulvectomy, *Obstet Gynecol* 55:716, 1980.

Farquharson DIM, Shingleton HM, Orr JW, et al: The short-term effect of radical hysterectomy on urethral and bladder function, *Br J Obstet Gynaecol* 94:351, 1987.

Fiorica JV, Roberts WS, Greenberg H, et al: Morbidity and survival patterns in patients after radical hysterectomy and postoperative adjuvant pelvic radiotherapy, *Gynecol Oncol* 36;343, 1990.

Forney JP: The effect of radical hysterectomy on bladder physiology, *Am J Obstet Gynecol* 138:374, 1980.

Green TM, Meigs JV, Ulfelder H, et al: Urologic complication of radical Wertheim hysterectomy: incidence, etiology, management and prevention, *Obstet Gynecol* 20:293, 1962.

Henriet MP, Neyra P, Elman B: Koch pouch procedures: continuing experience and evolution in 135 cases, *J Urol* 145:16, 1991.

Kadar N, Nelson JH: Treatment of urinary incontinence after radical hysterectomy, *Obstet Gynecol* 64:400, 1984.

Langmade CF, Oliver JA Jr: Partial colpocleisis, *Am J Obstet Gynecol* 154:1200, 1986.

Larson DM, Malone JM, Copeland LJ, et al: Ureteral assessment after radical hysterectomy, *Obstet Gynecol* 69:612, 1987.

Lee Y-N, Wang KL, Lin M-H, et al: Radical hysterectomy with pelvic lymph node dissection for treatment of cervical cancer: a clinical review of 954 cases, *Gynecol Oncol* 32:135, 1989.

Low JA, Mauger GM, Carmichael JA: The effect of Wertheim hysterectomy upon bladder and urethral function, *Am J Obstet Gynecol* 139:826, 1981.

Meigs JV: Radical hysterectomy with bilateral pelvic lymph node dissections. A report of 100 patients operated on five or more years ago, *Am J Obstet Gynecol* 62:854, 1951.

Mench H, Garfinkel L, Dodd GD: Preliminary report of the National Cancer Data Base, *CA Cancer J Clin* 41:7, 1991.

Monaghan JM, Ireland D, Mor-Yosef S, et al: Role of centralization of surgery in stage IB carcinoma of the cervix: a review of 498 cases, *Gynecol Oncol* 37:206, 1990.

Morley GW: Infiltrative carcinoma of the vulva: results of surgical treatment, *Am J Obstet Gynecol* 124:874, 1976.

Morley GW, Hopkins MP, Lindenauer SM, et al: Pelvic exenteration, University of Michigan: 100 patients at 5 years, *Obstet Gynecol* 74:935, 1989.

Morley GW, Seski JC: Radical pelvic surgery versus radiation therapy for stage I carcinoma of the cervix (exclusive of microinvasion), *Am J Obstet Gynecol* 126:785, 1976.

Narayan P, Broderick GA, Tanagho EA: Bladder substitution with ileocecal (Mainz) pouch. Clinical performance over 2 years, *Br J Urol* 68:588, 1991.

Parker RT, Wilbanks GD, Yowell RK, et al: Radical hysterectomy and pelvic lymphadenectomy with and without preoperative radiotherapy for cervical cancer, *Am J Obstet Gynecol* 99:933, 1967.

Penalver MA, Bejany DE, Averette HE, et al: Continent urinary diversion in gynecologic oncology, *Gynecol Oncol* 34:274, 1989.

Perez CA, Breaux S, Bedwinek JM, et al: Radiation therapy alone in the treatment of carcinoma of the uterine cervix, *Cancer* 54:235, 1984.

Photopulos GJ, Vander Zwaag R: Class II radical hysterectomy shows less morbidity and good treatment efficacy compared to Class III, *Gynecol Oncol* 40:21, 1991.

Ramon-Lopez JJ, Barclay DL: Bladder dysfunction following Schauta hysterectomy, *Am J Obstet Gynecol* 115:81, 1973.

Reid GC, DeLancey JOL, Hopkins MP, et al: Urinary incontinence following radical vulvectomy, *Obstet Gynecol* 75:852, 1990.

Roberts WS, Cavanagh D, Marsden DE, et al: Urinary tract fistulas following ligation of the internal iliac artery during radical hysterectomy, *Gynecol Oncol* 21:359, 1985.

Rotmensch J, Rubin SJ, Sutton HG, et al: Preoperative radiotherapy followed by radical vulvectomy with inguinal lymphadenectomy for advanced vulvar carcinomas, *Gynecol Oncol* 36:181, 1990.

Rubin SC, Young J, Mikuta JJ: Squamous carcinoma of the vagina: treatment complications and long-term follow-up, *Gynecol Oncol* 20:346, 1985.

Sasaki H, Yoshida T, Noda K, et al: Urethral pressure profiles following radical hysterectomy, *Obstet Gynecol* 59:101, 1982.

Scotti RJ, Bergman A, Bhatia NN, et al: Urodynamic changes in urethrovesical function after radical hysterectomy, *Obstet Gynecol* 68:111, 1986.

Seski JC, Diokno AC: Bladder dysfunction after radical abdominal hysterectomy, *Am J Obstet Gynecol* 128:643, 1977.

Shingleton HM, Fowler WC Jr, Pepper FD, et al: Ureteral strictures following therapy for carcinoma of the cervix, *Cancer* 24:7783, 1969.

Soisson AP, Soper JT, Clarke-Pearson DL, et al: Adjuvant radiotherapy following radical hysterectomy for patients with stage IB and IIA cervical cancer, *Gynecol Oncol* 37:390, 1990.

Tarkington MA, Dejter SW, Bresette JF: Early surgical management of extensive gynecologic ureteral injuries, *Surg Gynecol Obstet* 173:17, 1991.

Underwood PB, Wilson WC, Kreutner A, et al: Radical hysterectomy: a critical review of twenty-two years' experience, *Am J Obstet Gynecol* 134:889, 1979.

Vervest HAM, Barents JW, Haspels AA, et al: Radical hysterectomy and the function of the lower urinary tract, *Acta Obstet Gynecol Scand* 68:331, 1989.

Way S: *Malignant disease of the vulva*, Churchill Livingston, 1982, Edinburgh.

Wertheim E: The extended abdominal operation for carcinoma uteri, *Am J Obstet Gynecol* 66:169, 1912.

Westby M, Asmussen M: Anatomical and functional changes in the lower urinary tract after radical hysterectomy with lymph node dissection as studied by dynamic urethrocystography and simultaneous urethrocystometry, *Gynecol Oncol* 21:261, 1985.

Urologic Complications of Genital Cancer

Ball HG, Berman ML: Management of primary vaginal carcinoma, *Gynecol Oncol* 14:154, 1982.

Barclay DL: Carcinoma of the vagina after hysterectomy for severe dysplasia or carcinoma in situ of the cervix, *Obstet Gynecol* 8:1, 1979.

Coia L, Won M, Lanciano R, et al: The patterns of care outcome study for cancer of the uterine cervix, *Cancer* 66:2451, 1990.

Crowley AR, Byrne JC, Vaughan ED Jr, et al: The effect of acute obstruction on ureteral function, *J Urol* 143:596, 1990.

Dudley BS, Gershenson DM, Kavanaugh JV, et al: Percutaneous nephrostomy catheter use in gynecologic malignancy: MD Anderson Hospital experience, *Gynecol Oncol* 24:273, 1986.

Frohlich EP, Bex P, Nissenbaum MM, et al: Comparison between renal ultrasonography and excretory urography in cervical cancer, *Int J Gynecol Obstet* 34:49, 1990.

Henriksen E: The lymphatic spread of carcinoma of the cervix and of the body of the uterus, *Am J Obstet Gynecol* 58:924, 1949.

Koonings PP, Teitelbaum GP, Finck EJ, et al: Case report. Renal artery laceration secondary to percutaneous nephrostomy catheter placement, *Gynecol Oncol* 40:164, 1991.

Lerner HM, Jones HW III, Hill EC: Radical surgery for the treatment of early invasive cervical carcinoma (Stage IB): review of 15 years' experience, *Obstet Gynecol* 54:413, 1980.

McClinton S, Richmond P, Steyn JH: Spontaneous extravasation and urinoma formation secondary to cervical carcinoma, *Br J Urol* 64:100, 1989.

Soper JT, Blaszczyk TM, Oke E, et al: Percutaneous nephrostomy in gynecologic oncology patients, *Am J Obstet Gynecol* 158:1126, 1988.

Taussig FV: Cancer of the vulva: analysis of 155 cases, 1911-40, *Am J Obstet Gynecol* 40:764, 1940.

van Nagell JR Jr, Donaldson ES, Gay ER: Urinary tract involvement by invasive cervical cancer. In Buchsbaum HJ, Schmidt JD (eds): *Gynecologic and obstetric urology,* Philadelphia, 1982, WB Saunders.

Webb JAW, Reznek RH, White FE, et al: Can ultrasound and computerized tomography replace high-dose urography in patients with impaired renal function? *Q J Med* 53:411, 1984.

Urologic Complications of Radiation Therapy

Antonakopoulos GN, Hicks RM, Berry RJ: The subcellular basis of damage to the human urinary bladder induced by radiation, *J Pathol* 143:103, 1989.

Boronow RC, Rutledge FN: Vesicovaginal fistula, radiation and gynecologic cancer, *Am J Obstet Gynecol* 111:85, 1971.

Cushing RM, Tovell HMM, Liegner LM: Major urologic complications following radium and x-ray therapy for carcinoma of the cervix, *Am J Obstet Gynecol* 101:750, 1968.

Graham JB, Abad RS: Ureteral obstruction due to radiation, *Am J Obstet Gynecol* 99:409, 1967.

Hartman P, Diddle AW: Vaginal stenosis following irradiation therapy for carcinoma of the cervix uteri, *Cancer* 30:426, 1972.

Parkin DE, Davis JA, Symmonds RP: Urodynamic findings following radiotherapy for cervical carcinoma, *Br J Urol* 61:213, 1988.

Parliament M, Genest P, Girard A, et al: Obstructive ureteropathy

following radiation therapy for carcinoma of the cervix, *Gynecol Oncol* 33:237, 1989.

Rhamy RK, Stander RW: Postradiation ureteral stricture, *Surg Gynecol Obstet* 113:615, 1961.

Sklaroff DM, Gnaneswaran P, Sklaroff RB: Postirradiation ureteric stricture, *Gynecol Oncol* 6:538, 1978.

Slater JM, Fletcher GH: Ureteral strictures after radiation therapy for carcinoma of the uterine cervix, *Am J Radiat Ther Nuclear Med* 3:269, 1971.

Stryker JA, Bartholomew M, Velkley DE, et al: Bladder and rectal complications following radiotherapy for cervix cancer, *Gynecol Oncol* 29:1, 1988.

Taylor PM, Johnson RJ, Eddleston B, et al: Radiological changes in the gastrointestinal and genitourinary tract following radiotherapy for carcinoma of the cervix, *Clin Radiol* 41:165, 1990.

Urologic Complications of Chemotherapy

Kline Z, Gang M, Venditti JM: Protection with N-acetylcysteine (NAC) against isophosphamide (ISOPH, NSD-10924) host toxicity and enhancement of therapy in early murine leukaemia L1210, *Proc Am Assoc Cancer Res* 13:29, 1972.

Phillips FS, Sternberg SS, Cronin AP, et al: Cyclophosphamide and urinary bladder toxicity, *Cancer Res* 21:1577, 1961.

Safirstein R, Winston J, Goldstein M, et al: Cisplatinum nephrotoxicity, *Am J Kidney Dis* 8:356, 1988.

Sutton GP, Blessing JA, Photopulos G, et al: Gynecologic oncology group experience with ifosfamide, *Semin Oncol* 17:(suppl 4) 6, 1990.

Gynecologic Cancer, Treatment, and Hemorrhagic Cystitis

deVries CR, Freiha FS: Hemorrhagic cystitis: a review, *J Urol* 143:1, 1990.

Godec CJ, Geich P: Intractable hematuria and formalin, *J Urol* 130:688, 1983.

Goel AK, Rao MS, Bhagwat S, et al: Intravesical irrigation with alum for the control of massive bladder hemorrhage, *J Urol* 133:956, 1985.

Primack A: Amelioration of cyclophosphamide-induced cystitis, *J Natl Cancer Inst* 47:223, 1971.

Rubin JS, Rubin RT: Cyclophosphamide hemorrhagic cystitis, *J Urol* 96:313, 1966.

CHAPTER 27

The Urinary Tract in Pregnancy

Edward R. Newton

Anatomy and Physiology of the Urinary Tract in Pregnancy
    Anatomy
    Physiology
Urinary Tract Diseases in Pregnancy
    Urinary tract infection
    Renal disease in pregnancy
    Urologic disease

ANATOMY AND PHYSIOLOGY OF THE URINARY TRACT IN PREGNANCY

Anatomy

The kidneys and urinary tract play a major role in maternal adaptation to pregnancy. Consequently, the clinician must understand that observed differences in function cannot be judged by nonpregnant standards (Table 27-1).

The renal system increases in size and capacity during pregnancy. Intravenous pyelograms (IVPs) performed immediately postpartum demonstrate a 1 to 1.5 cm increase in renal length regardless of the size of the individual. Autopsy studies report an average kidney weight of 307 g in pregnant women, as compared to 259 g for kidneys in nonpregnant women. The increase in functional demand (a 50% increase in glomerular filtration rate [GFR]) stimulates renal cell hyperplasia and an increase in proximal tube length much like the renal growth that occurs after a unilateral nephrectomy. Additionally, increased water content explains a portion of the increase in the size and weight of the kidney.

The most striking anatomic change in the urinary tract is dilation of the ureters (Fig. 27-1). Bilateral dilation of the calyces, renal pelvis, and ureters can be seen early in the first trimester and is present in 90% of women in the late third trimester or early puerperium. The changes are usually more prominent on the right and may persist for 3 to 4 months. In 11% of women, ureteral dilation persists indefinitely. It is not known whether these patients suffer adverse sequelae, e.g., persistent asymptomatic bacteria from persistent ureteral dilation.

Vesicoureteric reflux is a sporadic, transient occurrence during pregnancy and has been demonstrated radiologically in 7 of 200 (3.5%) pregnant women; the authors felt this incidence represented an underestimate. The enlarging uterus displaces the ureters laterally, and the intravesical ureters are shortened and enter the bladder perpendicularly rather than obliquely. Consequently, the ureterovesical junction is less efficient in preventing reflux. This increased incidence of reflux may explain the high incidence of pyelonephritis during pregnancy; however, only one of 23 patients with asymptomatic bacteriuria ($\geq 10^5$ colonies/ml) had reflux. In a population of 321 preg-

TABLE 27-1   Urologic symptoms and measurements in pregnancy

	Trimester			
	First	**Second**	**Third**	**Postpartum**
Symptoms:				
Frequency				
Day ≥ 7	45%	61%	96%	17%
Night ≥ 2	22%	39%	64%	6%
Incontinence				
Stress	30%	31%	85%	6%
Urge	4%	13%	12%	8%
Hesitancy	24%	28%	22%	9%
Measurement:				
Urine output (ml)	1917	2020	1820	1475
Bladder capacity (ml)	410	460	272	410
Functional urethral length (mm)	—	30.3 ± 4.6	35.1 ± 5.1	27.6 ± 3.7
Bladder pressure (cm H_2O)	—	9 ± 3	20 ± 3	9 ± 2
Closure pressure (cm H_2O)	—	61 ± 14	73 ± 18	60 ± 14

Data from Stanton et al: *Br J Obstet Gynaecol* 87:897, 1980; Francis WJA: *J Obstet Gynaecol Br Commonw* 1960a, b; Iosif et al: *Am J Obstet Gynecol* 13:696, 1980.

nant and immediate postpartum patients, 24 had a history of pyelonephritis; 15 did not have reflux and three of the nine with reflux had a history of pyelonephritis. In summary, the transitory nature of vesicoureteral reflux and the necessary exposure to x-rays for study purposes hinders adequate evaluation of the problem. Nevertheless, vesicoureteric reflux plays only a small role in symptomatic or asymptomatic urinary tract infection.

The capacity of the urinary tract increases during pregnancy. Bladder volume during pregnancy increases to 450 to 650 ml, as compared to 400 ml in nonpregnant controls (Table 27-1), and the hydronephrotic ureters can hold as much as 200 ml of extra urine; however, no changes appear in the contraction patterns on retrograde cystometry. Depending on maternal position, uterine size, and position of the fetus, the functional volume of the bladder and ureters is dynamic in the third trimester. This increased functional volume, coupled with high urine flows (especially with fluid mobilization at night), causes frequent polyuria and nocturia in most pregnant women.

The etiology of ureteral and bladder dilation generates much discussion. Sharp termination of the ure-

teral dilation at the pelvic brim seen on IVP suggests an obstruction. When a woman is upright or supine, e.g., during the filming of an IVP, the pregnant uterus compresses the ureter against the pelvic rim and its overlying iliac vessels. On the left side, the ureter is somewhat protected by the iliac arteries and sigmoid colon and, as a result, is usually less dilated than the right ureter. Although mechanical obstruction plays a major role in ureteral dilation during pregnancy, the relative infrequency of ureteral obstruction by large ovarian tumors or fibroids in the nonpregnant state suggests additional factors. In addition, high urine production, as occurs in diabetes insipidus or pregnancy, is also associated with urinary tract dilation.

In the past, the elevated progesterone levels that accompany pregnancy were thought to cause smooth muscle relaxation and subsequent hypotonicity and hypomotility of the uterus—defects that would contribute to ureteral dilation. Contrary to the latter observation, the large doses of synthetic progesterone used in cancer chemotherapy do not cause ureteral dilation. Measurements of ureteral tone during pregnancy reveal an increase in ureteral tone and no decrease in frequency or amplitude of ureteral contrac-

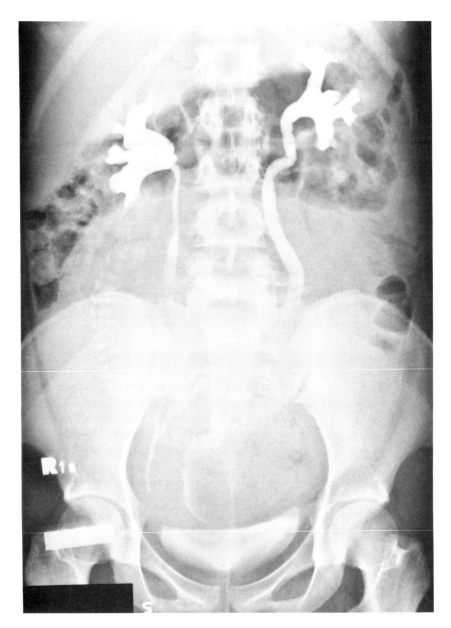

Fig. 27-1 Hydronephrosis and hydroureter associated with pregnancy.

TABLE 27-2 Diagnostic indices* for renal disease in pregnancy: normal values

	Pregnant	Nonpregnant
Blood		
Bicarbonate (mEq/l)	17-22	24-30
Arterial pH	7.40-7.45	7.38-7.44
BUN (mg/dl)	4-12	10-18
Uric acid (mg/dl)	2.6-3.4	2.6-6.6
Creatinine (mg/dl)	0.4-0.9	0.6-1.2
Creatinine clearance (ml/min)	89-222	46-136
Osmolarity (mosmol/kg)	275-285	275-295
Albumin (g/dl)	3.0-4.5	3.5-5.0
Hematocrit (%)	32-42	37-48
Renal threshold for glucose (mg/dl)	121-189	188-200
Urine		
Protein (mg/24 hr)	0-300	0-150
Alanine (μmol/24 hr)	673-2093†	101-429
Glycine (μmol/24 hr)	2216-7560†	614-2014
Phenylalanine (μmol/24 hr)	46-152†	0-77

*95% confidence intervals.
†Third trimester.

tions. Histologic study of the ureters of pregnant animals reveals smooth muscle hypertrophy and hyperplasia of the connective tissue. Thus progesterone probably plays a small role in ureteric dilation during pregnancy.

Physiology

The kidneys play a fundamental role in adaptation to pregnancy through regulation of body fluids. During pregnancy, the average healthy gravida accretes 6 to 8 liters of total body fluid, 950 mEq sodium, 2350 mEq potassium, and 400 ml red cell volume. Soon after conception, plasma osmolarity and thirst threshold fall to a level 10 mosmol/kg below the mean for nonpregnant women (Table 27-2). In nonpregnant women, this drop would shut off antidiuretic hormone (ADH) secretion, but in pregnancy the lower level of osmolarity is maintained and women dilute and concentrate their urine appropriately. In fact, ADH levels are higher in pregnant than in nonpregnant women.

The blood volume in a normal, singleton pregnancy increases from 2.38 ± 0.11 L/M^2 (nonpregnant) to 3.44 ± 0.2 L/M^2 (37 to 40 weeks' gestation). The most pronounced effect of these changes is a 30% to 50% increase in glomerular and effective renal plasma flow (ERPF). Fig. 27-2 depicts the changes in creatinine clearance by trimester. It is not clear whether the change results from a primary renal event or is secondary to peripheral vasodilation. An increase in blood volume occurs within a week or two of conception; however, the normal fall in mean arterial pressure occurs later in the mid-trimester of pregnancy. Late in pregnancy, a supine or a sitting position is associated with decreased ERPF, GFR, sodium excretion, and urine flow.

On the surface, pregnancy would appear to create a natriuretic state by producing: (1) a 50% increase in GFR and an additional 5000 to 10,000 mEq of filtered sodium, which must be reabsorbed; (2) increased progesterone values (blood levels are 10- to 100-fold higher in pregnancy) that cause natriuresis; (3) increased levels of natriuretic hormones such as ADH; and (4) physical factors such as decreased plasma albumin (decreased plasma oncotic pressure) and decreased vascular resistance (increased ERPF).

These natriuretic influences are opposed and, in fact, exceeded by the accretion of 950 mg of sodium through several mechanisms: (1) increased levels of renin, angiotensin, and aldosterone; (2) increased concentrations of other salt-retaining hormones such as estrogen, cortisol, placental lactogen, and prolactin; and (3) physical factors such as decreased mean arterial pressure (decreases ERPF), increased ureteral pressure, and an exaggerated antinatriuretic response to upright positions in pregnant women.

The elevated concentrations of renin, prorenin, angiotensin I, angiotensin II, and aldosterone seen in pregnancy would create severe hypertension, edema, and hypokalemia in the nonpregnant woman. Fortunately, the normal pregnant woman is highly resistant to the pressor effects of infused angiotensin. This resistance occurs early and seems specific to angiotensin II, as response to other pressors remains unaltered.

Interestingly, the decidua produce high concentrations of prorenin and renin, and production of these two hormones is enhanced by progesterone. The physiology of decidual renin is an area of active investi-

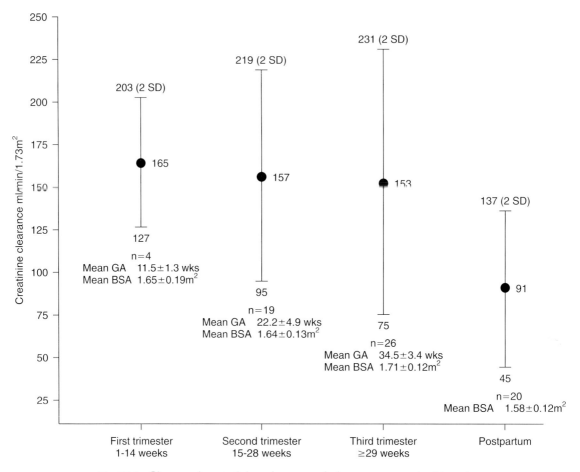

Fig. 27-2 Changes in creatinine clearance during pregnancy, by trimester.

gation. It is tempting to associate decidual renin pro-duction with the regulation of blood flow to the uterus and fetoplacental unit.

The expansion in blood volume affects the oxygen-carrying capacity of the blood. There is a rapid ex-pansion of the plasma volume (1250 to 1500 ml) with most of the increase occurring before 32 to 34 weeks. On the other hand, red cell mass increases from 1400 (nonpregnant) to 1800 ml (pregnant and receiving iron supplements), with the maximum being reached at 40 weeks. During the mid-trimester, the increase in plasma volume relative to red cell mass creates a phys-iologic anemia of pregnancy. During pregnancy, a hemoglobin <10 g/dl or a hematocrit <30% is con-sidered abnormal and warrants investigation and in-tervention.

The kidney is the major source of erythropoietin. Increased levels of erythropoietin are recognized in the first trimester and reach a maximum of 31 ± 16 mU/ml. This response correlates well with the phys-iologic anemia of pregnancy. Renal disease may limit erythropoietin production, and chronic, unresponsive anemia during pregnancy may be the initial symptom of that disease.

The characteristic increases in blood volume and subsequent increases in glomerular filtration result in clinically important laboratory values. These changes can be classified into two basic categories: (1) findings resulting from increased clearance and (2) urinary findings associated with a lowered renal threshold for reabsorption. These changes are included in Table 27-2.

URINARY TRACT DISEASES IN PREGNANCY

Diseases of the urinary tract and kidneys constitute a major portion of obstetric complications and may be classified as (1) infection, (2) renal disease, and (3) urologic disease.

Urinary Tract Infection
Pathophysiology

Fifteen percent to 20% of women will suffer one or more urinary tract infections during their lives. The physiologic changes of pregnancy increase the likelihood of symptomatic upper urinary tract disease, resulting in maternal and fetal morbidity and, occasionally, mortality. In fact, urinary tract infections represent the most frequent medical complication of pregnancy (Table 27-3). Thus, an understanding of the pathogenesis, clinical presentation, diagnosis, therapy, and prognosis is essential.

Although blood-borne organisms (e.g., staphylococcal bacteremia) may occasionally infect the renal parenchyma, the most common route of infection is ascension up the urinary tract. Female anatomy and behavior set the stage for inoculation of the bladder. The urethra is in close proximity to the vagina and rectum; both are fertile reservoirs for uropathogens. Indeed, the presence of *Enterobacteriaceae* at the vaginal vestibule is a predictor of asymptomatic bacteriuria. Pumping action by intravaginal coitus or urethral massage allows inoculation of the bladder.

Inoculation of the bladder does not always lead to colonization or symptomatic disease. Host-parasite interactions determine the likelihood of infection. The presence or absence of bacterial virulence factors may explain why some women with asymptomatic urinary tract infection go on to develop symptoms. These factors have been best defined for *Escherichia coli,* the most common uropathogen, and include increased adherence to uroepithelial cells, high quantities of K-antigen, the presence of aerobactin, and hemolysin production. Of these, adhesive properties seem to be the most important. *E. coli* pyelonephritis isolates adhere to uroepithelial cells better than do *E. coli* cystitis isolates, and urinary isolates tend to adhere better than do random fecal *E. coli* isolates. This adhesive capacity is mediated by the presence of "adhesins" on the bacterial cell surface. Often these adhesins are pili or fimbria. Pilus/fimbriae bind to the β-globoseries

TABLE 27-3 Incidence of urinary tract infection during pregnancy

Infection	Incidence (%)
Asymptomatic bacteriuria	2-11
Acute cystitis	1-2
Acute pyelonephritis	1-5

glycolipid receptors on the surface of the uroepithelial cells.

In nonpregnant women, 10% to 20% of *E. coli* strains isolated from patients with cystitis or asymptomatic bacteriuria express P-fimbriae. On the other hand, 80% to 90% of strains isolated from acute, nonobstructive, pyelonephritis express P-fimbriae. Recently, the same pattern has been shown in pregnant women.

Usually, the normal urinary tract resists colonization by bacteria and generally rapidly and efficiently eliminates microorganisms that gain access to the bladder. Urine possesses antibacterial activity, extremes in osmolarity, high urea concentrations, and low pH levels that inhibit the growth of uropathogens. However, pregnancy makes the urine more suitable for bacterial growth by increasing pH and normalizing osmolarity.

The flushing mechanism of the bladder adds an additional protective effect. The bladder mucosa has an active anti-adherence mechanism. A surface mucopolysaccharide, glycosaminoglycan, inhibits bacterial adherence. As a result, the bacteria remain in suspension and are more easily flushed out with urination. The impact of pregnancy on these mechanisms is unclear.

Diagnosis

The diagnosis of urinary tract infection has been based on the landmark studies by Kass (1956) and others (Elder et al, 1971) at Boston City Hospital. In a population of asymptomatic pregnant and nonpregnant women, a bacterial colony count of $\geq 10^5$ colony-forming units (cfu) per milliliter in two or more clean-catch midstream urine specimens reliably distinguished infection from contamination. Ten percent to 20% of pregnant women with an initial positive culture will have a second negative culture within a week, even without antibiotic therapy. Furthermore, 95% of patients with clinical pyelonephritis have persistent positive cultures at $\geq 10^5$ cfu/ml. Since these studies, most clinicians have used the criterion of 10^5 cfu/ml on a clean-catch midstream urine specimen to diagnose urinary tract infection. However, this criterion has not proven to be sufficiently predictive in nonpregnant women with acute dysuria, infections with fastidious organisms, or in catheterized patients.

Suprapubic or urethral aspiration of urine has been used to avoid vaginal contamination. In a series of classic articles, Stamm et al (1982, 1989) demonstrated the following in acutely dysuric nonpregnant women, (1) the correlation between midstream urine colony counts (MSU) and bladder bacteria (by suprapubic or urethral aspiration) was 0.78; (2) in women who were dysuric and whose bladders contained coliform bacteria, approximately 50% will have MSU $<10^5$ cfu/ml; and (3) an MSU with $\geq 10^2$ cfu/ml predicted most accurately a positive culture by bladder aspiration (sensitivity 0.95 and specificity 0.85). In contrast (1) an MSU with $\geq 10^5$ cfu/ml had a sensitivity of 0.51 and a specificity of 0.99; (2) pyuria (≥ 8 leukocytes/mm^3) on an unspun MSU specimen was highly sensitive (0.91), but not specific (0.5); (3) over one half of women will have an MSU culture positive for more than one organism; and (4) 48% of patients with more than one organism isolated on MSU, "a contaminated urine," will have coliform $\geq 10^2$ cfu/ml on bladder or urethral aspiration.

Using the criterion of $\geq 10^5$ cfu/ml, the urine culture cannot be viewed as a precise quantitative assay. The lack of precision is due to several causes including the following: (1) the type or stage of the disease, e.g., asymptomatic bacteriuria versus clinical pyelonephritis; (2) obstructions or abnormalities of the urinary tract; (3) perinephric abscess; (4) urolithiasis; (5) acidification of the urine; (6) hydration and diuresis; (7) polyuria; (8) collection methods, e.g., MSU versus suprapubic aspiration; (9) transport, storage, or culture methods; and (10) fastidious organisms.

Many women harbor fastidious organisms in their genitourinary tracts, which have been identified only through suprapubic aspiration and/or specialized microbiologic techniques. Stamm et al (1982) found that 37% of nonpregnant women with sterile pyuria have

Chlamydia trachomatis in their genitourinary tracts. Slowly growing fastidious bacteria were isolated from urine obtained by bladder aspiration in 10% to 15% of asymptomatic pregnant women. *Gardnerella vaginalis* and *Ureaplasma urealyticum* are the most common additional bacteria. The isolation of fastidious organisms such as *G. vaginalis* and *U. urealyticum* seems to be more common in patients with suspected renal disease (70%) than in normal pregnant women (26%).

Asymptomatic bacteriuria with aerobic organisms has been associated with adverse pregnancy outcome. Many of the preceding fastidious organisms in the vagina and/or cervix are also associated with adverse pregnancy outcome and, at least with group B streptococcus, a urinary tract infection is more often associated with adverse pregnancy outcome than is vaginal colonization alone. It is tempting to speculate that urinary tract infections with fastidious organisms may also predict adverse pregnancy outcome, but neither the correlation between vaginal and urinary tract colonization nor the correlation between fastidious organisms in the urinary tract and adverse pregnancy outcome has been studied.

The classic criterion of $\geq 10^5$ cfu/ml for diagnosing urinary tract infection is challenged in catheterized women. Stark and Mati (1984) demonstrated that 96% of patients with low levels of coliform bacteriuria ($<10^5$ cfu/ml) progressed to $\geq 10^5$ cfu/ml within 3 days if they did not receive antibiotics and remained catheterized. Although these observations help with the interpretation and management of positive urine cultures in catheterized patients, the questions of who and when to sample the urine in catheterized patients remain unanswered.

Urine cultures delay definitive diagnosis, are expensive ($40 to $60), and require microbiologic technology. Thus culture-independent diagnostic tools have appeal. The most commonly used tests include microscopic examination of urine, measurement of leukocyte esterase and nitrite, filter isolation of bacteria and white blood cells, and screening for bioluminescence.

For years, the technique for rapid diagnosis has been microscopic examination of the urine. A gram stain is performed by placing a drop of uncentrifuged urine on a slide. A positive Gram stain is ≥3 bacteria per oil immersion field (1000 × magnification). The sensitivity (84% to 94%) and specificity (68% to 97%) of this technique in predicting a culture positive at 10^5 cfu/ml compares favorably to other, newer tests. In addition, the Gram stain and examination of unstrained urinary sediment after centrifugation can identify the most probable pathogen (e.g., gram-negative rods) and the presence of upper urinary tract disease (e.g., white cell casts). The test takes about 5 minutes to perform and costs very little ($.20).

The least expensive and least labor-intensive of the other rapid tests is the test for nitrite and leukocyte esterase, Chemstrip LN (Biodynamics; Indianapolis, Ind). The plastic dipstick contains patches of color-responsive reagents that identify esterase and nitrite. The test takes 2 minutes to perform and costs approximately $.20 per test. At a threshold of ≥10^5 cfu/ml, the leukocyte esterase-nitrite strip has a sensitivity of 60% to 100% and a specificity of 60% to 98%. At a threshold of ≥10^3 cfu/ml, the strip has a sensitivity of 52% to 73% and specificity of 68% to 83%.

The filter isolation test, Bac-T-Screen (Marion Laboratories, Inc, Kansas City, Mo), uses an instrument ($2000) to filter 1 ml of urine. The attached bacteria and sediment (white blood cells) are stained and decolorized. The residual stain is proportional to the amount of bacteria and number of white blood cells in the urine. The test can be performed in 2 to 3 minutes and costs $.75 per test. At a culture threshold of ≥10^5 cfu/ml, the Bac-T-Screen has a sensitivity of 85% to 96% and a specificity of 38% to 81%. At a culture threshold of ≥10^3 cfu/ml, the sensitivity is 74% and specificity is 78%.

The bioluminescence tests (e.g., 3M LUMAC [Biocounter, 3M Company, St Paul, Minn]), are based on the principle that bacteria and mammals have distinct adenosine triphosphate (ATP) that can be destroyed selectively. After destruction of mammalian ATP, bacterial ATP can be detected by the bioluminescence produced in the firefly luciferin-luciferase reaction. The test takes about 30 minutes to produce a result, and the instrument costs $9000. The price of the reagents is approximately $1.40 per test. At a culture threshold of ≥10^5 cfu/ml, the test has a sensitivity of 93% to 99% and a specificity of 81% to 96%. At a culture threshold of ≥10^4 cfu/ml, the test has a sensitivity of 88% to 95% and a specificity of 81% to 95%.

The essential question is whether culture-independent tests are sufficiently robust to replace or enhance urine culture in the diagnosis of urinary tract infection. Table 27-4 depicts the efficiency of culture-independent tests at common prevalences of urinary infection at ≥10^5 cfu/ml: 5% to reflect the prevalence of asymptomatic bacteriuria in pregnancy and 50% to reflect the prevalence of positive culture in women with dysuria. A false-negative rate of 6% to 20% with the culture-independent test does not qualify them to supplant urine culture; however, many clinicians recommend that acutely dysuric nonpregnant women be treated without a culture. In pregnancy, the acutely dysuric women should always have a culture because 10% to 15% of positive cultures will have group B streptococcus, an organism that predicts adverse pregnancy outcome.

At a prevalence of 2% to 10%, as is seen in asymptomatic bacteriuria during pregnancy, the positive predictive values of culture-independent tests drop precipitously both in theory (Table 27-4) and practice and should not be used for diagnosis. On the other hand, the negative predictive value is ≥98% with any of these tests. In a low-risk population, urine testing for leukocyte esterase and nitrite on a clean-catch, first-void midstream specimen can supplant urine culture. In high-risk groups (see accompanying box), a culture should be obtained each trimester.

Asymptomatic Bacteriuria

A combination of host defense inefficiency, anatomy, behavior, and microbial virulence factors identifies a cohort of women who will have episodes of bacteriuria throughout their lifetimes. Cross-sectional prevalence studies identify 1% to 8% of women with asymptomatic bacteriuria. In longitudinal studies, 30% to 50% of nonpregnant women with bacteriuria will have symptomatic lower tract infections during 3 to 5 years of follow-up. Most episodes cluster over a 3- to 4-month period followed by an asymptomatic interval of variable length. Nine to 19-year follow-up studies on 60 asymptomatic bacteriuric school girls (6 to 10

TABLE 27-4 Culture independent tests for urinary tract infections

	Prevalence of $\geq 10^5$ cfu/ml					
	5%			50%		
Test	PP+	PP−	FN	PP+	PP−	FN
Gram stain	14	99	1	76	80	20
Leukocyte esterase/nitrite	22	99	1	84	81	19
Filter test	14	99	1	75	88	12
Bioluminescence	33	99	1	83	94	6

Gram stain: sensitivity 90%, specificity 75%.
Leukocyte esterase/nitrite: sensitivity 80%, specificity 85%.
Filter test: sensitivity 90%, specificity 70%.
Bioluminescence: sensitivity 95%, specificity 90%.
PP+, Positive predictive value; *PP−*, negative predictive value; *FN*, false negative.

Conditions that Place Patients at High Risk for Urinary Tract Infections During Pregnancy

Diabetes
Sickle cell disease or trait
Urinary tract abnormalities
Müllerian duct abnormalities
Renal disease
Urolithiasis
Hypertensive diseases
Chronic analgesic use
Genitourinary group B streptococcus
History of urinary tract infections
Severe ureteral reflux
Urinary infections as a child <4 years old

---

years old) were compared to studies on 38 nonbacteriuric control school girls matched for age, race, and school. Episodes of bacteriuria in the 5-year study period for infected girls, and controls were ≥5 episodes, 22% and 3%, and episodes during pregnancy, 64% and 27%, respectively. Interestingly, the children of bacteriuric women were more likely to have urinary tract infections than were the children of controls.

Twenty percent to 30% of women who are bacteriuric during pregnancy will be bacteriuric on long-term follow-up cultures when not pregnant. Radio-

logic examination at follow-up of women who were bacteriuric during pregnancy revealed abnormalities in 316 (41%) of 777 women (range, 5% to 75%). Chronic pyelonephritis was the most common radiologic diagnosis (47% of abnormalities). The incidence of bacteriuria during first pregnancies was significantly greater in women with (47%) than without (27%) renal scarring from childhood urinary infections. Similar controls who had not had childhood urinary infections had an incidence of 2%.

The cohort of women with chronic, episodic bacteriuria is identified by routine screening of urine cultures at the first prenatal visit. The prevalence of asymptomatic bacteriuria (≥2 cultures at ≥10⁵ cfu/ml) is increased by prior renal/urinary tract disease, diabetes, sickle cell trait/disease, poor hygiene, high parity, increased age, and lower socioeconomic status. The overall prevalence varies between 1.9% and 11.8%, with the lowest prevalence in primiparous patients of the upper socioeconomic class and the highest among indigent multiparas. Although most women with asymptomatic bacteriuria are identified shortly after entering prenatal care, approximately 1% to 2% will acquire bacteriuria later in pregnancy.

The microbiology of urinary tract infections in pregnancy is summarized in Table 27-5. The predominant organism is *E. coli*, and the identification markers and virulence traits from strains isolated from pregnant women with pyelonephritis do not differ

TABLE 27-5   Microbiology of urinary tract infections in pregnancy

Organisms	Percent
E. coli	60-90
K. pneumoniae-Enterobacter	5-15
Proteus sp.	1-10
Streptococcus faecalis	1-4
Group B streptococcus	1-4
Staphylococcus saprophyticus	1-11

significantly from those found in strains isolated from nonpregnant women with pyelonephritis. The pyelonephritic *E. coli* strains and strains from asymptomatic bacteriuria or cystitis patients differed in resistance to serum antibodies (83% vs 51%, $P < 0.05$) and epithelial adherence (63% vs 19%, $P < .001$).

The isolation and concentration of organisms other than gram-negative rods depends on preparation (cleansing the urethral orifice), collection methods (midstream versus suprapubic aspiration), and selective medium (Todd-Hewitt broth for group B streptococcus). Although *E. coli* and other gram-negative rods are associated with pyelonephritis during pregnancy, other organisms may be important in other adverse pregnancy outcomes. A large study that uses modern, comprehensive microbiologic techniques is needed to relate specific urinary tract pathogens to pregnancy outcome.

Uncomplicated, asymptomatic bacteriuria is a significant health risk for pregnant but not nonpregnant women. Asymptomatic bacteriuria has been associated with pyelonephritis, preterm birth, growth retardation, hypertension, and fetal neuropathology. The most consistent association is a greater likelihood of pyelonephritis. Sweet (1977) reviewed the relationship between asymptomatic bacteriuria and acute pyelonephritis. In 1699 patients with untreated asymptomatic bacteriuria (18 studies), pyelonephritis developed in 471 (27.8%, range 16% to 65%). In addition, placebo-controlled trials demonstrated a significant reduction (80%) in the frequency of pyelonephritis in asymptomatic bacteriuria that had been treated with antibiotics. The incidence of pyelonephritis in the treated groups ranged from 0 to 5.3%.

On the basis of these observations, treatment of asymptomatic bacteriuria in pregnancy is warranted to reduce the incidence of pyelonephritis.

The association between preterm birth and asymptomatic bacteriuria was first identified by Kass et al at Boston City Hospital between 1955 and 1960. As is true of many early studies, prematurity was defined as a birthweight of ≤ 2500 grams, a definition that would include 30% to 50% of growth-retarded term infants. His initial study reported that 32/179 (17.8%) of bacteriuric patients delivered low-birthweight (LBW) infants, whereas 88/1000 (8.8%) of nonbacteriuric patients delivered LBW infants. Since that report, many studies of small numbers and heterogenous populations have both supported and rejected this observation. Sweet and Gibbs (1990) reviewed 19 studies that related bacteriuria to LBW infants. In these studies, 3619 bacteriuric pregnant women delivered 400 (11%, range 4.4% to 23%) LBW infants. In these same studies, 31,277 nonbacteriuric women delivered 2725 (8.7%, range 3% to 13.5%) LBW infants. Some cohort studies designed to adjust for socioeconomic demographic variables failed to show a difference in LBW between women with and without asymptomatic bacteriuria. Perhaps asymptomatic bacteriuria is not associated with LBW per se, but is a marker for low socioeconomic status that does predict LBW.

On the other hand, when confounding variables are controlled, a strong relationship between asymptomatic bacteriuria and LBW remains. In 1989, Romero et al reported on the relationship between asymptomatic bacteriuria and LBW. A meta-analysis was performed to increase the statistical power for primary and secondary outcome variables and to improve estimations of the effect of sample size treatment trials. Previous cohort, case-controlled, and randomized antibiotic trials, many of which were also reviewed by Sweet, were analyzed for comparable and appropriate study design. Seventeen cohort studies met their criteria. The typical relative risk for a nonbacteriuric woman to deliver a LBW infant as compared to a bacteriuric woman was 0.65 (95% confidence interval 0.52, 0.72). One case-controlled study compared the prevalence of bacteriuria in women delivering at <36 weeks (33/404, 8.1%) to the prevalence of bacteriuria

TABLE 27-6   Consequences of asymptomatic renal infection

	Renal infection		Bladder infection	
	Bacteriuria n = 114	Control n = 114	Bacteriuria n = 134	Control n = 134
Preeclampsia	12%	15%	15%	14%
Hematocrit <30%	2.6%	2.6%	3.7%	1.5%
Delivery <37 wks	4%	14%	13%	12%
Small for gestational age	8%	6%	8%	10%

Adapted from Gilstrap LC et al: *Am J Obstet Gynecol* 141:709, 1981.

in women delivering at ≥37 weeks (15/404, 3.7%) ($P = 0.0036$) after matching for maternal race, age, parity, smoking habits, physical dimensions, and sex of the newborn infant. Eight randomized clinical trials of antibiotic therapy showed a significant reduction in the frequency of LBW after antibiotic therapy (typical relative risk of 0.56, with a 95% confidence interval of 0.429, 0.731). These analyses support the hypothesis that untreated asymptomatic bacteriuria is directly associated with a higher incidence of LBW. It is unclear whether the benefit from antibiotics results from a reduction in asymptomatic or symptomatic pyelonephritis or from beneficial changes in abnormal genital tract flora, which are associated with LBW.

The association between asymptomatic bacteriuria and other adverse pregnancy outcomes (hypertension, anemia, chronic renal disease, and fetal neuropathology) is controversial, being both supported and refuted by different cohort studies. Small sample size and heterogenous populations contribute to the conflicting results. Most studies are retrospective and fail to identify and control preexisting risk factors (e.g., prior obstetric or smoking history). Additionally, the portion of the population with prior renal disease and/or current renal involvement is not identified or controlled.

Renal involvement in urinary tract infections is determined by fever and costovertebral angle tenderness (acute pyelonephritis); elevated C-reactive protein or erythrocyte sedimentation rate; decreased renal concentration capacity; and/or the identification of renal bacteriuria by ureteral catheterization, bladder washout, or fluorescent antibody tests for antibody-coated

bacteria. Between 25% and 50% of pregnant women with asymptomatic bacteriuria will have evidence of asymptomatic renal involvement, and these women are twice as likely to relapse within 2 weeks after therapy as women with bladder bacteriuria alone.

Perhaps women with asymptomatic renal parenchymal involvement may be at higher risk for other adverse pregnancy outcomes. Harris et al (1976) found that 35 of 70 of women with asymptomatic bacteriuria ($\geq 10^5$ cfu/ml) had asymptomatic renal infection caused by antibody-coated bacteria. Asymptomatic renal infection was associated with decreased creatinine clearance, intrauterine growth retardation, and maternal hypertension.

On the other hand, Gilstrap et al (1981b) failed to note a difference in outcomes between asymptomatic women with and without renal infection, as defined by fluorescent antibody testing (Table 27-6). Two hundred forty-eight women with asymptomatic bacteriuria were compared to patients without bacteriuria who were matched for age, race, parity, and gestational age at enrollment. Forty-six percent of bacteriuric women had renal infections. Complication rates in women with asymptomatic renal infection were similar to those in women without renal infection and matched nonbacteriuric controls.

A variety of antimicrobial agents and treatment regimens have been used to treat asymptomatic bacteriuria during pregnancy. Most community-acquired pathogens associated with asymptomatic bacteriuria during pregnancy are sensitive to sulfa drugs (sulfisoxazole 1 g qid × 10 days), nitrofurantoin (100 mg qid × 10 days), or cephalosporins (cephalexin 500 mg qid × 10 days). Ampicillin (500 mg qid × 10 days) is a time-honored, safe, effective, and inexpensive therapy; however, there are a growing number of resistant *E. coli* strains.

Patient education should accompany any prescription for antibiotics to treat urinary tract infection. The essentials of behavior intervention include the following: (1) avoid the female superior position during sexual activity; (2) avoid anal intercourse before vaginal intercourse; (3) void within 15 minutes after sexual activity; (4) avoid bubble baths and oils; (5) avoid vaginal douching or deodorant sprays; and (6) always wipe the perineum, urethra, and anus from front to back. These interventions reduce the frequency of recurrent urinary tract infections in high-risk women.

Fihn and Stamm (1985) reviewed 62 treatment trials for uncomplicated urinary tract infections to assess whether methodologic problems compromised the validity of the study. These trials fulfilled an average of 56% of 12 standards necessary for accurate interpretation and comparability. The standards least often met were sufficient power to detect a meaningful difference (21%), double-blind assignment of treatment regimens (37%), and clear definitions of cure and failure (35%). Those deficiencies were especially true when comparing single versus multiple-dose therapy. None of 14 randomized controlled trials had sufficient power to prevent a type II error. In fact, when roughly comparable studies were pooled, single-dose amoxicillin (3 g) was significantly less effective than was conventional multidose therapy (69% vs 84%). Until a larger study is performed, single-dose therapy should not be used in the treatment of urinary tract infections in pregnancy.

Antibiotics will sterilize the urine in asymptomatic bacteriuria in 60% to 90% of women. The cure rate depends on compliance, length of regimen, preexisting risk factors, asymptomatic renal infection, and the sensitivity of the organism. A test of cure by culture within 2 weeks after the end of the antibiotic regimen will discriminate between relapse and reinfection.

Relapse (a positive test-of-cure culture) has been associated with complicated asymptomatic bacteriuria. These women may have urinary tract abnormalities, asymptomatic renal infection, or silent urolithiasis. Unusual organisms or antibiotic sensitivity patterns alert the clinician to a reservoir of partially protected bacteria, (e.g., renal abnormality, urolithiasis, or noncompliance). A urine pH >6.0 (*Proteus* sp.) and persistent hematuria are clues for an infection-related stone. During pregnancy, a renal ultrasound will help identify a renal stone as a cause for relapse. A postpartum IVP is warranted in any case of relapse. Relapse should be treated with another 10-day course of antibiotics chosen by the sensitivity pattern from the test-of-cure culture. The therapeutic regimen should be followed by suppressive therapy.

Suppressive antibiotic therapy is effective in reducing recurrent cystitis in nonpregnant women and recurrent pyelonephritis in pregnant women. The prophylactic efficacy depends on nightly bactericidal activity against sensitive reinfecting bacteria entering the bladder urine. Vaginal colonization with uropathogenic *Enterobacteriaceae* continues unabated, depending on the regimen chosen. The rectal reservoir for potential uropathogens is rarely sterilized by either therapeutic or prolonged suppressive regimens. One danger of suppressive therapy is the emergence of antibiotic-resistant strains. High-dose (500 mg qid) cephalexin, but not low-dose cephalexin (250 mg qid), induces resistant *E. coli* strains.

Nitrofurantoin macrocrystals (100 mg qhs) neither reduces the prevalence of *Enterobacteriaceae* in rectal or periurethral flora nor induces antibiotic resistance. Trimethoprim 40 mg plus sulfamethoxazole 200 mg qhs reduces the incidence of *Enterobacteriaceae* in rectal and periurethral flora, but it is also not associated with antibiotic resistance, although Lincoln et al (1970) reported resistant urinary infections resulting from sulfonamide suppression therapy.

In motivated patients, a combination of patient education and urine testing biweekly for leukocyte esterase and nitrite is just as effective as prophylactic antibiotic suppression in reducing the incidence of recurrent pyelonephritis after an initial episode during pregnancy. The incidence of recurrent pyelonephritis in the antibiotic suppression group was 7% versus 8% in the close surveillance group. The latter surveillance regimen may be further enhanced by antibiotic prophylaxis (nitrofurantoin macrocrystals, 100 mg, or cephalexin monohydrate, 500 mg) after each episode of sexual intercourse or masturbation.

Acute Cystitis

Acute cystitis occurs in 0.3% to 2% of pregnancies. The reported frequency is only minimally greater than the frequency of cystitis in sexually active nonpregnant women. Unfortunately, the diagnosis is more difficult to make during pregnancy. Most pregnant women have urgency, frequency, and/or suprapubic discomfort. Suprapubic discomfort in pregnancy often results from pressure from the presenting fetal part or early labor. Nevertheless, suprapubic discomfort from cystitis is unique, and most women with a history of acute cystitis can discriminate accurately between cystitis and pregnancy-related discomfort. The most reliable findings are dysuria and hematuria. Acute dysuria may also result from labial or perivaginal irritation from vaginitis, vulvitis, herpes simplex, condylomata acuminatum, or genital ulcers. Due to the separate pregnancy risks encumbered with these factors, an inspection of the vulva and vagina is warranted in patients with acute cystitis during pregnancy.

Preterm labor and threatening second trimester loss often presents with signs and symptoms similar to those of acute cystitis. As the lower uterine segment expands and the presenting fetal part descends, hesitancy, urgency, frequency, and suprapubic discomfort occur. A bloody vaginal discharge may contaminate and confuse urine testing and may lead to misdiagnosis of urinary tract infection. Pelvic examination is warranted in patients presenting with signs and symptoms of lower urinary tract infection to rule out preterm labor.

The pathophysiology of acute cystitis is similar to that of asymptomatic bacteriuria rather than pyelonephritis. Acute cystitis has sociodemographic and behavioral risk factors similar to those of asymptomatic bacteriuria. *Enterobacteriaceae,* especially *E. coli,* are the most common uropathogens. Acute cystitis is associated with a high prevalence of uropathogens in the periurethral flora. *E. coli* serotypes are associated with more epithelial cell adherence, hence virulence, than are fecal strains. The presence of antibody-coated bacteria, indicative of renal infection, is present in only 5% of acute cystitis, as compared to 45% for asymptomatic bacteriuria and 65% for acute pyelonephritis. This difference may be due to earlier identification and treatment of the patient in

these latter conditions because of the intense discomfort that accompanies cystitis.

Treatment of acute cystitis is similar to that of asymptomatic bacteriuria: nitrofurantoin 100 mg qid × 7 days, a cephalosporin 500 mg qid × 7 days, or a sulfonamide 1 g qid × 7 days. As these patients are symptomatic, therapy is initiated as soon as a midstream, clean-catch urine culture has been obtained. A test-of-cure culture is obtained within 2 weeks after therapy is complete. Between 10% and 20% will have a positive test-of-cure culture, representing a relapse. These women should be retreated with another antibiotic, as determined by bacterial sensitivities. Subsequent to retreatment, these patients should be placed on suppressive antibiotic therapy. Without suppressive therapy, an additional 20% to 30% of women will develop another urinary tract infection—a reinfection—during the remainder of her pregnancy and puerperium. Because of the risk of recurrence, patients with cystitis should be followed intensively with a urine screen biweekly for nitrite and leukocyte esterase.

The delivery process comprises a significant risk period for symptomatic urinary tract infections. Trauma to the urethra, periurethra, and labia creates swelling and pain that inhibits frequent and complete voiding. Multiple vaginal examinations and the pumping action of the fetal head in the second stage inoculate the urine with periurethral flora. Urinary retention is exacerbated by epidural anesthesia and perineal trauma. Interventions such as simple in-and-out catheterization to relieve urinary retention pose a 10% to 15% risk of bacteriuria. As a result, 10% to 25% of all pyelonephritis associated with pregnancy occurs in the first 14 days postpartum.

Acute Pyelonephritis

Acute pyelonephritis is the most common serious medical complication of pregnancy. The modern incidence of pyelonephritis is 1% to 5%. Often these patients present for prenatal care late in pregnancy with the signs and symptoms of pyelonephritis. Only 40% to 67% of pyelonephritis occurs in patients with a known history of asymptomatic bacteriuria. Three fourths of women with pyelonephritis present in the antepartum period, 5% to 10% in labor, and 15% to

20% postpartum. Antepartum pyelonephritis occurs mainly after the first trimester: 10% to 20% during the first trimester, 45% to 70% during the second trimester, and 8% to 45% during the third trimester. The predominance of pyelonephritis in late pregnancy and the puerperium relates to the partial obstruction caused by the growing uterus and to trauma or interventions at birth.

The diagnosis of acute pyelonephritis is based on clinical presentation: temperature $\geq 38°$ C, costovertebral angle (CVA) tenderness, and either bacteriuria or pyuria. Among patients meeting these criteria (n = 656), 12% had temperatures $\geq 40°C$; CVA tenderness was on the right side in 54%, on the left side in 16%, and bilateral in 27%. Chills and back pain were a presenting complaint in 82% of patients, whereas only 40% had dysuria, frequency, urgency, or hematuria. Twenty-four percent had nausea and vomiting.

Enterobacteriaceae cause a majority of the cases of pyelonephritis: *E. coli,* 72% to 90%; *Klebsiella-enterobacter* sp. 5% to 23%; and *Proteus* sp., 2% to 4%. Blood cultures are positive in 15% of cases. Infection of the kidney has a profound effect on function. About 50% of patients will have an endogenous creatinine clearance ≤ 100 ml/min/1.73M^2 and 20% will be ≤ 70 ml/min/1.73M^2. Twenty percent will have a serum creatinine >1 mg/dl. This dysfunction is a direct result of endotoxic injury to both kidneys. After appropriate antibiotic treatment, renal function returns to normal by 3 to 8 weeks.

Endotoxins produced by *Enterobacteriaceae* have adverse consequences on multiple organ systems as well as the kidneys. The injuries include thermoregulatory instability (fever and chills), destruction of blood cells (leukocytopenia, thrombocytopenia, anemia), hypercoagulability (disseminated intervascular coagulation), endothelial injury (adult respiratory distress syndrome), cardiomyopathy (pulmonary edema), and myometrial irritability (preterm labor).

Overt septic shock and/or adult respiratory distress syndrome occurs in 1% to 2% of pregnant women with acute pyelonephritis. Clinical clues to the development of these life-threatening complications are leukocytopenia (<6000 cells/ml^2), hypothermia ($\leq 35°$ C), elevated respiratory rate, and widened pulse

pressure. In the late stages, hypothermia, mental confusion, and symptomatic hyperstimulation of the sympathetic nervous system (cold, clammy extremities) herald a scenario that often leads to maternal and/or fetal death. In all cases, the mother and fetus should be treated in facilities having the expertise and equipment to handle critically ill mothers and infants.

All pregnant women with pyelonephritis should be hospitalized due to the additional fetal and maternal risks of acute pyelonephritis in pregnancy. Intravenous antibiotics (cefazolin 2 g IV q6h, ampicillin 2 g plus sulbactam 1 g IV q6h, cefamandole 2 g IV q8h or mezlocillin 4 IV q6h) should be initiated as soon as possible after urine and blood cultures are obtained. Because many patients are dehydrated due to nausea and vomiting, careful rehydration is started. The degree of endothelial damage in the lungs may not be apparent, so careful attention to fluid intake and output and vital signs, especially respiratory rate, is imperative. Respiratory symptoms (e.g., an increased respiratory rate), peripheral cyanosis, and/or mental confusion prompt an immediate x-ray study and measurement of arterial blood gases. Colloid oncotic pressure and serum albumin measurements are important in the fluid management of these critically ill patients.

Endotoxins stimulate cytokine and prostaglandin production by decidual macrophages and fetal membranes. The ensuing preterm contractions raise concern for preterm birth. Three major problems confront the physician at this point. First, although pyelonephritis is often a clear diagnosis, the presence of lower abdominal pain and contractions raises the possibility of intraamniotic infection, a diagnosis that precludes tocolytic therapy. The presence of white blood cells and bacteria on an unspun Gram stain of amniotic fluid is sufficiently sensitive in the diagnosis of intraamniotic infection to preclude the use of tocolysis. Second, premature contractions do not necessarily indicate labor. Often uterine irritability will cease after hydration and administration of antibiotics. On the other hand, if contractions are of sufficient frequency and strength to change the cervix on serial pelvic examinations (≥ 2 cm in dilation, ≤ 1 cm in length and $\geq 50\%$ effacement), the diagnosis of preterm labor is made. Third, preterm labor must be treated with an appropriate tocolytic agent if no other contraindication to tocolysis is present (e.g., intraamniotic infection, fetal lung maturity, fetal abnormalities, or rupture of membranes). Ritodrine hydrochloride, the only tocolytic approved by the Food and Drug Administration, will exacerbate the cardiovascular effects of endotoxemia. The risk of pulmonary edema, cardiac toxicity, and adult respiratory distress is increased. Magnesium sulfate (4 g IV slow bolus, followed by 2 to 4 g/hr) is the tocolytic of choice. However, serum magnesium levels (≤ 10 mEq/L) and physical signs of toxicity (loss of deep tendon reflexes) are especially important to follow, as one half of patients with acute pyelonephritis will have renal dysfunction.

Maternal hyperthermia ($\geq 38.3°$C) should be aggressively treated with antipyretics such as acetaminophen. Maternal hyperthermia, hence fetal hyperthermia (an additional 0.5°C), increases the metabolic demand of the fetus. Glucocorticoids should not be used to enhance fetal lung maturity, as they may exacerbate maternal infection.

Eighty percent to 90% of patients will become afebrile within 48 hours, an additional 5% to 15% by 72 hours, and 5% to 10% will be classified as initial treatment failures. In patients with a significant deterioration of their condition after the first 18 hours of therapy or in patients with temperatures >38°C at 48 hours of therapy, gentamicin, 1.5 mg/kg every 8 hours, should be added. The dosing frequency is lengthened for serum creatinine >1.0 mg/dl (8 × serum creatinine). Antibiotic therapy should be continued until the patient is afebrile (<37°C) for more than 24 hours. The patient should finish a 14-day course of antibiotics with oral medication (nitrofurantoin, 100 mg qid or cephalosporin, 500 mg qid). A test-of-cure urine culture should be performed 2 weeks after therapy. Reinfection is common in these patients; 20% have asymptomatic bacteriuria and 23% have recurrent pyelonephritis. Frequent surveillance (nitrite/leukocyte esterase testing biweekly) and/or suppressive antibiotic therapy (nitrofurantoin, 100 mg qhs) is warranted. With either regimen the risk of recurrent pyelonephritis is less than 10%.

The differential diagnosis in patients with persistent fever and CVA tenderness at 72 hours of therapy includes a resistant organism, urolithiasis, renal abscess, complete ureteral obstruction, or another source of infection (e.g., appendicitis or intraamniotic infection). A radiologic evaluation of the urinary tract is warranted after reexamination of the patient and review of culture and sensitivity reports. Many radiologists have undue concern regarding the fetal dangers of IVPs during pregnancy and will advocate renal ultrasound. A renal ultrasound is useful for evaluating renal abscess, but not for evaluating function or ureteral abnormalities, the more common issues associated with antibiotic failure. A "one-shot" IVP (no plain film and one 20-minute film) is appropriate (Fig. 27-3).

Renal Disease in Pregnancy

A wide variety of diseases and injuries can occur in the kidneys and urinary tract during pregnancy. The diagnosis and management of renal disease is unchanged, except for the recognition of four principles of medical care during pregnancy.

1. No ordinarily performed radiologic examination should be withheld if the results will change management and if other less invasive techniques (e.g., ultrasound) will not give the clinician as reliable or valid information. A delay in radiologic study until after 13 weeks' gestation and limited use of fluoroscopy are prudent.

2. The clinician must remember the fetus is his patient. Any disease and/or procedure has the potential for fetal compromise and/or early delivery. If delivery occurs at a medical center with certified maternal-fetal medicine and neonatal specialists, intact survival is frequent (>50%) after 25 weeks or ≥ 750 g birthweight. Consultation with a maternal-fetal medicine specialist is usually prudent.

3. The fetus is remarkably tolerant to noxious drugs after the first trimester; however, each medication should be scrutinized for fetal effects and risk must be weighed against the benefits to the mother.

4. Hypertension is a major manifestation of renal parenchymal disease, especially in pregnancies

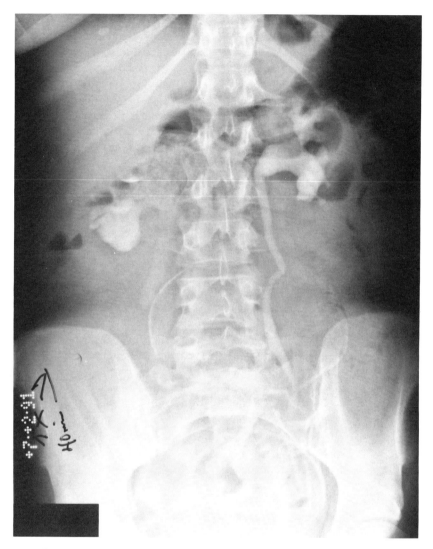

Fig. 27-3 "One-shot" IVP can be used to examine the kidneys and ureters in pregnant women with pyelonephritis who fail to respond to appropriate antibiotic therapy.

where antecedent renal disease increases the risk of preeclampsia, abruptio placentae, fetal growth retardation, and fetal death.

Urologic Disease

Four areas of urologic disease deserve closer scrutiny: urolithiasis during pregnancy, delivery in patients who

have had previous urologic surgery, complete obstruction by a gravid uterus, and urologic injuries during delivery.

Urolithiasis

Urolithiasis occurs in 0.03% to 0.5% of pregnancies, usually in the last two trimesters. Between 30% and

60% of women with urolithiasis during pregnancy will have a history of urolithiasis. Although pregnancy does not appear to increase the risk of urolithiasis over any 9-month period in susceptible persons, recurrent urolithiasis may indicate primary renal disease (medullary sponge kidney), transport diseases (renal tubular acidosis), or metabolic diseases (hyperparathyroidism). The fetal or maternal risk may reflect these systemic diseases rather than urolithiasis alone.

Most stones (70%) pass in the second or third trimester, with equal distribution between the right and left sides. The presentation is more obscure during pregnancy, the most common signs being severe flank pain, nausea, and vomiting. Renal colic is less common after the first trimester because of ureteral dilation. Likewise, gross hematuria is less common, but microscopic hematuria occurs in 60% to 90% of cases.

The differential diagnosis includes premature labor, appendicitis, and, most commonly, pyelonephritis. Premature labor is diagnosed by contractions and cervical dilation. Urolithiasis is more likely than appendicitis when the patient has no fever, the abdominal pain is not localized to the right lower quadrant, and no peritoneal signs are present. The most difficult differentiation is between pyelonephritis and urolithiasis. Indeed, they may coexist.

IVP is the diagnostic technique of choice. In pregnancy, the protocol and frequency of IVP are curtailed. The IVP should be limited to a 20-minute film and, if there is delayed excretion, a 60-minute film. Fluoroscopy is not used except in very exceptional circumstances. An IVP is indicated when the patient has (1) renal colic and gross hematuria, (2) persistent fever or a positive culture after 48 hours of parenteral antibiotic therapy, (3) persistent nausea and vomiting after 48 hours of conservative therapy, or (4) evidence of a complete obstruction (e.g., increasing levels of blood urea nitrogen and serum creatinine).

Urolithiasis in pregnancy is treated conservatively with bed rest, hydration, and analgesics. Seventy percent of patients will pass the stone spontaneously. Urolithiasis during pregnancy does not increase the likelihood of abortion, prematurity, or hypertension; but the incidence of symptomatic urinary tract disease is higher in pregnancies complicated by a history of urolithiasis (20% to 65%). Parenteral antibiotics (ce-

fazolin 2 g IV q6h) are added to conservative management when infection is likely.

When conservative management is unsuccessful (complete obstruction, persistent pain, or sepsis), surgical intervention is indicated. The choice of procedure depends on the size and location of the stone. The usual procedures include basket extraction or retrograde stent placement at cystoscopy. Percutaneous nephrostomy under ultrasound guidance also has been used as a temporizing procedure. Rarely and with considerably more fetal and maternal morbidity, ureterolithotomy, pyelolithotomy/pyelotomy, or partial nephrectomy can be performed. Extracorporeal lithotripsy has gained popularity in the management of renal calculi outside of pregnancy, but its safety during pregnancy has not been established. This technique should not be used in pregnancy until more information is available.

Previous Urologic Surgery

An increasing number of women are becoming pregnant who were born with urinary tract abnormalities that were corrected surgically. These operations include urinary diversion procedures (ileal conduit and ureterosigmoidostomy), augmentation cystoplasty, and ureteral reimplantation for vesicoureteral reflux. The changes in pelvic anatomy caused by the enlarging uterus create the potential for infection, obstruction, and trauma at cesarean section.

Pregnancy in patients with a urinary diversion is complicated by premature delivery, 20% to 50%; symptomatic urinary tract infections, 15%; urinary obstruction, 10%; and intestinal obstruction, 10%. Cesarean delivery should be reserved for obstetric indications, except for ureterosigmoidostomy. In this case, the integrity of the anal sphincter must be preserved and cesarean delivery is indicated.

In the past 20 years, the management of patients with abnormal urinary tracts has changed from cutaneous diversion to continent internal diversion with the popularization of intermittent catheterization and augmentation cystoplasty. These operations include vesical neck reconstruction or artificial sphincter placement and may place the patient at risk for the development of incontinence after vaginal delivery.

Hill et al (1990) reviewed 15 pregnancies in 15

women after augmentation cystoplasty. Eight of 13 were continent before, during, and after pregnancy. One patient who was continent before delivery became incontinent after vaginal delivery. Four patients became incontinent during the last trimester, but regained continence postpartum. The pregnancies were complicated by urinary tract infections (60%), preterm labor (20%), and urinary obstruction (7%). Five cesarean deliveries were performed, three electively for vesical neck or artificial sphincter construction. One cesarean operation was complicated by extensive anterior uterine adhesions. Although stretching of the mesentery by the enlarging uterus has the potential risk of vascular compromise, this complication was not seen among the 15 patients.

Ureteral reimplantation has been performed routinely for severe primary vesicoureteral reflux for many years. Austenfeld and Snow (1988) reviewed 64 pregnancies in 34 women after ureteroneocystostomy for primary reflux. The overall infection rate before pregnancy was 48%. During pregnancy, 57% experienced a urinary tract infection. Pyelonephritis was more common during pregnancy (17%) than before pregnancy (4%). Eight of the 64 pregnancies were lost between 9 and 21 weeks, and six were associated with a urinary tract infection. The authors did not report the route of delivery and the difficulty of cesarean section.

The latter reviews of pregnancies in women with urinary tract surgery suggests the following obstetric management: (1) close monitoring for preterm labor (patient education, frequent office visits, frequent pelvic examinations), (2) suppressive antibiotic therapy (nitrofurantoin 100 mg, qhs), (3) monthly blood urea nitrogen and serum creatinine evaluation, (4) vigilance for ureteral obstruction, (5) vaginal delivery except for obstetric indications and patients with urinary diversion to the sigmoid and bladder neck/sphincter surgery, and (6) urologic consultation at cesarean section for patients with a history of complex urologic surgery, especially augmentation cystoplasty.

Urinary Tract Obstruction by Gravid Uterus

Occasionally, the enlarging uterus completely obstructs both ureters and causes azotemia. Risk factors for obstruction include previous urologic surgery, uni-

lateral absence of a kidney, polyhydramnios, multiple gestation, and ovarian or uterine neoplasia. Patients usually present in the third trimester with flank pain and minimal signs of infection. The differential diagnosis includes pyelonephritis, renal calculi, or papillary necrosis. Serum creatinine is elevated (3.8 to 11.6 ml/dl), but urinary sediment does not indicate intrinsic renal disease or prerenal azotemia. The diagnosis is confirmed by IVP and/or renal ultrasound.

Ultimately, delivery relieves the obstruction and postpartum recovery is complete. In cases remote from term, fetal risk from preterm delivery outweights the risks of urologic management. In one case, conservative management with decubitus positioning and bed rest resulted in an immediate increase in urine output (36 ml/hr to 200 ml/hr) and a fall in serum creatinine (from 6.6 mg/dl to 2.0 mg/dl) after 60 hours of hospitalization. Conservative management for 12 to 24 hours is warranted before more aggressive therapy is initiated, including amniocentesis (in cases with polyhydramnios), cystoscopically placed ureteral stents, or percutaneous nephrostomy under ultrasound guidance.

Lower Urinary Tract Injuries During Delivery

Injury to the urethra and/or bladder trigone from prolonged, obstructed labor or difficult operative deliveries is rare in modern obstetrics. On the other hand, the dramatic increase in cesarean deliveries from 5% to 25% in the last 20 years has increased the rates of bladder dome and ureteral injury. Recently, a large, descriptive study reported injury to the bladder in 0.19% of primary and 0.6% of repeat cesarean deliveries. Most bladder injuries are associated with postsurgical (cesarean) adhesions between the bladder and the lower uterine segment. The risk of bladder injury is increased among patients with four or more uterine incisions (1.5%) and cesarean hysterectomy (1.7%).

Ureteral injury occurs in 0.09% to 0.6% of cesarean operations and usually occurs in association with late second-stage dystocia, deep uterine/cervical/vaginal lacerations, or cesarean hysterectomy. Two thirds of urinary tract injuries are identified at the time of surgery. In difficult cases, evaluation for injury should be routine. Bladder injury can be identified by the instillation of sterile infant formula into the bladder through a three-way Foley catheter. Ureteral function is documented by the efflux of blue-green tinged urine from the ureters after intravenous injection of indigo carmine. The technique and management of bladder and ureteral injury repair are described in Chapter 25.

BIBLIOGRAPHY

Anatomy and Physiology of the Urinary Tract in Pregnancy

Bailey RR, Rolleston GL: Kidney length and ureteric dilatation in the puerperium, *J Obstet Gynaecol Br Commonw* 78:55, 1971.

Beguin Y, Lipscei G, Oris R, et al: Serum immunoreactive erythropoietin during pregnancy and in the early postpartum, *Br J Haematol* 70:545, 1990.

Davison JM, Hytten FE: Glomerular filtration during and after pregnancy, *Am J Obstet Gynecol* 81:588, 1974.

Davison JM, Shiells EA, Phillips et al: Influence of humoral and volume factors on altered osmoregulation of normal human pregnancy, *Am J Physiol* 81:588, 1974.

Dure-Smith P: Pregnancy dilatation of the urinary tract: the iliac sign and its significance, *Radiology* 96:545, 1970.

Fainstat T: Ureteral dilatation in pregnancy: a review, *Obstet Gynecol Surv* 18:845, 1963.

Francis WJA: Disturbances in bladder function in relation to pregnancy, *J Obstet Gynaecol Br Commonw* 67:353, 1960a.

Francis WJA: The onset of stress incontinence, *J Obstet Gynaecol Br Commonw* 67:89, 1960b.

Gant NF, Daley GL, Chand S, et al: A study of angiotensin II presser response throughout primigravid pregnancy, *J Clin Invest* 52:2682, 1973.

Hedrick WP, Mattingly RF, Amberg JR: Vesicoureteral reflux in pregnancy, *Obstet Gynecol* 29:571, 1967.

Iosif S, Ingermarsson I, Ulmsten U: Urodynamic studies in normal pregnancy and puerperium, *Am J Obstet Gynecol* 137:696, 1980.

Lindheimer MD, Katz AI: The kidney in pregnancy, *N Engl J Med* 283:1095, 1970.

Marchant DJ: Alterations in anatomy and function of the urinary tract during pregnancy, *Clin Obstet Gynecol* 21:855, 1978.

Mattingly RF, Borkouf HI: Clinical implications of ureteral reflux in pregnancy, *Clin Obstet Gynecol* 21:863, 1978.

Rubi RA, Sala NL: Ureteral function in pregnant women. III. Effect of different position and fetal delivery upon ureteral tone, *Am J Obstet Gynecol* 101:230, 1968.

Sala NL, Rubi RA: Ureteral function in pregnant women. II. Ureteral contractibility during normal pregnancy, *Am J Obstet Gynecol* 99:228, 1967.

Shah DM, Higuchi K, Inagama T, et al: Effect of progesterone on renin secretion in endometrial stromal, chorionic trophoblast, and mesenchymal monolayer cultures, *Am J Obstet Gynecol* 164:1145, 1991.

Sheehan HL, Lynch JB: *Pathology of toxemia of pregnancy,* New York, 1973, Churchill-Livingstone.

Stanton SL, Kerr-Wilson R, Harris VG: The incidence of urological symptoms in normal pregnancy, *Br J Obstet Gynaecol* 87:897, 1980.

van Geelen JM, Lermeus WAJG, Eskes TKAB, et al: The urethral pressure profile in pregnancy and after delivery in healthy nulliparous women, *Am J Obstet Gynecol* 144:636, 1982.

Weinberger MH, Kramer NJ, Grim CE, et al: The effect of posture and saline loading on plasma renin activity and aldosterone concentration in pregnant, nonpregnant and estrogen-treated women, *J Clin Endocrinol Metab* 44:69, 1977.

Weir RJ, Doig A, Fraser R, et al: Studies in the renin angiotensin aldosterone system, cortisol, DOC and ADH in normal and hypertensive pregnancy. In Lindheimer AI, Katz MS, Zuspan FP (eds): *Hypertension in pregnancy,* New York, 1976, John Wiley and Sons.

Zuspan FP, Nelson GH, Ahlquist RP: Epinephrine infusion in normal and toxemic pregnancy, *Am J Obstet Gynecol* 90:88, 1964.

Urinary Tract Disease in Pregnancy

Andriole VT, Patterson TF: Epidemiology, natural history and management of urinary tract infections in pregnancy, *Med Clin North Am* 75:359, 1991.

Austenfeld MS, Snow BW: Complication of pregnancy in women after reimplantation for vesicoureteral reflux, *J Urol* 140:1103, 1988.

Bran JL, Levison ME, Kaye D: Entrance of bacteria into the female urinary bladder, *N Engl J Med* 286:626, 1972.

Buckley RM, McGuckin M, MacGregor RR: Urine bacterial counts after sexual intercourse, *N Engl J Med* 298, 1978.

Campbell-Brown M, McFadyen IR, Seal DV, et al: Is screening for bacteriuria in pregnancy worthwhile? *Br Med J* 294:1579, 1987.

Coe FL, Parks JH, Lundheimer MD: Nephrolithiasis during pregnancy, *N Engl J Med* 298:324, 1978.

Cox CE, Hinman F: Experiments with induced bacteriuria, vesical emptying and bacterial growth on the mechanism of bladder defense to infection, *J Urol* 86:739, 1961.

Cunningham FG, Morris GB, Mickal A: Acute pyelonephritis of pregnancy: a clinical review, *Obstet Gynecol* 42:112, 1973.

Eisenkop SM, Richman R, Platt LD, et al: Urinary tract injury during cesarean section, *Obstet Gynecol* 60:591, 1982.

Elder HA, Santamarine BAG, Smith S, et al: The natural history of asymptomatic bacteriuria during pregnancy: the effect of tetracycline on the clinical course and the outcome of pregnancy, *Am J Obstet Gynecol* 111:44, 1971.

Fihn ST, Stamm WE: Interpretation and comparison of treatment studies for uncomplicated urinary tract infections in women, *Rev Infect Dis* 7:468, 1985.

Gilbert GL, Garland SM, Fairley KF, et al: Bacteriuria due to ureaplasmas and other fastidious organisms during pregnancy: prevalence and significance, *Pediatr Infect Dis* 5:239, 1986.

Gillenwater JY, Harrison RB, Kunin CM: Natural history of bacteriuria in schoolgirls, *N Engl J Med* 301:396, 1979.

Gilstrap LC, Cunningham FG, Whalley PJ: Acute pyelonephritis in pregnancy: an anterospective study, *Obstet Gynecol* 57:409, 1981a.

Gilstrap LC, Leveno KJ, Cunningham FG, et al: Renal infection and pregnancy outcome, *Am J Obstet Gynecol* 141:709, 1981b.

Harris RE: Correlation of postpartum intravenous pyelograms with clinical localization of antepartum pyelonephritis, *Am J Obstet Gynecol* 141:105, 1981.

Harris RE: The significance of eradication of bacteriuria during pregnancy, *Obstet Gynecol* 53:71, 1979.

Harris RE, Gilstrap LC: Cystitis during pregnancy: a distinct clinical entity, *Obstet Gynecol* 57:578, 1981.

Harris RE, Thomas VL, Shelokov A: Asymptomatic bacteriuria in pregnancy: antibody-coated bacteria, renal function, and intrauterine growth retardation, *Am J Obstet Gynecol* 126:20, 1976.

Hedegarrd CK, Wallace D: Percutaneous nephrostomy: current indications and potential uses in obstetrics and gynecology, *Obstet Gynecol Surv* 42:671, 1987.

Hill DE, Chantigian PM, Kramer SA: Pregnancy after augmentation cystoplasty, *Surg Gynecol Obstet* 170:485, 1990.

Hill DE, Kramer SA: Management of pregnancy after augmentation cystoplasty, *J Urol* 140:457, 1990.

Homans DC, Blake GD, Harrington JT, et al: Acute renal failure caused by ureteral obstruction by a gravid uterus, *JAMA* 246:1230, 1981.

Horowitz E, Schmidt JD: Renal calculi in pregnancy, *Clin Obstet Gynecol* 28:324, 1985.

Johnson JR, Moseley SL, Roberts PL, et al: Aerobactin and other virulence factor genes among strains of *Escherichia coli* causing urosepsis: association with patient characteristics, *Infect Immun* 56:405, 1988.

Kass EH: Asymptomatic infections of the urinary tract, *Trans Assoc Am Physicians* 69:56, 1956.

Kellogg JA, Manzella JP, Shaffer SN, et al: Clinical relevance of culture versus screens for the detection of microbial pathogens in urine specimens, *Am J Med* 83:739, 1987.

Komaroff AL: Acute dysuria in women, *N Engl J Med* 310:368, 1984.

Latham RH, Wong ES, Larson A, et al: Laboratory diagnosis of urinary tract infection in ambulatory women, *JAMA* 254:3333, 1985.

Lattan ZI, Cook WA: Urinary calculi in pregnancy, *Obstet Gynecol* 56:462, 1980.

Leigh DA, Gruneberg RN, Brumfit W: Long-term follow-up of bacteriuria in pregnancy, *Lancet* 1:603, 1968.

Lenke RR, van Dorsten JP, Schifin BS: Pyelonephritis in pregnancy: a prospective randomized trial to prevent recurrent disease evaluating suppressive therapy with nitrofurantoin and close surveillance, *Am J Obstet Gynecol* 146:953, 1983.

Leveno KJ, Harris RE, Gilstrap LC et al: Bladder versus renal bacteriuria during pregnancy: recurrence after treatment, *Am J Obstet Gynecol* 139:403, 1981.

Lincoln K, Lidin-Janson G, Winberg J: Resistant urinary infections resulting from changes in resistance pattern of fecal flora induced by sulphonamide and hospital environment, *Br Med J* 3:305, 1970.

Lindheimer MD, Katz AI: The kidney in pregnancy, *N Engl J Med* 283:1095, 1970.

Little PJ, McPherson DR, Wardener HE: The appearance of the intravenous pyelogram during and after acute pyelonephritis, *Lancet* 1:186, 1965.

Lomberg H, Hellstrom M, Jodal U: Properties of *Escherichia coli* in patients with renal scarring, *J Infect Dis* 159:579, 1989.

Lumsden L, Hyner GC: Effects of an educational intervention on the rate of recurrent urinary tract infections in selected female outpatients, *Women Health* 310:79, 1985.

McDowall DRM, Buchanan JD, Fairley KF, et al: Anaerobic and other fastidious microorganisms in asymptomatic bacteriuria in pregnant women, *J Infect Dis* 144:114, 1981.

McNeeley SG, Baselski VS, Ryan GM: An evaluation of two rapid bacteriuria screening procedures, *Obstet Gynecol* 69:550, 1987.

McNeeley SG: Treatment of urinary tract infections during pregnancy, *Clin Obstet Gynecol* 31:480, 1988.

Man PD, Jodal U, Svanborg C: Dependence among host response parameters used to diagnose urinary tract infection, *J Infect Dis* 163:331, 1991.

Martinell J, Jodal U, Lidin-Janson G: Pregnancies in women with and without renal scarring after urinary infection in childhood, *Br Med J* 300:840, 1990.

Meijer-Severs GJ, Aarnoudse JG, Mensing WFA, et al: The presence of antibody-coated anaerobic bacteria in asymptomatic bacteriuria during pregnancy, *J Infect Dis* 140:653, 1979.

Miller RD, Kakkis J: Prognosis, management and outcome of obstructive renal disease in pregnancy, *J Reprod Med* 27:199, 1982.

Needham CA: Rapid detection methods in microbiology: are they right for your office? *Med Clin North Am* 71:591, 1987.

Ojerskog B, Kock NG, Philipson BM, et al: Pregnancy and delivery in patients with a continent ileostomy, *Surg Gynecol Obstet* 167:61, 1988.

Romero R, Oyarzun E, Mazor M, et al: Meta-analysis of the relationship between asymptomatic bacteriuria and preterm delivery/low birthweight, *Obstet Gynecol* 73:576, 1989.

Ronald AR, Cutler RE, Turck M: Effect of bacteriuria on renal concentrating mechanisms, *Ann Intern Med* 70:723, 1969.

Sandberg T, Kaijser B, Lidin-Janson G, et al: Virulence of *Escherichia coli* in relation to host factors in women with symptomatic urinary tract infection, *J Clin Microbiol* 26:1471, 1988.

Schumann GB, Greenberg NF: Usefulness of macroscopic urinalysis as a screening procedure, *Am J Clin Pathol* 452, 1977.

Smith LH: The medical aspects of urolithiasis: an overview, *J Urol* 141:707, 1988.

Soisson AP, Watson WJ, Benson WL, et al: Value of a screening urinalysis in pregnancy, *Obstet Gynecol* 30:586, 1985.

Stamey T: Recurrent urinary tract infections in female patients: an overview of management and treatment, *Rev Inf Dis* 9:195, 1987.

Stamm WE, Counts GW, Running KR, et al: Diagnosis of coliform infection in acutely dysuric women, *N Engl J Med* 307:463, 1982.

Stamm WE, Hooton TM, Johnson JR, et al: Urinary tract infections: from pathogenesis to treatment, *J Infect Dis* 159:400, 1989.

Stark RP, Maki DG: Bacteriuria in the catheterized patient, *N Engl J Med* 311:559, 1984.

Stenqvist K, Dahlen-Nillson I, Lidin-Janson G, et al: Bacteriuria in pregnancy, *Am J Epidemiol* 129:372, 1989.

Stenqvist K, Sandberg T, Lidin-Janson G, et al: Virulence factors of *Escherichia coli* in urinary isolates from pregnant women, *J Infect Dis* 156:870, 1987.

Strom BL, Collins M, West SL, et al: Sexual activity, contraceptive use, and other risk factors for symptomatic and asymptomatic bacteriuria, *Ann Intern Med* 107:816, 1987.

Sweet RL, Gibbs RS: Urinary tract infections. In *Infectious diseases of the female genital tract*, Baltimore, 1990, Williams & Wilkins.

Sweet RL: Bacteriuria and pyelonephritis during pregnancy, *Semin Perinatol* 1:25, 1977.

Thomsen AC, Morup L, Brogaard Hansen K: Antibiotic elimination of group B streptococci in prevention of preterm labor, *Lancet* 1:591, 1987.

Turck M, Anderson KN, Petersdorf RG: Relapse and reinfection in chronic bacteriuria, *N Engl J Med* 275:70, 1966.

Turck M, Goffe B, Petersdorf RG: The urethral catheter and urinary tract infection, *J Urol* 88:834, 1962.

Vosti KL: Recurrent urinary tract infection: prevention by prophylactic antibiotics after sexual intercourse, *JAMA* 231:934, 1975.

Whalley PJ, Cunningham FG, Martin FG: Transient renal dysfunction associated with acute pyelonephritis of pregnancy, *Obstet Gynecol* 46:1747, 1975.

Wong ES, McKevitt M, Running K, et al: Management of recurrent urinary tract infections with patient-administered single-dose therapy, *Ann Intern Med* 102:302, 1985.

Zinner SH, Kass EH: Long-term (10 to 14 years) follow-up of bacteriuria of pregnancy, *N Engl J Med* 235:820, 1971.

CHAPTER 28

Geriatric Issues in Female Incontinence

Pat D. O'Donnell

The Aging Population
Pathophysiology of Incontinence in Elderly Women
Medications in the Elderly
Nonsurgical Treatment in Elderly Women
  Biofeedback
  Pelvic muscle exercises
  Prompted voiding
  Electrical stimulation
  Pharmacologic therapy
Incontinence Surgery in the Elderly

Urinary incontinence is one of the most serious problems affecting elderly women, and the economic, social, and medical impact of incontinence on their lives is immense. At the present time, over 38 million Americans are over 60 years of age. Of the elderly individuals who are community dwelling and live independently, approximately 38% of women experience urinary incontinence, and approximately 19% of men in this group experience urinary incontinence. Of elderly people in chronic-care facilities, over 55% experience urinary incontinence. There are more than twice as many elderly women in nursing homes than elderly men. The total direct health care cost of urinary incontinence in the elderly in this country in 1987 was approximately $10.3 billion. The annual cost of man-agement of urinary incontinence in the elderly is more than the combined annual costs of all coronary artery bypass surgery and renal dialysis performed in the United States. Although the medical, economic, and social impact of urinary incontinence in the elderly is enormous, the cause of incontinence in this group remains unclear, and the approach to management has not been well established.

With the shift of the population in America to an elderly society, it is essential for physicians to better understand the problems of the elderly and the kind of treatment goals that are reasonable to manage this group. As a result of improved health care, elderly people are living longer with each passing decade (Fig. 28-1). However, the life span of every individual has a limit and the treatment goals of the elderly must involve not only survival but also quality of life and functional status.

In the future, when surgery is necessary to improve the quality of life of the elderly person, it will be required that physicians are able to perform surgery in older people with minimal risk and reasonable surgical outcomes. With the changes in the age of the population of our society and the expectations of patients, management decision guidelines must be more clearly established and techniques developed for successful surgical management of problems in older people.

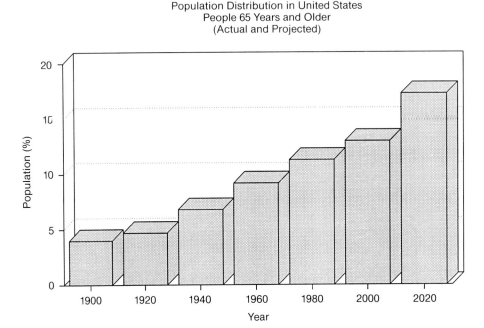

Population Distribution in United States
People 65 Years and Older
(Actual and Projected)

Fig. 28-1 Throughout this century, the percent of the population in the United States 65 years of age and older has continued to increase. Not only is the total population of our society increasing, but also the percent of older people within the society is increasing.

THE AGING POPULATION

Urinary incontinence in the elderly is primarily a problem of older women. The incidence of urinary incontinence in women increases with age. The expected survival at birth of women is much longer than that of men (Fig. 28-2). The incidence of urinary incontinence in women is at least twice the incidence of incontinence in men. The elderly population 80 years of age and older represents the fastest growing segment of our society (Fig. 28-3). By age 80, there are approximately 40 men for every 100 women. In this age group, there are 2½ times as many women as men (Fig. 28-4), and the incidence of incontinence in women is more than twice that of men. As a result, there are millions of older women in our society who suffer from urinary incontinence, and the number is growing at an exceedingly rapid rate. One of the most

debilitating medical problems in our society during the next one to two decades will be urinary incontinence in older women. Research in the pathophysiology of incontinence in elderly women has been extremely limited which seriously compromises a rational approach to the therapeutic management of incontinence in older women.

PATHOPHYSIOLOGY OF INCONTINENCE IN ELDERLY WOMEN

There is a steady decline in maximum urethral closing pressure with aging. This means that the intrinsic properties of the urethra that contribute to continence decrease as women become older. In addition, as women become older, they develop more irritative bladder symptoms. Urinary frequency and nocturia

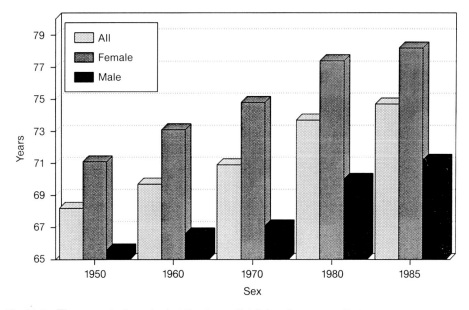

Fig. 28-2 The expected survival at the time of birth has been steadily increasing throughout this decade. The most significant increases have occurred in the past few decades with women having a considerably longer life expectancy at birth than men.

are the most noticeable urinary symptoms that occur in older women.

Clinical observations in the management of urinary incontinence in older women suggest that there may be an interaction between sphincteric incompetence and irritative voiding symptoms. The most common among these is the observation that patients who have surgery for stress urinary incontinence will not only have relief of the symptoms of stress incontinence, but also will have improvement in frequency, urgency, and nocturia. Therefore, in patients who have symptoms of stress incontinence and urge incontinence, it is likely that each component of incontinence makes the other component of incontinence worse. Also, as women become older, it appears clinically that there may be a difference in the urge characteristic of incontinence compared with younger women.

Research in urinary incontinence in elderly men may provide significant insight into the pathophysiology of incontinence in older women. Sphincteric incompetence as a cause of urinary incontinence in elderly men is almost nonexistent in the absence of previous prostate or pelvic surgery. Therefore the complexity of the interaction of sphincteric incompetence and urge incontinence is not present in elderly men as it is in elderly women. Thus the isolated component of bladder dysfunction in aging can be studied in this population. In studies of elderly men with urinary incontinence, it has been shown that a wide variation within patients in the volume of involuntary urine loss occurs with each incontinence episode. In addition, there is a wide variation within individual patients in the time interval between incontinence episodes. Residual urine volume measurements have been done to determine the role of bladder emptying in the observed variations in incontinence volume.

Population Distribution in United States
People 85 Years and Older
(Actual and Projected)

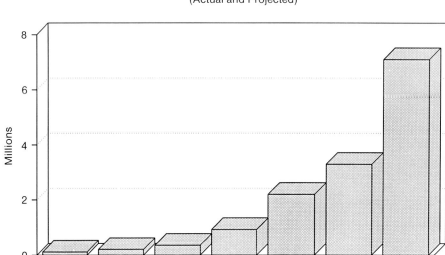

Fig. 28-3 People 85 years old and above are often considered the "very old" and represent the most rapidly growing segment of our population.

The residual urine volume after incontinence episodes showed a wide variation among incontinence episodes within individual patients. The total bladder volume at the time of an incontinence episode, which was the incontinence volume plus the residual urine volume, showed wide variation in volume within patients. It was concluded from these observations that the occurrence of an incontinence episode in elderly men is independent of the accumulated volume of urine in the bladder at the time of the episode. It is postulated that the origin of an incontinence episode is in the central nervous system control of the bladder in elderly men.

In elderly men with urinary incontinence, those patients considered to have severe incontinence will have approximately 5 to 10 episodes of incontinence per day. However, an important characteristic of this population is that even in the patients with severe

incontinence, most voiding occurs voluntarily. In both elderly incontinent men and women, nocturia occurs more frequently than in patients who are continent. This means that the patient has the capacity to perceive a need to void while asleep. Sleep arousal occurs while continence is being maintained and voluntary voiding occurs. Although nocturia occurs in elderly incontinent people, nocturnal enuresis also occurs with some of the voiding episodes. On these occasions, incontinence usually occurs with little warning of a need to void.

In both older men and older women the most common description of an incontinence episode is the occurrence of incontinence with no warning. In these patients, voluntary voiding occurs both day and night in which the need to void is perceived well in advance of voluntary voiding. On other occasions, involuntary voiding occurs with no warning to the patient that a

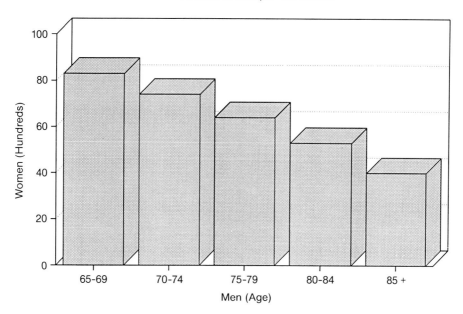

Fig. 28-4 As a result of the longer life expectancy of women, the number of men per 100 women has a steady decline with aging. This means that issues involving community dwelling elderly, chronic care elderly, and the medical problems of the older patient will affect women more often than men.

bladder contraction is going to occur. As described previously, the stimulus for the involuntary bladder contraction appears to be independent of the accumulated volume of urine in the bladder at the time of the episode. Therefore in older people the occurrence of incontinence resulting from involuntary detrusor contractions appears to be more than an uninhibited normal bladder contraction. Incontinence resulting from an involuntary detrusor contraction probably is an abnormal bladder contraction, which appears to originate within the central nervous system most likely occurring at a midbrain level. Incontinence in older people that results from involuntary detrusor contractions shows a coordinated EMG activity, which suggests that the origin of the detrusor contraction is a suprapontine level. The fact that the involuntary de-

trusor contraction is not perceived until it is actually in progress suggests that it occurs independent of the cortical control of the bladder and that it may not be due to lack of cortical inhibition of bladder function.

There are two neurophysiologic mechanisms involved in these observations: the sensory-motor balance of the central nervous system control of the bladder and the facilitory-inhibitory balance of the central nervous system involved in micturition. Since the patients describe an absence of sensation of a need to void before the onset of an incontinence episode, there may be a perception sensory deficit associated with urge incontinence of older people. The impairment of sensory function appears to alter the facilitory-inhibitory balance of the central nervous system control of micturition, which results in a failure of the normal unconscious inhibition of the bladder. It is important to recognize that normal inhibition of a bladder contraction appears to occur at a subcortical level. For example, people do not consciously inhibit their bladder during normal daily activities. Rather, the bladder is inhibited automatically both when the patient is awake and asleep. It is only when the sensation of a need to void is perceived that voluntary inhibition of the bladder may be required and becomes a cortical function. In the elderly, incontinence episodes do not appear to occur as a result of failure of cortical inhibition of detrusor contractions, but rather a failure of cortical perception of an involuntary bladder contraction until it is in progress.

Another important clinical observation that is commonly seen in elderly men may also be a factor in incontinence in older women. In younger patients who present to a clinic for any type of voiding dysfunction, a urine specimen can be provided by the patient in almost every case regardless of how short a time it may have been since the patient voided. Therefore voluntary voiding in younger people will normally occur under almost any circumstance. However, that is not true of older people and especially of older people with urinary incontinence. It is common to request a urine sample from an older patient and have the patient unable to provide the urine specimen. Paradoxically, it is common for an older patient with urinary incontinence to have an incontinent episode within minutes after being unable to voluntarily void. Therefore the elderly patient appears to have an impairment of the ability to voluntarily initiate voiding. Thus the older patient not only has an impairment of the ability to prevent a bladder contraction but also they have an impairment of the ability to voluntarily initiate a bladder contraction. These concepts are very important in understanding the reasons for success and failure after surgery in older women and in applying treatment programs such as prompted voiding and pelvic floor exercises in older people which target these particular deficits. Prompted voiding is one of the most commonly used behavioral therapy interventions in management of bladder control in older people. The mechanism for efficacy of this treatment has been unclear in the past. However, it appears to target a

common impairment of older people which is the inability to voluntarily initiate voiding.

Behavioral therapy, such as pelvic floor exercises and biofeedback therapy, appears to target the common impairment in the elderly of an inability to prevent an involuntary detrusor contraction. In addition, these behavioral therapies provide training for the individual in voluntary control of bladder function. These types of treatment programs stabilize the central nervous system control of bladder function. It appears that the facilitory-inhibitory balance within the central nervous system is stabilized by these activities which also result in improvement in the ability of the individual to prevent an involuntary detrusor contraction.

Although the pathophysiology of incontinence in women has been addressed in previous chapters, the previous discussion was provided to allow a better understanding of the complexity of incontinence in older women especially as it relates to involvement of the aging central nervous system. The physician is not only dealing with mixed incontinence of an urge and stress component, but the urge and stress components in the elderly are different from those in younger people. In older women, sphincteric incompetence has more of an intrinsic urethral dysfunction rather than an anatomic defect as seen in younger women. However, in many cases of incontinence in older women, both components of intrinsic and anatomic incontinence are combined to produce the symptoms of stress incontinence. In addition, the problem of urge incontinence in older women appears to be different from the younger woman who has urgency and involuntarily leaks urine on the way to the bathroom. In the older woman the first sensation of a need to void is often the actual involuntary loss of urine with no warning of an impending bladder contraction.

MEDICATIONS IN THE ELDERLY

Many elderly women who present with voiding dysfunctions have multiple other medical problems and are currently receiving numerous medications. It is important that the physician carefully review all of these medications to determine which have effects on the bladder and urethra. Many cardiac drugs affect urethral function and contribute to urinary incontinence. It is important for the primary care physician or the geriatrician who is managing the medical problems of the patient to review all medications to determine if each is necessary. One of the most common problems in older people is too many different medications. When a medication can be eliminated, in most cases it should be eliminated. Recommendations can be made to the primary care physician regarding changes in medications that are likely to improve bladder and urethral function.

In older women who have mild stress urinary incontinence, changing the medications sometimes can improve their incontinence. However, in most cases, changing the medication will have minimal impact on the problem of incontinence especially in patients who have more severe incontinence. It is always important for physicians working with older patients to review their medications since so many problems occur in older people as a result of side effects of medications.

In considering medications in the treatment of bladder dysfunctions in older people the physician treating the bladder problem can contribute to the problems of side effects of drugs in the older population by treating the bladder problem. For example, drugs such as oxybutynin are frequently prescribed for older patients with irritative bladder symptoms. Older people have a low tolerance for cholinolytic medications and often have side effects such as confusion at relatively low doses of medication. In addition, the therapeutic effect of these drugs in older people tends to be much less than in younger people. For this reason, a trial of pharmacologic therapy for incontinence in older patients is recommended, but a great deal of caution should be used with each drug trial.

Drugs having α-adrenergic activity, such as phenylpropanolamine or imipramine, may have beneficial effects in the treatment of incontinence in older women, but the use of these drugs should be done very carefully. Use of α-adrenergic drugs in older patients may precipitate cardiac complications. In many cases, these drugs should be used only with the approval of a cardiologist who is managing the patient.

As is mentioned in other chapters, estrogen is efficacious for use in the treatment of incontinence in the elderly female and should always be considered when there are no contraindications to its use.

NONSURGICAL TREATMENT IN ELDERLY WOMEN

Nonsurgical therapy is preferred as primary treatment in elderly women who have urgency, urge incontinence, or mild sphincteric incompetence or patients who are not candidates for any surgical procedure because of general health status. Postoperative problems in elderly women require active participation in the management of the problems by the patient. This means that patients with compromised mental status or compromised functional status may not be able to manage the problems that occur after surgery. In many cases the spouse or the family may be able to offer assistance. If the functional status of the patient and the environment in which the patient lives will not support the required involvement of the patient in postoperative management of a surgical approach to incontinence, then nonsurgical approaches should be considered initially.

Many physicians consider a nonsurgical approach to sphincteric incompetence as the first treatment option to be considered with surgery as a last resort. Although this is reasonable, sphincteric incompetence responds best to surgical management over the long term. Nonsurgical treatments have shown efficacy in patients who appear to have sphincteric incompetence, although in practice the long-term results often do not seem to be as good as those reported. The decision regarding management of incontinence in elderly women is not a simple one and depends on the complexity of the bladder dysfunction, the mental status and functional status of the patient, and the family and social support that is available in the environment.

The mental and functional status of a patient can be evaluated reasonably well in the office by the physician. A Mini-Mental Status Exam (MMSE) is a commonly used scale for assessment of mental status. Generally, any patient scoring less than 20 on the MMSE is difficult to manage with most nonsurgical interventions and would be extremely difficult to manage surgically. Many investigators recommend an

MMSE score of 23 or above for behavioral interventions such as biofeedback therapy. The functional status of the patient can be evaluated with a Modified Katz Activities of Daily Living (ADL) Scale. Any significant compromise in activities of daily living of the elderly patient makes the individual extremely difficult to manage with any surgical or behavioral intervention.

Biofeedback

Biofeedback therapy has been used extensively in the elderly as a nonsurgical intervention for the treatment of urinary incontinence. Biofeedback is especially useful in training patients to learn the specific muscles to be used in pelvic muscle exercises. Biofeedback of the pelvic muscles has many advantages and disadvantages. The advantages are that the treatment is safe and can be used specifically to teach older people how to voluntarily contract pelvic muscles with a precise skill-acquisition technique. The patients can continue to exercise pelvic muscles after biofeedback therapy using standard pelvic muscle exercise programs. Biofeedback can be used as an initial therapeutic approach in elderly patients and maintenance therapy following the initial biofeedback therapy can be done with pelvic muscle exercises.

The problems with biofeedback are numerous. The first major problem is lack of standardization in biofeedback therapy techniques. There are many people who use biofeedback for treatment of incontinence who have little understanding of the pathophysiology of incontinence in older people. The signal sources used for feedback of performance to the patient vary widely. The concept of biofeedback therapy is that the patient must be aware of their own performance through feedback in order to improve their performance. If the signal source is inaccurate or inappropriate, the patient will have no basis for learning the skill that is required. Therefore one of the most limiting factors in the efficacy of biofeedback therapy is a lack of standardization of the biofeedback technique which is necessary for efficacy of the treatment.

Another disadvantage of biofeedback is that it is labor intensive. It requires skilled personnel to administer biofeedback therapy. In elderly people, learning a skill may occur at a fairly slow rate. Therefore

the treatment program may be longer and require much more intensive work with the patient to accomplish the desired outcome than in the younger patient.

Pelvic Muscle Exercises

Although pelvic muscle exercise is described in Chapter 13, it is mentioned here because success with pelvic muscle exercises in elderly women is more difficult to achieve than in younger women. The elderly woman has more difficulty learning which muscles to contract and how to contract them. This is where biofeedback therapy initially can be of some assistance in the use of pelvic muscle exercises in elderly women. Another difficulty in the elderly woman is maintaining a schedule that is consistent from day to day. Finally, elderly women often will discontinue pelvic muscle exercises after a short time of treatment. Although the mechanism of treatment efficacy of pelvic muscle exercises in elderly women is not completely clear, numerous studies in older women with urinary incontinence demonstrate the efficacy of pelvic muscle exercises in the treatment of incontinence of older women.

Prompted Voiding

Prompted voiding or timed voiding is one of the most commonly used behavioral therapies. In community dwelling patients the patient is instructed to void on a schedule during the waking hours. The most commonly recommended schedule is a 2-hour timed voiding schedule. Some patients may complain of frequency and void more often than every 2 hours. In these cases, it still can be efficacious for the patient to learn a timed voiding schedule. As described previously, this technique seems to teach the older patient the ability to voluntarily initiate voiding, which is an important part of bladder control.

In chronic care patients, prompted voiding is done by the nursing staff. Again, the schedule recommended is a 2-hour prompted voiding schedule during the waking hours of the patient. A timed voiding schedule or prompted voiding treatment program for elderly incontinent women is easy to implement and has no side effects. In community dwelling elderly incontinent women, it is important to involve the spouse or family in assisting with the timed voiding schedule. This is especially important if any significant compromise exists in the mental status of the patient.

The overall results of timed voiding and prompted voiding programs uniformly demonstrate an improvement in incontinence. It is important to recognize that the outcome of treatment in these patients is rarely complete continence. In the elderly incontinent woman who is not a candidate for any surgical procedure the treatment outcome must be realistic and the goals must be recognized and appreciated by the physician, the patient, and the family. For example, if an elderly incontinent woman requires six pads each day for containment of her incontinence, a reduction of incontinence episodes to a level of three pads each day is a significant improvement in the quality of life of the patient. The cost of absorbent pads is reduced by one half. The inconvenience to the patient is significantly reduced. Although many people would consider a patient wearing three pads each day a treatment failure, realistic treatment outcomes need to be recognized and appreciated.

Electrical Stimulation

Electrical stimulation for treatment of incontinence has been done for many years with good success in most studies. Studies of treatment efficacy of electrical stimulation in elderly women are lacking. Electrical stimulation can be provided with integrated vaginal devices or with the use of a transcutaneous electrical nerve stimulator (TENS). The TENS unit may be used in conjunction with behavioral therapy interventions. The electrodes may be placed along the S2 dermatome posteriorly. The amplitude of the stimulation is usually increased until a slight tingling can be felt by the patient. The device has rechargeable batteries and can be worn 24 hours each day. It is usually recommended that at least 1 to 3 months of therapy be used to determine if a response occurs. The TENS units can be rented from a physical therapist at the request of a physician. The patient should be advised against purchasing one of the devices until it has been determined clinically that a response to the device has occurred. The advantage of the TENS unit in elderly incontinent women is the low incidence of side effects. The major problem in treatment of incontinence in the elderly woman is balancing the risks and benefits of treatment.

Pharmacologic Therapy

Pharmacologic therapy of urinary incontinence in elderly women is generally less effective than in younger women. As described previously, there appears to be differences in the cause of incontinence in elderly women, both in those with sphincteric incompetence and those with urge incontinence. Sphincteric incompetence tends to have a greater component of intrinsic urethral dysfunction in elderly women, which may also be associated with an anatomic abnormality in some of these patients. Urge incontinence associated with detrusor instability in the elderly tends to be characterized by the patient as having a minimal warning before an incontinence episode occurs.

In the pharmacologic management of sphincteric incompetence, exogenous estrogen therapy can be used with significant improvement and few side effects. The α-adrenergic drugs such as phenylpropanolamine, which is commonly used in younger women, are less effective in the elderly incontinent woman. A trial of α-adrenergic drugs for stress incontinence in elderly women can be given to determine their effectiveness in a particular patient with close monitoring of the patient for side effects. It may be that the lower urethral pressure in older women and the greater component of intrinsic urethral dysfunction causes the α-adrenergic drugs to be somewhat less effective than in younger women. However, comparison studies of effectiveness of drugs stratified according to age are lacking. The other problem with α-adrenergic drugs is drug side effects which is a problem with any kind of pharmacologic therapy in the elderly. Thus urinary incontinence in older women resulting from sphincteric incompetence has a relatively poor response to pharmacologic management except for the response to exogenous estrogen.

Elderly women who have symptoms of urge incontinence may be treated with cholinolytic drugs. As described previously, oxybutynin is one of the most common drugs used for treatment of urge incontinence. Again, the type of urge incontinence experienced by the elderly woman tends to be less responsive to cholinolytic drugs. Cholinolytic drugs such as oxybutynin have a high incidence of side effects in older women, which not only include the common side effects experienced by younger women but also includes confusion. Women with any significant compromise in mental function on the MMSE evaluation are more likely to experience confusion with even low doses of cholinolytic drugs.

INCONTINENCE SURGERY IN THE ELDERLY

The issue of surgical treatment of urinary incontinence in elderly women has many unanswered questions at this time. Of elderly women with urinary incontinence, who should be considered for surgery? Is the risk of surgery in older women worth the benefit that may result? Should patients who have sphincteric incompetence and detrusor instability be considered for surgery? Is combination surgical treatment and nonsurgical treatment an option in this population?

In considering surgery in older women, the risk of surgery and the problems associated with surgery vary considerably within the population. Older women are a much more heterogenous population relative to their general health status than younger women. In addition, the complexity of the problem of incontinence is much greater in older women. Therefore the results of surgery for incontinence are less predictable in the elderly than in younger women. For this reason, incontinence surgery in elderly women requires a careful overall approach. First, the evaluation of older women regarding the cause of incontinence must be complete. It is important for the physician to be able to predict with some degree of accuracy the outcome of the surgical procedure and the associated problems that are likely to occur. Being able to predict the outcome of surgery based on the preoperative evaluation is important for both the physician and the patients in order for patients and their families to have reasonable expectations of the surgical outcome and to be prepared for some of the problems that may occur. In addition, it is important for the physician to have a network of other physicians such as cardiologists, internists, geriatricians, rehabilitation medicine specialists, and anesthesiologists to work with the patient to reduce the risk of surgery and restore the patient to a preoperative functional status as quickly as possible. These concepts are essential in the success of surgery in elderly women.

It is important for the physician who performs a surgical procedure in elderly women with urinary incontinence that the technique used is expedient and successful in correcting the problem of sphincteric incompetence. The anesthesia must be done smoothly and postoperative medical problems must be managed promptly and correctly. If significant ambulatory impairment exists preoperatively, it is essential that rehabilitation begin as soon as possible after surgery in order that the patient is restored to the preoperative ambulatory status as quickly as possible. If an elderly woman with ambulatory impairment is allowed to lie in bed for a week after surgery, the rehabilitation of that patient to a preoperative functional status is an enormous problem requiring prolonged hospitalization.

Physicians who perform incontinence surgery in elderly women also will need extensive nursing support during the postoperative period. Elderly women who have postoperative urinary retention may require long-term, intermittent self-catheterization and may feel that it is impossible for them to perform. Although many physicians would disagree, almost every elderly woman can perform long-term, intermittent self-catheterization after surgery if it is necessary. The success depends on the motivation of the physician and nursing person working with the patient, the motivation of the patient, and the support of the family. An elderly continent woman requiring long-term, intermittent self-catheterization almost always has a better quality of life than when she was incontinent. However, it is essential that the patient and the family are prepared for long-term, intermittent self-catheterization when it is required.

The other problem after surgery for incontinence in older women that is extremely difficult to manage is postoperative irritative bladder syndromes. A difficult surgical outcome in older women with mixed incontinence of sphincteric incompetence and urge incontinence is a patient whose problem of sphincteric incompetence is corrected surgically and persistent urge incontinence remains. Persistant urge incontinence after surgical correction of sphincteric incompetence is one of the most perplexing outcomes of surgical management of incontinence in older women. Generally, an adequate amount of time should be allowed for the patient to stabilize their bladder function after surgery. This usually will occur in 2 to 3 months after surgery. If urge incontinence persists, a consideration at that point is to completely reevaluate the patient in every aspect. If sphincteric incompetence has been corrected and an elevated residual urine volume is not a factor, involuntary detrusor contractions are almost always the cause of the incontinence.

Management of postoperative urinary incontinence in elderly women resulting from involuntary detrusor contractions is an extremely difficult problem. Because this problem responds so poorly to treatment, it may be a consideration to use behavioral therapy, pharmacologic therapy, and electrical stimulation simultaneously in these patients. Behavioral therapy can include pelvic muscle exercises, biofeedback, and prompted voiding. Generally, prompted voiding and pelvic muscle exercises can be used simultaneously. Pharmacologic therapy has a major limitation in older people of drug side effects. However, with the use of multiple drugs at low doses, the side effects can be minimized and the efficacy often can be used. Electrical stimulation is probably easiest done using a transcutaneous electrical nerve stimulation unit (TENS) with surface electrodes placed at the S2 dermatome. A physician can develop a working relationship with a physical therapist who can apply the electrodes and teach the patient how to use the unit. The physician should encourage the patient to persist in using the unit for 2 or 3 months before considering it to be ineffective.

The surgical management of urinary incontinence in elderly women is much more complex than surgery in younger women. First, the causes of incontinence in older women are more complex. Second, the risk of surgery is greater and surgical management needs to be tailored to the health status of the patient. Finally, the postoperative problems are more difficult to manage in the elderly. The physician must be persistent in managing postoperative urine retention and postoperative irritative syndromes. Although one cannot expect the kind of surgical outcome in elderly women that is seen in younger women, surgery for incontinence in older women can be a gratifying experience for the physician and the patient with major improvement in the quality of life of the individual as long as the limitations of surgery are recognized and managed.

SUMMARY

Population studies show that America is rapidly becoming an aging society. Much of the practice of medicine related to urinary incontinence in the future will involve treatment of older women. The incidence of incontinence in older women is at least twice that of older men. The number of older women is approximately twice that of older men because of the longer survival of women. The complexity of incontinence in older women is considerably greater than incontinence in younger women. In the elderly woman, stress incontinence and urge incontinence often coexist within an individual patient and each component seems to make the other worse. The characteristics and pathophysiology of both stress and urge incontinence in the elderly woman may be somewhat different from younger women. The general health status, the mental status, and the functional status of the elderly woman are extremely important in decisions regarding the management of incontinence. Social and psychologic factors related to the environment and family are important considerations in the management of incontinence in this group. With the changing attitudes regarding health care in older people, the expectations of older women are changing, which reflects a demand for a higher quality of life. The demands of the aging population for a higher quality of life translates to a challenge for physicians to meet these desired high standards of health care for the future in an expanding group of older people that are much more difficult to achieve an excellent treatment outcome than in the younger population.

BIBLIOGRAPHY

Aging america: Trends and projections, Rockville, Md, 1987-1988, US Department of Health and Human Services, Publ. No. LR 3377 188 D 12198.

Barker JC, Mitteness LS: Nocturia in the elderly, *J Gerontol Soc Am* 28:99, 1988.

Burgio KL: Behavioral training for stress and urge incontinence in the community, *Gerontology* 36(suppl 2):36:27, 1990.

Burgio KL, Burgio LD: Behavior therapies for urinary incontinence in the elderly, *Clin Geriatr Med* 2:809, 1986.

Burgio KL, Engel BT: Biofeedback-assisted behavioral training for elderly men and women, *JAGS* 38:338, 1990.

Burns PA, Pranikoff K, Nochajski T, et al: Treatment of stress incontinence with pelvic floor exercises and biofeedback, *JAGS* 38:341, 1990.

Burton JR, Pearce KL, Burgio KL, et al: Behavioral training for urinary incontinence in elderly ambulatory patients, *JAGS* 36:693, 1988.

Constantinou CE: Resting and stress urethral pressures as a clinical guide to the mechanism of continence in the female patient, *Urol Clin North Am* 12:247, 1985.

Diokno AC, Brock BM, Brown MB, et al: Prevalence of urinary incontinence and other urological symptoms in the noninstitutionalized elderly, *J Urol* 136:1022, 1986.

Ehrman JS: Correspondence from Washington, use of biofeedback to treat incontinence, *J Am Geriatr Soc* 31:182, 1983.

Engel BT, Burgio LD, McCormick KA, et al: Behavioral treatment of incontinence in the long-term care setting, *JAGS* 38:361, 1990.

Fall M: Does electrostimulation cure urinary incontinence, *J Urol* 131:664, 1984.

Ferguson KL, McKey PL, Bishop KR, et al: Stress urinary incontinence: effect of pelvic muscle exercise, *Obstet Gynecol* 75(4):671, 1990.

Fossburg E, Sorensen S, Ruutu M, et al: Maximal electrical stimulation in the treatment of unstable detrusor and urge incontinence, *Eur Urol* 18:120, 1990.

Hu T-W, Igou JF, Kaltreider L, et al: A clinical trial of a behavioral therapy to reduce urinary incontinence in nursing homes, *JAMA* 261(18):2656, 1989.

Janez J, Plevnik S, Vrtacnik P: Maximal electrical stimulation for female urinary incontinence. In Zinner N, Sterling A, editors: *Female Incontinence* New York, 1981, Alan R Liss.

Kegel AH: Progressive resistance exercise in the functional restoration of the perineal muscles, *Am J Obstet Gynecol* 56(2):238, 1948.

Kegel AH: Physiologic therapy for urinary stress incontinence, *JAMA* 146(10):915, 1951.

Kegel AH: Stress incontinence of urine in women: physiologic treatment, *J Int Coll Surg* 25(4):487, 1956.

McGuire EJ: Urinary dysfunction in the aged: neurological considerations, *Bull NY Acad Med* 56:275, 1980.

McGuire EJ, Shi-Chun Z, Horwinski ER, et al: Treatment of motor and sensory detrusor instability by electrical stimulation, *J Urol* 129:78, 1983.

McGuire EJ: Urinary incontinence in the elderly, *J Arkansas Med Soc* 81:640, 1985.

McGuire EJ: Identifying and managing stress incontinence in the elderly, *Geriatrics* 45(6):44, 1990.

Mitteness LS: The management of urinary incontinence by community-living elderly, *The Gerontologist* 27(2):185, 1987.

O'Donnell PD: The pathophysiology of urinary incontinence in the elderly. In Lytton B et al, editors: *Advances in urology*, Chicago, 1991, Mosby–Year Book.

O'Donnell PD: Combined Raz urethral suspension and McGuire pubovaginal sling for treatment of complicated stress urinary incontinence, *J Arkansas Med Soc* 88(8):389, 1992.

O'Donnell PD: The continence interval in elderly incontinent men, *Neurourol Urodyn* 8:1, 1989.

O'Donnell PD, Beck CM, Finkbeiner AE: Incontinence volume measurements in elderly inpatient men, *J Urol* 33(6):499, 1990.

O'Donnell PD, Beck CM: Incontinence volume patterns in elderly inpatient men, *J Urol* 38(2):128, 1991.

O'Donnell PD, Calandro V: Incontinence management scale in elderly inpatient men, *J Urol* 37(3):220-223, 1991.

O'Donnell PD, Beck CM, Walls RC: Serial incontinence assessment in elderly inpatient men, *J Rehab Res Dev* 27(1):1, 1990.

O'Donnell PD, Doyle R: Biofeedback therapy technique for treatment of urinary incontinence, *J Urol* 37(5):432, 1991.

O'Donnell PD, Hannish H: Telemetric electromyographic monitoring in elderly inpatient men, *Neurourol Urodyn* 11(2):115, 1992.

Plevnik S, Janez J: Maximal electrical stimulation for urinary incontinence, *J Urol* 14(6):639, 1979.

Resnick NM, Yalla SV, Laurino E: Urinary incontinence among elderly persons, *N Engl J Med* 320:1421, 1989.

Schnelle JF, Traughber B, Sowell VA, et al: Prompted voiding treatment of urinary incontinence in nursing homes patients, *JAGS* 37:1051, 1989.

Schnelle JF: Treatment of urinary incontinence in nursing home patients by prompted voiding, *JAGS* 38:356, 1990.

Taylor K, Henderson J: Effects of biofeedback and urinary stress incontinence in older women, *J Gerontol Nurs* 12(9):25, 1986.

Urinary incontinence in adults: *National Institutes of Health Consensus Development Conference Statement* 7:1, 1988.

Wells TJ, Brink CA, Diokno AC, et al: Pelvic muscle exercise for stress urinary incontinence in elderly women, *JAGS* 39:785, 1991.

Woodside JR: Stress urinary incontinence in men, *J Urol* 128:1246, 1982.

CHAPTER **29**

Bladder Drainage and Urinary Protective Methods

Carmen J. Sultana

Bladder Drainage
  Transurethral catheterization
  Suprapubic catheterization
  Intermittent self-catheterization
  General catheter care
  Catheter and drainage bag management
Urine Loss Appliances
  Pads and pants
  External collecting devices

Short- or long-term bladder drainage is required in a variety of situations. Patients with areflexic bladders, voiding dysfunction, or intractable incontinence may require indwelling or intermittent catheterization for long-term management. Postoperative urinary retention may be managed over the short term with similar techniques.

Long-term use of indwelling catheters can lead to infection and reduced bladder capacity; in incontinent patients who fail treatment and in whom urinary diversion is not used, protective garments and urinary loss appliances are helpful. They may be preferable when treatment is more risky or objectionable to the patient than is continued leaking. This chapter discusses three catheterization methods—transurethral catheterization, suprapubic catheterization and inter-

mittent self-catheterization—as well as various types of incontinence devices and protective garments.

BLADDER DRAINAGE

The gynecologist most often encounters the need for bladder drainage in patients after surgery for genuine stress incontinence or severe pelvic prolapse. These procedures commonly increase urethral resistance to flow and place the patient at risk for postoperative retention requiring prolonged bladder drainage. The risk of this complication after vaginal and retropubic procedures ranges from 3% to 25% and may be substantially higher for suburethral sling procedures. Adequate postoperative bladder drainage is important because overdistention may lead to postoperative infection and difficulty in resuming normal voiding. Bladder drainage can be accomplished by transurethral and suprapubic catheters and by intermittent self-catheterization.

Transurethral Catheterization

The first self-retaining transurethral catheter was described in 1937 by Foley. A saline-inflated intravesical balloon holds the catheter in place. The ease of insertion of the Foley catheter has led to its use in a variety of situations where bladder drainage or monitoring of urine output is required. It is commonly used after many gynecologic procedures.

A major difficulty with long-term use of transurethral drainage is the potential for infection. Bacterial colonization of even a closed system is unavoidable, with a rate of 5% to 10% per day. Prophylactic antibiotics do not prevent bacteriuria or cystitis in the presence of a catheter, although they may postpone their onset. Other problems with prolonged use of transurethral catheters include periurethral discomfort and irritation of the trigone, against which the balloon rests. Once the catheter is removed, repeated catheterization will be required if the patient fails to void spontaneously. These drawbacks have led to the widespread use of alternatives, such as suprapubic catheters, after incontinence procedures.

The major gynecologic indications for use of a transurethral Foley catheter are bladder drainage after operative procedures with little or no involvement of the urethra (such as vaginal hysterectomy). It can also be used when the need for drainage is expected to be less than 5 days or for a short time before beginning intermittent self-catheterization.

The mini-catheter, as advocated by O'Leary and O'Leary, is a variation on transurethral drainage, which has not been widely used. It is an 8 to 10 French plastic catheter that is sutured to the urethral meatus. The small diameter permits voiding around the catheter and causes less urethral irritation.

Suprapubic Catheterization

Hodgkinson and Hodari demonstrated a lower incidence of bacteriuria and shorter time to reestablish normal voiding with suprapubic bladder drainage, compared to transurethral drainage, after surgical procedures for incontinence. Other studies have supported these findings. Suprapubic catheters also improve patient comfort and ease of nursing care. They allow patients to control voiding trials, and they avoid the need for repeated transurethral catheterization to check postvoid residual urine volumes.

The disadvantages of suprapubic catheterization include infection, although to a lesser degree than transurethral drainage; leakage around the catheter; and reduced bladder capacity with prolonged use. Urinary deposits and blood clots may obstruct the smaller-caliber catheters, necessitating frequent irrigation.

TABLE 29-1   Types of suprapubic catheters and self-catheterization catheters

Name	Catheter type and size	Procedure	Manufacturer
Bonanno	Loop; 14 gauge	Inserted over a needle obturator	Becton Dickinson, Rutherford, NJ
Argyle-Ingram	Balloon; 12, 16F	Inserted over a needle obturator	Sherwood Med Co, St Louis, Mo
Stamey	Malecot; 10, 12, 14, 16F Loop; 8, 10, 12, 14F	Inserted over a needle obturator	Cook Urological Inc, Spencer, Ind
Sof-flex	Loop; 10, 12, 14F	Inserted over a needle obturator	Cook Urological Inc, Spencer, Ind
Rutner	Balloon; 10, 12, 16F	Inserted over a needle obturator	Cook Urological Inc, Spencer, Ind
Pigtail suprapubic	Pigtail; 7F	Inserted through a needle cannula	Cook Urological Inc, Spencer, Ind
Cystocath	Straight; 8F	Inserted through a cannula and trocar	Dow Corning, Midland, Mich
Robertson	Loop; 15F	Inserted through a transurethral trocar	Mentor Corp, Goleta, Calif
Self-cath	5 to 18F	—	Mentor Corp, Santa Barbara, Calif

The invasive nature of insertion can lead to rare complications such as hematuria, cellulitis, bowel injury, urine extravasation, and catheter fracture. Despite these potential problems, suprapubic catheters are preferred to transurethral catheters when prolonged drainage is anticipated or when significant dissection around the urethra has been performed.

The major catheter types available are listed in Table 29-1 and shown in Fig. 29-1. All are refinements of the original catheter used by Hodgkinson and Hodari and are inserted through a sharp trocar cannula or over a needle obturator. A Foley catheter introduced through a Robertson cystotrocar also can be used.

Suprapubic catheters can be inserted using either an open or closed technique. Cystotomy into the bladder dome under direct visualization at the end of a retropubic procedure is the safest method. It is preferred when distention of the bladder is difficult, when gross hematuria is present, when there has been a recent cystotomy, or in the presence of malignancy. Any of the catheter types listed in Table 29-1, as well as a Foley catheter, can be used for open cystotomy. The catheter is brought out alongside the incision through a second skin puncture and sutured in place.

Percutaneous or closed insertion also can be performed using a variety of catheters. In addition to the catheter types listed in Table 29-1, insertion of a Foley catheter by using a peel-away sheath and guide wire (Cook Urological, Spencer, Ind) has been reported by O'Brien. To insert a catheter percutaneously, the sur-

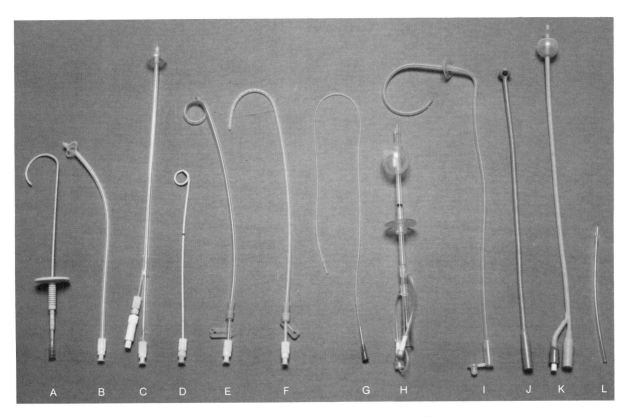

Fig. 29-1 Suprapubic and self-catheterization bladder drainage catheters. **A**, Bonanno, 14 gauge. **B**, Stamey Malecot, 12 or 14F. **C**, Rutner balloon, 16F. **D**, Pigtail, 7F. **E**, Sof-flex loop, 14F. **F**, Stamey loop, 12F. **G**, Cystocath, 8F. **H**, Argyle-Ingram, 12 or 16F. **I**, Robertson, 15F. **J**, Malecot. **K**, Foley. **L**, Mentor Self-Cath, 14F. *(From Hurt WG:* Obstet Gynecol Rep *2:307, 1990.)*

geon should place the patient in the Trendelenburg position and fill the bladder through a transurethral catheter with at least 500 ml of sterile saline or water until the bladder is easily palpable abdominally. This positioning will help ensure that no bowel lies between the bladder and the anterior abdominal wall. After the usual skin prepping, the needle or trocar should be inserted through the skin and fascia into the bladder, at a point no more than 3 cm above the pubic symphysis and at an angle directed downward toward the pubic symphysis (Fig. 29-2, *A*). The trocar or needle is removed (Fig. 29-2, *B*), and the catheter secured. The transurethral catheter is then removed.

A third method of suprapubic insertion of a Foley or Malecot catheter is to insert a perforated urethral sound transurethrally into the bladder. The tip of the sound is directed anteriorly, and the bladder dome and abdominal wall are tented upward by the sound (Fig. 29-3, *A*). An abdominal incision is made into the bladder at this site. The catheter is sutured to the sound and pulled backward to the urethral meatus, where the suture is removed (Fig. 29-3, *B*). The balloon is then inflated after the catheter is withdrawn into the bladder.

Intermittent Self-Catheterization

The technique of clean, intermittent self-catheterization (ISC) was evaluated initially by Lapides in patients with incontinence or voiding dysfunction because of neurogenic bladder disease. ISC allows the patient to insert a short plastic catheter, such as a 14 French Self-Cath catheter (Mentor Corp, Santa Barbara, Calif) into the urethra as needed to empty the bladder.

The rationale for nonsterile, clean ISC is based on the theory that functional abnormalities of the lower urinary tract lead to infection. Decreased blood flow, resulting from overdistention, is cited as one of the most common causes. The benefits of eliminating overdistention outweigh the disadvantages of intermittent insertion of a nonsterile catheter. Although Kass and Schneiderman have stated that each catheterization event carries a 3% to 4% infection rate, clinical studies of ISC have shown its safety with long-term follow-up of 255 children with neurogenic bladder dysfunction. Ninety percent of these children were

---

Instructions to Patient on Intermittent Self-Catheterization

1. Wash your hands with soap and water.
2. Use a clean (soap and water) catheter, with water-soluble lubricant if needed.
3. Attempt to empty your bladder before catheterization
4. Position yourself lying in bed or straddling a toilet.
5. Spread the labia with the fourth and index fingers of one hand, and use the middle finger to locate the urethra.
6. Insert the catheter 1 to 2 inches, and drain until all urine flow stops.
7. Measure and record the amount of urine ("residual") obtained.

---

free of major kidney infection after 10 years, despite a 56% rate of intermittent bacteriuria. Since then, ISC has been evaluated in patients with spinal cord injury and multiple sclerosis. Elderly persons have experienced low infection rates (one per 8 months) with ISC. The complication rate for postoperative use of ISC should be even lower because it is seldom used longer than 6 weeks.

ISC can be started in the immediate postoperative period, usually the second postoperative day. A Foley catheter can be used for the first 24 hours. To use ISC the patient must have the manual dexterity and mental ability to perform catheterization. The bladder capacity should be at least 100 ml. Complications other than infection are rare; they include retention of the catheter and perforation of the urethra to create a false passage.

The technique of ISC can be taught to patients preoperatively or postoperatively by direct demonstration (Fig. 29-4) (see box above). The patient should be supplied with a device to measure urine and with short plastic or rubber catheters. She should be instructed to carry them with her at all times, with separate containers for clean and used catheters. Sterile catheters are not required. Home sterilization with a microwave oven has been described, but whether this technique will be of any clinical significance in preventing bacteriuria and infection remains to be

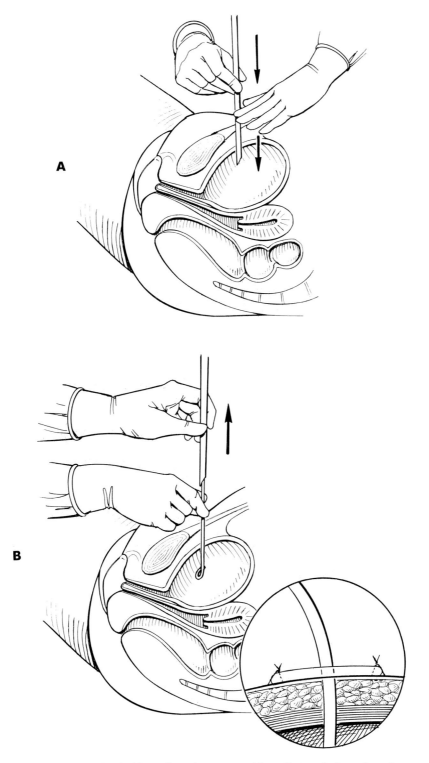

Fig. 29-2 Typical method of insertion of a suprapubic catheter. **A**, Insertion of suprapubic Cystocath catheter via trochar. **B**, Withdrawal of trochar. *Inset*, Catheter sutured to skin.

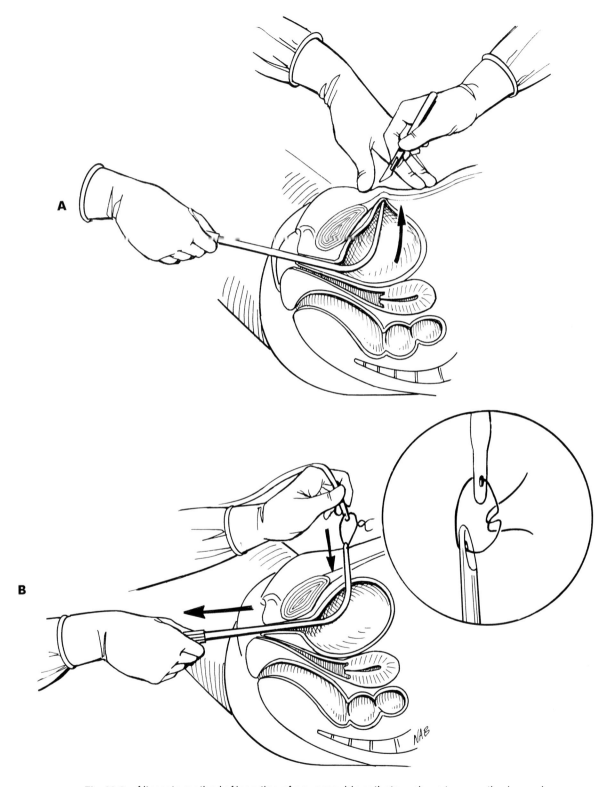

Fig. 29-3 Alternate method of insertion of a suprapubic catheter using a transurethral sound. **A**, Tenting of abdominal wall in preparation for incision. **B**, Pulling catheter into bladder. *Inset*, Demonstration of temporary suture.

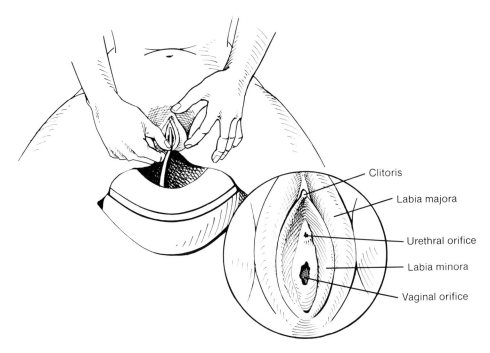

Fig. 29-4   Illustration of self-catheterization for patient instruction.

studied. Catheterization can be performed anywhere, and the importance of emptying the bladder frequently enough to keep the urine volumes obtained less than 300 ml should be stressed to the patient.

Most patients catheterize every 3 to 4 hours and then as needed during the night. The need to catheterize should take priority over the availability of soap and water. The urethra does not need to be cleansed before catheterization. Voiding should be attempted before every catheterization, and the residual urine volume measured and recorded, if possible. When residual volumes are consistently less than 20% of the total voided volume, ISC can be stopped. Prophylactic antibiotics can be given, if desired, for short periods of ISC, although equivocal benefit has been shown in patients using ISC for a long time.

General Catheter Care

A Foley catheter inserted transurethrally after uncomplicated surgical procedures can be removed on the first postoperative day. If the patient has difficulty voiding, intermittent catheterization can be used until normal voiding is established. Bladder training (i.e., intermittent clamping and unclamping of the catheter without voiding attempts) does not decrease the time required to reestablish normal voiding.

When a suprapubic catheter is used, the patient should drink at least 2 liters of fluid per day. Some hematuria on the first day is common. Narrow-diameter catheters may require periodic irrigation to remove blood clots. The catheter is left to straight drainage until the second or third postoperative day. It should be clamped in the morning, and the patient allowed to void with the catheter clamped at least every 2 to 4 hours. If the patient cannot void, the clamp is opened, the bladder drained, and the catheter reclamped until the next voiding trial. If the patient seems to be voiding well, a postvoid residual urine volume can be obtained by unclamping the tube for 15 minutes after a voiding episode and measuring the amount of urine obtained. When the residual volume is less than 20% of the total voided volume, the catheter can be removed or clamped overnight and removed the next day. If voiding trials are unsuccessful, the patient should be discharged with the catheter and given written instructions to continue the voiding trials at home.

Catheter and Drainage Bag Management

In general, care of the drainage bag is similar for both suprapubic and transurethral catheters. To prevent ascending infection, disconnection of the catheter and bag should be avoided. A bag with a urometer helps to break the urine column between the bag and catheter. The bag should be below the level of the bladder at all times, and the drainage port should be kept clean. Prophylactic antibiotics are of no benefit in preventing colonization of the system.

URINE LOSS APPLIANCES

Pads and Pants

Patients whose incontinence is not correctable with bladder training, medical therapy, or surgical therapy or patients who simply would rather use protective undergarments have a variety of choices. These options range from shields resembling ordinary sanitary pads to disposable briefs to washable garments designed to hold pads. The accompanying box lists the types and brands available in the United States.

Several different brands of disposable shields have become available in recent years. These are shaped like sanitary pads but contain a powder (such as sodium polyacrylate) that absorbs liquid to form a gel, thus preventing clothing wetness. They are available in different absorbencies and are ideal for patients who experience small amounts of urine loss (for example, only with severe exercise). Specially made, reusable panties that will hold disposable pads or shields snugly against the perineum are available.

Disposable fitted briefs are suitable for moderate to heavy leaking and are available in a variety of absorbencies. Undergarments are less bulky than fitted briefs because they do not wrap around the hips. They are held in place with front-to-back reusable elastic straps. For severe incontinence, rubber and vinyl panties to wear over regular panties, as well as reusable, washable absorbent panties with waterproof outer barriers are available.

Types of Urine Loss Appliances

Shields

Serenity Guards (Johnson & Johnson, McNeil-PPC Inc, Milltown, NJ)
Depends (Kimberly-Clark, Neenah, Wis)
Tranquility (Principle Business Enterprises, Dunbridge, Ohio)
Suretys (ICD Products, Inc, King of Prussia, Pa)

Undergarments/briefs

Depends (Kimberly-Clark)
Attends (Proctor & Gamble, Cincinnati, Ohio)
Tranquility (Principle Business Enterprises)
Suretys (ICD Products, Inc)
Promise (Scott Paper Co, Philadelphia, Pa)
Comply (Duraline Medical Products, Leipsic, Ohio)

Pad and pants systems

Tranquility (Principle Business Enterprises)
Suretys (ICD Products, Inc)
Promise (Scott Paper Co)
Dignity (Humanicare International, North Brunswick, NJ)

Rubberized garments

Priva (Med-I-Pant, Inc, Champlain, NY)

External Collecting Devices

Attempts at creating devices to control female incontinence that could be worn like a male condom catheter have come and gone. In 1981, the British Science Research Council concluded that there was no satisfactory, commercially available external urinary incontinence device for women. Female anatomy poses many problems that need to be solved to create such a device. These problems include securing the device against the vulva with minimal skin irritation, making application and cleaning easy, fitting for different body types, and minimizing leaking.

In a recent review by Pieper et al, the following attempts at creating external collecting devices were noted. In 1971, Crowley et al described a vestibulovaginal device that used a suction developed by the drainage of urine. A device introduced in 1975 used a wide, rubber-necked funnel held by straps. During the same year, Fielding and Wells described a cup with a vaginal locator that was held in place by a special panty. Unfortunately, pressure on and erosion of the vulvar soft tissue was noted.

The Misstique device (Shield Health Care Center, Inc, South Gate, Calif) was introduced in 1982 and consists of a cup held over the urethra with stoma adhesives. It had a valve to prevent urine backflow. The Femex device was similarly held with an adhesive and marketed for a short time in 1982.

In 1986, Hollister marketed an external device held in place over the urethra by a form-fitting pericup with a vaginal portion to help retain it in place (Hollister, Inc, Libertyville, Ill). The company also makes an adhesive urinary pouch that fits over the vulva. In nursing tests by Johnson et al, the device kept 49% of patients dry for 48 hours, with 14% requiring replacement for unacceptable leakage.

BIBLIOGRAPHY

Bergman A, Matthews L, Ballard CA, et al: Suprapubic vs. transurethral bladder drainage after surgery for stress urinary incontinence, *Obstet Gynecol* 69:546, 1987.

Bump RC: Prevention and management of complications following continence surgery. In Ostergard DR, Bent AE (eds): *Urogynecology and urodynamics,* ed 3, Baltimore, 1991, Wilkins & Wilkins.

Cottenden AM, Stocking B, Jones NB, et al: Biomedical engineering priorities for research in external aids, *J Biomed Eng* 3:325, 1981.

Crowley IP, Cardozo LJ, Lawrence LC: Female incontinence: a new approach, *Br J Urol* 43:492, 1971.

Fielding P, Wells T: Urinary collecting device: a clinical trial among female geriatric patients, *Nurs Times* 71:136, 1975.

Foley FEB: A self-retaining bag catheter, *J Urol* 38:140, 1937.

Harlass FE, Magelssen DJ: Benefits of posturethropexy bladder conditioning—fact or fiction? *J Reprod Med* 33:961, 1988.

Hodgkinson CP, Hodari AA: Trocar suprapubic cystotomy for postoperative bladder drainage in the female, *Am J Obstet Gynecol* 96:773, 1966.

Hurt WG: Bladder drainage after incontinence surgery, *Obstet Gynecol Rep* 2:307, 1990.

Johnson DE, Muncie HL, O'Reilly JL, et al: An external urine collection device for incontinent women—evaluation of long-term use, *J Am Geriatr Soc* 38:1016, 1990.

Kass EH, Schneiderman LJ: Entry of bacteria into the urinary tracts of patients with inlying catheters, *N Engl J Med* 256:556, 1957.

Kass EJ, Koff SA, Diokno AC, et al: The significance of bacilluria in children on long-term intermittent catheterization, *J Urol* 126:223, 1981.

Lapides J, Diokno AC, Silber SJ, et al: Clean, intermittent self-catheterization in the treatment of urinary tract disease, *J Urol* 107:458, 1972.

Lian CJ, Bracken RB: Urinary catheter sterilization with microwave oven, *Int Urogynecol J* 2:94, 1991.

Maynard FM, Diokno AC: Urinary infection and complications during clean intermittent catheterization following spinal cord injury, *J Urol* 132:943, 1984.

O'Brien WM: Percutaneous placement of a suprapubic tube with peel away sheath introducer, *J Urol* 145:1015, 1991.

O'Leary JR, O'Leary JA: The mini-catheter, a reliable in-dwelling catheter substitute, *Obstet Gynecol* 36:141, 1970.

Pieper B, Cleland V, Johnson DE, et al: Inventing urine incontinence devices for women, *Image* 21:205, 1989.

Pierson CA: Pad testing, nursing interventions, and urine loss appliances. In Ostergard DR, Bent AE (eds): *Urogynecology and urodynamics,* ed 3, Baltimore, 1991, Wilkins & Wilkins.

Segal AI, Corlett RC: Postoperative bladder training, *Am J Obstet Gynecol* 133:366, 1979.

Terpenning MS, Allada RA, Kauffman CA: Intermittent urethral catheterization in the elderly, *J Am Geriatr Soc* 37:411, 1989.

Warren JW: Catheter-associated urinary tract infections, *Infect Dis Clin North Am* 1:823, 1987.

Webb RJ, Lawson AL, Neal DE: Clean intermittent self-catheterization in 172 adults, *Br J Urol* 65:20, 1990.

Wyndaele JJ, Maes D: Clean intermittent self-catheterization: a 12-year follow-up, *J Urol* 143:906, 1990.

APPENDIX: The Standardisation of Terminology of Lower Urinary Tract Function Recommended by the International Continence Society

CONTENTS

1. Introduction
2. Clinical Assessment
   2.1 History
   2.2 Frequency/volume chart
   2.3 Physical examination
3. Procedures related to the evaluation of urine storage
   3.1 Cystometry
   3.2 Urethral pressure measurement
   3.3 Quantification of urine loss
4. Procedures related to the evaluation of micturition
   4.1 Measurement of urine flow
   4.2 Bladder pressure measurements during micturition
   4.3 Pressure flow relationships
   4.4 Urethral pressure measurements during micturition
   4.5 Residual urine
5. Procedures related to the neurophysiological evaluation of the urinary tract during filling and voiding
   5.1 Electromyography
   5.2 EMG findings
   5.3 Nerve conduction studies
   5.4 Reflex latencies
   5.5 Evoked responses
   5.6 Sensory testing
6. Classification of lower urinary tract dysfunction
   6.1 The storage phase
   6.2 Bladder capacity
   6.3 The voiding phase
7. Units of measurement
8. Symbols

1. INTRODUCTION

The International Continence Society (ICS) established a committee for the standardisation of terminology of lower urinary tract function in 1973. Five of the six reports from this committee, approved by the Society, have been published (1-5). The fifth report on "Quantification of urine loss" was an internal ICS document but appears, in part, in this document.

These reports are revised, extended and collated in this monograph. The standards are recommended to facilitate comparison of results by investigators who use urodynamic methods. These standards are recommended not only for urodynamic investigations carried out on humans but also during animal studies. When using urodynamic studies in animals the type of any anesthesia used should be stated. It is suggested

From Abrams P, Blaivas JG, Stanton SL, Andersen JT: *Int Urogynecol J* 1:45, 1990.

that acknowledgement of these standards in written publications be indicated by a footnote to the section "Methods and Materials" or its equivalent, to read as follows: "Methods, definitions and units conform to the standards recommended by the International Continence Society, except where specifically noted."

Urodynamic studies involve the assessment of the function and dysfunction of the urinary tract by any appropriate method. Aspects of urinary tract morphology, physiology, biochemistry and hydrodynamics affect urine transport and storage. Other methods of investigation such as the radiographic visualisation of the lower urinary tract is a useful adjunct to conventional urodynamics. This monograph concerns the urodynamics of the lower urinary tract.

2. CLINICAL ASSESSMENT

The clinical assessment of patients with lower urinary tract dysfunction should consist of a detailed history, a frequency/volume chart and a physical examination. In urinary incontinence, leakage should be demonstrated objectively.

2.1 History

The general history should include questions relevant to neurological and congenital abnormalities as well as information on previous urinary infections and relevant surgery. Information must be obtained on medication with known or possible effects on the lower urinary tract. The general history should also include assessment of menstrual, sexual and bowel function, and obstetric history.

The urinary history must consist of symptoms related to both the storage and the evacuation functions of the lower urinary tract.

2.2 Frequency/Volume Chart

The frequency/volume chart is a specific urodynamic investigation recording fluid intake and urine output per 24 hour period. The chart gives objective information on the number of voidings, the distribution of voidings between daytime and nighttime and each voided volume. The chart can also be used to record episodes of urgency and leakage and the number of incontinence pads used. The frequency/volume chart is very useful in the assessment of voiding disorders, and in the follow-up of treatment.

2.3 Physical Examination

Besides a general urologic and, when appropriate, gynecologic examination, the physical examination should include the assessment of perineal sensation, the perineal reflexes supplied by the sacral segments S2-S4, and anal sphincter tone and control.

3. PROCEDURES RELATED TO THE EVALUATION OF URINE STORAGE

3.1 Cystometry

Cystometry is the method by which the pressure/volume relationship of the bladder is measured. All systems are zeroed at atmospheric pressure. For external transducers the reference point is the level of the superior edge of the symphysis pubis. For catheter mounted transducers the reference point is the transducer itself. Cystometry is used to assess detrusor activity, sensation, capacity and compliance.

Before starting to fill the bladder the residual urine may be measured. However, the removal of a large volume of residual urine may alter detrusor function especially in neuropathic disorders. Certain cystometric parameters may be significantly altered by the speed of bladder filling (See compliance, 6.2.1).

During cystometry it is taken for granted that the patient is aware, unanesthetized and neither sedated nor taking drugs that affect bladder function. Any variations should be specified.

3.1.1. General Information. The following details should be given:

1. Access (transurethral or percutaneous).
2. Fluid medium (liquid or gas).
3. Temperature of fluid (state in degrees Celsius).
4. Position of patient (e.g., supine, sitting, or standing).
5. Filling method—may be by diuresis or catheter. Filling by catheter may be continuous or incremental; the precise filling rate should be stated. When the incremental method is used the volume increment should be stated. For general discussion, the following terms for the range of filling rate may be used:

a) up to 10 ml per minute is *slow fill cystometry* ("physiological" filling).

b) 10-100 ml per minute is *medium fill cystometry*.

c) over 100 ml per minute is *rapid fill cystometry*.

3.1.2. Technical Information. The following details should be given:

1. Fluid-filled catheter—specify number of catheters, single or multiple lumens, type of catheter (manufacturer), size of catheter.
2. Catheter tip transducer—list of specifications.
3. Other catheters—list specifications.
4. Measuring equipment.

3.1.3. Definitions. Cystometric terminology is defined as follows:

Intravesical pressure is the pressure within the bladder.

Abdominal pressure is taken to be the pressure surrounding the bladder. In current practice it is estimated from rectal or, less commonly, extraperitoneal pressure.

Detrusor pressure is that component of intravesical pressure that is created by forces in the bladder wall (passive or active). It is estimated by subtracting abdominal pressure from intravesical pressure. The simultaneous measurement of abdominal pressure is essential for the interpretation of the intravesical pressure trace. However, artifacts on the detrusor pressure trace may be produced by intrinsic rectal contractions.

Bladder sensation. Sensation is difficult to evaluate because of its subjective nature. It is usually assessed by questioning the patient in relation to the fullness of the bladder during cystometry.

Commonly used descriptive terms include:

First desire to void.

Normal desire to void—defined as the feeling that leads the patient to pass urine at the next convenient moment, but voiding can be delayed if necessary.

Strong desire to void—defined as a persistent desire to void without the fear of leakage.

Urgency—defined as a strong desire to void accompanied by fear of leakage or fear of pain.

Pain (the site and character of which should be specified). Pain during bladder filling or micturition is abnormal.

The use of objective or semi-objective tests for sensory function, such as electrical threshold studies (sensory testing), is discussed under Sensory Testing (See 5.6).

The term "Capacity" must be qualified as follows:

Maximum cystometric capacity, in patients with normal sensation, is the volume at which the patient feels he/she can no longer delay micturition. In the absence of sensation the maximum cystometric capacity cannot be defined in the same terms and is the volume at which the clinician decides to terminate filling. In the presence of sphincter incompetence the maximum cystometric capacity may be significantly increased by occlusion of the urethra e.g. by Foley catheter.

The *functional bladder capacity,* or voided volume, is more relevant and is assessed from a frequency/volume chart (urinary diary).

The *maximum (anesthetic) bladder capacity* is the volume measured after filling during a deep general or spinal/epidural anaesthetic, specifying fluid temperature, filling pressure, and filling time.

Compliance indicates the change in volume for a change in pressure. Compliance is calculated by dividing the volume change (ΔV) by the change in detrusor pressure (ΔP_{det}) during that change in bladder volume ($C = \Delta V / \Delta P_{det}$). Compliance is expressed as milliliters per centimeters of water pressure. (See also Compliance, 6.2.1).

3.2. Urethral Pressure Measurement

It should be noted that the urethral pressure and the urethral closure pressure are idealised concepts which represent the ability of the urethra to prevent leakage (See Urinary Incontinence, 6.2.3). In current urodynamic practice the urethral pressure is measured by a number of different techniques which do not always yield consistent values. Not only do the values differ with the method of measurement but there is often lack of consistency for a single method. For example the effect of catheter rotation when urethral pressure is measured by a catheter mounted transducer.

Intraluminal urethral pressure may be measured:

At rest, with the bladder at any given volume
During coughing or straining
During the process of voiding (See section on voiding urethral pressure profile, 4.4)

Measurements may be made of one point in the urethra over a period of time, or at several points along the urethra consecutively forming a *urethral pressure profile* (UPP).

Two types of UPP may be measured in the *storage phase:*

1. Resting urethral pressure profile—with the bladder and subject at rest.
2. Stress urethral pressure profile—with a defined applied stress (e.g., cough, strain, valsalva).

In the storage phase the *urethral pressure profile* denotes the intraluminal pressure along the length of the urethra. All systems are zeroed at atmospheric pressure. All systems are zeroed at atmospheric pressure. For external transducers the reference point is the superior edge of the symphysis pubis. For catheter mounted transducers the reference point is the transducer itself. Intravesical pressure should be measured to exclude a simultaneous detrusor contraction. The subtraction of intravesical pressure from urethral pressure produces the *urethal closure pressure profile.*

The simultaneous recording of both intravesical and intra-urethral pressures are essential during stress urethral profilometry.

3.2.1 *General Information.* The following details should be given:

1. Infusion medium (liquid or gas).
2. Rate of infusion.
3. Stationary, continuous or intermittent withdrawal.
4. Rate of withdrawal.
5. Bladder volume.
6. Position of patient (supine, sitting or standing).

3.2.2. *Technical Information.* The following details should be given:

1. Open catheter—specify type (manufacturer), size, number, position and orientation of side or end hole.
2. Catheter mounted transducers—specify manufacturer, number of transducers, spacing of transducers along the catheter, orientation with respect to one another; transducer design, e.g., transducer face depressed or flush with catheter surface; catheter diameter and material. The orientation of the transducer(s) in the urethra should be stated.
3. Other catheters, e.g., membrane, fiberoptic—Specify type (manufacturer), size, and number of channels as for microtransducer catheter.
4. Measurement technique: For stress profiles the particular stress employed should be stated, e.g., cough or valsalva.
5. Recording apparatus: Describe type of recording apparatus. The frequency response of the total system should be stated. The frequency response of the catheter in the perfusion method can be assessed by blocking the eyeholes and recording the consequent rate of change of pressure.

3.2.3. *Definitions.* Terminology referring to profiles measured in storage phase (See Fig. 1) is defined as follows:

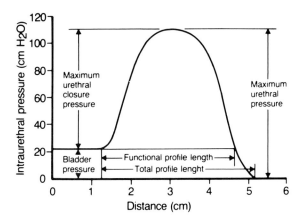

Fig. 1 Diagram of a female urethral pressure profile (static) with ICS recommended nomenclature.

Maximum urethral pressure is the maximum pressure of the measured profile.

Maximum urethral closure pressure is the maximum difference between the urethral pressure and the intravesical pressure.

Functional profile length is the length of the urethra along which the urethral pressure exceeds intravesical pressure.

Functional profile length (on stress) is the length over which the urethral pressure exceeds the intravesical pressure on stress.

Pressure transmission ratio is the increment in urethral pressure on stress as a percentage of the simultaneously recorded increment in intravesical pressure. For stress profiles obtained during coughing, pressure transmission ratios can be obtained at any point along the urethra. If single values are given the position in the urethra should be stated. If several pressure transmission ratios are defined at different points along the urethra a pressure "transmission" profile is obtained. During "cough profiles" the amplitude of the cough should be stated if possible. *Note:* The term "transmission" is in common usage and cannot be changed. However transmission implies a completely passive process. Such an assumption is not yet justified by scientific evidence. A role for muscular activity cannot be excluded.

Total profile length is not generally regarded as a useful parameter.

The information gained from urethral pressure measurements in the storage phase is of limited value in the assessment of voiding disorders.

3.3. Quantification of Urine Loss

Subjective grading of incontinence may not indicate reliably the degree of abnormality. However it is important to relate the management of the individual patients to their complaints and personal circumstances, as well as to objective measurements.

In order to assess and compare the results of the treatment of different types of incontinence in different centres, a simple standard test can be used to measure urine loss objectively in any subject. In order to obtain a representative result, especially in subjects with variable or intermittent urinary incontinence, the test should occupy as long a period as possible; yet it

must be practical. The circumstances should approximate to those of everyday life, yet be similar for all subjects to allow meaningful comparison. On the basis of pilot studies performed in various centres, an internal report of the ICS (5th) recommended a test occupying a one-hour period during which a series of standard activities was carried out. This test *can* be extended by further one hour periods if the result of the first one hour test was not considered representative by either the patient or the investigator. Alternatively the test can be repeated having filled the bladder to a defined volume.

The total amount of urine lost during the test period is determined by weighing a collecting device such as a nappy, absorbent pad or condom appliance. A nappy or pad should be worn inside waterproof underpants or should have a waterproof backing. Care should be taken to use a collecting device of adequate capacity. Immediately before the test begins the collecting device is weighed to the nearest gram.

3.3.1. *Typical Test Schedule*

1. Test is started without the patient voiding.
2. Preweighed collecting device is put on and first one hour test period begins.
3. Subject drinks 500 ml sodium-free liquid within a short period (max. 15 min), then sits or rests.
4. Half-hour period: subject walks, including stair climbing equivalent to one flight up and down.
5. During the remaining period the subject performs the following activities:
   a) Standing up from sitting, 10 times.
   b) Coughing vigorously, 10 times.
   c) Running on the spot for 1 min.
   d) Bending to pick up small object from floor, 5 times.
   e) Wash hands in running water for 1 min.
6. At the end of the one hour test the collecting device is removed and weighed.
7. If the test is regarded as representative the subject voids and the volume is recorded.
8. Otherwise the test is repeated preferably without voiding.

If the collecting device becomes saturated or filled during the test it should be removed and weighed, and replaced by a fresh device. The total weight of urine lost during the test period is taken to be equal to the gain in weight of the collecting device(s). In interpreting the results of the test it should be born in mind that a weight gain of up to 1 gram may be due to weighing errors, sweating or vaginal discharge.

The activity programme may be modified according to the subject's physical ability. If substantial variations from the usual test schedule occur, this should be recorded so that the same schedule can be used on subsequent occasions.

In principle the subject should not void during the test period. If the patient experiences urgency, then he/she should be persuaded to postpone voiding and to perform as many of the activities in section (e) as possible in order to detect leakage. Before voiding the collection device is removed for weighing. If inevitable voiding cannot be postponed then the test is terminated. The voided volume and the duration of the test should be recorded. For subjects not completing the full test the results may require separate analysis, or the test may be repeated after rehydration.

The test result is given as grams urine lost in the 1-hour test period in which the greatest urine loss is recorded.

3.3.2. Additional Procedures. Provided that there is no interference with the basic test, additional procedures intended to give information of diagnostic value are permissible. For example, additional changes and weighing of the collecting device can give information about the timing of urine loss; the absorbent nappy may be an electronic recording nappy so that the timing is recorded directly.

3.3.3. Presentation of Results. The following details should be given:

1. Collecting device
2. Physical condition of subject (ambulant, chairbound, bedridden)
3. Relevant medical conditions of subject
4. Relevant drug treatments
5. Test schedule

In some situations the timing of the test (e.g., in relation to the menstrual cycle) may be relevant.

Findings: Record weight of urine lost during the test (in the case of repeated tests, greatest weight in any stated period). A loss of less than one gram is within experimental error and the patients should be regarded as essentially dry. Urine loss should be measured and recorded in grams.

Statistics: When performing statistical analysis of urine loss in a group of subjects, non-parametric statistics should be employed, since the values are not normally distributed.

4. PROCEDURES RELATED TO THE EVALUATION OF MICTURITION

4.1. Measurement of Urinary Flow

Urinary flow may be described in terms of *rate* and *pattern* and may be *continuous* or *intermittent*. *Flow rate* is defined as the volume of fluid expelled via the urethra per unit time. It is expressed in ml/s.

4.1.1. General Information. The following details should be given:

1. Voided volume.
2. Patient environment and position (supine, sitting, or standing).
3. Filling:
   a) By diuresis (spontaneous or forced: specify regimen).
   b) By catheter (transurethral or suprapubic).
4. Type of fluid.

4.1.2. Technical Information. The following details should be given:

1. Measuring equipment.
2. Solitary procedure or combined with other measurements.

4.1.3. Definitions. The terminology referring to urinary flow is defined as follows:

1. *Continuous flow* (Fig. 2):
   Voided volume is the total volume expelled via the urethra.
   Maximum flow rate is the maximum measured value of the flow rate.
   Average flow rate is voided volume divided by flow

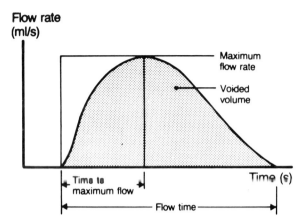

Fig. 2 Diagram of a continuous urine flow recording with ICS recommended nomenclature.

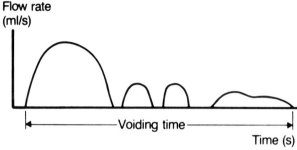

Fig. 3 Diagram of an interrupted urine flow recording with ICS recommended nomenclature.

time. The calculation of average flow rate is only meaningful if flow is continuous and without terminal dribbling.

Flow time is the time over which measurable flow actually occurs.

Time to maximum flow is the elapsed time from onset of flow to maximum flow.

The flow pattern must be described when flow time and average flow rate are measured.

2. *Intermittent flow* (Fig. 3):

The same parameters used to characterise continuous flow may be applicable if care is exercised in patients with intermittent flow. In measuring flow time the time intervals between flow episodes are disregarded.

Voiding time is total duration of micturition, i.e. includes interruptions. When voiding is completed without interruption, voiding time is equal to flow time.

4.2. Bladder Pressure Measurements During Micturition

The specifications of patient position, access for pressure measurement, catheter type and measuring equipment are as for cystometry (See 3.1).

4.2.1. Definitions. The terminology referring to bladder-pressure during micturition is defined as follows (Fig. 4):

Opening time is the elapsed time from initial rise

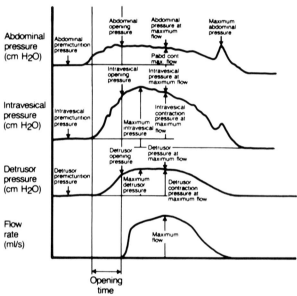

Fig. 4 Diagram of a pressure-flow recording of micturition with ICS recommended nomenclature.

in detrusor pressure to onset of flow. This is the initial isovolumetric contraction period of micturition. Time lags should be taken into account. In most urodynamic systems a time lag occurs equal to the time taken for the urine to pass from the point of pressure measurement to the uroflow transducer.

The following parameters are applicable to measurements of each of the pressure curves: intravesical, abdominal and detrusor pressure.

Premicturition pressure is the pressure recorded immediately before the initial isovolumetric contraction.

Opening pressure is the pressure recorded at the onset of measured flow.

Maximum pressure is the maximum value of the measured pressure.

Pressure at maximum flow is the pressure recorded at maximum measured flow rate.

Contraction pressure at maximum flow is the difference between pressure at maximum flow and pre-micturition pressure.

Postmicturition events (e.g., after contraction) are not well understood and so cannot be defined as yet.

4.3. Pressure Flow Relationships

In the early days of urodynamics the flow rate and voiding pressure were related as a "urethral resistance factor". The concept of a resistance factor originates from rigid tube hydrodynamics. The urethra does not generally behave as a rigid tube as it is an irregular and distensible conduit whose walls and surroundings have active and passive elements and hence, influence the flow through it. Therefore a resistance factor cannot provide a valid comparison between patients.

There are many ways of displaying the relationships between flow and pressure during micturition, an example is suggested in the ICS [3] (Fig. 5). As yet available data do not permit a standard presentation of pressure/flow parameters.

When data from a group of patients are presented, pressure-flow relationships may be shown on a graph as illustrated in Fig. 5. This form of presentation allows lines of demarcation to be drawn on the graph to separate the results according to the problem being studied. The points shown in Fig. 5 are purely illustrative to indicate how the data might fall into groups. The group of equivocal results might include either an unrepresentative micturition in an obstructed or an unobstructed patient, or underactive detrusor function with or without obstruction. This is the group which invalidates the use of "urethral resistance factors."

4.4. Urethral Pressure Measurements During Voiding

The voiding urethral pressure profile VUPP is used to determine the pressure and site of urethral obstruction. Pressure is recorded in the urethra during voiding.

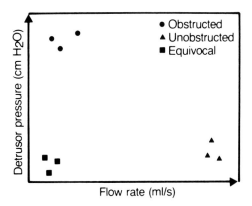

Fig. 5 Diagram illustrating the presentation of pressure flow data on individual patients in three groups of 3 patients: obstructed, equivocal, and unobstructed.

The technique is similar to that used in the UPP measured during storage (the resting and stress profiles; see 3.2.).

General and technical information should be recorded as for UPP during storage (See 3.2).

Accurate interpretation of the VUPP depends on the simultaneous measurement of intravesical pressure and the measurement of pressure at a precisely localised point in the urethra. Localisation may be achieved by radio opaque marker on the catheter which allows the pressure measurements to be related to a visualised point in the urethra. This technique is not fully developed and a number of technical as well as clinical problems need to be solved before the VUPP is widely used.

4.5. Residual Urine

Residual urine is defined as the volume of fluid remaining in the bladder immediately following the completion of micturition. The measurement of residual urine forms an integral part of the study of micturition. However voiding in unfamiliar surroundings may lead to unrepresentative results, as may voiding on command with a partially filled or overfilled bladder. Residual urine is commonly estimated by the following methods:

1. Catheter or cystoscope (transurethral, suprapubic).
2. Radiography (excretion urography, micturition cystography).

3. Ultrasonics.
4. Radioisotopes (clearance, gamma camera).

When estimating residual urine the measurement of voided volume and the time interval between voiding and residual urine estimation should be recorded: this is particularly important if the patient is in a diuretic phase. In the condition of vesicoureteric reflux, urine may re-enter the bladder after micturition and may falsely be interpreted as residual urine. The presence of urine in bladder diverticula following micturition present special problems of interpretation, since a diverticulum may be regarded either as part of the bladder cavity or as outside the functioning bladder.

The various methods of measurement each have limitations as to their applicability and accuracy in the various conditions associated with residual urine. Therefore it is necessary to choose a method appropriate to the clinical problems. The absence of residual urine is usually an observation of clinical value, but does not exclude infravesical obstruction or bladder dysfunction. An isolated finding of residual urine requires confirmation before being considered significant.

5. PROCEDURES RELATED TO NEUROPHYSIOLOGICAL EVALUATION OF THE URINARY TRACT DURING FILLING AND VOIDING

5.1. Electromyography

Electromyography (EMG) is the study of electrical potentials generated by the depolarization of muscle. The following refers to striated muscle EMG. The functional unit in EMG is the motor unit. This is comprised of a single motor neurone and the muscle fibers it innervates. A motor unit action potential is the recorded depolarization of muscle fibres which results from activation of a single anterior horn cell. Muscle action potentials may be detected either by needle electrodes, or by surface electrodes.

Needle electrodes are placed directly into the muscle mass and permit visualization of the individual motor unit action potentials.

Surface electrodes are applied to an epithelial surface as close to the muscle under study as possible. Surface electrodes detect the action potentials from groups of adjacent motor units underlying the recording surface.

EMG potentials may be displayed on an oscilloscope screen or played through audio amplifiers. A permanent record of EMG potentials can only be made using a chart recorder with a high frequency response (in the range of 10 KHz).

EMG should be interpreted in the light of the patients symptoms, physical findings and urological and urodynamic investigations.

5.1.1. General Information. The following details should be given:

1. EMG (solitary procedure, part of urodynamic or other electrophysiological investigation).
2. Patient position (supine, standing, sitting or other).
3. Electrode placement:
   a) Sampling site (intrinsic striated muscle of the urethra, periurethral striated muscle, bulbocavernosus muscle, external anal sphincter, pubococcygeus or other). State whether sites are single or multiple, unilateral or bilateral. Also state number of samples per site.
   b) Recording electrode: define the precise anatomical location of the electrode. For needle electrodes, include site of needle entry, angle of entry and needle depth. For vaginal or urethral surface electrodes state method of determining position of electrode.
   c) Reference electrode position. *Note:* ensure that there is no electrical interference with any other machines, e.g., x-ray apparatus.

5.1.2. Technical Information. The following details should be given:

1. Electrodes:
   a) Needle electrodes—design (concentric, bipolar, monopolar, single fibre, other); dimensions (length, diameter, recording area); electrode material (e.g., platinum).
   b) Surface electrodes—type (skin, plug, catheter, other); size and shape; electrode material; mode

of fixation to recording surface; conducting medium (e.g., saline, jelly).
2. Amplifier (make and specifications).
3. Signal processing (data: raw, averaged, integrated, or other).
4. Display equipment (make and specifications to include method of calibration, time base, full scale deflection in microvolts and polarity).
   a) Oscilloscope.
   b) Chart recorder.
   c) Loudspeaker.
   d) Other.
5. Storage (make and specifications)
   a) Paper.
   b) Magnetic tape recorder.
   c) Microprocessor.
   d) Other.
6. Hard copy production (make and specifications)
   a) Chart recorder.
   b) Photographic/video reproduction of oscilloscope screen.
   c) Other.

5.2. EMG Findings

5.2.1. Individual motor unit action potentials. Normal motor unit potentials have a characteristic configuration, amplitude and duration. Abnormalities of the motor unit may include an increase in the amplitude, duration and complexity of waveform (polyphasicity) of the potentials. A polyphasic potential is defined as one having more than 5 deflections. The EMG findings of fibrillations, positive sharp waves and bizarre high frequency potentials are thought to be abnormal.

5.2.2. Recruitment patterns. In normal subjects there is a gradual increase in "pelvic floor" and "sphincter" EMG activity during bladder filling. At the onset of micturition there is complete absence of activity. Any sphincter EMG activity during voiding is abnormal unless the patient is attempting to inhibit micturition. The finding of increased sphincter EMG activity, during voiding, accompanied by characteristic simultaneous detrusor pressure and flow changes is described by the term, detrusor-sphincter-dyssynergia. In this condition a detrusor contraction occurs concurrently with an in appropriate contraction of the urethral and or periurethral striated muscle.

5.3. Nerve Conduction Studies

Nerve conduction studies involve stimulation of a peripheral nerve, and recording the time taken for a response to occur in muscle, innervated by the nerve under study. The time taken from stimulation of the nerve to the response in the muscle is called the "latency." Motor latency is the time taken by the fastest motor fibres in the nerve to conduct impulses to the muscle and depends on conduction distance and the conduction velocity of the fastest fibers.

5.3.1. General Information. Also applicable to reflex latencies and evoked potentials (See below). The following details should be given:

1. Type of investigation:
   a) Nerve conduction study (e.g., pudendal nerve).
   b) Reflex latency determination (e.g., bulbocavernosus).
   c) Spinal evoked potential.
   d) Cortical evoked potential.
   e) Other.
2. Is the study a solitary procedure or part of urodynamic or neurophysiological investigations?
3. Patient position and environmental temperature, noise level and illumination.
4. Electrode placement: Define electrode placement in precise anatomical terms. The exact interelectrode distance is required for nerve conduction velocity calculations.
   a) Stimulation site (penis, clitoris, urethra, bladder neck, bladder or other).
   b) Recording sites (external anal sphincter, periurethral striated muscle, bulbocavernosus muscle, spinal cord, cerebral cortex or other).
      When recording spinal evoked responses, the sites of the recording electrodes should be specified according to the bony landmarks (e.g., L4). In cortical evoked responses the sites of the recording electrodes should be specified as in the International 10-20 system (6). The sampling techniques should be specified (single or multiple, unilateral or bilateral, ipsilateral or contralateral, or other).
   c) Reference electrode position.
   d) Grounding electrode site. Ideally this should be between the stimulation and recording sites to reduce stimulus artifact.

5.3.2. Technical Information. Also applicable to reflex latencies and evoked potential (See 5.4). The following details should be given:

1. Electrodes (make and specifications). Describe separately stimulus and recording electrodes as below:
   a) Design (e.g., needle, plate, ring, and configuration of anode and cathode where applicable).
   b) Dimensions.
   c) Electrode material (e.g., platinum).
   d) Contact medium.
2. Stimulator (make and specifications):
   a) Stimulus parameters (pulse width, frequency, pattern, current density, electrode impedance in Kohms). Also define in terms of threshold (e.g., in case of supramaximal stimulation).
3. Amplifier (make and specifications):
   a) Sensitivity (mV-μV).
   b) Filters—low pass (Hz) or high pass (kHz).
   c) Sampling time (ms).
4. Averager (make and specifications):
   a) Number of stimuli sampled.
5. Display equipment (make and specifications to include method of calibration, time base, full scale deflection in microvolts and polarity):
   a) Oscilloscope.
6. Storage (make and specifications):
   a) Paper.
   b) Magnetic tape recorder.
   c) Microprocessor.
   d) Other.
7. Hard copy production (make and specification):
   a) Chart recorder.
   b) Photographic/video reproduction of oscilloscope screen.
   c) XY recorder.
   d) Other.

5.3.3. Description of Nerve Conduction Studies. Recordings are made from muscle and latency of response of the muscle is measured. The latency is taken as the time to onset, of the earliest response.

To ensure that response time can be precisely measured, the gain should be increased to give a clearly defined takeoff point. (Gain setting at least 100 μV/div and using a short time base, e.g., 1-2 ms/div).

Additional information may be obtained from nerve conduction studies, if, when using surface electrodes to record a compound muscle action potential, the amplitude is measured. The gain setting must be reduced so that the whole response is displayed and a longer time base is recommended (e.g., 1 mV/div and 5 ms/div). Since the amplitude is proportional to the number of motor unit potentials within the vicinity of the recording electrodes, a reduction in amplitude indicates loss of motor units and therefore denervation. (*Note:* A prolongation of latency is not necessarily indicative of denervation).

5.4. Reflex Latencies

Reflex latencies require stimulation of sensory fields and recordings from the muscle which contracts reflexly in response to the stimulation. Such responses are a test of reflex arcs which are comprised of both afferent and efferent limbs and a synaptic region within the central nervous system. The reflex latency expresses the nerve conduction velocity in both limbs of the arc and the integrity of the central nervous system at the level of the synapse(s). Increased reflex latency may occur as a result of slowed afferent or efferent nerve conduction or due to central nervous system conduction delays.

5.4.1. General Information and Technical Information. The same technical and general details apply as discussed above under Nerve Conduction Studies.

5.4.2. Description of Reflex Latency Measurements. Recordings are made from muscle and the latency of response of the muscle is measured. The latency is taken as the time to onset, of the earliest response.

To ensure that response time can be precisely measured, the gain should be increased to give a clearly defined take-off point. (Gain setting at least 100 μV/div and using a short time base, e.g., 1-2 ms/div).

5.5. Evoked Responses

Evoked responses are potential changes in central nervous system neurones resulting from distant stimulation usually electrical. They are recorded using averaging techniques. Evoked responses may be used to test the integrity of peripheral, spinal and central nervous pathways. As with nerve conduction studies, the conduction time (latency) may be measured. In addition, information may be gained from the amplitude and configuration of these responses.

5.5.1. General Information and Technical Information. See above Nerve Conduction Studies (5.3).

5.5.2. Description of Evoked Responses. When describing the presence or absence of stimulus evoked responses and their configuration the following details should be given:

1. Single or multiphasic response.
2. Onset of response—defined as the start of the first reproducible potential. Since the onset of the response may be difficult to ascertain precisely, the criteria used should be stated.
3. Latency to onset—defined as the time (ms) from the onset of stimulus to the onset of response. The central conduction time relates to cortical evoked potentials and is defined as the difference between the latencies of the cortical and the spinal evoked potentials. This parameter may be used to test the integrity of the corticospinal neuraxis.
4. Latencies to peaks of positive and negative deflections in multiphasic responses (Fig. 6). P denotes positive deflections, N denotes negative deflections. In multiphasic responses, the peaks are numbered consecutively (e.g., P1, N1, P2,

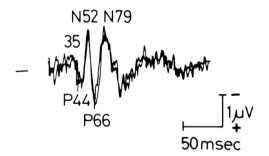

Fig. 6 Multiphasic evoked response recorded from the cerebral cortex after stimulation of the dorsal aspect of the penis. The recording shows the conventional labelling of negative (N) and positive (P) deflections with the latency of each deflection from the point of stimulation in milliseconds.

N2 . . .) or according to the latencies to peaks in milliseconds (e.g., P44, N52, P66 . . .).
5. The amplitude of the responses is measured in microvolts.

5.6. Sensory Testing

Limited information, of a subjective nature, may be obtained during cystometry by recording such parameters as the first desire to micturate, urgency or pain. However, sensory function in the lower urinary tract, can be assessed by semi-objective tests by the measurement of urethral and/or vesical sensory thresholds to a standard applied stimulus such as a known electrical current.

5.6.1. General Information. The following details should be given:

1. Patient's position (supine, sitting, standing, other)
2. Bladder volume at time of testing
3. Site of applied stimulus (intravesical, intraurethral)
4. Number of times the stimulus was applied and the response recorded. Define the sensation recorded, e.g., the first sensation or the sensation of pulsing.
5. Type of applied stimulus
   a) electrical current—is usual to use a constant current stimulator in urethral sensory measurement. State electrode characteristics and placement as in section on EMG (5.2); electrode contact area and distance between electrodes if applicable; impedance characteristics of the system; type of conductive medium used for electrode/epithelial contact. *Note: Topical anesthetic agents should not be used.* Also state stimulator make and specifications; and stimulation parameters (pulse width, frequency, pattern, duration, current density).
   b) Other (e.g., mechanical, chemical).

5.6.2. Definition of Sensory Thresholds. The vesical/urethral sensory threshold is defined as the least current which consistently produces a sensation perceived by the subject during stimulation at the site under investigation. However, the absolute values will vary in relation to the site of the stimulus, the characteristics of the equipment and the stimulation parameters. Normal values should be established for each system.

6. A CLASSIFICATION OF URINARY TRACT DYSFUNCTION

The lower urinary tract is composed of the *bladder* and *urethra*. They form a functional unit and their interaction cannot be ignored. Each has two functions, the bladder to store and void, the urethra to control and convey. When a reference is made to the hydrodynamic function or to the whole anatomical unit as a storage organ—the vesica urinaria—the correct term is the *bladder*. When the smooth muscle structure known as the m.detrusor urinae is being discussed then the correct term is *detrusor*. For simplicity the bladder/detrusor and the urethra will be considered separately so that a classification based on a combination of functional anomalies can be reached. Sensation cannot be precisely evaluated but must be assessed. This classification depends on the results of various objective urodynamic investigations. A complete urodynamic assessment is not necessary in all patients. However, studies of the filling and voiding phases are essential for each patient. As the bladder and urethra may behave differently during the storage and micturition phases of bladder function it is most useful to examine bladder and urethral activity separately in each phase.

Terms used should be objective and definable, ideally should be applicable to the whole range of abnormality. When authors disagree with the classification presented below, or use terms which have not been defined here, their meaning should be made clear.

Assuming the absence of inflammation, infection and neoplasm, *lower urinary tract dysfunction* may be caused by:

1. Disturbance of the pertinent nervous or psychological control system.
2. Disorders of muscle function.
3. Structural abnormalities.

Urodynamic diagnoses based on this classification should correlate with the patients symptoms and signs. For example the presence of an unstable contraction in an asymptomatic continent patient does not warrant a diagnosis of detrusor overactivity during storage.

6.1. The Storage Phase

6.1.1. Bladder Function During Storage. This may be described according to:

Detrusor activity
Bladder sensation
Bladder capacity
Compliance

6.1.2. Detrusor Activity. In this context detrusor activity is interpreted from the measurement of detrusor pressure (P_{det}). Detrusor activity may be:

Normal
Overactive

In Normal detrusor function the bladder volume increases without a significant rise in pressure (accommodation). No involuntary contractions occur despite provocation. A normal detrusor so defined may be described as "stable."

Overactive detrusor function is characterised by involuntary detrusor contractions during the filling phase, which may be spontaneous or provoked and which the patient cannot completely suppress. Involuntary detrusor contractions may be provoked by rapid filling, alterations of posture, coughing, walking, jumping and other triggering procedures. Various terms have been used to describe these features and they are defined as follows:

The *unstable detrusor* is one that is shown objectively to contract, spontaneously or on provocation, during the filling phase while the patient is attempting to inhibit micturition. Unstable detrusor contractions may be asymptomatic or may be interpreted as a normal desire to void. The presence of these contractions does not necessarily imply a neurological disorder. Unstable contractions are usually phasic in type (Fig. 7a). A gradual increase in detrusor pressure without subsequent decrease is best regarded as a change of compliance (Fig. 7b).

Detrusor hyperreflexia is defined as overactivity due to disturbance of the nervous control mechanisms. The term detrusor hyperreflexia should only be used when there is objective evidence of a relevant neu-

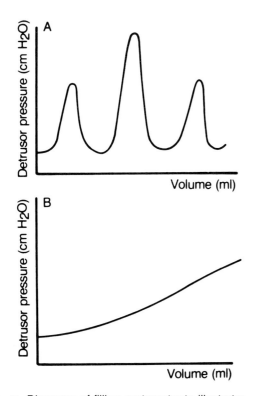

Fig. 7 Diagrams of filling cystometry to illustrate:
A: Typical phasic unstable detrusor contraction
B: The gradual increase of detrusor pressure with filling characteristic of reduced bladder compliance.

rological disorder. The use of conceptual and undefined terms such as hypertonic, systolic, uninhibited, spastic and automatic should be avoided.

6.1.3. Bladder sensation. During filling bladder sensation can be classified in qualitative terms (See 3.1) and by objective measurement (See Sensory Testing, 5.6). Sensation can be classified broadly as follows:

Normal
Increased (hypersensitive)
Reduced (hyposensitive)
Absent

6.2. Bladder Capacity. (See Cystometry, 3.1.)

6.2.1. Compliance. This is defined as: $\Delta V / \Delta p$ (See 3.1.).

Compliance may change during the cystometric examination and is variably dependent upon a number of factors including:

1. Rate of filling.
2. The part of the cystometrogram curve used for compliance calculation.
3. The volume interval over which compliance is calculated.
4. The geometry (shape) of the bladder.
5. The thickness of the bladder wall.
6. The mechanical properties of the bladder wall.
7. The contractile/relaxant properties of the detrusor.

During normal bladder filling little or no pressure change occurs and this is termed "normal compliance". However at the present time there is insufficient data to define normal, high and low compliance. When reporting compliance, specify:

1. The rate of bladder filling
2. The bladder volume at which compliance is calculated
3. The volume increment over which compliance is calculated
4. The part of the cystometrogram curve used for the calculation of compliance.

6.2.2. Urethral Function During Storage. The urethral closure mechanism during storage may be:

Normal
Incompetent

The *normal urethral closure mechanism* maintains a positive urethral closure pressure during filling even in the presence of increased abdominal pressure. Immediately prior to micturition the normal closure pressure decreases to allow flow.

An *incompetent urethral closure mechanism* is defined as one which allows leakage of urine in the absence of a detrusor contraction. Leakage may occur whenever intravesical pressure exceeds intraurethral pressure (Genuine stress incontinence) or when there is an involuntary fall in urethral pressure. Terms such as "the unstable urethra" await further data and precise definition.

6.2.3. Urinary Incontinence. This as is defined involuntary loss of urine which is objectively demonstrable and a social or hygienic problem. Loss of urine through channels other than the urethra is extraurethral incontinence.

Urinary incontinence denotes:

1. A symptom.
2. A sign.
3. A condition.

The symptom indicates the patients statement of involuntary urine loss, the sign is the objective demonstration of urine loss, and the condition is the urodynamic demonstration of urine loss.

6.2.4. Symptoms. These can be defined as follows:
Urge incontinence—the involuntary loss of urine associated with a strong desire to void (urgency). *Urgency* may be associated with two types of dysfunction:

Overactive detrusor function *(motor urgency)*
Hypersensitivity *(sensory urgency)*

Stress incontinence—the symptom indicates the patient's statement of involuntary loss of urine during physical exertion.
"Unconscious" incontinence—Incontinence may occur in the absence of urge and without conscious recognition of the urinary loss.
Enuresis—any involuntary loss of urine. If the term is used to denote incontinence during sleep, it should always be qualified with the adjective "nocturnal".
Post micturition dribble and *continuous leakage*—denote other symptomatic forms of incontinence.

6.2.5. Signs. The sign stress incontinence denotes the observation of loss of urine from the urethra synchronous with physical exertion (e.g. coughing). Incontinence may also be observed without physical exercise. Post-micturition dribble and continuous leakage denotes other signs of incontinence. Symp-

toms and signs alone may not disclose the cause of urinary incontinence. Accurate diagnosis often requires urodynamic investigation in addition to careful history and physical examination.

6.2.6. Conditions. These can be defined as follows:
Genuine stress incontinence—the involuntary loss of urine occurring when, in the absence of a detrusor contraction, the intravesical pressure exceeds the maximum urethral pressure.

Reflex incontinence—loss of urine due to detrusor hyperreflexia and/or involuntary urethral relaxation in the absence of the sensation usually associated with the desire to micturate. This condition is only seen in patients with neuropathic bladder/urethral disorders.

Overflow incontinence—any involuntary loss of urine associated with over-distension of the bladder.

6.3. The Voiding Phase

6.3.1. The Detrusor During Voiding. During micturition the detrusor may be:

Acontractile
Underactive
Normal

The acontractile detrusor is one that cannot be demonstrated to contract during urodynamic studies. *Detrusor areflexia* is defined as acontractility due to an abnormality of nervous control and denotes the complete absence of centrally coordinated contraction. In detrusor areflexia due to a lesion of the conus medullaris or sacral nerve outflow, the detrusor should be described as *decentralised*—not denervated, since the peripheral neurones remain. In such bladders pressure fluctuations of low amplitude, sometimes known as "autonomous" waves, may occasionally occur. The use of terms such as "atonic," "hypotonic," "autonomic," and "flaccid" should be avoided.

Detrusor underactivity is defined as a detrusor contraction of inadequate magnitude and/or duration to effect bladder emptying with a normal time span. Patients may have underactivity during micturition and detrusor overactivity during filling.

Normal detrusor contractility. Normal voiding is achieved by a voluntarily initiated detrusor contraction that is sustained and can usually be suppressed voluntarily. A normal detrusor contraction will effect complete bladder emptying in the absence of obstruction. For a given detrusor contraction, the magnitude of the recorded pressure rise will depend on the degree of outlet resistance.

Urethral Function During Micturition. During voiding urethral function may be:

Normal
Obstructive
    overactivity
    mechanical

Normal. The normal urethra opens to allow the bladder to be emptied.

Obstruction. This occurs when the urethral closure mechanism contracts against a detrusor contraction or fails to open at attempted micturition.

Synchronous detrusor and urethral contraction is *detrusor/urethral dyssynergia*. This diagnosis should be qualified by stating the location and type of the urethral muscles (striated or smooth) which are involved. Despite the confusion surrounding "sphincter" terminology the use of certain terms is so widespread that they are retained and defined here. The term *detrusor/external sphincter dyssynergia or detrusor-sphincter-dyssynergia (DSD)* describes a detrusor contraction concurrent with an involuntary contraction of the urethral and/or periurethral striated muscle. In the adult, detrusor sphincter dyssynergia is a feature of neurological voiding disorders. In the absence of neurological features the validity of this diagnosis should be questioned. The term *detrusor/bladder neck dyssynergia* is used to denote a detrusor contraction concurrent with an objectively demonstrated failure of bladder neck opening. No parallel term has been elaborated for possible detrusor/distal urethral (smooth muscle) dyssynergia.

Overactivity of the striated urethral sphincter may occur in the absence of detrusor contraction, and may prevent voiding. This is not detrusor/sphincter dyssynergia.

Overactivity of the urethral sphincter may occur during voiding in the absence of neurological disease and is termed *dysfunctional voiding*. The use of terms such as "non-neurogenic" or "occult neuropathic" should be avoided.

Mechanical obstruction. This is most commonly anatomical, e.g., urethral stricture.

Using the characteristics of detrusor and urethral function during storage and micturition an accurate definition of lower urinary tract behaviour in each patient becomes possible.

Summary

Using the characteristics of detrusor and urethral function during storage and micturition an accurate definition of lower urinary tract behavior in each patient becomes possible.

7. UNITS OF MEASUREMENT

In the urodynamic literature pressure is measured in cm H_2O and *not* in millimeters of mercury. When Laplace's law is used to calculate tension in the bladder wall, it is often found that pressure is then measured in dyne cm^{-2}. This lack of uniformity in the systems used leads to confusion when other parameters, which are a function of pressure, are computed, for instance, "compliance", contraction force, velocity etc. From these few examples it is evident that standardisation is essential for meaningful communication. Many journals now require that the results be given in SI Units. This section is designed to give guidance in the application of the SI system to urodynamics and defines the units involved. The principal units to be used are listed in Table 1.

8. SYMBOLS

It is often helpful to use symbols in a communication. The system in Table 2 has been devised to standardise a code of symbols for use in urodynamics. The rationale of the system is to have a basic symbol representing the physical quantity with qualifying subscripts. The list of basic symbols largely conforms to international usage. The qualifying subscripts relate to the basic symbols to commonly used urodynamic parameters.

TABLE 1   Recommended units of measurement

Quantity	Acceptable unit	Symbol
Volume	milliliter	ml
Time	second	s
Flow rate	milliliters/second	ml/s
Pressure	centimeters of water[a]	cmH_2O
Length	meters or submultiples	m, cm, mm
Velocity	meters/second or sub-multiples	m/s, cm/s
Temperature	degrees Celsius	°C

The SI Unit is the pascal (Pa), but it is only practical at present to calibrate our instruments in cm H_2O. One centimetre of water pressure is approximately equal to 100 pascals (1 cmH_2O = 98.07 Pa = 0.098 kPa).

TABLE 2   List of symbols

Basic symbols		Urologic qualifiers		Value	
Pressure	P	Bladder	ves	Maximum	max
Volume	V	Urethra	ura	Minimum	min
Flow rate	Q	Ureter	ure	Average	ave
Velocity	v	Detrusor	det	Isovolumetric	isv
Time	t	Abdomen	abd	Isotonic	ist
Temperature	T	External	ext	Isobaric	isb
Length	l	Stream	ext	Isometric	ism
Area	A				
Diameter	d				
Force	F				
Energy	E				
Power	P				
Compliance	C				
Work	W				
Energy per unit volume	e				

P_{det}, max   = maximum detrusor pressure
e_{ext} = kinetic energy per unit volume in the external stream

REFERENCES

1. Abrams P, Blaivas JG, Stanton SL et al. Sixth report on the standardisation of terminology of lower urinary tract function. Procedures related to neurophysiological investigations: Electromyography, nerve conduction studies, reflex latencies, evoked potentials and sensory testing. *World J Urol* 1986; 4:2-5; *Scand J Urol Nephrol* 1986; 20:161-164; *Br J Urol* 1987; 59:300-307.

2. Bates P, Bradley WE, Glen E et al. First report on the standardisation of terminology of lower urinary tract function. Urinary incontinence. Procedures related to the evaluation of urine storage—cystometry, urethral closure pressure profile, units of measurement. *Br J Urol* 1976; 48:39-42; *Eur Urol* 1976; 2:274-276; *Scand J Urol Nephrol* 1976; 11:193-196; *Urol Int* 1976; 32:81-87.

3. Bates P, Glen E, Griffiths D et al. Second report on the standardisation of terminology of lower urinary tract function. Procedures related to the evaluation of micturition: Flow rate, pressure measurement, symbols. *Acta Urol Jpn* 1977; 27:1563-1566; *Br J Urol* 1977; 49:207-210; *Eur Urol* 1977; 3:168-170; *Scand J Urol Nephrol* 1977; 11:197-199.

4. Bates P, Bradley WE, Glen E et al. Third report on the standardisation of terminology of lower urinary tract function. Procedures related to the evaluation of micturition: Pressure flow relationships, residual urine. *Br J Urol* 1980; 52:348-350; *Eur Urol* 1980; 6:170-171; *Acta Urol Jpn* 1980; 27:1566-1568; *Scand J Urol Nephrol* 1980; 12:191-193.

5. Bates P, Bradley WE, Glen E et al. Fourth report on the standardisation of terminology of lower urinary tract function. Terminology related to neuromuscular dysfunction of lower urinary tract. *Br J Urol* 1981; 52:333-335; *Urology* 1981; 17:618-620; *Scand J Urol Nephrol* 1981; 15:169-171; *Acta Urol Jpn* 1981; 27:1568-1571.

6. Jasper HH. Report to the committee on the methods of clinical examination in electroencephalography. *Electroencephalogr Clin Neurophysiol* 1958; 10:370-75.

Index

A

Abdominal approach to urinary sphincter implantation, 221
Abdominal film, 134
Abdominal hysterectomy, 358-360
Abdominal pressure, 167-168
Abdominal repair
    of cystocele, 230-231
    of enterocele, 241, 242, 243, 244
    of urinary tract fistulas, 338-339
Abdominal sacral colpopexy, 255-258
Ablation, 349
    in suburethral diverticula repair, 351-352
Abscess
    suburethral sling operaiton and, 216
    tubo-ovarian, 358
    urethral, 344, 345
Accommodation, 24, 63, 151-152
Acetaminophen, 402
Acetylcholine
    bladder emptying and, 26-27
    detrusor and, 20, 21
    pudendal cortical pathways and, 22
    urethra and, 20
Acidification of urine, 319
Acquired suburethral diverticula, 343-344
Adnexal surgery, 355-358
Adrenergic agents
    agonist
        bladder emptying and, 27
        ganglia and, 19-20
        in stress incontinence, 173-174
        urethra and, 20
        urinary tract function and, 26, 50
        voiding dysfunction and, 304
    blocker
        bladder emptying and, 27
        in stress incontinence, 175
        in urethral syndrome, 288
        urinary tract function and, 26, 50

Adrenergic agents—cont'd
    blocker—cont'd
        in voiding dysfunction, 307
    elderly and, 415, 417
Adult respiratory distress syndrome, 401
Agenesis, renal, 6
Air in cystoscopy, 127
Allantois formation, 3
Allis clamp, 247
Alpha-adrenergic agonsits
    bladder emptying and, 27
    ganglia and, 19-20
    in stress incontinence, 173-174
    urethra and, 20
    urinary tract function and, 26, 50
    voiding dysfunction and, 304
Alpha-adrenergic blockers
    bladder emptying and, 27
    in urethral syndrome, 288
    urinary tract function and, 26, 50
    in voiding dysfunction, 307
Alpha-motor neurons, 18
Alpha-sympathetic blockers
    bladder emptying and, 27
    in detrusor-sphincter dyssynergia, 305
Alpha-sympathomimetics, 171
Ambulatory monitoring, 71
Amifloxacin, 320
Aminocaproic acid, 385
Ammoniacal dermatitis, 334
Amoxicillin, 322
Amphetamines, 304
Ampicillin
    in bacteriuria, 399
    in pyelonephritis, 401
    in urinary tract infection, 320, 321
Amplitude in electromyelography, 116
AMS 800 artificial urinary sphincter, 219-220
Anal canal, 15

Anal plug electrode, 106
Anal reflex, 51
Anal sphincter, 14-15
    postpartum pelvic injury and, 157
Analgesia
    in urethrocystoscopy, 128
    in urinary tract infection, 319
Anatomic bladder outlet obstruction, 131
Anatomic stress incontinence, 43, 44
Ancillary equipment for endoscopy, 127
Anesthesia
    in urethrocystoscopy, 128
    in urinary tract fistulas, 334-335
    in vesicovaginal fistulas, 331
    voiding dysfunction and, 304
Anteroposterior films in cystourethrography, 139
Antibiotics
    in cystitis, 322, 400
    in diverticulectomy, 349
    in pyelonephritis, 326, 401, 402
    in ureteroneocystostomy, 364
    in urinary tract infection, 288, 399
        catheter-associated, 326
    in urolithiasis, 404
    in vesicovaginal fistulas, 331
Anticholinergics
    in detrusor instability, 276-278
    in interstitial cystitis, 294
    in sensory urgency, 292
    in urethral syndrome, 288
    urinary tract function and, 26, 50
    voiding dysfunction and, 304
Anticholinesterase inhibitors, 307
Antidepressants, 50
Antidromic conduction, 111
Antihistamines
    in interstitial cystitis, 295
    voiding dysfunction, 304
Antiinflammatories
    in buttock pain, 252
    in interstitial cystitis, 294, 295
Antimicrobials, 320
    in bacteriuria, 398-399
    prophylactic, 311
    in pyelonephritis, 326
    suppressive, 311
    in urethral syndrome, 288
    in urinary tract infection, 325
Antipsychotics, 50
Antispasmodics
    in interstitial cystitis, 294
    in voiding dysfunction, 304
Arcus tendineus fasciae pelvis, 14
Areflexia, detrusor, 302-303
    in multiple sclerosis, 265
    voiding phase and, 42

Argyle-Ingram catheter, 422, 423
Arnold-Breuning intercordal injection set, 217
Artifact
    electromyography and, 108
    stimulus, 111
Ascending infection in urinary tract, 312, 313
Aseptic technique in cystoscopy, 128
Aspiration, bladder, 394
Asymptomatic bacteriuria, 320-321
    in pregnancy, 395-399
Atrophy, urethral mucosal, 130
Atropine-like agents, 304
Augmentation cystoplasty
    in detrusor instability, 280
    pregnancy and, 405
Autoimmune system, 292-293
Automatic bladder; *see* Detrusor, instability of
Automatic integrated functional electrical stimulation,
        175
Autonomic nervous system
    bladder filling/storage and voiding and, 24
    lesions of, 304
    lower urinary tract and, 18-21
Azathioprine, 294, 295

B

Babcock clamp, 247
Bac-T-Screen, 395, 396
Baclofen
    in detrusor-sphincter dyssynergia, 305
    in urinary tract function, 26
Bacteria
    adherence of, 313-314
    persistence of, 312
Bacteriuria, 311, 315-318
    asymptomatic, 320-321
        in pregancy, 395-399
    laboratory tests in, 54
    urethrocystoscopy and, 132
    urinary tract and, 323, 325, 326
Bactrim, 320
Balloon catheter
    in cystometry, 66
    in urethral pressure profilometry, 89-90
Barium
    in cystography, 139
    in cystourethrography, 138
Basal ganglia, 22
Bead-chain cystourethrography, 52-53
Bedwetting
    detrusor instability and, 267
    unstable bladder and, 58
Behavioral management in stress incontinence, 163-171
    elderly and, 414
    implementing, 171

Beta-adrenergic agents
  agonist
    in detrusor instability, 279
    urethra and, 20
    urinary tract function and, 26, 50
  blocker, 175
Beta-sympathetic blocker, 171
Bethanechol chloride
  in supersensitivity testing, 117
  of detrusor instability, 273
  in urinary tract function, 27
  in voiding dysfunction, 307
Biofeedback
  in detrusor instability, 275-276
  in incontinence
    elderly and, 414, 416
    stress, 164, 166-168, 170-171
  in urethral syndrome, 288
Bioluminescence test, 395-396
Biopsy
  bladder, 294
  forceps for, 127
  urethrocystoscopy and, 129
Birth trauma, 343
Bladder, 6-8, 130-132
  aspiration of, 394
  automatic; *see* Detrusor, instability
  biopsy of, 294
  cervical cancer and, 376
  continence and, 151-152
  contraction of
    cystometry and, 269
    cystourethrography in, 140
    decreasing, 27-28
    pressure-flow study in, 84
  control of, 299
  cystourographic findings of, 139, 141
  in detrusor instability, 280
  distention of, 22
    detrusor instability and, 279
    interstitial cystitis and, 295
  drainage of, 421-429
  elderly and, 413-414
  emptying of, 26-28
  filling of
    abnormalities of, 71
    cystometry and, 66, 68
    detrusor responses to, 73
    in genital prolapse, 228
    incontinence and, 55-56, 59
    mechanisms in, 24-25
    sensations in, 63
  high volume, 74
  hyperreflexic; *see* Detrusor, instability of hypertonic; *see* Detrusor, instability of hysterectomy and
    abdominal, 359

Bladder—cont'd
  hyperreflexic—cont'd
    radical, 379-380
  infection of, 304, 398
  inflammation of, 304
  injury to
    delivery and, 405
    prevention of, 364
    repair of, 370-371
    suburethral sling operation and, 216
  irrigation of, 322
  low compliance, 269
  low volume, 74
  mucosa of, 267
  neurologic pathways of, 22
  nonneurogenic neurogenic, 305
  outlet obstruction of, 131
    detrusor hyperreflexia and, 266
  pregnancy and, 389
  retraining of, 273-275
  sensory abnormalities of, 71, 73
  spastic; *see* Detrusor, instability of
  storage in, 22, 23, 24-25
    disorders of, 40-46
  stress incontinence and, 155
  systolic; *see* Detrusor, instability of
  trabeculations of, 141, 142
  training of, 166
  tumor of, 142
  ultrasonography of, 144-145
  uninhibited; *see* Detrusor, instability of
  unstable; *see* Detrusor, instability of
  in ureteral injury, 368-369
  voiding of, 55-56
    mechanisms in, 25
Bladder neck
  bladder filling and, 25
  elevation test of, 56
  fistulas of, 338
  incontinence and, 152-153
  stress incontinence and, 43, 44
  surgery of
    laparoscopic retropubic, 201-202
    pressure-flow studies in, 83
    voiding dysfunction and, 305
  ultrasound evaluation of, 145
Blastema, renal, 5
Bleeding, 257
Blood volume in pregnancy, 390-391
Bonnano catheter, 422, 423
Bonnar mechanical device, 178
Brain
  lesions of, 304
  tumors of, 266
Brain stem, 23
  lesions of, 118, 303

Brain stem—cont'd
　micturition reflex and, 25
Briesky-Navratil retractors, 247, 248
Bromocriptine
　in sensory urgency, 292
　in urinary tract function, 26
Bulbocavernosus reflex, 51
Bulk-enhancing agents, 216-218
Burch colposuspension, 205, 206
　in cystocele repair, 230-231
　enterocele and, 207
　hysterectomy and, 207
　results of, 202-204, 233
　in stress incontinence, 197-198, 199
Burch procedure in abdominal sacral colpopexy, 255
Burch urethropexy, 189-191
Buttock pain, 252

C

C-SSL; *see* Coccygeus-sacrospinous ligament
Caffeine, 166
Calcium-channel blockers
　in detrusor instability, 277, 279
　urinary tract function and, 26, 50
　voiding dysfunction and, 304
Cancer, 373-387
　vaginal
　　urologic complications of, 376-377
　　vaginectomy in, 382-383
　vulvar, 377
　　radical vulvectomy in, 381-382
　　urologic complications of, 376
Candidal infection, 318
Cannon's law of denervation, 117
Carbenicillin, 321
Carbon dioxide
　in cystography, 139
　in cystometry, 66
　in cystoscopy, 127
　in urethrocystometry, 129
Carcinoma; *see* Cancer
Cardiac drugs, 414-415
Catheter
　in adnexal surgery, 355-356
　in bladder drainage, 427-428
　in colporrhaphy, 361
　in cystometry, 66-67, 68
　double-balloon
　　in diverticulectomy, 349
　　in urinary tract infection, 318
　in endoscopy, 127
　Foley; *see* Foley catheter
　ureteral, 363, 367
　in urethral pressure profilometry, 89-90
　urinary tract infection and, 325-326

Catheterization
　suprapubic, 422-424, 425, 426
　transurethral, 421-422
　in urinary incontinence, 218
Cauda equina, 114
　electrophysiologic testing and, 120-121
　injury to, 116-117
Cefazolin, 401
Cefmandole, 401
Central nervous system
　elderly and, 413-414
　modulation of, 21-23
　urinary tract and, 17-18
Cephalexin
　in bacteriuria, 398-399
　in urinary tract infection, 321, 324
Cephalosporins
　in bacteriuria, 398-399
　in cystitis, 322, 400
　in pyelonephritis, 402
　in urinary tract infection, 323
Cerebellum, 22-23
Cerebral cortex, 299
Cerebrovascular accident, 303
Cerebrovascular disease, 265-266
Cervical cancer, 374-376
　radical hysterectomy in, 378
Cesarean section
　incontinence and, 31-32
　urinary tract injury and, 362
　vaginal hysterectomy and, 361
Chemotherapy, 384
Childbirth; *see also* Cesarean section; Vaginal delivery
　trauma in, 343
　urinary incontinence and, 31-32
Chlamydial infection
　in periurethral duct, 344
　urethral syndrome and, 286, 288
Cholinergic agents
　in detrusor innervation, 20
　voiding dysfunction, 307
Cholinesterase agents, 27
Cholinolytics, 417-418
Cinoxacin, 324
Ciprofloxacin, 320
Cisplatin, 384
Clamp
　Allis, 247
　Babcock, 247
　ureteral, 359, 360
Clenbuterol, 279
Clitoris, 117
Cloaca, 3, 4
Clorpactin; *see* Oxychlorosene
CMAP; *see* Compound muscle action potential
Coagulation, 355

Coccygeus muscle, 13
Coccygeus-sacrospinous ligament, 245
Collecting devices for urine loss, 428-429
Collecting system of kidney, 135
Colpectomy, 254-255
Colpocleisis
    Latzko technique of, 338
    LeFort technique of, 252-254
Colpopexy, abdominal sacral, 255-258
Colporrhaphy, 234
    cystocele and, 229-230
    indications for, 233
    in perineal relaxation and rectocele, 231
    results of, 189-191, 233
    vaginal hysterectomy and, 361-362
Colposuspension
    Burch; *see* Burch colposuspension
    detrusor instability and, 280
    vaginal, 188-189, 190
Compliance, bladder, 269
Complicated, defined, 311-312
Compound fistula, 333
Compound muscle action potential, 111
Compressor urethrae, 20
Concentric needle electromyography, 108-110
Conductance, urethral, 290
Conduction studies in electrophysiologic testing, 111-113
Conductive fluids in cystopscopy, 127
Conduits in genital malignancy, 382
Cones, weighted vaginal, 170-171
Congenital anomalies of urinary tract, 6
Congenital enterocele, 238
Congenital suburethral diverticula, 343
Connective tissue defects, 237
Constipation, 166
Contigen, 217, 218
Continence, 151-154
Continent urinary diversion in genital malignancy, 382
Contraception, 315, 325
Contractility
    bladder, decreasing, 27-28
    detrusor
        bladder filling and, 24-25
        hyperactivity with impaired, 267
        uroflowmetric parameters and, 80
Cook continence ring, 178
Corpus uteri cancer, 378
Cortical evoked response, 114
Cortical lesion
    electrophysiologic testing and, 117-119
    urinary retention and, 303
Cortical pathways, 21-22
Corticosteroids, 295
Corynebacteria, 286
Cost of urinary incontinence, 36-37
Cough pressure profile, 93, 94, 95, 96

Cough-provoked detrusor instability, 269, 270, 271
Cranial nerves, 18
Creatinine clearance in pregnancy, 392
CTX; *see* Cyclophosphamide
Cube pessary, 258
Culdoplasty, McCall, 239-241
Culture, urine, in detrusor instability and hyperreflexia, 268-269
Cutaneous ureterostomy, 369-370
Cyclophosphamide, 384, 385
Cyst of periurethral duct, 344-345
Cystectomy, 296, 385
Cystitis, 310-311, 315, 321-322; *see also* Urinary tract infection
    hemorrhagic, 131, 384-385
    interstitial, 130-131, 292-296
    laboratory tests in, 54
    in pregnancy, 400
Cystocath catheter, 422, 423
Cystocele, 228
    pelvic organ prolapse and, 225
    postpartum pelvic injury and, 157
    surgical repair for, 229-231
Cystography, 139
Cystokon; *see* Sodium acetrizoate
Cystolysis, 296
Cystometry, 63-68, 69, 71-74, 75
    in detrusor instability and hyperreflexia, 269, 270, 271
    in interstitial cystitis, 293
    in urethral syndrome, 287
Cystoplasty, augmentation
    in detrusor instability, 280
    pregnancy and, 405
Cystoscopy, 124-125
    in bladder injury, 364
    flexible fiberoptic, 126
    in interstitial cystitis, 293-294
    in ureteral injury, 364
    in urethral syndrome, 288
    in vesicovaginal fistulas, 334
    in voiding dysfunction, 307-308
Cystotomy
    in bladder dissection, 356-357
    in cesarean section, 361
    in vaginal hysterectomy, 370-371
Cystourethrography, 136-143
    bead-chain, 52-53
    findings in, 139-143
    voiding, 140-141
        in suburethral diverticula, 347, 348
        in urethral diverticula, 136
        in urinary tract infection, 318
Cystourethroscopy
    suburethral sling procedure and, 213
    in urethral syndrome, 287
    in urinary tract infection, 317-318
Cytologic smears, vaginal, 228

D

Dantrolene
  in detrusor-sphincter dyssynergia, 305
  in urinary tract function, 26
DDAVP; *see* 1-Desamino-8-[e2]D[/e2]-arginine vasopressin
Delivery systems for endoscopy, 127
Dementia, 266
Denervation
  Cannon's law of, 117
  pelvic muscle, 164
Denonvilliers, fascia of, 226
Dermatitis, ammoniacal, 334
Dermatomes, sensory, 52
DES; *see* Diethylstilbestrol
1-Desamino-8-[e2]D[/e2]-arginine vasopressin, 279
Deschamps ligature carrier, 247, 248
Detrusor
  areflexia of, 265, 302-303
    testing in, 117
    voiding phase and, 42
  contractility of
    bladder filling and, 24-25
    cystometry and, 270
    uroflowmetric parameters and, 80
  elderly and, 413-414
  filling and, 73
  hyperactivity of, 267
  hyperreflexia of, 41, 263-266; *see also* Detrusor, instability of
    in multiple sclerosis, 265
    neurologic disease and, 265-266
  hypoactivity of, 117
  incontinence and, 41
  innervation of, 20
  instability of, 263-284
    multichannel urethrocystometry in, 72
    retropubic surgical procedures and, 206-207
    sling procedures and, 211, 216
    transvaginal needle suspension procedures and, 192
    urgency and, 290
  outlet obstruction of, 79
  urinary retention and, 306-307
  voiding and, 42, 301, 303
Detrusor-sphincter dyssynergia, 106-108
  multichannel urodynamic tracing of, 274
  in multiple sclerosis, 265
  uroflowmetric parameters and, 80
  voiding dysfunction and, 305
Diabetics, 315
Diaphragm
  as contraceptive, 315, 325
  pelvic, 12-14
  urogenital, 14
Diary
  bladder, 164, 165, 166
  urinary, 51
Diathermy instruments, 127

Diatrizoate, 137-138
Diazepam
  in detrusor-sphincter dyssynergia, 305
  in sensory urgency, 292
Dicyclomine hydrochloride
  bladder emptying and, 27
  in detrusor instability, 277, 278
Diet in stress incontinence, 166
Diethylstilbestrol, 377
Dilation
  in LeFort partial colpocleisis, 253
  in urethral syndrome, 288, 289
  vesicovaginal fistulas and, 335
  in voiding dysfunction, 307-308
Dilator, Hegar, 221
Dimethyl sulfoxide
  in interstitial cystitis, 295
  in urinary tract function, 26
Displacement cystocele, 225
Dissection
  in abdominal hysterectomy, 358-359
  in abdominal sacral colpopexy, 257
  in adnexal surgery, 356-357
  in anterior colporrhaphy, 229
  in diverticulectomy, 350, 351
  in LeFort partial colpocleisis, 253
  in retropubic space, 184, 198
  in sacrospinous fixation, 247
Dissemination, hematogenous, 312, 313
Distal pudendal neuropathy, 121-122
Distal ureteral repair, 365-569
Distention
  bladder
    in detrusor instability, 279
    interstitial cystitis and, 295
  cystocele, 225
    abdominal repair of, 231
Distigmine bromide, 307
Diuretics, 50
Diurnal frequency, 58
Diversion, urinary; *see* Urinary diversion
Diverticula
  bladder, 131
    cystourethrography in, 141
  suburethral; *see* Suburethral diverticula
  urethral, 136
Diverticulectomy, 348, 349-351
DMSO; *see* Dimethyl sulfoxide
Donut pessary, 258
L-Dopa, 304
Dopamine
  bladder emptying and, 27
  somatic movements and, 22
Double-balloon catheter
  in diverticulectomy, 349
  in urinary tract infection, 318

Double ureter, 6
Doxycycline, 288
Drainage, bladder, 421-429
Duplication of collecting system of kidney, 135
Dyssynergia, detrusor-sphincter; *see* Detrusor-sphincter dyssynergia
Dysuria
  sexually transmitted diseases and, 318, 319
  urethrocystoscopy and, 132

E

Ectopic ureter, 6
Edwards pubovaginal spring, 178
Efferent fiber lesion, 118
Elderly
  bladder infection and, 325
  incontinence in; *see* Geriatric issues in incontinence
Electric conductance, urethral, 290
Electrical stimulation
  elderly incontinence and, 417
  functional
    in detrusor instability, 276
    in interstitial cystits, 295-296
    in stress incontinence, 175-178
Electrodes in electromyography, 105-108
Electromyelography, 115-117
Electromyography
  concentric needle, 108-110
  in detrusor instability, 273, 274
  in detrusor-sphincter dyssynergia, 305
  in electrophysiologic testing, 104-111
  needle, 108
  single fiber, 110-111
  surface electrodes in, 105-108
  vaginal delivery and pudendal nerve damage and, 158-159
Electrophysiologic testing, 102-123
Elmiron, 295
Elsberg syndrome, 306
Emepronium
  in detrusor instability, 278
  in sensory urgency, 292
EMG; *see* Electromyography
Endocrine etiology in voiding dysfunction, 305
Endometrial cancer
  radical hysterectomy in, 378
  urologic complications of, 377-378
Endometrial implants, 358
Endometriosis, 357-358
Endopelvic fascia, 14
  Pereyra procedure and, 184, 185
  sutures and, 183
Endoscopy, 124-125
  in detrusor instability, 273
  in genital prolapse, 228
  in interstitial cystitis, 296

Endoscopy—cont'd
  in suburethral diverticula, 347
  of urinary tract; *see* Urinary tract
Endosonography, 145
Endotoxins in pyelonephritis, 401-402
Enkephalin, 20, 22
Enoxacin, 320
Enterobacter
  antimicrobials and, 321
  in urinary tract infection, 315
Enterobacteriaceae in pyelonephritis, 401
Enterocele, 228, 238-241
  rectocele with, 226
  rectovaginal examination for, 227
  surgical repair of, 238-241, 242, 243, 244
Enterococcus, 321
Ephedrine, 173-174
Epidemiology of urinary incontinence; *see* Incontinence
Epidural anesthesia, 304
Epinephrine, 252
Episiotomy, 157-158
Epithelium, 8, 10
  interstitial cystitis and, 293
Equipment for endoscopy, 125-128
Erythromycin, 288
Erythropoietin, 392
Escherichia coli
  antimicrobials and, 321
  in pregnancy, 393
  in urinary tract infection, 312, 313, 314, 315
Estradiol, 307
Estriol, 172-173
Estrogen
  in ammoniacal dermatitis, 334
  bladder emptying and, 27-28
  in detrusor instability, 280
  elderly and, 415
  in stress incontinence, 171-173, 174
  urethral function and, 32-33
  in urethral syndrome, 286-287, 288
  in urinary dysfunction, 307, 308
  urinary tract function and, 26
  in vaginal stenosis, 252
  in vaginal vault fixation, 245
Eversion of vagina; *see* Vaginal vault prolapse
Evoked response in electrophysiologic studies, 113-115
Examination
  neurologic, 287
  physical
    for detrusor instability and hyperreflexia, 268
    incontinence and, 49-51, 52
    pelvic organ prolapse and, 226-228
  rectovaginal, 227
Exenteration, pelvic, 382
Exercise, pelvic, 164
  elderly and, 414, 416

Exercise, pelvic—cont'd
in stress incontinence, 168-170
Exstrophy, bladder, 6

F

F wave, 113
Fallopian tube cancer, 377-378
Fascia
of Denonvilliers, 226
endopelvic, 14
in sling procedures, 212, 213, 214, 215
sutures and, 183
Fecal flora, 314, 323, 324
Fecal incontinence, 13
Femoral nerve injury, 193
FES; *see* Functional electrical stimulation
Fiber cables, 126
Fiberoptic cystoscope, flexible, 126
FIGO; *see* International Federation of Gynecology and Obstetrics
Filling, bladder; *see* Bladder, filling of
Filling media in cystometry, 66
Filter test, 316-317, 395, 396
Fimbriae, 393
Fistula
after suburethral sling operation, 216
of bladder neck, 338
urachal, 6
urethral, 338
urinary tract; *see* Urinary tract, fistulas of
vaginal, 364-365
vesicouterine, 142, 143
vesicovaginal, 132
cystourethrography in 142, 143
Fixation of vaginal vault to sacrospinous ligament, 245-254
Flap-splitting technique, 331
Flavoxate hydrocholoride
bladder emptying and, 27
in detrusor instability, 277, 278
Flexible fiberoptic cystoscope, 126
Flow curve patterns in uroflowmetry, 78, 79-80
Fluid-filled cables, 126
Foley catheter
in adnexal surgery, 355-356
in bladder drainage, 421-422, 423
in colporrhaphy, 361
transurethral, 66
Foley catheter ring electrode, 107
Forceps, biopsy, 127
Formalin, 385
Frequency syndromes, 291
unstable bladder and, 267
uroflowmetry and, 81
Frontal gyrus-septal lesion, 117-119
FUL; *see* Functional urethral length
Functional electrical stimulation
in detrusor instability, 276

Functional electrical stimulation—cont'd
in intersitital cystitis, 295-296
in stress incontinence, 175-178
Functional incontinence, 44-45
Functional urethral length, 93

G

GABA; *see* Gamma-amniobutyric acid
Gamma-amniobutyric acid, 22-23
Gamma-motor neurons, 18
Ganglia, 18-20
Ganglionic blockers, 304
Gas
in cystometry, 66
in cystoscopy, 127
Gehrung pessary, 258
Gellhorn pessary, 258
Genital cancer, 374-378
Genital herpes, 306
Genital tubercle formation, 3
Gentamicin
in pyelonephritis, 402
in urinary tract infection, 321
Geriatric issues in incontinence, 409-420
Gittes procedure, 186-187, 190
Glomerular filtration rate in pregnancy, 391, 392
Gonococcus, 344, 345
Graft
in abdominal sacral colpopexy, 255
Martius, 337, 371-372
in vesicovaginal fistula, 379
Gram stain in urinary tract infection, 316, 396
Granular urethral trigonitis, 311
Granuloma formation, 218
Gravid uterus, 405
Gynecologic cancer, 373-387
Gynecologic examination, 51
Gyrus-septal lesion, 117-119

H

H reflex, 113
Halban procedure, 241, 243
in abdominal sacral colpopexy, 257
Heaney retractors, 247, 248
Hegar dilator, 221
Hemacytometer, 316
Hematocrit, 398
Hematogenous dissemination, 312, 313
Hematuria, 54
urinary tract infection and, 316
Hemorrhage
sacrospinous fixation and, 251-252
transvaginal needle suspension procedures and, 192
Hemorrhagic cystitis, 131
gynecologic cancer and, 384-385
Hemostasis, 257

Heparin, 296
Herniation of peritoneum; *see* Enterocele
Herpes
  dysuria and, 318
  urinary retention and, 306
High volume bladder, 74
The HIP Report, 166
Histamine, 20
Hodge pessary, 258
Hormones, 171
Horseshoe kidney, 6
Host defense mechanisms, 313
Host susceptibility, 313-315
Hunner ulcers, 131
Hydration, 318
Hydrocortisone, 296
Hydronephrosis, 390
Hydrostatic bladder distention, 295
Hydroureter
  intravneous pyelogram in, 137
  pregnancy and, 390
Hypaque; *see* Diatrizoate
Hyperreflexia
  detrusor, 41; *see also* Detrusor, instability of
    defined, 263-264
    neurologic disease and, 265-266
Hypersensitive bladder, 71, 73
Hypertension, 402
Hyperthermia, 402
Hypertonic bladder; *see* Detrusor, instability of
Hypnotics, 50
Hypochondriasis, 286
Hypoestrogenism, 286-287
Hypogastric plexus, 19
Hyposensitive bladder, 71, 73
Hypothalamus, 22
Hypothermia, 401
Hysterectomy
  abdominal, 358-360
  radical, 358-360, 378-380, 381
  in treatment of incontinence, 207
  vaginal
    cystotomy in, 370-371
    urinary tract injury and, 360-362
  vaginal vault prolapse and, 241-242, 243
  vesicovaginal fistulas and, 332
  voiding dysfunction after, 303-304
Hysteria, 286

I

Iatrogenic enterocele, 238
ICS; *see* International Continence Society
Idiopathic detrusor instability, 264-265
Ifosfamide
  hemorrhagic cystitis and, 385
  urologic complications of, 384

Ileal conduit, 382
Ileal transplant in ureteral injury, 370
Ileococcygeus muscles, 12-13
Ilioinguinal nerve injury, 192-193
Imipramine
  bladder emptying and, 27
  in detrusor instability, 277, 278-279, 280
  in stress incontinence, 171, 174-175
Immunogenicity, 218
Immunosuppressives, 295
Implant
  excision of endometrial, 358
  urinary sphincter replacement, 218-222
Impulse transmission, 102
Incision
  in abdominal sacral colpopexy, 255-257
  in adnexal surgery, 356
  in anterior colporrhaphy, 229
  in bladder dissection, 356-357
  in diverticulectomy, 349
  in gynecologic surgery, 355
  in perineal relaxation and rectocele, 231-232
  in retropubic surgical procedures, 197
  in sacrospinous fixation, 247
  in sling procedures, 212, 213
  in urinary sphincter implantation, 222
  in vesicovaginal fistula repair, 335-336, 338
Incontinence, 49-61
  algorithm for clinical assessment of, 56-58
  cystourethrography and, 139-140
  defined, 41-42
  detrusor instability and, 280
  differential diagnosis of, 44-45
  economic issues of, 36-37
  in elderly, 417
  fecal, 15
  functional, 44-45
  geriatric issues in; *see* Geriatric issues in incontinence
  hysterectomy in, 207
  motor urge; *see* Detrusor, instability of
  organizations on, 166
  overflow, 42
    needle suspension procedures and, 193
  postoperative, 193
    retropubic surgical procedures and, 206
    transvaginal needle suspension procedures and, 193
  prevalence and incidence of, 29-30
  prolapse and, 228
  psychosocial impact of, 33-36
  reflex, 42
  risk factors for, 30-33
  sling procedures and, 215
  stress; *see* Stress incontinence
  urge
    in elderly, 417
    unstable bladder and, 58

Incontinent urinary diversion, 382
Infection
    after suburethral sling operations, 216
    ascending, 312, 313
    bladder, 304
    suburethral diverticula and, 343, 344
    transurethral drainage and, 422
    transvaginal needle suspension procedures and, 191
    urethral syndrome and, 285-286
    urinary tract; see Urinary tract infection
Inflammation
    detrusor instability and, 267
    voiding dysfunction and, 304
The Informer, 100
Infrapontine lesions, 303
Ingelman-Sundberg procedure in detrusor instability, 280
Innova intravaginal functional electrical stimulator, 177
Intercellular nerve conduction, 103
Intercourse
    after incontinence sugery, 234
    urinary tract infection and, 314-315, 325
Interference pattern, 109
Intermittent self-catheterization
    bladder drainage and, 424, 427
    in voiding dysfunction and retention, 308
International Continence Society, 40-42
    on classfication of voiding dysfunction, 302-303
    on definition of urgency, 289
    on terminology for pressure-flow studies, 81, 82
International Federation of Gynecology and Obstetrics
    cervical cancer and, 374, 375
    corpus uteri cancer and, 378
    vaginal cancer and, 377
    vulvar cancer and, 377
Interrupted pattern in uroflowmetry, 79, 80
Interstitial cystitis, 130-131, 292-296
Intraabdominal pressure, 43, 153, 155-156
Intracellular nerve conduction, 103
Intraembryonic mesoderm formation, 3
Intraurethral pressure, resting, 152
Intravenous pyelography, 134-136, 137
    in abdominal hysterectomy, 358
    in adnexal surgery, 355
    in genital prolapse, 228
    in pyelonephritis, 402, 403
    in urinary tract infection, 318
    in urolithiasis, 404
Intravesical pressure, 24-25
Involuntary detrusor contractions, 270
Iodine, 137
Ionic distribution, 102
Irrigation, bladder, 322
ISC; see Intermittent self-catheterization
Ischiococcygeus muscle, 156
IVP; see Intravenous pyelography

J

Jackknife position, 335
Jejunal conduit, 382
Juxta-urethral fistula, 333
Juxtacervical fistula, 333, 338

K

Kidney; see also Renal disease in pregnancy
    duplication of collecting system of, 135
    horseshoe, 6
    pelvic, 6
    ureteral obstruction and, 375
Klebsiella
    antimicrobials and, 321
    in urinary tract infection, 314, 315

L

Laboratory tests, 54
Lamina propria, 10
Laparoscopic retropubic bladder neck surgery, 201-202
Laparotomy, 255-256
Laser, Nd:YAG, 296
Lateral films in cystourethrography, 139
Latzko technique of partial colpocleisis, 338
Lead pipe urethra, 43
LeFort partial colpocleisis, 252-254
Lembert suture, 361-362
Leukocyte esterase, 396
Levator ani, 12-14
    in urinary continence, 153
    vaginal delivery and, 156, 157
Levator plate, 14
Lidocaine
    in LeFort partial colpoclesis, 252
    in urethrocystoscopy, 128
    in urinary incontinence, 217
Ligature carrier
    Pereyra, 185
    in sacrospinous fixation, 247-279
Light sources and cables for endoscopy, 126
Limbic system in temporal lobes, 22
Lithotomy position
    in sacrospinous fixation, 246
    in suburethral sling procedure, 212
Low birth weight, 397-398
Low compliance bladder, 269
Low volume bladder, 74
Lumbar vertebrae, 115
Lumbosacral cord lesion, 118
Lymph node dissection, 358-359
Lymphatics, 313

M

M Wave, 111, 113
Macrodantin, 320
Magnesium sulfate, 402

Magnetic resonance imaging, 145
Malecot catheter, 423
Marshall-Marchetti-Krantz procedure, 56, 202, 205-208
  in stress incontinence, 198-199, 200
  urethral injury and, 364
Martius graft, 337, 371-372
Massive fistula, 333
Maximum urethral pressure, 92, 93
McCall culdoplasty, 239-241
Mecamylamine, 304
Media
  distention, 127
  filling, 66
Menopause
  urinary incontinence and, 32-33
  voiding dysfunction and, 307
Mentor catheter, 423
Mesoderm, intraembryonic, 3
Methantheline bromide, 277
Methenamine, 319
Methylene blue dye
  in diverticulectomy, 349
  vesicovaginal fistulas and, 333-334
Metoclopramide, 27
Metzenbaum scissors
  in enterocele repair, 238-239
  in vaginal entry, 184
Mezlocillin, 401
Microbiology of urinary tract infections, 315
Microgyn II stimulation device, 177
Microtransducer catheter
  in cystometry, 66-67, 68
  in urethral pressure profilometry, 90
Micturition; *see also* Voiding
  nervous system in, 117, 188
  neurophysiology of, 299-301
  reflexes in, 23, 25
Mid-vaginal fistula, 333
Midodrine, 173-174
Mini-Mental Status Exam, 415-416
Minnesota Multiphasic Personality Inventory, 286, 287
Misstique device, 429
Mixed incontinence, 280
Miya hook ligature carrier, 249
MMPI; *see* Minnesota Multiphasic Personality Inventory
MMSE; *see* Mini-Mental Status Exam
Monitoring
  ambulatory, 71
  in behavioral managment, 170-171
Monopolar needle electromyography, 108
Moorhuate sodium, 216
Moschcowitz procedure
  in abdominal enterocele repair, 241, 242
  in abdominal sacral colpopexy, 257
Motor neurons, 18
Motor system evaluation, 51

Motor unit, 104
Motor unit action potential, 104, 105
  polyphasic, 109
Motor urge incontinence; *see* Detrusor, instability of
Motor urgency, 41
  defined, 289
  unstable bladder and, 267
MRI; *see* Magnetic resonance imaging
MS; *see* Multiple sclerosis
MUAP; *see* Motor unit action potential
Mucosa
  bladder, 267
  urethral, 130
Multichannel cystometry, 65, 199
  subtracted, 68
Multichannel urethrocystometry
  in combined detrusor instability and stress incontinence, 72
  subtracted
    detrusor instability and, 272, 273
    technique of, 67-68, 69
Multichannel urodynamic tracing
  of cough-provoked detrusor instability, 269, 271
  of detrusor-external sphincter dyssynergia, 274
Multiple peak pattern in uroflowmetry, 79, 80
Multiple sclerosis, 265
MUP; *see* Maximum urethral pressure
Muscarinic receptors, 19
Muscle action potential, 111
Muscle relaxants
  in detrusor instability, 277, 278
  in detrusor-sphincter dyssynergia, 305
  in urethral syndrome, 288
Muscles, bladder, 8
Musculotropic relaxants
  in detrusor instability, 277, 278
  in urinary tract function, 26
  voiding dysfunction and, 304
Muzsnai procedure, 188-189, 190, 191
Mycoplasma hominis, 286

N

N-acetylcysteine sulphonate, 384
Nalidixic acid, 325
Narcotics, 294
Nd:YAG laser, 296
Necrosis, 332
Needle electrobyography, 108-110
Needle suspension procedure,183, 233; *see also* Transvaginal needle suspension procedures
Needle urethropexy, 230
Neisseria gonorrhoeae, 318
Neomycin, 322
Neoplasia, 266
Neoureter formation with bladder flap, 368-369
Nephrostomy tube, 376
Nerve conduction, 102-104

Nerve fiber classification, 104
Nerve injury
  needle suspension procedures and, 192-193
  sacrospinous fixation and, 252
  sling procedures and, 216
Nervous system
  in micturition, 117, 118
  in urinary tract control, 18-23
Neurectomy, 280
Neurogenic bladder, nonneurogenic, 305
Neurologic conditions
  cystourethrography and, 140
  detrusor hyperreflexia and, 265-266
  radical hysterectomy and, 379
  urinary retention and, 306
  uroflowmetry and, 81
  voiding dysfunction and, 303-304
Neurologic examination
  in incontinence, 51, 52
  in urethral syndrome, 287
Neurologic lesion, 303
Neurons, motor, 18
Neuropathy
  in cauda equina, 120-121
  in pelvic floor disorders, 113
  pudendal, 121-122
Neuropeptide agents, 20
Neurophysiology of urinary tract; *see* Urinary tract
Neurotransmitters, 20
Nicotinic acetylcholine receptors, 19
Nifedipine, 277
Nitritie test, 316
Nitrofurantoin
  in bacteriuria, 398
  in cystitis, 322, 400
  in pyelonephritis, 402
  in urinary tract infection, 320, 321, 323, 324, 325
  in urinary tract surgery, 204
Nocturia, 267
Nocturnal frequency, 58
Nodes of Ranvier, 103
Nonconductive fluids in cystoscopy, 127
Nonneurogienic neurogenic bladder, 305
Nonsteroidal antiinflammatory agents, 294
Norepinephrine, 19, 20
Norfenefrine, 173-174
Norfloxacin, 320, 321, 324
Nuclei, central nervous system, 17

O

Obesity, 33
Oblique straining film, 139
Obstetric delivery, 156-160
Obstruction
  ureteral, 137

Obstruction—cont'd
  urethral
    stenosis and, 286
    urinary retention and, 306
  urinary tract, 405
  voiding, 304-305
    pattern of, 79-80
Obturator nerve injury, 193
Office urine kits, 316-317
Operative urethrocystoscopy, 129
Opioid antagonists, 26
Orgasm, 267
Orthodromic conduction, 111
Osteitis pubis, 207
Outpatient urethrocystoscopy, 128-129
Ovary
  cancer of, 377-378
  tumors of, 356-357
Overdistention, 305
Overflow incontinence
  defined, 42
  needle suspension procedures and, 193
Oxybutynin
  bladder emtpying and, 27
  in detrusor instability, 277, 278, 280
Oxygchlorocine, 295
Oxychlorosene, 295

P

Pads for urine loss, 428
Pain
  sacrospinous fixation and, 252
  sling procedures and, 216
Palpation of ureter, 359, 360
Paracentral lobule lesion, 118
Parasympathomimetic agents, 26
Paraurethral glands, 343, 344
Paravaginal procedure in stress incontinence, 199-201
Parity, 31-32
Parkinson's disease, 266
Parovarian tumors, 356-357
Partial ablation, 351-352
Partial colpocleisis, 338
Partial cystectomy, 296
Pefloxacin, 320
Pelvic floor
  abdominal hysterectomy and, 360
  anatomy of, 12-14
  childbirth and, 156-160
  disorders of, 113
  elderly and, 414
  nerves of, 154
Pelvic kidney, 6
Pelvic muscles
  caudal, 20-21

Pelvic muscles—cont'd
exercise of
in elderly incontinence, 416
in stress incontinence, 168-170
stress incontinence and, 164, 167, 168
Pelvic nerves
blockade of sacral, 280
filling bladder capacity and, 25
Pelvic organ prolapse, 225-260; *see also* Vaginal vault prolapse
Pelvic plexus, 19
injury to, 121
Pelvic radiotherapy
hemorrhagic cystitis and, 384-385
vesicovaginal fistulas and, 332-333
Pelvic relaxation classification, 228
Pelvic surgery
detrusor instability after, 267
pressure-flow studies in, 83
uroflowmetry and, 81
vesicovaginal fistulas and, 332
voiding dysfunction after, 303-304
Pelvic ureter, 8-10
Pelvis, 12-14
adnexal surgery and, 356
exenteration of, 382
Penicillin, 322, 323
PeNTML: *see* Perineal nerve terminal motor latency
Peptides, 22
Pereyra ligature carrier, 185
Pereyra procedure, 183-185, 186, 189-191
Perfusion catheter, 66
Perfusion techniques in urethral pressure profilometry, 90
Perineal nerve, 21
Perineal nerve terminal motor latency, 112
Perineal pad tests, 53-54
Perineum
membrane of, 14
relaxation of, 231-234
sensory dermatomes of, 52
urinary tract infection and, 313
vaginal delivery and, 157-158
Periodic voiding, 313
Peripheral innervation
lesions, of 304
of lower urinary tract, 19
micturition and, 301
Peripheral nervous system, 18
Peripheral neuropathy, 113
Perirectal space, 247
Peritoneal herniation; *see* Enterocele
Periurethral colonization, 313
Periurethral duct cyst, 344-345
Periurethral injection of bulk-enhancing agents, 216-218
Periurethral muscles, 10-11
continence and, 153
nerves of, 154

Periurethral muscles—cont'd
somatic motor control of, 21
striated, 20, 22
Peroneal nerve injury, 193
Pessary
in stress incontinence, 178
vaginal, 258
Pharmacology
in detrusor instability, 276-279
in incontinence, 417-418
urinary tract and, 25-28
in voiding dysfunction, 304, 307
Phenazopyridine hydrochloride
in urinary tract infection, 319
in vaginal wetness test, 54
Phenol
in cystitis, 385
in detrusor instability, 280
Phenothiazines, 304
Phenoxybenzamine
in detrusor-sphincter dyssynergia, 305
in voiding dysfunction, 307
Phenylephrine, 173-174
Phenylpropanolamine
in incontinence
elderly, 417
stress, 171, 173-174
Physical examination
detrusor instability and, 268
incontinence and, 49-51, 52
pelvic organ prolapse and, 226-228
Pigtail suprapubic catheter, 422, 423
Pilus, urinary tract, 314, 393
Plication of bladder neck, 253-254
PM; *see* Pelvic muscles
PNTML; *see* Pudendal nerve terminal motor latency
Polyphasic motor unit action potential, 109
Polysynaptic inhibitors, 26
Polytetrafluoroethylene, 216, 217, 218
Pons lesion, 120
Pontine reticular formation, 299-301
Position
in abdominal sacral colpopexy, 255
in cystometry, 269
in enterocele repair, 238
in fistula surgery, 334-335
in McCall culdoplasty, 239
in sling procedure, 212
Positive pressure urethrography, 144
Postoperative incontinence
retropubic surgical procedures and, 206
transvaginal needle suspension procedures and, 193
Posturethrocystoscopy care, 132
PPA; *see* Phenylpropanolamine
Prazosin, 305
Preeclampsia, 398

Preganglionic fibers, 18-19
Pregnancy
    after retropubic surgery, 207-208
    asymptomatic bacteriuria in, 321, 395-599
    cystitis in, 400
    pyelonephritis in, 400-402, 403
    renal disease in, 391, 402-403
    urinary tract in; *see* Urinary tract, in pregnancy
    urolithiasis in, 403-404
    urologic disease in, 403-406
    urologic symptoms and measurements in, 389
Prematurity, 397
Pressure-flow studies, 81-87
Pressure transmission, 133-136
    ratio of, 93, 94
Proctotomy, 234
Profilometry, urethral pressure; *see* Urethral pressure
    profilometry
Progesterone, 389-390
Prolapse, pelvic organ; *see* Pelvic organ prolapse
Prompted voiding, 416-417
Propantheline
    in detrusor instability, 277-278
    in sensory urgency, 292
Prophylactic antimicrobial therapy, 311
Propranolol hydrochloride, 171
Prostaglandins
    inhibitors of, 26
    urethra and, 20
    in urinary tract function, 26
    in voiding dysfunction, 307
Protein, Tamm-Horsfall, 313
Proteus
    antimicrobials and, 321
    in urinary tract infection, 314, 315, 318
Pseudoephedrine hydrochloride, 171
Pseudomonas
    antimicrobials and, 321
    in urinary tract infection, 315, 320
Psoas hitch, 368
Psychiatric testing, 287
Psychogenic etiology
    in urethral syndrome, 286
    in voiding dysfunction, 305, 306
Psychosomatic detrusor instability, 266
Psychotherapy in detrusor instability, 276
Psychotropic agents, 50
PTFE; *see* Polytetrafluoroethylene
Pubocervical fascia, 183
Pubococcygeus muscle, 12-13
    vaginal delivery and, 156
Puborectalis muscle, 12-13, 14-15
Pubourethral ligaments, 11, 12
    sutures and, 183
Pubovaginal spring, 178
Pudendal cortical pathways, 22

Pudendal electrodes, 108
Pudendal nerve, 21
    damage to, 158-160
    neuropathy of, 121-122
Pudendal nerve terminal motor latency, 158
    in electrophysiologic studies, 111-112
Pulley stitch in sacrospinous fixation, 250
Pulsion enterocele, 238
Purinergic receptors, 20
Pyelography, intravenous; *see* Intravenous pyelography
Pylonephritis, 311, 315, 326
    pregnancy and, 399, 400-402, 403
Pyridium; *see* Phenazopyridine hydrochloride
Pyuria
    urethral syndrome and, 288
    urinary tract infection and, 316, 318

Q
Q-tip test, 53
Quinolones, 320, 323

R
Radiation therapy, 383-384
Radical hysterectomy
    urinary tract injury and, 358-360
    urologic complications of, 378-380, 381
Radical pelvic surgery, 303-304
Radical vulvectomy, 381-382
Radiology
    in genital prolapse, 228
    in interstitial cystitis, 293
    of lower urinary tract; *see* Urinary tract
    in suburethral diverticula, 346-347
    in urinary tract infections, 318
Radiotherapy
    hemorrhagic cystitis and, 384-385
    vesicovaginal fistulas and, 332-333
Ranvier, nodes of, 103
Raz procedure, 186, 187, 190
Rectal injury, 252
Rectocele, 225-228
    enteroceles and, 238
    postpartum pelvic injury and, 157
    surgical repair in, 231-234
Rectovaginal septum, 227
    pelvic injury and, 157
Rectum, 15
    partitioning of cloaca in, 3, 4
Recurrent urinary tract infection, 322-325
Recurrent vaginal wall prolapse, 252
Reflex
    anal, 51
    bulbocavernosus, 51
    in electrophysiologic studies, 115-117
    H, 113
    micturition, 25

Reflex—cont'd
  skeletal muscle, 18
  somatic pathways of, 18
  spinal, 21
  urine storage and evacuation, 23
Reflex incontinence, 42
Reflex, vesicoureteral, 140-141
Reinfection, defined, 312
Relapse, 312
  of urinary tract infection, 323
Relaxation, urethral; *see* Urethra, instability of
Renal agenesis, 6
Renal blastema, 5
Renal disease in pregnancy, 391, 398, 402-403
Renal function tests, 384
Renal stones, 399, 403-404
Renal ultrasound in genital prolapse, 228
Renshaw cells, 18
Residual urine measurement, 80
Respiratory distress, 401
Resting urethral pressure, 152, 155-156
Retention, urinary, 301-305, 306-307
  after suburethral sling operations, 216
Reticular formatin, pontine, 299-301
Retractors
  Briesky-Navratil, 247, 248
  Heaney, 247, 248
Retrograde bladder filling, 59
Retrograde ureteral stents, 355
Retrograde urinary tract infection, 312, 313
Retropubic space dissection, 184
Retropubic surgical procedures, 196-209
  Burch colposuspension in, 197, 198, 199-201, 202-204, 205-207
  indications for, 197
  mechanisms of cure and, 204-205
  pregnancy after, 207-208
Rigid endoscopes, 125
Ring pessary, 258
Risser pessary, 258
Ritodrine hydrochloride, 402
Robertson catheter, 422, 423
Rutner catheter, 422, 423

S

Sacral colpopexy, 255-258
Sacral neurectomy, 280
Sacral pelvic nerve block, 280
Sacral spinal cord
  electrophysiologic testing and, 120
  micturition and, 301
Sacrospinous ligament fixation, 245-254
St. Mark's disposable pudendal electrodes, 108
Saline, 296
Saphenous nerve injury, 193

Saprophyte, 315
Sciatic nerve
  injury to, 193
  sacrospinous fixation and, 252
Scissors, Metzenbaum
  in enterocele repair, 238-239
  in vaginal entrance, 184
Sclerosing solution, 216
Sedatives
  in sensory urgency, 292
  urinary tract function and, 50
Self-cath catheter, 422, 423
Self-catheterization, intermittent
  bladder drainage and, 424, 427
  in voiding dysfunction and retention, 308
Self-examination in stress incontinence, 170-171
Self-start intermittent therapy, 324-325
Sensitivity testing, 317
Sensory abnormalities of bladder, 71, 73
Sensory dermatomes, 52
Sensory function
  elderly and, 413-414
  incontinence and, 51
Sensory innervation
  of urethra, 20
  of urinary tract, 21, 22
Sensory lesion, 118
Sensory study in electrophysiologic testing, 115-117
Sensory urgency, 289-292
  unstable bladder and, 58, 267
Septic shock, 401
Septra, 320
Serratia marcescens
  antimicrobials and, 321
  in urinary tract infection, 315
Sexual changes of incontinence, 35-36
Sexual intercourse
  after incontinence surgery, 234
  urinary tract infection and, 314-315, 325
Sexually transmitted diseases, 318
SFEMG; *see* Single fiber electromyography
Sheath of cystoscope, 125-126
Shock, septic, 401
Sholum procedure, 349
Sigmoid colon conduit, 382
Silver chloride electrodes, 107
Silver nitrate, 295
Single-channel cystometry, 64, 65
Single fiber electromyography, 110-111
Sinus, urogenital, 3, 4, 5
Sinus tract after suburethral sling operations, 216
Skeletal muscle reflex, 18
Skeletal muscle relaxants
  in urethral syndrome, 288
  in urinary tract function, 26
Skene's gland, 343, 344

Sling procedures, suburethral, 211-216
Smears, vaginal cytologic, 228
Smith pessary, 258
Smith-Hodge pessary, 178
Smoking, 33
Smooth muscle, urethral, 10
Smooth muscle relaxants
  bladder emptying and, 27
  in detrusor instability, 277, 278
Social changes of incontinence, 33-35; *see also* Incontinence
Sodium acetrizoate, 138
Sodium iodine, 137
Sodium pentosanpolysulfate, 294-295
Sof-flex catheter, 422, 423
Somatic nervous system
  urethra and, 20-21
  voiding and, 24
Somatic reflex pathway, 18
Somatosensory evoked responses, 114
Sonography in subrethral diverticula, 347
Spasms, urethral sphincter, 286
Spastic bladder; *see* Detrusor, instability of
Spence procedure, 348-349, 352
Sphincter
  anal, 14-15
    postpartum pelvic injury and, 157
  dysfunction of; *see* Stress incontinence
  dyssynergia of
    multichannel urodynamic tracing of, 274
    in multiple sclerosis, 265
    uroflowmetric parameters and, 80
  implantation of urinary, 218-222
  incompetence of; *see* Stress incontinence
  urethral, 10-11, 20
    incompetence of, 154-156
    spasms of, 286
Spinal cord
  injury to, 119-120
  lesions of, 304
  micturition and, 301
  tumors of, 266
  urinary tract and, 23
Spinal nerve control, 18
Spinal reflex, 21
Stamey catheter, 422, 423
Stamey procedure, 185-186, 187, 190
  results of, 191
  sutures in, 183
Staphylococcus
  antimicrobials and, 321
  urethral syndrome and, 286
  urinary tract infection and, 314, 315
Static urethral pressure profilometry, 91-92
Stenosis
  urethral, 130, 286
  vaginal, 252

Stents
  in adnexal surgery, 355
  in cervical cancer, 376
Sterilization of instruments, 127-128
Steroids, 294
Stimulation, functional electrical
  in detrusor instability, 276
  in interstitital cystitis, 295-296
  in stress incontinence, 175-178
Stimulus artifact, 111
Stones
  bladder, 132
  renal, 399, 403-404
  in suburethral diverticula, 343-344
  ureteral, 138
Stop test, 83, 86
Stress incontinence, 41-44, 151-181
  detrusor instability and, 280
  diagnosis of, 197
  in elderly, 417
  hysterectomy and, 207
  LeFort partial colpocleisis and, 252-253
  multichannel urethrocystometry in, 72
  pressure-flow studies in, 83-87
  prevalence of, 30, 31
  retropubic surgical procedures in; *see* Retropubic surgical procedures
  sacrospinous fixation and, 252
  sling procedures and, 211
  surgical correction of, 210-224
  urethral pressure profilometry in, 93-97
  urodynamic diagnosis of, 75
  vulvectomy and, 381
Striated muscle
  urethral, 10-11
  urogenital, 11
  urogenital sphincter, 20
Stricture, ureteral, 383-384
Suarez continence ring, 178
Substance P, 20, 21, 22
Subtracted cystometry, 64, 65
  multichannel, 68
Subtracted urethrocystometry, multichannel
  detrusor instability and, 272, 273
  technique of, 67-68, 69
Suburethral diverticula, 130, 342-353
  urethral pressure profilometry in, 99-100
Suburethral sling procedures, 211-216
Sulbactam, 401
Sulfa drugs, 398
Sulfamethoxazole and trimethoprim
  in cystitis, 322
  in pyelonephritis, 326
  in urinary tract infection, 320, 321, 324, 325
Sulfisoxazole, 398

Sulfonamides
  in cystitis, 400
  in urinary tract infection, 320, 323, 325
Super-flow pattern, 79, 80
Superinfection, defined, 312
Supersensitivity test
  in detrusor instability, 273
  in electrophysiologic studies, 117
Suppressive antimicrobial therapy, defined, 311
Suprapubic catheterization, 422-424, 425, 426
Suprasacral cord, 119-120
Surface electrodes, 105-108
Surgery
  adnexal, 355-358
  bladder neck
    pressure-flow studies in, 83
    voiding dysfunction and, 305
  in detrusor instability or hyperrflexia, 279-280
  in enterocele, 238-241, 242, 243
  in incontinence, 418-419
  in interstitial cystitis, 296
  pelvic; *see* Pelvic surgery
  retropubic; *see* Retropubic surgical procedures
  in stress incontinence; *see* Stress incontinence
  in suburethral diverticula, 348-352
  transvaginal needle suspension procedures and, 183-189
  urethral pressure profilometry in, 96-97
  in urinary tract fistulas, 334-339
  urinary tract injury in; *see* Urinary tract, injury to
  urologic complications of, 378-383
  in voiding dysfunction and retention, 307-308
Sympathtic blockers
  bladder emptying and, 27
  in detrusor-sphincter dyssynergia, 305
  in stress incontinence, 171
Sympathomimetics, 171
Synaptic vesicles, 20
Systolic bladder; *see* Detrusor, instability of

T

Tamm-Horsfall protein, 313
Tancer procedure, 349
Temporal lobes, 22
TENS; *see* Trancutaneous electrical nerve stimulation
Terbutaline, 279
Terminal bladder contraction, 269
Terodiline
  in detrusor instability, 277, 279
  in sensory urgency, 292
Tetracycline
  in urethral syndrome, 288
  in urinary tract infection, 320, 321, 323
Theophylline, 304
Tibial nerve, 114
TMP-SMX; *see* Trimethoprim and sulfamethoxazole
Trabeculations, bladder, 141, 142

Traction enterocele, 238
Tranquilizers, 294
Transcutaneous electrical nerve stimulation, 417, 419
Transection, bladder, 280
Transient incontinence, 56
Transureteroureterostomy, 369
Transurethral catheterization
  in bladder drainage, 421-422
  in cystometry, 66
Transvaginal approach to urinary sphincter implantation, 221-222
Transvaginal diverticulectomy, 348
Transvaginal needle suspension procedures, 182-195
  anatomy and terminology in, 182-183
  complications of, 191-193
  indications for, 183
  procedure of, 183-189
  results of, 189-191
Transverse conduit, 382
Trendelenburg position
  in McCall culdoplasty, 239
  in vesicovaginal fistula repair, 335
Trichomonas
  in periurethral duct infection, 344
  in urinary tract infection, 318
Tricyclic antidepressants
  bladder emptying and, 27
  in detrusor instability, 277, 278-279
  in stress incontinence, 171
  urinary tract function and, 26
  voiding dysfunction and, 304
Trigone, 4-9, 20
Trigonitis, 311
Trimethoprim and sulfamethoxazole
  in cystitis, 322
  in pyelonephritis, 326
  in urinary tract infection, 320, 321, 324, 325
Tubo-ovarian abscess, 358
Tumor
  bladder
    cystourethrography in, 142
    dysfunction and, 266

U

UEC; *see* Urethra, electric conductance of
Ulcer, Hunner, 131
Ultrasonography
  in genital prolapse, 228
  in suburethral diverticula, 347
  in urethral mobility, 53
  of urinary tract, 144-145
Uninhibited bladder; *see* Detrusor, instability of
Uninhibited urethral relaxation; *see* Urethra, instability of
Unstable bladder; *see* Detrusor, instability of
Unstable detrusor, 41
Urachal fistula, 6
Ureaplasma urealyticum, 286

Urecholine; *see* Bethanechol cloride
Uremia, 376
Ureter
  catheterization of, 367
  dilation of, 388
  double, 6
  ectopic, 6
  injury to
    abdominal hysterectomy and, 358-360
    delivery and, 406-407
    intravenous pyelography and, 136, 137
    prevention of, 362-364
    repair of, 365-370
    vesicovaginal fistulas and, 332
  obstruction of
    Burch colposuspension and, 206
    cervical cancer and, 374-376
  pelvic, 8-10
  reimplantation of, 405
  stones of, 138
  stricture of, 383-384
Ureteral catheter
  cystotomy and, 363
  duration of, 367
  in endoscopy, 127
Ureteral stents
  in adnexal surgery, 355
  in cervical cancer, 376
Ureteric bud formation, 4, 5
Ureteroneocystostomy, 365-368, 379
Ureterosigmoidostomy, 339
Ureterostomy, 369-370
Ureterovaginal fistula, 379
Ureterovesicotrigonal complex, 9
Urethography, 346-347, 348
Urethra, 3-12, 20
  abscess of, 344, 345
  bladder filling and, 25
  continence and, 152-154
  cystourographic findings of, 139
  dilation of
    in urethral syndrome, 288, 289
    in voiding dysfunction, 307-308
  diverticula of, 136; *see also* Suburethral diverticula
  electric conductance of, 290
  fistulas of, 338
  function of
    after prolapse, 229
    storage and, 41
  granular trigonitis of, 311
  injury to, 216
    prevention of, 364
    repair of, 371-372
  innervation of, 153
  instability of, 74
    pressure-flow study in, 84, 85

Urethra—cont'd
  instability of—cont'd
    pressure profilometry in, 97-99
  lead pipe, 43
  mobility of
    incontinence and, 58-59
    measurement of, 51-53
    stress incontinence and, 44
  mucosa of, 130
  obstruction of
    urethral syndrome and, 286
    urinary retention and, 306
    voiding dysfunction and, 304-305
  pathology of, 129-130
  postpartum pelvic injury and, 157
  radical hysterectomy and, 380
  relaxation of; *see* Urethra, instability of
  stenosis of, 130
  stress incontinence and, 43, 155
    continence and, 152-153
  ultrasound evaluation of, 145
  urine in, 266-267
  uroflowmetric parameters and, 80
  voiding and, 25, 301, 303
Urethral coaptation, 153-154
Urethral pressure
  detrusor instability and, 273
  fluctuations in, 97, 99
  stress incontinence and, 44, 154, 155-156
Urethral pressure profilometry, 89-101
  in detrusor instability, 269-273
  in suburethral diverticula, 347-348
Urethral sphincter
  dysfunction of; *see* Stress incontinence
  spasms of, 286
Urethral syndrome, 285-289
  diagnosis of, 130
Urethritis, 311
urethrocystometry
  carbon dioxide, 129
  multichannel
    detrusor instability and, 272, 273
    in stress incontinence, 72
    technique of, 67-68, 69
Urehtrocystoscopy, 128-129, 129; *see also* Cystoscopy
Urethrography, 144
Urethropexy
  Burch, 189-191
  needle, 230
  retropubic, 204
Urethroscope, 125, 126
Urethrovaginal sphincter, 20
Urge incontinence
  in elderly, 417
  unstable bladder and, 58
Urgency, 289

Urgency—cont'd
  motor, 41, 267, 289
  sensory, 289-292
  suburethral sling operations and, 216
  unstable bladder and, 267
  uroflowmetry and, 81
Urinalysis
  in detrusor instability, 268-269
  in genital prolapse, 228
Urinary diversion
  in detrusor instability, 280
  in genital malignancy, 382
  hemorrhagic cystitis and, 385
  pregnancy and, 404
  urinary tract fistulas and, 339
Urinary incontinence; *see* Incontinence
Urinary retention, 301-305
  acute, 306
  after suburethral sling operations, 216
  chronic, 306-307
Urinary sphincter implantation, 218-222
Urinary stream interruption, 22
Urinary tract, 3-12
  cancer and, 374-376; *see* Gynecologic cancer
  dysfunction of, 40-43
  endoscopy of, 124-133
  fistulas of, 132, 330-341
  function of,
    standardisation of terminology of, 430-446
  infection of; *see* Urinary tract infection
  injury to, 354-362
    colporrhaphy and, 316
    during delivery, 405-406, 406-407
    repair of, 365-372
    transvaginal needle suspension procedures and, 192
  neurophysiology of, 17-28
  peripheral innervation of, 19
  in pregnancy, 388-408
  radiology of, 134-147
Urinary tract infection, 310-324
  after suburethral sling operations, 216
  catheter-associated, 325-326
  culture tests for, 393-395, 396
  instrumentation and, 326
  laboratory tests in, 54
  management of, 318-325
  in pregnancy, 393-402, 403
    bacteriuria and, 395-399
    cystitis and, 400
    diagnosis of, 393-395, 396
    incidence of, 393
    microbiology of, 397
    pathophysiology of, 393
    pyelonephritis and, 400-402, 403
    risk for, 396
  pyelonephritis in, 326

Urinary tract infection—cont'd
  recurrent, 322-325
  sexual intercourse and diaphragm use and, 325
  urethral syndrome and, 287-288
Urine
  acidification of, 319
  aspiration of, 394
  collection of, 315-316
  culture of
    in urinary tract infection, 317, 393-394
  evacuation of, 40-46
  examination of, 333
  flow of, 302
  residual measurement of, 80
  storage of
    disorders in, 40-46
    reflexes in, 23
    therapeutic facilitation in, 27-28
  in urethra, 266-267
  urinary tract infection and, 313
Urine kits, 316-317
Urine loss appliances, 428-429
Urine microscopy, 316
Urodynamic studies, 62
  in detrusor instability and hyperreflexia, 269-273
  in genital prolapse, 228
  in incontinence, 59-60
  in multiple sclerosis, 265
  in urethral syndrome, 287
  in urinary tract infections, 318
Urodynamic tracing, multichannel
  cough-provoked detrusor instability and, 269, 271
  detrusor-sphincter dyssynergia and, 274
Uroflowmetry, 77-81
  in urethral syndrome, 287
Urogenital diaphragm, 14
Urogenital hiatus, 13
Urogenital sinus, 3, 4, 5
Urolithiasis, 399, 403-404
Urologic complications of gynecologic cancer, 378-384
Urologic disease in pregnancy, 403-406
Urorectal septum formation, 3, 4
Urteropelvic prolapse, 258
Uterosacral ligament plication, 241, 244
Uterovaginal prolapse, 242
Uterus
  gravid, 405
  postpartum pelvic injury and, 157
  prolapse of, 228

V

Vagina, 12
  after suburethral sling operations, 216
  axis of, 237
  cancer of
    urologic complications of, 376-377

Vagina—cont'd
  cancer of—cont'd
    vaginectomy in, 382-383
  fistulas of, 333, 364-365
  prolapse of, 258
    nonsurgical treatment in, 258
  stenosis of, 252
  urinary tract infection and, 313
Vaginal colposuspension, 188-189, 190
Vaginal cones, 170-171-171
Vaginal cytologic smears, 228
Vaginal delivery
  incontinence and, 31-32
  pelvic floor damage and, 156-157
  perineal damage and, 157-158
  pudendal nerve damage and, 158-160
Vaginal enterocele repair, 238-239
Vaginal hysterectomy
  cystotomy in, 370-371
  lower urinary tract injury and, 360-362
Vaginal pessary, 258
Vaginal silver chloride electrodes, 107
Vaginal ultrasonography, 347
Vaginal vault prolapse, 228, 241-258
Vaginal wall
  massage of, 288, 289
  prolapse of; see also Pelvic organ prolapse
    posterior, 227
    recurrent anterior, 252
  stress urinary incontinence and, 44
  urethral support and, 11-12
Vaginectomy, 382-383
Vaginitis, 318
Valsalva maneuver, 85
Vasoactive intestinal polypeptide
  detrusor instability and, 264-265
  urethra and, 20
Vertebrae, lumbar, 115
Vesical neck plication, 229-230
Vesicocervical fistula, 333
Vesicoureteral reflux
  cystourethrography in, 140-141
Vesicoureteric reflux
  pregnancy and, 388
Vesicouterine fistula, 333
  cystourethrography in, 142, 143
Vesicovaginal fistula, 132, 332, 333; see also Urinary tract,
    fistulas of
  cystourethrography in, 142, 143
  radiation and, 383
  radical hysterectomy and, 379

Vest-over-pants technique, 350, 351
Video-urodynamic testing, 68-70
  in stress incontinence, 44
  in urinary tract infection, 318
Videocystourethrography, 52, 144
VIP; see Vasoactive intestinal polypeptide
Voided volume chart, 269
Voiding; See also Micturition
  after coporrhaphy, 234
  difficulty in
    detrusor instability and, 267-268
    retropubic surgical procedures and, 206
  dysfunction of, 42-43, 299-309
    radical hysterectomy and, 380
    transvaginal needle suspension procedures and, 192
    uroflowmetry and, 80-81
  evaluation of, 55-56
  failure in, 42; see also Incontinence
  in genital prolapse, 228
  mechanisms of, 25
  neurologic pathways in, 22
  obstructed, 79-80
  periodic, 313
  pressure/flow studies and, 83
  prompted, 416-417
  sling procedures and, 215
  studies of, 77-88
Voiding cystourethrography, 140-141
  in suburethral diverticula, 347, 348
  in urethral diverticula, 136
  in urinary tract infection, 318
VOS procedure, 199-201
Vulva
  cancer of
    radical vulvectomy in, 381-382
    staging for, 376, 377
    urologic complications in, 376
Vulvectomy, 381-382

W

Waldeyer's sheath, 8, 9, 10
Water perfusion catheter, 66
Weighted vaginal cones, 170-171
Wein and Barrett functional classification of incontinence, 42
Wound abscess, 216

Z

Zero-degree urethroscope, 125, 126
Zinc oxide, 334